Urolithiasis
CLINICAL AND BASIC RESEARCH

Urolithiasis

CLINICAL AND BASIC RESEARCH

Edited by

Lynwood H. Smith

Mayo Clinic
Rochester, Minnesota

William G. Robertson

The General Infirmary
Leeds, England

and

Birdwell Finlayson

University of Florida
Gainesville, Florida

SPRINGER SCIENCE+BUSINESS MEDIA, LLC

Library of Congress Cataloging in Publication Data

International Symposium on Urolithiasis Research, 4th, Williamsburg, Va., 1980.
Urolithiasis, clinical and basic research.

"Proceedings of the Fourth International Symposium on Urolithiasis Research, held June 22-26, 1980, Williamsburg, Virginia."
Includes bibliographical references and index.
I. Calculi, Urinary–Congresses. I. Smith, Lynwood H. II. Robertson, William G. III. Finlayson, Birdwell, 1932- . IV. Title. [DNLM: 1. Kidney–Physiology–Congresses. 2. Urinary calculi–Congresses. W3 IN924XA 4th 1980u/WJ 356 I62 1980u]
RC916.I58 1980 616.6'22 80-27716
ISBN 978-1-4684-8979-8 ISBN 978-1-4684-8977-4 (eBook)
DOI 10.1007/978-1-4684-8977-4

Proceedings of the Fourth International Symposium on Urolithiasis Research, held June 22–26, 1980, in Williamsburg, Virginia

Organizing Committee
L. Cifuentes Delatte, A. deVries, B. Finlayson, H. Fleisch, J. Gillenwater, F. Knox, J. Lemann, Jr., G. H. Nancollas, C. Y. C. Pak, W. G. Robertson, and H. E. Williams.

Secretary: L. H. Smith

Originally published by Plenum Press, New York in 1981
Softcover reprint of the hardcover 1st edition 1981
A Division of Plenum Publishing Corporation
233 Spring Street, New York, N.Y. 10013

PREFACE

In 1968 Drs. B. E. C. Nordin and A. Hodgkinson organized the First International Symposium on Urolithiasis Research in Leeds, England. One hundred and five participants from continental Europe, Great Britain, and the United States met to review their work and exchange ideas regarding the formation of urinary calculi. This meeting achieved several important goals. It pulled together a nidus of workers in the many scientific disciplines that relate to urolithiasis. This nidus served as the seed for research growth in a complex, interdisciplinary field. It established a forum for continuing communication in urolithiasis research with subsequent symposia being held every 4 years.

The Williamsburg Symposium was the fourth in the Leeds-Madrid-Davos series involving 186 participants from throughout the world. A stated emphasis was on clinical research under way in the field. There were no invited speakers and for the first time the 41 papers that were presented orally at the meeting were selected from 184 submitted abstracts. A total of 134 papers were presented in the poster sessions in the afternoons where informal exchange between interested participants and investigators could occur without the restrictions of a plenary session. Virtually all areas of urolithiasis research from the most fundamental physical chemistry to clinical patterns of disease and specific modes of treatment were presented, reviewed and discussed during the meeting.

This volume presents the Proceedings of the Symposium and includes 40 papers that were presented orally in the plenary sessions and 120 papers presented as posters. An additional paper that was the product of a committee of experts on standardized nomenclature for crystal formation is included in the section on Crystal Formation and Physical Chemistry.

The meeting was made possible by the generous support from the National Institute of Arthritis, Metabolism, and Digestive Diseases, NIH; Burroughs Wellcome, Wellcome Foundation, and Deutsche Wellcome; Merck Sharp and Dohme; Smith Kline and French. Eaton Laboratories;

Willen Drug; Beach Pharmaceuticals; P. Keppler Verlag; and Blaine Company. The Organizing Committee wishes to express their thanks for this most critical support.

Behind any successful meeting are special people who play a critical role in the planning, organization, and conduct of the meeting. Mrs. Sherry Linander filled this role with the Williamsburg meeting. She also typed the entire proceedings of the meeting for publication. To her goes our special gratitude and admiration.

Lynwood H. Smith
W. G. Robertson
Birdwell Finlayson

Williamsburg, Virginia
June 22-26, 1980

ACKNOWLEDGMENTS

This Symposium was supported by:

1. The National Institute of Arthritis, Metabolism and Digestive Diseases, National Institutes of Health, Public Health Service, Department of Health, Education and Welfare, Bethesda, Maryland, U.S.A. Grant No. AM 26949.

2. Burroughs Wellcome Company
   Research Triangle Park, North Carolina, U.S.A.

   Wellcome Foundation, LTD., Sweden.

   Deutsche Wellcome, Burgwedel, West Germany.

3. Merck Sharp and Dohme
   West Point, Pennsylvania, U.S.A.

4. Smith Kline & French
   Philadelphia, Pennsylvania, U.S.A.

5. Eaton Laboratories
   Norwich, New York, U.S.A.

6. Willen Drug Company
   Baltimore, Maryland, U.S.A.

7. Beach Pharmaceuticals
   Tampa, Florida, U.S.A.

8. P. Keppler Verlag
   Heusenstomm, West Germany

9. Blaine Company, Inc.
   Ft. Mitchell, Kentucky, U.S.A.

CONTENTS

I. CLINICAL UROLITHIASIS

EVALUATION

CLINICAL DISORDERS

TREATMENT

IV. INHIBITORS AND PROMOTERS

VIII. STONE MORPHOLOGY AND STRUCTURE

IX. ANALYTICAL METHODS

I. CLINICAL UROLITHIASIS EVALUATION

THE MAIN RISK FACTOR FOR CALCIUM OXALATE STONE DISEASE IN MAN: HYPERCALCIURIA OR MILD HYPEROXALURIA?

W. G. Robertson, M. Peacock, D. Ouimet,
P. J. Heyburn, and A. Rutherford
M.R.C. Mineral Metabolism Unit
The General Infirmary
Leeds LS1 3EX, United Kingdom

For over 40 years now it has been considered by many workers that hypercalciuria is the main cause of idiopathic calcium oxalate stone disease in man. Indeed it is a frequent biochemical finding in most series of calcium stone-formers[1-7]. Other investigators, however, have failed to find any increase in urinary calcium excretion in this group of patients and do not consider it to be of importance either in the initiation[8-11] or in the recurrent formation[12] of these stones. They emphasize that many recurrent calcium oxalate stone-formers are not hypercalciuric and, even of those who initially present as being hypercalciuric, many continue to form stones even after normalization of their urinary calcium. Furthermore, there are many hypercalciuric individuals, including normal subjects and patients with some metabolic disorder, predisposing to a high urinary calcium excretion, who never form stones at all. The importance, therefore, of hypercalciuria in stone-formation is far from clear.

Only within the last decade have a few investigators begun to consider the alternative possibility that the formation of idiopathic calcium oxalate stones may be due to an increase in the urinary excretion of oxalate rather than of calcium[13-16]. Historically, the reason for this is that most laboratories have been able to measure calcium in urine much more readily than oxalate. Indeed the inability to measure urinary oxalate accurately and precisely undoubtedly accounts for many of the apparent discrepancies between those investigators who have found a significant increase in urinary oxalate amongst idiopathic stone-formers[13,14,17-21] and those who have been unable to do so[22-26]. Another reason is that the increases observed are relatively small in comparison with those found in patients with the more striking congenital or enteric hyperoxaluria in which urinary oxalate is usually greater than 0.8 mmol/day and where there is a high risk of nephrocalcinosis, multiple, small calcium oxalate stones and renal impairment[16]. We propose that this intermediate condition, in which urinary oxalate excretion lies between the upper limit of the normal range (about 0.5 mmol/day) and the lower limit of the congenital hyperoxaluric range (about 0.8 mmol/day) be termed "mild hyperoxaluria".

The object of this paper is to determine the incidence of mild hyperoxaluria in idiopathic calcium stone-formers, to examine the relative importance of hypercalciuria and mild hyperoxaluria in the formation of calcium oxalate stones and to attempt to identify the mechanism by which each influences the risk of forming such stones.

The Prevalence of Hypercalciuria and Mild Hyperoxaluria in Idiopathic Calcium Stone Disease

In a study of this nature it is important to define the terms "hypercalciuria" and "mild hyperoxaluria". In this report we define "hypercalciuria" and "mild hyperoxaluria" as states in which the 95% upper confidence limits of urinary calcium and oxalate in the normal male population are exceeded. These limits are 10 mmol/day and 0.46 mmol/day respectively.

The mean values (±SEM) of urinary calcium and oxalate in the 24-hour urines of normal men and male idiopathic stone-formers on a "free diet" are shown in Table 1. The stone-formers are divided into those who have had only a single stone episode (SSF) and those who have had recurrent episodes of the disorder (RSF). The results from two studies are shown, the first on patients when they initially attended the Urology Department Clinics soon after their stone episode(s) and the second on patients attending our own departmental Stone Clinic. This latter group consists almost entirely of stone-formers referred to us after initial consultation with the urologists and generally are seen by us some time after their stone episode(s).

Table 1 shows firstly that the severity of the disorder appears to be related to both urinary calcium and oxalate excretion since there is a progressive increase in the mean value of both variables according to the series normal <SSF<RSF. Secondly, in our own departmental series of patients, the prevalence of hypercalciuria and mild hyperoxaluria is approximately the same. Thirdly, in the patients attending the Urology Clinics the prevalence of hypercalciuria is almost identical to that when they subsequently attended our departmental Stone Clinic. The prevalence of mild hyperoxaluria, however, in the patients is approximately double that found in patients attending our Stone Clinic. This was also observed in a paired test in individuals who attended both clinics[27]. It would appear, therefore, that mild hyperoxaluria at a stage near to the time of formation of the stone is much more common than

Table 1. The Urinary Excretion of Calcium and Oxalate in Stone-Formers and Normals

Source	Group	n	Calcium (mmol/day)			Oxalate (mmol/day)			Correlation Between Urinary Calcium and Oxalate	
			mean±SEM	P*	%>10 mmol/day	mean±SEM	P*	%>0.46 mmol/day	r	P
Hospital Staff	Male normals	60	5.95±0.35	-	3	0.33±0.01	-	2	0.320	<0.05
Urology Clinics	Male SSF**	55	6.80±0.38	ns	11	0.41±0.02	<0.01	27	0.442	<0.001
	Male RSF***	53	8.23±0.38	<0.001	28	0.48±0.02	<0.001	43	0.392	<0.01
Mineral Metabolism Clinics	Male SSF**	30	7.45±0.50	<0.05	13	0.37±0.02	<0.05	13	0.370	<0.05
	Male RSF***	30	8.93±0.63	<0.001	30	0.43±0.02	<0.001	23	0.375	<0.05

* P significance of difference from normal

** SSF = single episode stone-former

*** RSF = recurrent stone-formers

hypercalciuria. It is not clear, however, what causes such transient increases in oxalate excretion.

The Relative Importance of Hypercalciuria and Mild Hyperoxaluria for Stone-Formation

According to our risk factor model of stone-formation the most important urinary factors in the genesis of stones are a decrease in volume and an increase in oxalate excretion. The weakest risk factor is an increase in urinary calcium. This is supported by the data in Figure 1 which shows that the severity of stone recurrence is highly related to the excretion of oxalate but is at most only weakly related to the excretion of calcium in the same patients.

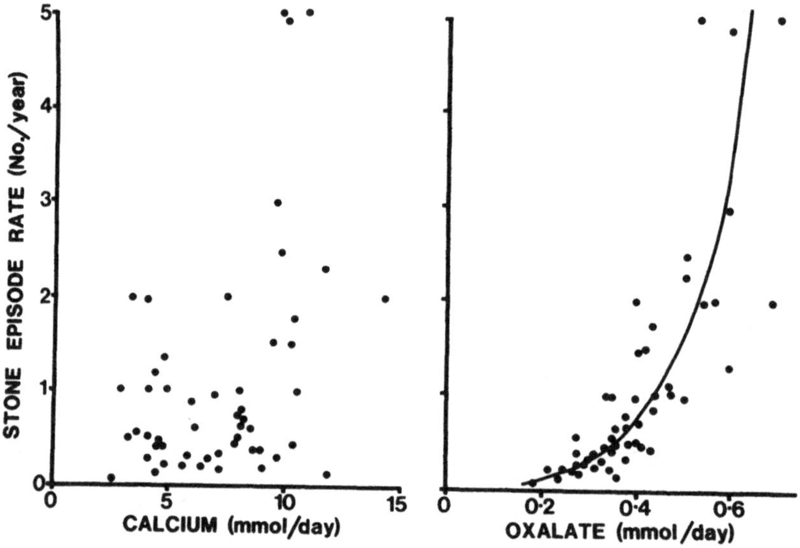

Figure 1. The stone episode rate of recurrent calcium oxalate stone-formers in relation to their daily excretion of (left) calcium and (right) oxalate.

There are at least two reasons for the strong relationship between the risk of stones and urinary oxalate excretion: one is the marked effect which an increase in the latter has on the supersaturation of urine with calcium oxalate compared with an increase in calcium excretion[27]; and the other is the effect which, at a constant level of supersaturation, an increase in oxalate has on the oxalate/calcium ratio in urine[28]. In turn, both these effects serve to increase the volume of calcium oxalate crystals excreted in urine (Figures 2 and 3) and therefore the percentage of large particles of crystal aggregates produced (Figure 4). It is the increase in the latter which determines the increase in the risk of stones.

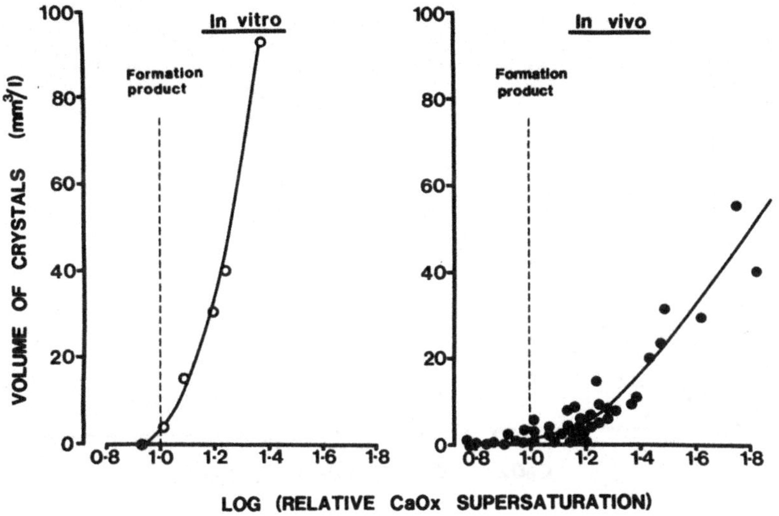

Figure 2. The volume of calcium oxalate crystals in urine in relation to the log relative calcium oxalate supersaturation (left) in vitro and (right) in vivo.

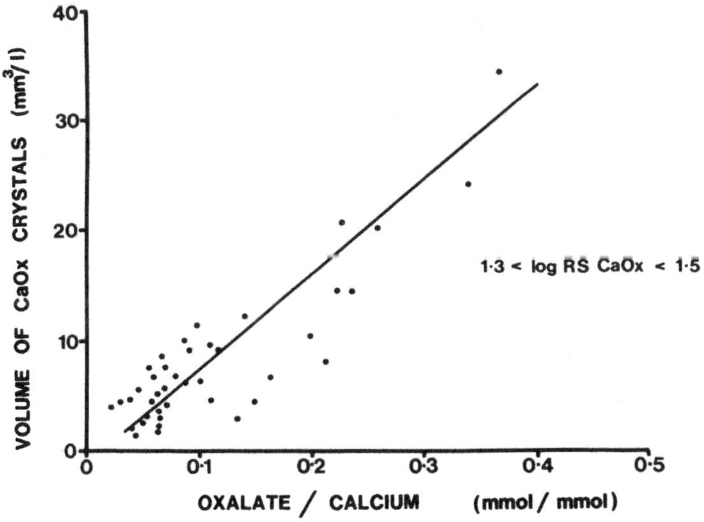

Figure 3. The volume of calcium oxalate crystals in urine in relation to the oxalate/calcium ratio at constant level of supersaturation.

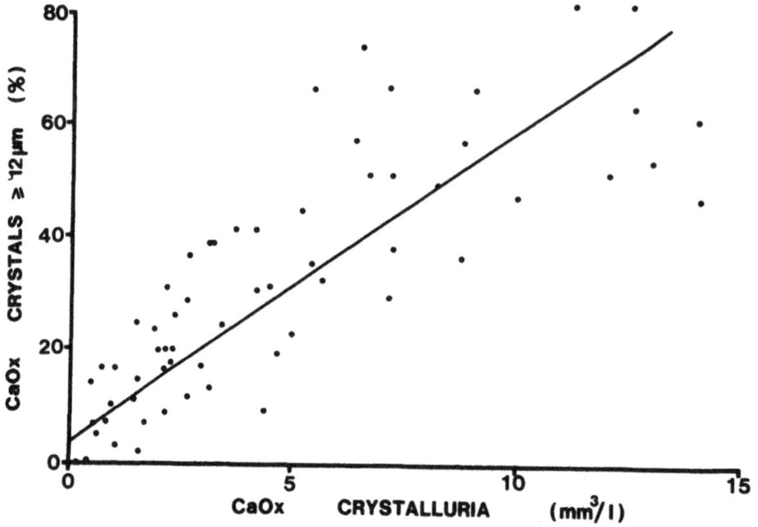

Figure 4. The percentage of large calcium oxalate crystals in urine in relation to the volume of calcium oxalate crystals.

Neglect of the effect of increases in the [Ox]/[Ca] ratio of urine (at a constant [Ca]x[Ox] product) explains why Hallson and Rose[29] have failed to find any relationship between crystalluria and urine saturation.

Figures 5 and 6 show how much more important mild hyperoxaluria is than hypercalciuria in causing the increases in calcium oxalate crystalluria and the percentage of large particles produced. In both cases the relationships are quadratic with respect to oxalate concentration. The reason for this is that over the range of calcium [Ca] and oxalate [Ox] concentrations in urine the volume of calcium oxalate crystals (V_{CaOx}) is proportional to both the product ([Ca] x [Ox]) (Figure 2) and, at a constant product, to the ratio ([Ox]/[Ca]) (Figure 3). Combination of these relationships yields the equation:

$$V_{CaOx} = b\ [Ox]^2 \qquad (1)$$

where b is a constant. Best fit analysis shows b to have a value of

44 $(mm^3/l)/(mmol/l)^2$ (Figure 5).

Since the percentage of large calcium oxalate crystals (% large V_{CaOx}) is proportional to V_{CaOx} (Figure 4) then it follows that:

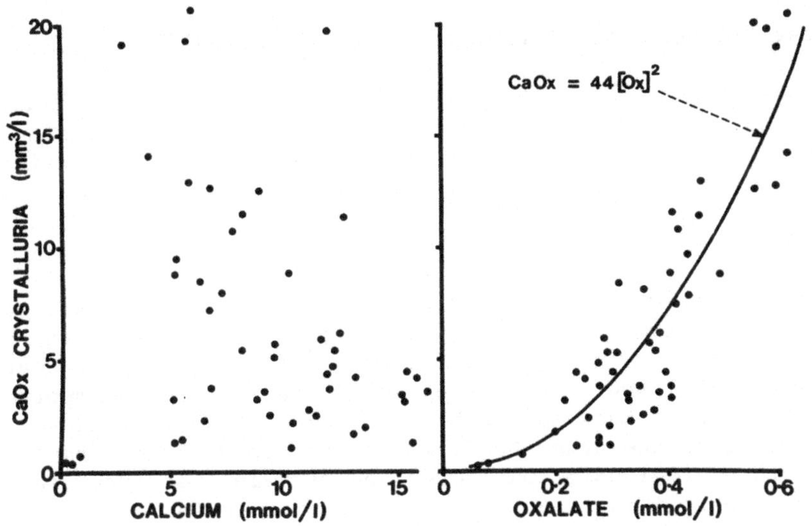

Figure 5. The volume of calcium oxalate crystals in the urine of recurrent stone-formers in relation to their (left) calcium and (right) oxalate concentrations.

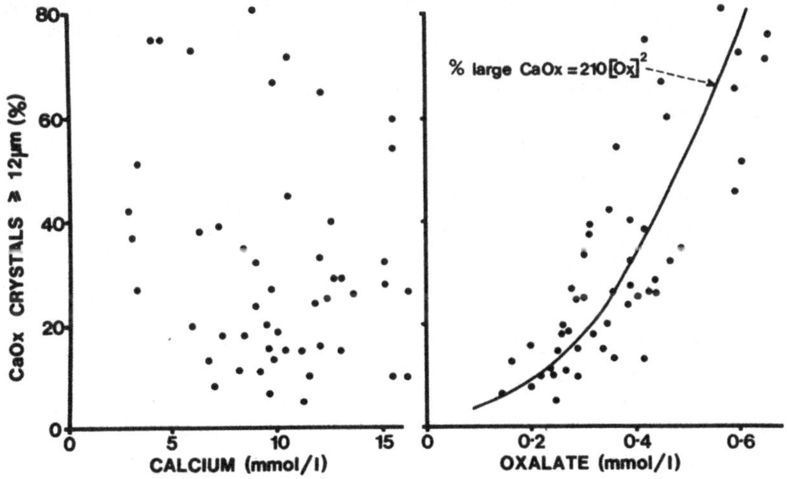

Figure 6. The percentage of large calcium oxalate crystals in the urine of recurrent stone-formers in relation to their (left) calcium and (right) oxalate concentrations.

$$\% \text{ large } V_{CaOx} = c[Ox]^2 \quad (2)$$

where best fit analysis shows c to be 210 (%)/(mmol/1)^2.

Figures 5 and 6 also show that there is little or no relationship between either the amount of calcium oxalate crystalluria or the proportion of large particles and the concentration of urinary calcium, even at the highest values of the latter.

DISCUSSION

Is hypercalciuria then of no significance in the genesis of calcium oxalate stones? Certainly from the above evidence and from the risk factor study previously reported[21] it would appear that, at least chemically, hypercalciuria by itself may not be as important in the initiation of stones as has been hitherto thought by many. Mild hyperoxaluria, on the other hand, would seem to be considerably more important than previously considered and certainly of more significance than hypercalciuria as a risk factor for the disorder.

There is, however, one possible way in which hypercalciuria may be linked to the formation of stones through an indirect mechanism. It has been reported by a few workers that there is a correlation between urinary oxalate and urinary calcium excretion when the data from normal subjects, idiopathic stone-formers and hyperparathyroid stone-formers are plotted together[13,30,31], although the relationship is less strongly significant within each of these sub-groups. In this present study the correlation between urinary oxalate and urinary calcium is highly significant ($p<0.001$) when all the data from the groups in Table 1 are plotted together. Moreover, the intra-group correlations are also significant. The currently accepted explanation for this observation is that the hypercalciuria and, indirectly, the mild hyperoxaluria are both due to the hyperabsorption of calcium from the intestinal tract, a common feature of both idiopathic and hyperparathyroid stone-formers[5,7]. The correlation between urinary oxalate and the hyperabsorption of calcium derives from the fact that the greater proportion of calcium absorbed from the bowel, the more oxalate (normally bound to intestinal calcium) is released. This free oxalate then becomes available for passive absorption lower down the gastro-intestinal tract[31-34]. The additionally absorbed oxalate is finally excreted in the urine. This secondary hyperabsorption hypothesis is supported by the observations that reduction of the calcium/oxalate ratio of the diet[35] or binding of calcium in the intestine by administration of cellulose phosphate[36] or diphosphonates[37], similarly increase oxalate absorption and excretion in the urine.

In conclusion, it would seem that hypercalciuria plays, at most, only a secondary role in the genesis of calcium stones compared with mild hyperoxaluria. Hypercalciuria may, in fact, only be a reflection of an abnormality (namely, the hyperabsorption of calcium) whose indirect effect (to increase oxalate absorption and excretion in urine) is chemically more critical to the formation of stones than it is itself. It would perhaps be more appropriate in the future, for investigators to direct their attention towards defining more closely the origins and control of mild hyperoxaluria.

REFERENCES

1. R. H. Flocks, J. Urol. 43:214 (1940).
2. F. Albright, P. Henneman, P. H. Benedict, and A. P. Forbes, Proc. Roy. Soc. Med. 46:1077 (1953).
3. A. Hodgkinson and L. N. Pyrah, Brit. J. Surg. 46:10 (1958).
4. W. G. Robertson, M. Peacock, and B. E. C. Nordin, Clin. Sci. 34:579 (1968).
5. B. E. C. Nordin, M. Peacock, and R. Wilkinson, Clinics Endocrin. and Metab. 1:169 (1972).
6. F. L. Coe, J. M. Canterbury, J. J. Firpo, and E. Reiss, J. Clin. Invest. 52:134 (1973).
7. C. Y. C. Pak, M. Ohata, E. C. Lawrence, and W. Snyder, J. Clin. Invest. 54:387 (1974).
8. J. E. Lathem and J. S. King, J. Urol. 89:541 (1963).
9. F. S. Jorgensen, Scand. J. Urol. Nephrol. 9:243 (1975).
10. S. G. Welshman and M. G. McGeown, Brit. J. Urol. 47:237 (1975).
11. R. S. Malek, R. M. Wilkiemeyer, and W. H. Boyce, J. Urol. 116:11 (1976).
12. V. Marshall, R. H. White, M. Chaput de Saintonge, G. C. Tressider, and J. P. Blandy, 47:117 (1975).
13. P. M. Zarembski and A. Hodgkinson, Clin. Chim. Acta. 25:1 (1969).
14. W. G. Robertson, M. Peacock, and B. E. C. Nordin, Clin. Sci. 40:365 (1971).
15. J. Thomas, J.-M. Melon, E. Thomas, A. Steg, P. Desgrez, and P. Aboulker, Ann. Urol. 6:31 (1972).
16. H. E. Williams, in:"Urolithiasis Research," H. Fleisch, W. G. Robertson, L. H. Smith and W. Vahlensieck, ed. Plenum Press, New York (1976).
17. V. Revusova, V. Zvara, and J. Gratzlova, Urol. Int. 26:277 (1971).
18. A. Hodgkinson, Clin. Sci. Mol. Med. 46:357 (1974).
19. B. Pinto, G. Crespi, F. Sole-Balcells, and P. Barcelo, Kid. Int. 5:285 (1974).
20. W. G. Robertson, M. Peacock, R. W. Marshall, D. H. Marshall, and B. E. C. Nordin, N. Engl. J. Med. 294:249 (1976).
21. W. G. Robertson, M. Peacock, P. J. Heyburn, D. H. Marshall, and P. B. Clark, Brit. J. Urol. 50:449 (1978).
22. E. Takasaki and E. Shimano, Invest. Urol. 5:303 (1967).
23. H.-G. Tiselius, Invest. Urol. 15:5 (1977).
24. C. Y. C. Pak, C. Fetner, J. Townsend, L. Brinkley, C. Northcutt, D. E. Barilla, M. Kadesky, and P. Peters, Amer. J. Med. 64:979 (1978).

25. P. O. Schwille, M. Paulus, D. Scholz, and A. Sigel, Urologe A17:217 (1978).
26. R. Galosy, L. Clarke, D. L. Ward, and C. Y. C. Pak, J. Urol. 123:320 (1980).
27. W. G. Robertson, M. Peacock, P. J. Heyburn, R. W. Marshall, A. Rutherford, R. E. Williams, and P. B. Clark, in:"Oxalate in Human Biochemistry and Clinical Pathology," G. A. Rose, W. G. Robertson, and R. W. E. Watts, ed., Wellcome Foundation, London (1980).
28. W. G. Robertson, D. S. Scurr, and C. M. Bridge, J. Cryst. Growth (in press).
29. P. C. Hallson and G. A. Rose, Brit. J. Urol. 50:442 (1978).
30. M. Peacock, R. W. Marshall, W. G. Robertson, and C. K. Varnavides, in:"Colloquium on Renal Lithiasis," B. Finlayson, and W. C. Thomas, Jr., eds., University Presses of Florida, Gainesville, Florida (1976).
31. A. Hodgkinson, Clin. Sci. Mol. Med. 54:291 (1978).
32. M. Peacock and W. G. Robertson, in:"Proceedings of VIIth International Congress of Nephrology," M. Bergeron, ed., Karger, Basel (1978).
33. B. Pinto and J. L. Paternain, Invest. Urol. 15:502 (1978).
34. K. Cooper, A. Broadus, R. Lang, H. Rasmussen, H. Binder, and J. Dobbins, Clin. Res. 27:364 (1979).
35. R. W. Marshall, M. Cochran, and A. Hodgkinson, Clin. Sci. 43:91 (1972).
36. R. W. Marshall and H. Barry, in:"Urinary Calculi," L. Cifuentes-Delatte, A. Rapado, and A. Hodgkinson, eds., Karger, Basel (1973).
37. W. G. Robertson, M. Peacock, R. W. Marshall, and F. Knowles, Clin. Sci. Mol. Med. 47:13 (1974).

PREDICTION OF STONE RECURRENCE

S. Ljunghall, B. G. Danielson, R. Källsen, and
A. Fritjofsson
Departments of Internal Medicine and Urology,
University Hospital
S-750 14 Uppsala, Sweden

SUMMARY

A prospective study was carried out among 52 patients presenting with their first attack of renal stones. During a 4-year followup period half of them developed recurrent stones. This occurred more often in males than in females and particularly in individuals with a high urinary calcium. However, the overlap between the two groups was large and in the individual patient determinations of serum and urinary electrolytes could not predict the risk of recurrence.

INTRODUCTION

The risk factor profile in the patients with recurrent renal stones has been thoroughly investigated[1]. The importance of a high urinary calcium, oxalate and urate and a low excretion of glycosaminoglycans in a concentrated urine has been emphasized. Few prospective studies of stone patients after their first renal stone seem to have been performed although it appears desirable to identify patients at particular risk of recurrences early in the course of the disease.

In this study we have carried out a metabolic investigation in patients who were diagnosed with their first renal stone and have re-evaluated the clinical course of stone disease after four years in relation to the initial metabolic findings.

PATIENTS AND METHODS

During a 3 month period 52 patients presented with their first attack of renal stones; 49 of these were followed for 4 years. There were 42 males and 10 females with a mean age (± standard deviation) of 40 ± 14 years. In all patients serum samples were taken during their first visit to the emergency department and analyzed for calcium. When the acute attack had subsided they were requested to collect 24 h urine samples and to return for further investigation. This was performed according to our standard out-patient protocol[2] which includes the determination of serum and urinary electrolytes. A follow-up study concentrating on the subsequent history of stones was performed after 4 years.

RESULTS

At the time of the initial investigation one patient was found to have primary hyperparathyroidism, one had hyperoxaluria secondary to an intestinal by-pass operation and a 19-year-old boy was suspected to have Cushing's disease, which was later verified. These 3 patients were not included in the evaluation of the natural history of untreated stone disease.

Of the remaining 46 patients who could be followed-up, 23 had formed a recurrent stone after 4 years. Among these were 22 males and only one female. Recurrences appeared equally distributed over that time. During each year after the first stone, 5 or 6 patients experienced their first recurrent stone.

Patients who developed recurrences had, at the initial examination, a higher urinary calcium than the others and also a higher serum urate concentration. No other differences could be detected between the patients with recurrences and those without (See Table 1).

DISCUSSION

We have previously found in epidemiological studies that recurrences are common among patients with renal stones and that the risk of stone formation is related to the urinary calcium output[3]. In this study during four years half of all the patients formed at least one recurrent stone. Thus it appears that, in general, the formation of a stone is not a singular event but given enough time most patients will have relapses[3,4]. However, at least in this study several patients lost interest in a metabolic investigation as soon as they were relieved of their acute symptoms. An investigation of stone formers at this stage will thus have to be performed with little time and expense. Also for practical reasons, since stones are so common in the population, only simple screening procedures will be possible in any larger number of individuals.

Urinary calcium was significantly increased among the patients who were to develop recurrent stones. However, since there was a large overlap between the two groups in this respect, urinary calcium alone was not a sensitive indicator of future stone formation.

Table 1. Results of laboratory investigations (mean values ± S.D.) in patients with their first renal stone, separated according to recurrences during a 4-year follow-up period.

	Recurrences during follow-up	No recurrences
Number of patients	23	23
Males/females	22/1	15/8
Age (years)	40 ± 12	39 ± 15
Serum values		
calcium (mmol/l)	2.45 ± 0.09	2.43 ± 0.08
phosphate (mmol/l)	0.90 ± 0.18	0.98 ± 0.21
magnesium (mmol/l)	0.80 ± 0.06	0.84 ± 0.06
urate (μmol/l)	292 ± 98**	190 ± 58
Urinary values		
volume (l/24h)	1.3 ± 0.6	1.1 ± 0.5
calcium (mmol/24h)	7.0 ± 3.1*	4.9 ± 2.4
magnesium (mmol/24h)	4.3 ± 2.1	3.5 ± 1.3
urate (mmol/24h)	3.4 ± 1.0	3.7 ± 0.9
oxalate (μmol/24h)	140 ± 90	140 ± 100

*) $p < 0.05$; **) $p < 0.01$ compared to the recurrent-free group.

Serum urate was also higher in the group with recurrences but the level among these patients was not higher than among stone-free control subjects[5]. Urinary urate excretion was not higher in those with recurrent stones despite the differences in the serum levels.

When we compared the outcome of this study of patients with their first stone episode with our experiences from over 5 years with an out-patient clinic for patients with recurrent stones, where over 600 patients have been investigated, it is evident that detailed metabolic studies will be primarily indicated in those patients with frequent recurrences or when the clinical picture has been complicated. A simple screening procedure, including a clinical examination should, however, be performed in all patients with a renal stone since not infrequently a treatable important disorder can be diagnosed.

REFERENCES

1. W. G. Robertson, M. Peacock, P. J. Heyburn, D. H. Marshall, and P. B. Clark, Br. J. Urol. 50:499 (1978).
2. U. Backman, B. G. Danielson, G. Johansson, S. Ljunghall, and B. Wikstrom, Br. J. Urol. 51:175 (1979).

3. S. Ljunghall, Scand. J. Urol. Nephrol. Suppl. 41:6 (1977).
4. R. E. Williams, Br. J. Urol. 35:416 (1963).
5. B. Fellström, U. Backman, B. G. Danielson, G. Johansson, S. Ljunghall, and B. Wikström, Scand. J. Urol. Nephrol. Suppl. 54: (in press)

CRYSTALLURIA

P. G. Werness, J. H. Bergert, and L. H. Smith

Mayo Clinic

Rochester, Minnesota 55901

The human urinary tract may contain crystals of a variety of compositions and habits. Although there is not a one to one correspondence between crystalluria and urolithiasis, the presence of crystalluria is proof that a state of supersaturation exists or existed somewhere in the urinary tract. In addition, crystalluria can reflect the state of the urine with respect to factors such as inhibitors of aggregation and growth which are important to urinary stone formation. Quantitation of changes in crystalluria can be used to evaluate the effectiveness of various forms of treatment. Using a previously described method for the evaluation of crystalluria[1], we have studied 4835 voidings in 162 patients, both on and off treatment. A quantitative evaluation of crystalluria and supersaturation for calcium oxalate monohydrate and brushite in four groups of patients before and after treatment is presented.

The type of crystalluria observed is shown in Figure 1. The groups studied included normal subjects and patients with primary hyperparathyroidism (1° HPT) with and without stones, primary hyperoxaluria (1° HOx), and idiopathic calcium urolithiasis (ICU). None of the subjects were on treatment when studied. The most common crystals seen were hydroxyapatite (HAP), calcium oxalate monohydrate (COD), uric acid (UA) and brushite (BRU). Crystal identification was by petrographic microscopy and scanning electron microscopy with energy dispersive x-ray analysis.

The degree of crystalluria is shown in Figure 2. Quantitation of the degree of crystalluria for each voiding was by petrographic microscopy. Crystalluria found in each voiding was graded from 0 to 3+ (0 = neg; 1+ = 1-200 crystals/filter; 2+ = 200-500 crystals/ filter; 3+ = >500 crystals/filter). A semi-quantitative score was

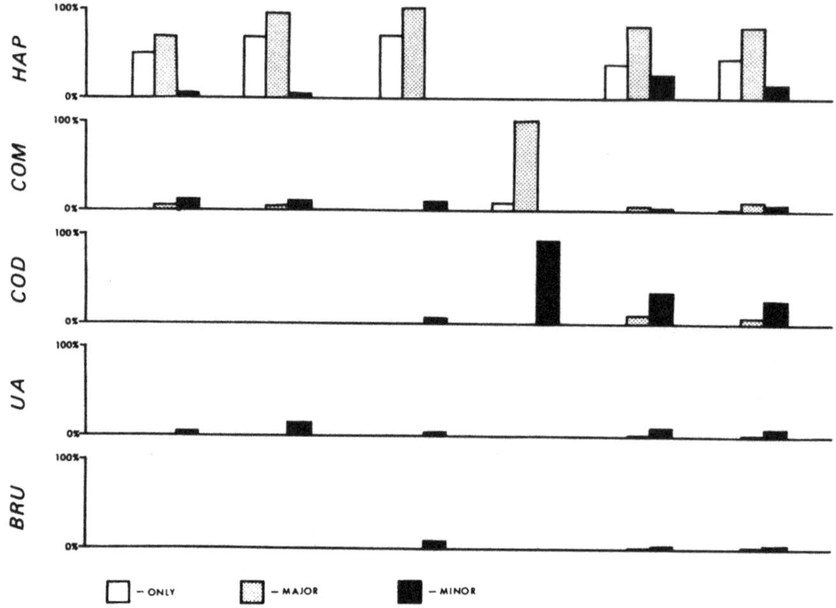

Figure 1. Type of crystalluria.

assigned to each voiding (0 = 0; 1+ = 1; 2+ = 3; and 3+ = 5). The sum of the scores from the individual voidings divided by the number of voidings during the 24-hour collection provided the crystalluria score, a gross quantitation of the degree of crystalluria.

The crystalluria score (the bottom line at Figure 2) was significantly higher ($p < .05$) for all patient groups before treatment compared to the normal subjects. Changes in crystalluria score with effective treatment is shown in Figure 3. Treatment for patients with primary hyperparathyroidism was parathyroid surgery. Patients with primary hyperoxaluria were treated with orthophosphate and pyridoxine. Orthophosphate or thiazide diuretics were used to treat patients with idiopathic calcium urolithiasis. In all patient groups, treatment reduced the crystalluria score to a level not different from that observed in normal subjects. The effect of treatment on supersaturation (SS) for calcium oxalate monohydrate (CaOx) and brushite ($CaHPO_4$) in the same patients is shown in Figure 4. Supersaturation is defined as (Activity Product - Solubility Product)/Solubility Product so that a SS of zero indicates a urine at saturation, negative numbers represent undersaturated urines and positive numbers represent supersaturated urines. Supersaturation for calcium oxalate is significantly reduced by treatment in all groups to the levels seen in normal subjects or less. Calcium phosphate supersaturation is reduced in patients with hyperparathyroidism

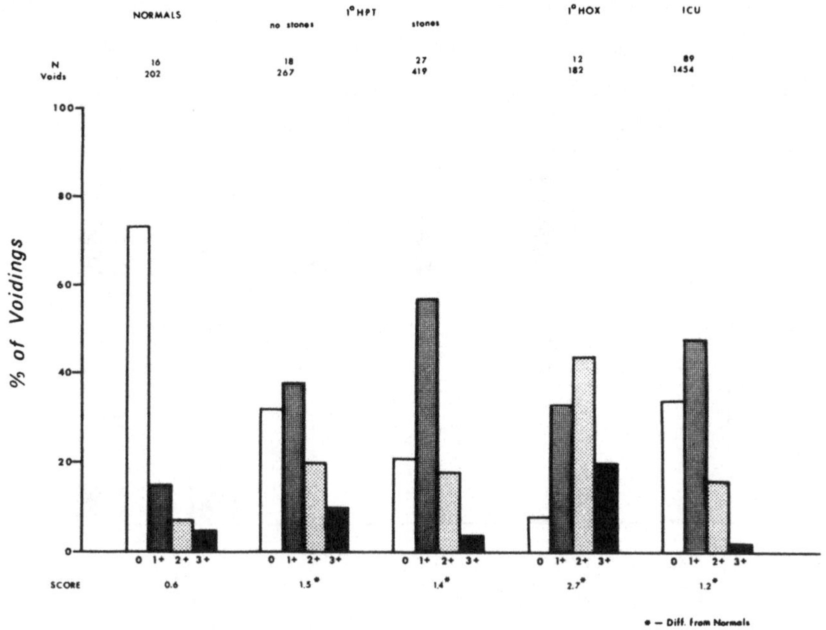

Figure 2. Degree of crystalluria.

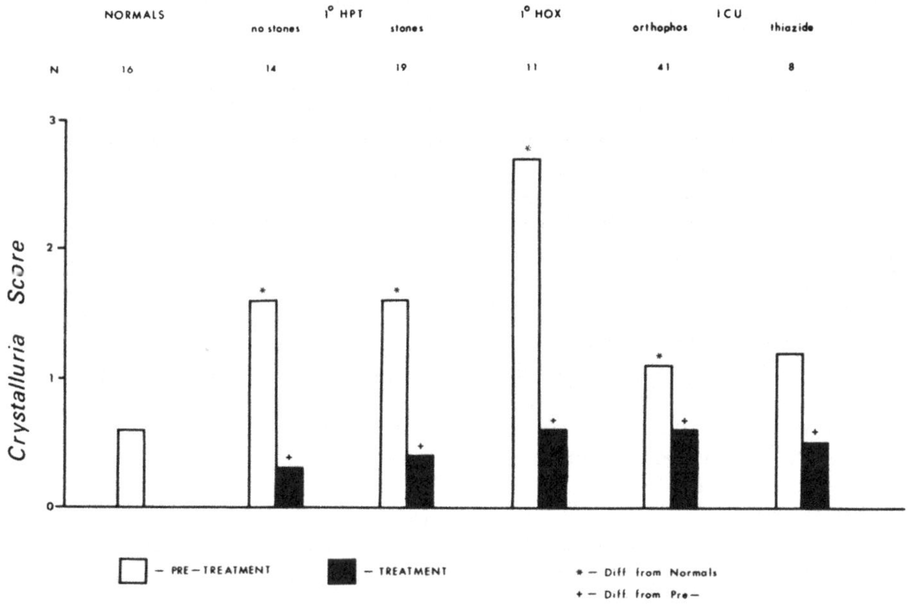

Figure 3. Effect of treatment on crystalluria score.

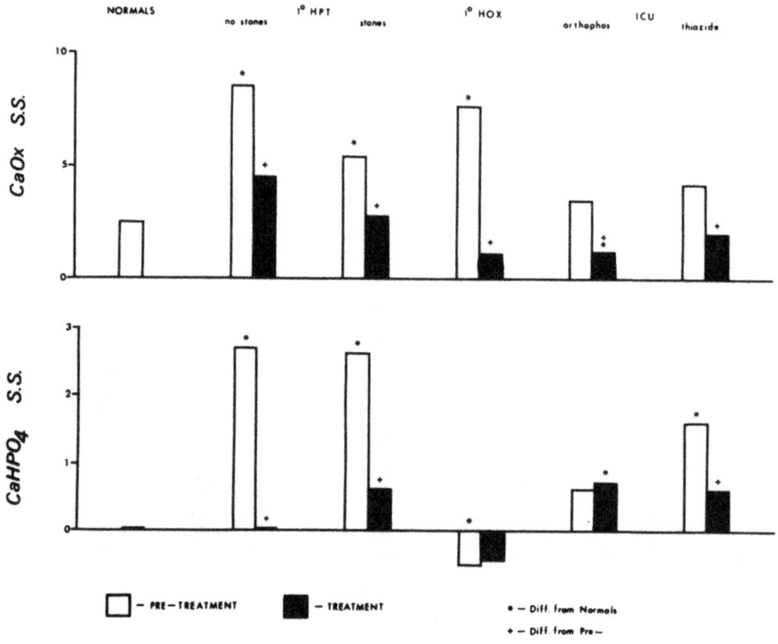

Figure 4. Effect of treatment on supersaturation.

following surgery and in patients with idiopathic calcium urolithiasis treated with thiazides.

We conclude that as a group, stone-forming patients have a greater number of crystals in their urine than normal subjects and that effective therapy results in a decrease in crystalluria to the levels seen in normal subjects (Figures 2 and 3). However, normal subjects may exhibit marked crystalluria in some voidings and patients with hyperparathyroidism who have never formed a urinary stone have as much crystalluria as those who do form stones. It is not possible to identify a stone-forming individual only on the basis of crystalluria. Evaluation of crystalluria can, however, provide an index of the efficacy of treatment. Effective treatment was accompanied by a decrease of crystalluria score in 93% of the patients. The five patients who responded to therapy with an increase in crystalluria had crystalluria scores within the normal range before and after treatment. Since the changes in crystalluria score occur soon after effective treatment is begun, it may be possible to monitor therapy rapidly and relatively easily with observations of crystalluria. The measurement of numerous other metabolic and urinary factors certainly provides valuable information on the stone forming potential of a subject, but stone disease is a complicated disorder involving many factors. Examination of crystalluria has the distinct advantage that it reflects the state of the urine with respect to a large number of factors, known and unknown, which affect stone formation and growth.

REFERENCES

1. C. J. Van Den Berg, T. M. Cahill, and L. H. Smith, in: "Urolithiasis Research," H. Fleisch, W. G. Robertson, L. H. Smith, and W. Vahlensieck, eds., Plenum Press, New York (1976).

ACKNOWLEDGMENTS

This investigation was supported in part by research grants, AM 20605 and RR 585 from the National Institutes of Health, Public Health Service.

STUDY OF CALCIUM CRYSTALS IN PATIENTS WITH KIDNEY STONES

L. Brandes, D. G. Oreopoulos, H. Husdan, and
P. Crassweller
Department of Medicine and Urology, Toronto Western
Hospital and University of Toronto
Toronto, Canada

INTRODUCTION

An important factor in the formation of calcium-containing kidney stones is the supersaturation of urine with calcium salts. However, we have been unable to find any difference in the saturation of calcium oxalate between stone-formers and normals, whereas the saturation of octocalcium phosphate was indeed higher in the stone formers although there was a considerable overlap[1].

An alternative method of studying the saturation of urine with various salts is the study of crystals. Crystals will not be formed unless the urine has been supersaturated and the various factors which prevent their formation (inhibitors) have been low (relatively or absolutely). Accordingly, formation of crystals is an indication that the balance between the two opposing forces has been disturbed in favor of precipitation.

In this paper we describe the results of our studies on urine calcium crystals in a group of normals and stone formers. In the latter group the crystalluria was studied before and after treatment.

MATERIALS AND METHODS

Since there is no difference between crystals of random and a concentrated (after 12-h overnight fast) sample[2], we included only random samples. The samples were voided in a Thermos flask and maintained at 37°C during the counting procedure.

The controls and the patients consisted of adult men (20-55 years old). The patients were investigated either during their initial assessment or while on treatment. In 43 of them serial measurements were available. The therapeutic regimens that were used were either hydrochlorothiazide (50 mg b.i.d.), or phosphate (500 mg b.i.d. or t.i.d.) or allopurinol (300 mg/day). A total of 23 samples from normals and 278 samples from stone formers were studied. We followed the technique described by Robertson et al.[3]. The model T_A Coulter Counter (Coulter Electronics Inc, Hialeh, FL) was used to measure the volume of the calcium crystals particles, with diameter 5 to 40 μm. With this method all calcium crystals are measured and no attempt was made to differentiate them. The results were expressed as either the volume of all calcium crystals present (V_T) or the volume of only the large (> 12μm) crystals or crystals aggregate (V_L).

Finally we measured the concentration of acid mucopolysaccharide (AMPS) in a fasting urine sample obtained 3 days after the crystal measurement was performed[4]. Statistical analysis of the data was performed using the Wilcoxon's rank test.

RESULTS

(a) Frequency of Crystalluria

Since there is a seasonal variation in urine crystalluria[5], we divided our results into two periods i.e. October-March (Winter) and April-September (Summer). In the normals we had data available only during the summer period. Among the patients there was an increased percentage of samples containing crystals (V_T) during the summer months (88% vs 71%), ($p < 0.005$), but the reverse was observed for the large crystals (V_L) i.e. 51% of the winter samples contained crystals but only 38% of the summer samples ($p < 0.05$). Among normals, 82% of the samples had crystals (V_T) and only 26% of them had crystals larger than 12 μm (V_L). This difference was not statistically significant from the summer patients.

The seasonal variation was further investigated among 35 pairs of urine samples of stone formers who had their urine tested twice. The summer samples had higher mean values for both total and large crystal volumes but the differences reached statistical significance ($p < .01$) for the total volumes only (summer $V_T = 3.87 \pm 5.82 \times 10^6$ vs winter $V_T = 2.15 \pm 3.33 \times 10^6 \frac{\mu m^3}{ml}$).

Comparison Between Normals and Stone Formers

Figure 1 shows the total crystal volumes in a group of normals and 4 groups of stone formers (untreated and after allopurinol, hydrochlorothiazide or phosphates). Untreated stone formers had significantly ($p < 0.001$) higher values than normal controls. After treatment these values remained high for the allopurinol-and

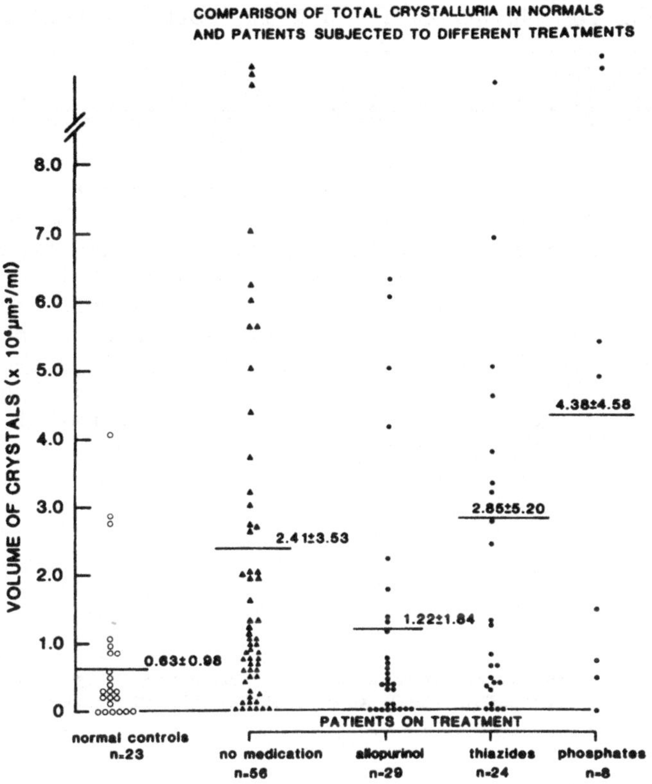

Figure 1. Comparison of total crystalluria in normals and patients undergoing different treatments.

chlorothiazide-treated groups, whereas those treated with phosphates showed even higher values ($p < 0.02$).

A study was carried out on the total crystal volume and the volume of large crystals only in a group of untreated stone formers who had sequential measurement over 6 to 12 month periods. There was a statistically significant increase ($p < 0.001$) in the volume of total crystals (V_T) with passage of time. However the increase in the volume of large crystals (V_L) was not statistically significant. This increase in the volume of crystals with passage of time was not observed in the group of treated patients.

An attempt was made to correlate the amount of crystals present in urine with the saturation level of either calcium oxalate or octocalcium phosphate of fasting urine samples obtained within 15 days of the crystalluria test. We were unable to observe any correlation (for non-treated patients (n = 15) calcium oxalate r =

0.0961, octocalcium phosphate r = 0.0051, both statistically insignificant).

Correlation of Crystal Volumes with the Concentration of Acid Mucopolysaccharide.

An attempt was made to correlate the concentration of acid mucopolysaccharide and the amount of crystals. In 38 samples, both of these were measured, but in 22 of them the large crystals were absent at the time of investigation. Accordingly this correlation was performed only in 16 in whom both parameters were present. Figure 2 shows that there was a statistically significant positive correlation between the total volume of crystals (V_T) and the concentration of AMPS ($p < 0.001$) performed in the semi-logarithmic transformation, and a negative one between the volume of large crystals (V_L) and AMPS ($p < 0.05$).

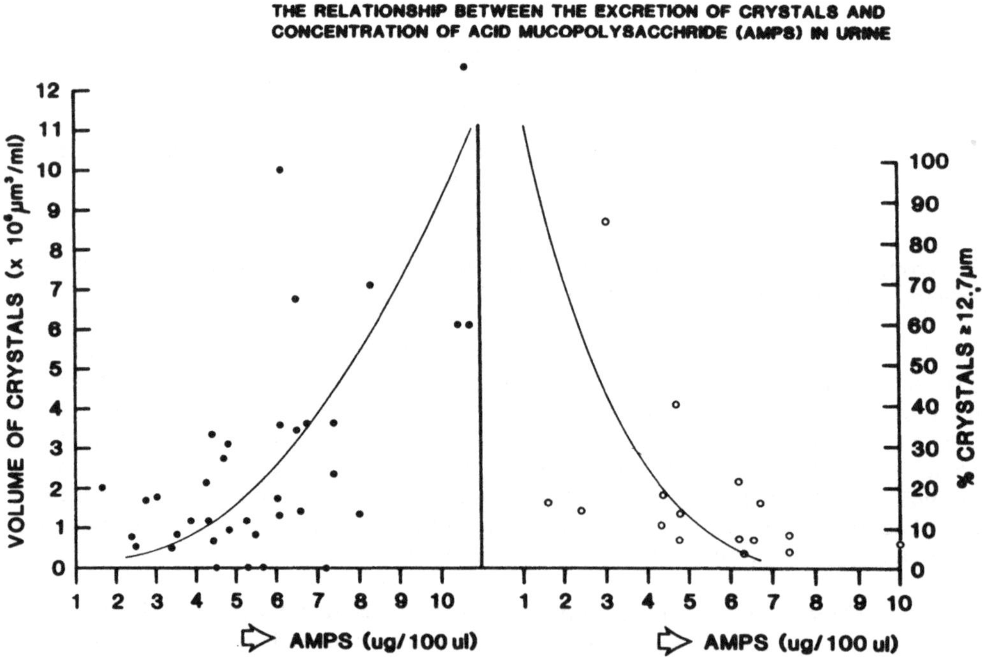

Figure 2. Correlation between crystal volumes and concentration of acid mucopolysaccharide (AMPS) in urine.

DISCUSSION

Our observation that during the summer period there is an increase in the amount of crystals present in the urine agrees with a previous observation[5]. This may be due to an increase in saturation of urine with calcium oxalate salts during the summer. Our inability to confirm a correlation between crystals and activity products, however, may suggest that the activity products, as we measure them, may not be an accurate index of the urine saturation. This is supported by our previous observation that there was no difference in the saturation level of calcium oxalate between normals and stone formers[1]. The fact that the large crystals do not follow the same changes in volume as that of the total crystals indicates that crystal growth and aggregation are two distinct phases governed by different control mechanisms. This may be reflected with the positive correlation between total crystals and AMPS, whereas the large crystals showed an inverse correlation. The latter observation suggests that AMPS is mainly an inhibitor of aggregation of crystals, while may not prevent nucleation.

The increase in total volume of crystals but not of the large ones, among patients treated with phosphates indicates that the increased phosphate concentration enhances crystal formation (especially calcium phosphate) but the simultaneous increase in urine pyrophosphate, prevents their aggregation to large crystals.

The results of the follow-up studies on treatment were surprising; according to these results the only effect that various treatments had was to prevent the increase in the volume of total crystals which the untreated patients show with passage of time. None of the treatments led to the normalization of crystalluria, and actually, those treated with phosphates had an increase in total volumes. This observation cast some doubt on the usefulness of this test in the studies of patients with renal stones and their response to various treatments.

REFERENCES

1. P. O. Crassweller and D. G. Oreopoulos, J. Urol. 120:6 (1978).
2. P. O. Crassweller, L. Brandes, A. Katirtzoglou, and D. G. Oreopoulos, Can. J. of Surg. 22:527 (1979).
3. W. G. Robertson, Clin. Chem. Acta. 26:105 (1969).
4. P. Whiteman, Biochem. J. 131:343 (1973).
5. P. C. Hallson and G. A. Rose, Br. J. Urol. 49:277 (1977).

ACKNOWLEDGMENT

This work was supported by the Medical Research Council of Canada (Grant No. MA-3889).

METABOLIC INVESTIGATIONS IN 407 RECURRENT STONE-FORMERS AND HEALTHY CONTROLS ON CONDITION OF INDIVIDUAL AS WELL AS STANDARD DIET

W. Vahlensieck, D. Bach, A. Hesse, and W. Schneeberger

Section for Urolithiasis Research, Department of Urology, University Hospital, Bonn, West-Germany

Recurrent stone-formers require a detailed and standardized metabolic investigation to gain a better understanding about the pathogenesis of the stone formation in order to determine treatment to prevent stone recurrences. Since 1977 we have investigated lithogenic and inhibitory substances in serum and urine in 407 recurrent stone-formers and a group of 18 healthy controls. Both groups had been as in-patients for a period of 12 days.

METHOD

Prior to hospitalization serum and a 24-hour urine was collected from each of the study subjects on their normal diet (basic investigation). For the following 12 days the patients received a standard diet with 1.1 l liquid supply. Serum constituents were measured on day one, five and ten, while urinary substances were determined daily in the 24-hour urine from day one through eight. (See Table 1). On days nine and ten urine was collected in 3-hour specimens over 48 hours. In case of pathological deviations of values after 10 days on the condition of a standard diet compared to the initial basic investigations special loading tests were performed on days eleven and twelve.

RESULTS

Serum constituents did not change during the time on the standard diet. The results of calcium and magnesium shown in Figure 1 are representative of all measured serum components. The mean urine pH was 6.0 and the specific gravity ranged from 1001 to 1005 on the standard diet. All data generated from the study of

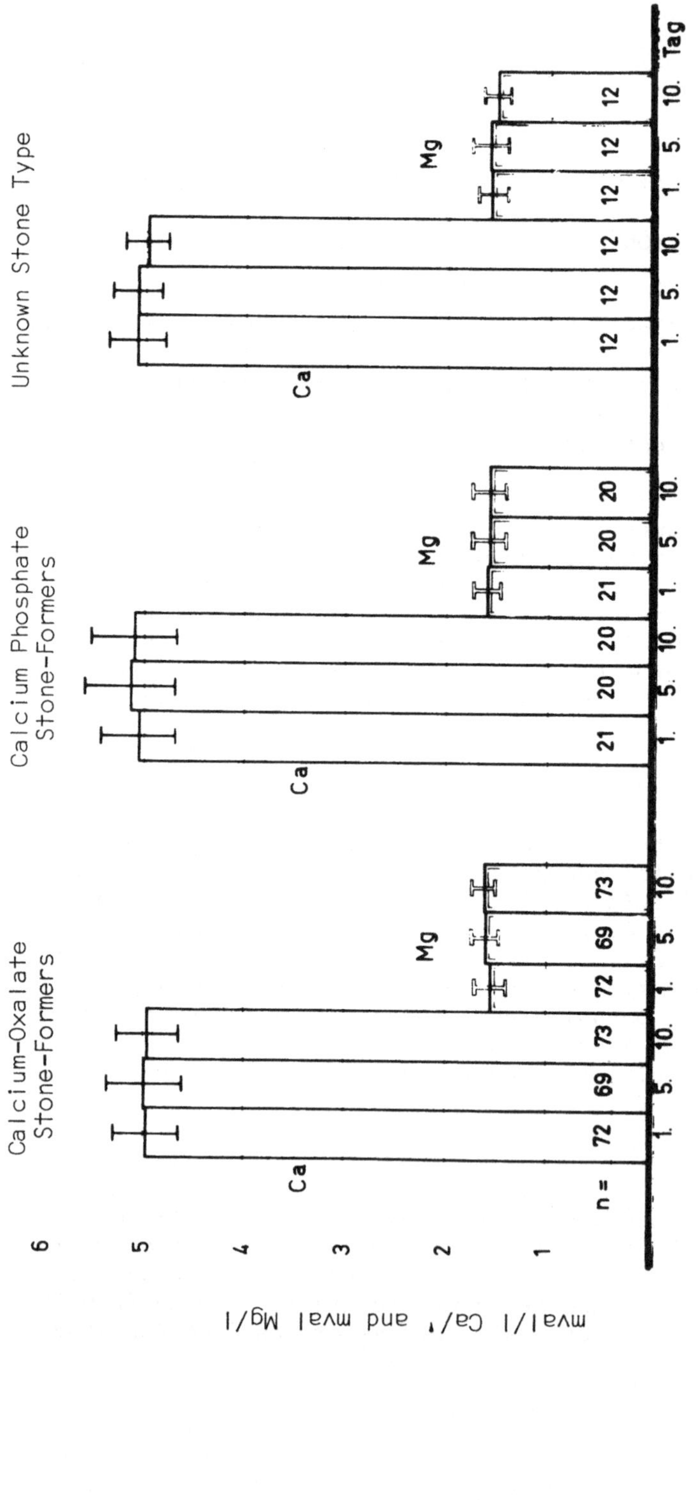

Figure 1. Calcium and magnesium concentration in the serum (mval/l) in calcium-oxalate stone-formers, calcium phosphate stone-formers and stone-formers with unknown type of calculus. Investigations were made on day 1, 5 and 10 on conditions of a 12 day standard diet.

Table 1. Investigations in Serum and Urine

Serum	Urine		Optional
Sodium	Sodium	pH	Loading Tests (LT)
Potassium	Potassium	Density	Ammonium-Chloride LT
Calcium	Calcium	Uric acid	Uric acid LT
Magnesium	Magnesium	Citric acid	Calcium LT
Zinc	Zinc	Oxalic acid	Oxalic acid LT
Chloride	Chloride	Cystine	
Phosphate	Phosphate	Urinalysis	Miscellaneous
Sulphate	Sulphate	Bacteriologic-	
Creatinine	Creatinine	Investigation	Bone densitometry
Uric acid			Bone marrow biopsy
Parathormone			
Vitamin D			

urine composition cannot be presented. Selected observations of importance are outlined below.

A steady state on the standard diet appeared to be reached from days 5 to 7 based on the urine results. An example of this is shown in Figure 2. The calcium and magnesium concentration decreased during the investigation on the standard diet (Figure 3). Deviation from this pattern occurred only in those patients where factors other than diet determine the excretion of calcium and magnesium.

Investigations of the effect of the standard diet on the 3-hour urine fractions over a 48-hour period (day nine and ten) showed in both stone-formers and controls sinusoid curves in excretion and concentration of lithogenic substances, which are correlating with food and liquid supply.

The curves showing the calcium-excretion and concentration of 17 calcium-oxalate stone formers is a typical example (Figure 4). While the concentration is decreasing during the morning (due to breakfast and increased liquid supply) and the first half of the night (due to supper and "liquid for the night") it is increasing after lunch (caused by increased electrolyte intake) and in the last part of the night (caused by low drinking). Also the excretion and concentration of citric acid showed a typical sinusoid rhythm. The mean citric acid concentration and excretion is higher in the controls (n = 18) compared to calcium oxalate stone-formers (n = 20) (Figures 5a and b). Here the minimum concentration between 8 p.m. and 2 a.m. seems to be of special importance, since this is the time when the calcium concentration is found at its highest.

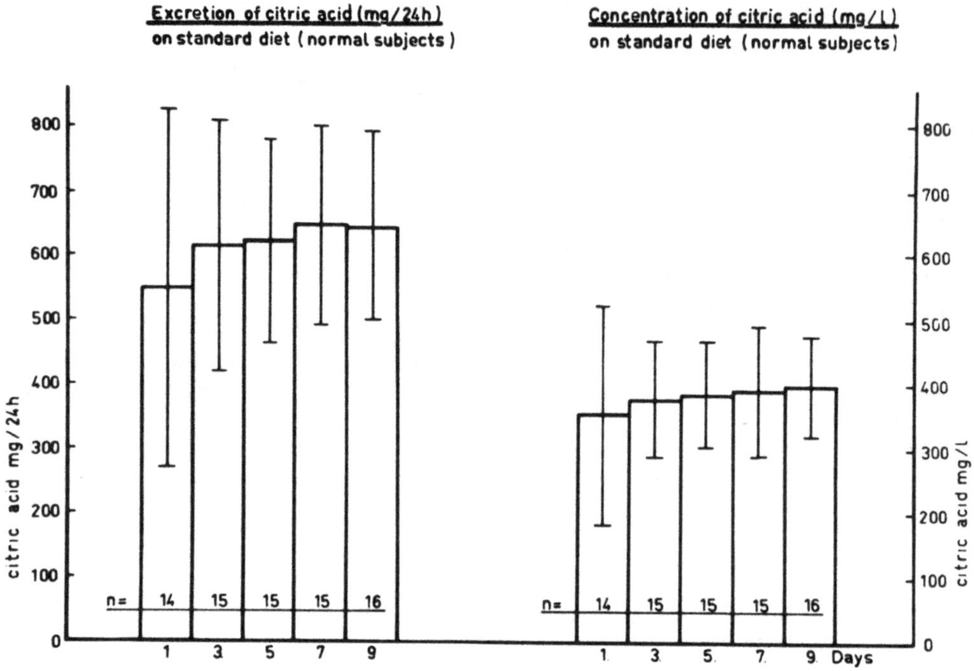

Figure 2. Excretion and concentration of citric acid in healthy controls (n = 16) on condition of a 12 day standard diet.

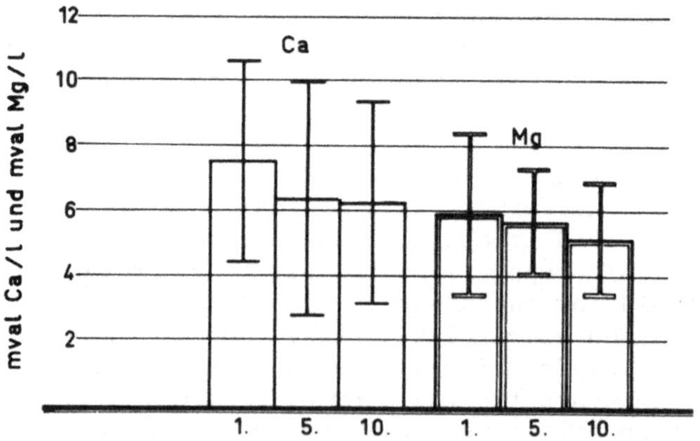

Figure 3. Concentration of calcium and magnesium (mval/l) in 24-hour urine in 21 calcium phosphate stone-formers on condition of a 12 day standard diet.

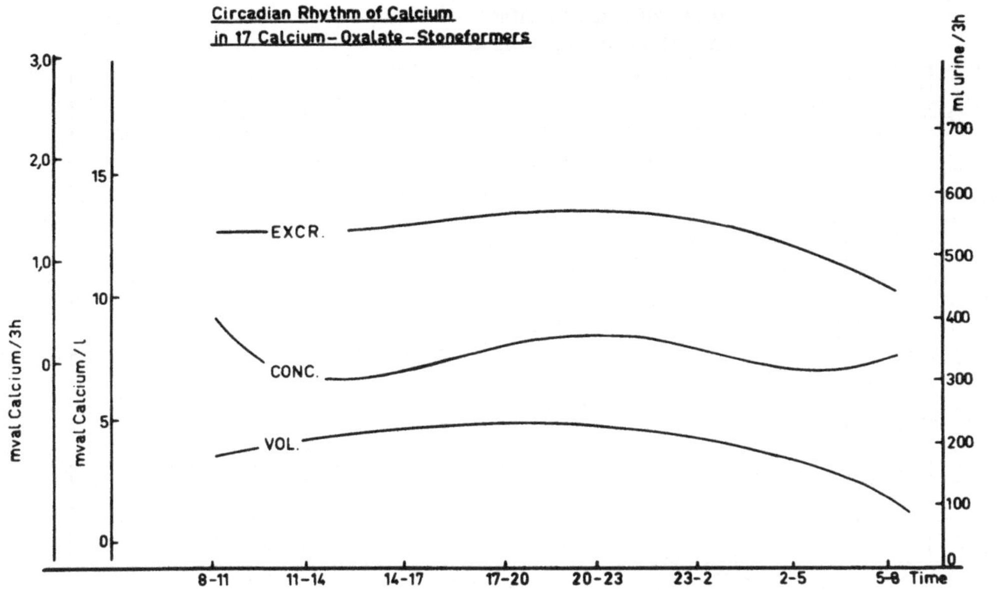

Figure 4. Circadian rhythm of calcium in 17 calcium oxalate stone-formers at the day nine and ten on condition of standard diet.

DISCUSSION

Our standardized program for the investigation of recurrent stone-formers enables us to define pathogenic features that cannot be observed in patients on a free diet. On the standard diet a so-called "steady state" in the urinary excretion and concentration of lithogenic and inhibitory substances is reached within 5 to 7 days. When initial values are above "steady state" values, then evidence of overconsumption of lithogenic substances in the free diet is present. In patients where a "steady state" is not reached, the causal factors for stone-formation seems to be non-dietary. The investigation of the circadian rhythm of excretion and concentration of lithogenic substances as well as the subsequent loading tests lead to further diagnostic knowledge. This investigation model provides information regarding the influence of different foods, liquids and drugs on the excretion of lithogenic and inhibitory substances in the urine.

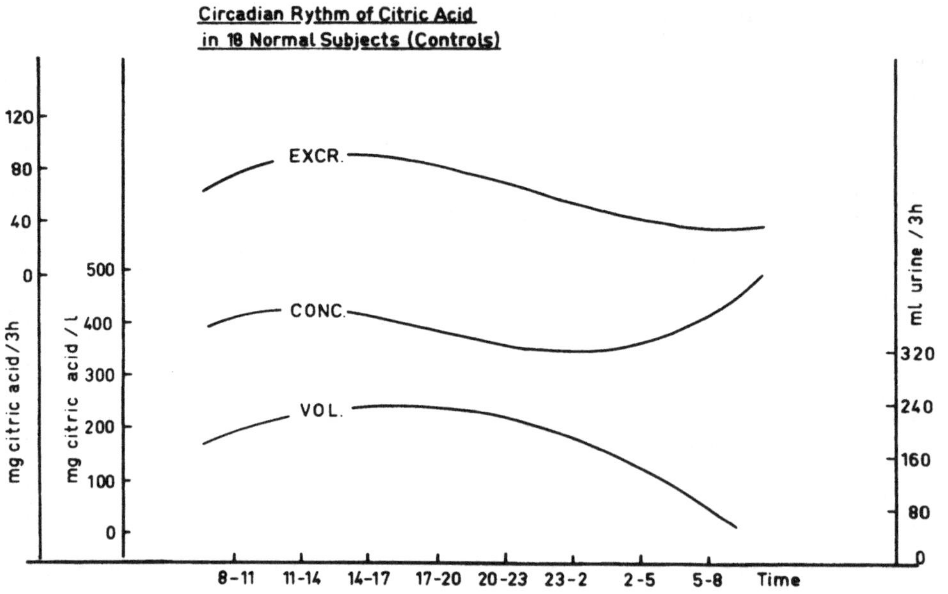

Figure 5a. Circadian rhythm of citric acid in 18 healthy controls on condition of standard diet (day 9 and 10).

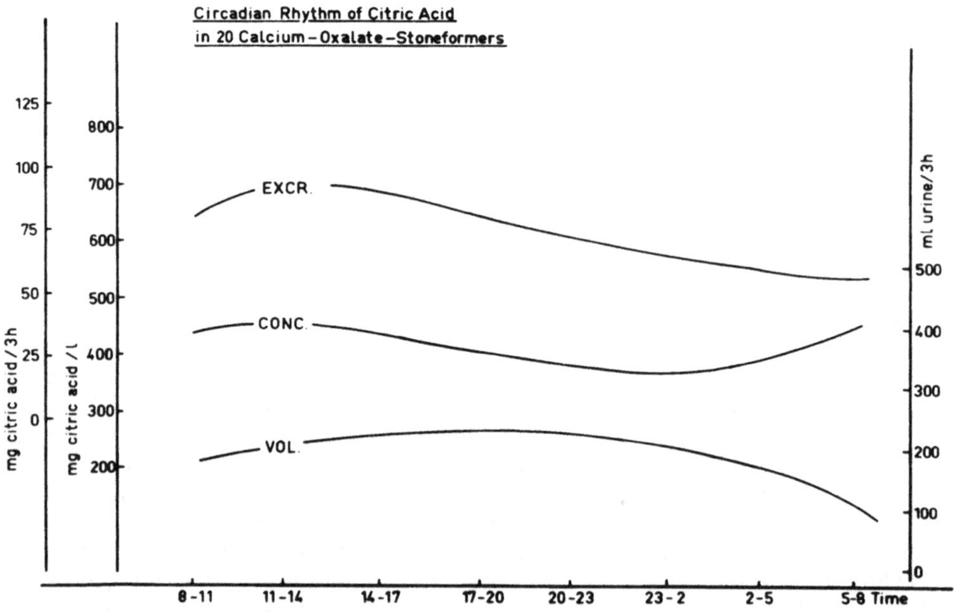

Figure 5b. Circadian rhythm of citric acid in 20 calcium oxalate stone-formers on condition of standard diet (day 9 and 10).

CLASSIFICATION OF STONE-PATIENTS AND HEALTHY PERSONS ON THE BASIS OF THE URINARY ANALYSIS

R. Hartung, P. Leskovar, J. Riedel,
H. Schneider, A. Siebert, and M. Kratzer
Urologische Klinik und Poliklinik rechts der Isar der Technischen Universität München
München, Federal Republic of Germany

INTRODUCTION

There are many reports on the differences between the urine of stone-formers and that of healthy controls. Some authors have emphasized, however, that the main difference is not between healthy persons and stone-patients in general but between the single and multiple (recurrent) stone-formers. It should not be overlooked that the reported differences represent the differences between the mean values of the groups whereas the mean values of individuals within each group and the values of the individual urinary sample may be scattered widely around the mean value of the group, producing a broad overlap between patients and controls. This may be demonstrated in the case of the urinary magnesium measured every day for eighteen days in a group of 16 recurrent stone-formers and 11 healthy controls.

Figure 1 shows the mean (± 1 SD) values in both groups of their morning (A), midday (B), evening (C) and 12 h urines. There is a clear difference in the Mg concentration in all daily urine portions. If, however, the corresponding 18-day mean values for the individual subjects are examined, the overlap becomes more evident.

The question arises whether or not a single urinary analysis allows a clear, unequivocal separation and classification of stone-formers and healthy controls. We have therefore set out to determine if a single urinary analysis gives a sufficient information to allow unequivocal separation of stone-patients and healthy persons.

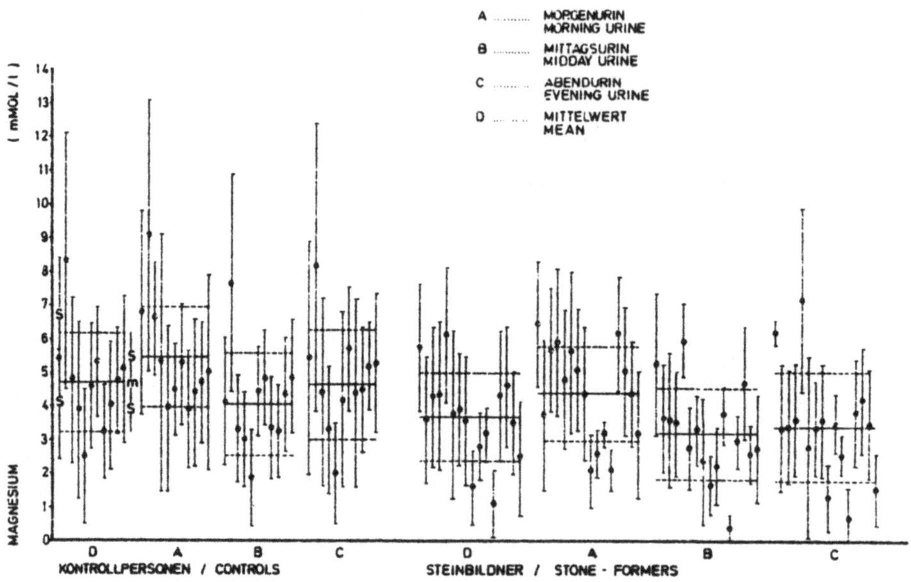

Figure 1. Individual mean values and standard deviations of the Mg-concentration in recurrent stone-patients and controls after 18 days of observation. The wide overlap-zone is obvious.

MATERIAL AND METHODS

In the morning (A), midday (B), evening (C) and 12 h urines of eleven recurrent stone-formers and 10 controls the following variables were analyzed during a period of 6 days: calcium (total), magnesium and sodium (by AAS 400/Perkin & Elmer), ionized calcium (by Ca^{2+}-selective electrode Orion 93 - 20, combined with Orion Ionalyzer 801 A, both Colora Meßtechnik/Lorch), citric acid (by Boehringer test combination 139076), ammonia (by NH_4^+-sensitive electrode Orion 95 - 10), titratable acidity (by pH meter E 510/ Impulsomat E 473/Dosimat E 535, all Metrohm/Herisau), crystalluria (by Coulter Counter ZF/Size Distribution Analyzer P 128), osmolarity (by vapour pressure osmometer 5130, Wescor/Logan) and microscopic hematuria both by Sangur test (Boehringer/Mannheim) and by the light-microscopic evaluation (Leitz/Wetzlar) of urinary sediment.

RESULTS

The basic idea was to combine, in the form of quotients, all those urinary parameters that proved to be different between the stone-patients and their healthy controls. In this way, the minimal differences in the single urinary parameters could be amplified and the overlap between the individual 6-day mean values could be

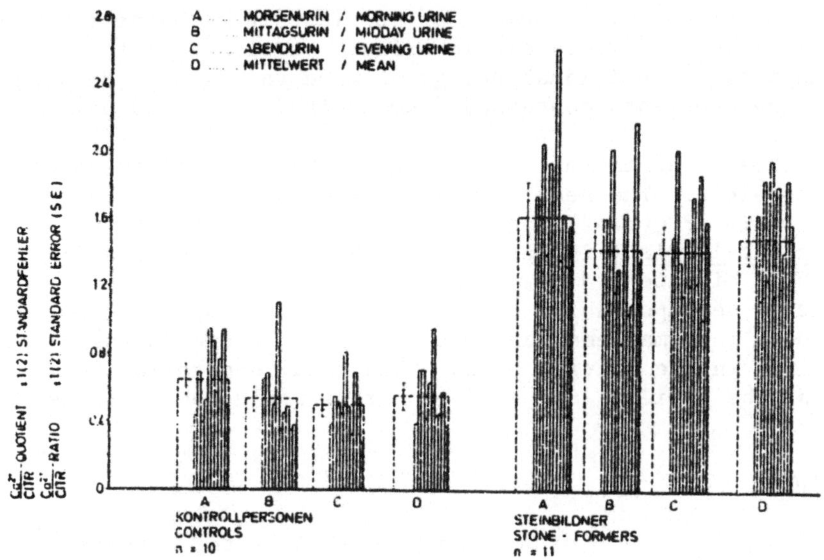

Figure 2. Individual and group mean values of the Ca^{2+}/citrate-quotient in the group of recurrent stone-formers and their controls.

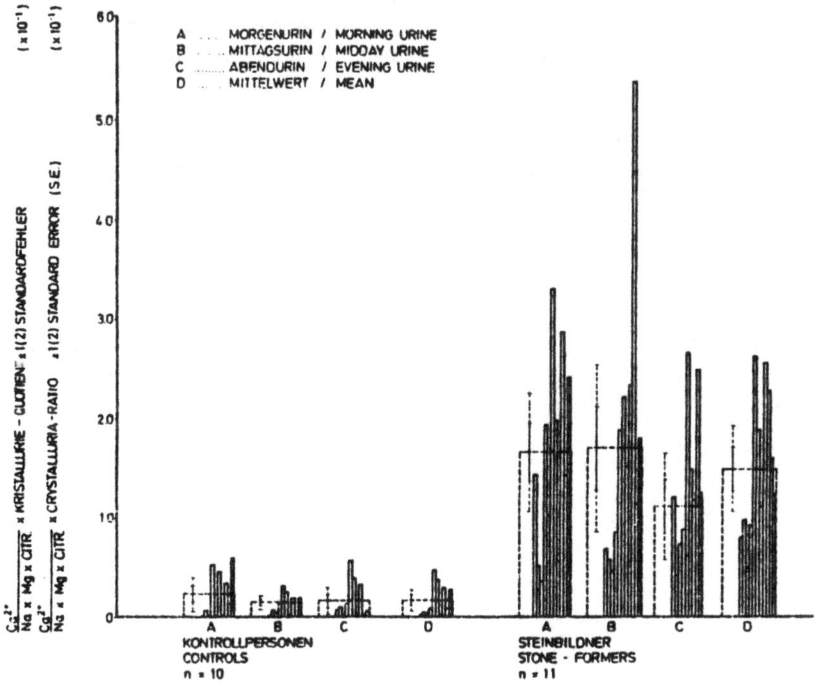

Figure 3. One of the most "favorable" quotients is the (Ca^{2+} x crystalluria)/(Na x Mg x citrate)-quotient.

considerably reduced. A number of quotients used by various authors were calculated for every single urinary sample separately and from them the various individual and group mean values were derived. Some of the quotients contained "osmolarity"-corrected parameters.

In this presentation, a detailed comment on all the quotients is not possible. The best simple quotient appeared to be the Ca^{2+}/citrate ratio (Figure 2) and the best complex quotient was $\frac{Ca^{2+} \times \text{crystalluria}}{Na \times Mg \times \text{citrate}}$ (Figure 3). A total separation of both groups appeared to be impossible. If, however, microscopic hematuria could be included in a mathematically correct form there is the problem of zero values in the control group, then total separation between the values of the patients and their controls would appear to be possible.

CONCLUSION

From our data it can be concluded that by the systematic combination of urinary variables which are different in stone-patients and healthy persons, small differences between the groups can be amplified and the large overlap zone reduced to a minimum. The additional introduction of a term to cover microscopic hematuria would allow total, unequivocal separation of patients and controls. The problem however, is how to include in a mathematically correct manner, the zero values for microscopic hematuria found in many normal individuals.

One additional experience is that a single measurement of each variable is insufficient to separate stone-formers from normals. The individuals must be observed for at least 3 - 6 days to provide the characteristic pattern of urinary excretion.

ACKNOWLEDGMENT

The authors would like to thank Mrs. D. Scherm, Mr. K.-L. Schade, Mrs. H. Richter and Mr. M. Gottinger (München) for their kind technical assistance.

URINARY EXCRETION OF CITRATE IN NORMAL SUBJECTS AND PATIENTS WITH UROLITHIASIS

Hans-Göran Tiselius

Department of Urology
University Hospital
S-581 85 Linköping, Sweden

In previous investigations it has been demonstrated that citrate has two different roles in urine with respect to calcium-oxalate stone formation: (a) a complex formation between calcium and citrate resulting in a decreased ion activity product for calcium-oxalate, and (b) a direct inhibitory influence on the crystallization of calcium-oxalate.

Contradictory results concerning citrate excretion have been reported in stone forming patients[1], and the present investigation was undertaken in order to obtain information on citrate excretion in normal subjects and stone formers, to compare citrate excretion in men and women and furthermore to study the inhibition of calcium oxalate crystal growth by citrate.

METHODS

Twenty-four hour urine samples were collected from 132 normal men with an age of 43 ± 10 years (mean ± SD), 30 normal women 40 ± 12 years, 83 male patients 46 ± 11 years and 30 female patients 46 ± 17 years.

Urine was collected in plastic bottles without any preservative. During the collection period all subjects ate their ordinary diet. The urine samples were immediately brought to the laboratory and frozen until analyzed. Samples containing bacteria were discarded. Citrate was determined with a method described by Greenbaum and Pace[2], and creatinine was analyzed by an alkaline picrate method.

Inhibition of calcium oxalate crystal growth was analyzed by measuring the loss of ^{14}C-oxalate following addition of seed crystals to a crystallization system with a composition mainly as described by Robertson et al.[3] The process was run during 120 minutes and crystals were removed by filtration through a Millipore filter (0.22 µm).

RESULTS

From Figure 1 it is evident that citrate is a potent inhibitor of calcium oxalate crystal growth. Therefore, urinary excretion of citrate might be of fundamental importance for the crystallization properties of urine.

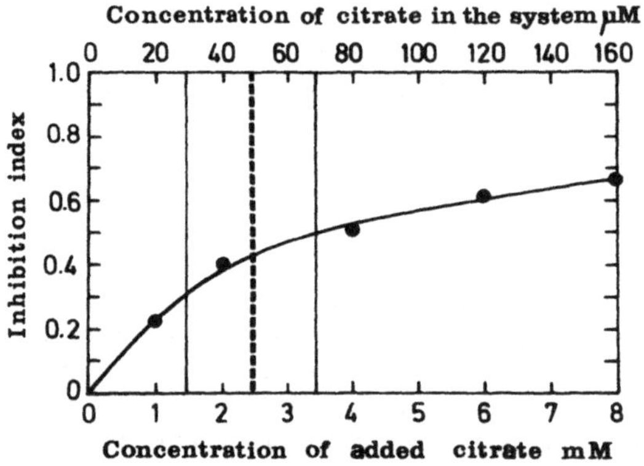

Figure 1. Inhibition of calcium oxalate crystal growth by different concentrations of citrate in the crystallization system. The normal mean citrate concentration (± SD) in urine is indicated in the figure.

The cumulative frequency distribution curves for urinary citrate during 24 hours in normal men and male patients with calcium oxalate stone disease (Figure 2) demonstrate a lower citrate excretion in male patients than in normal men. The mean excretion was 2.48 ± 0.99 mmol (± SD) and 3.16 ± 1.10 mmol respectively. The difference is statistically significant ($p < 0.001$).

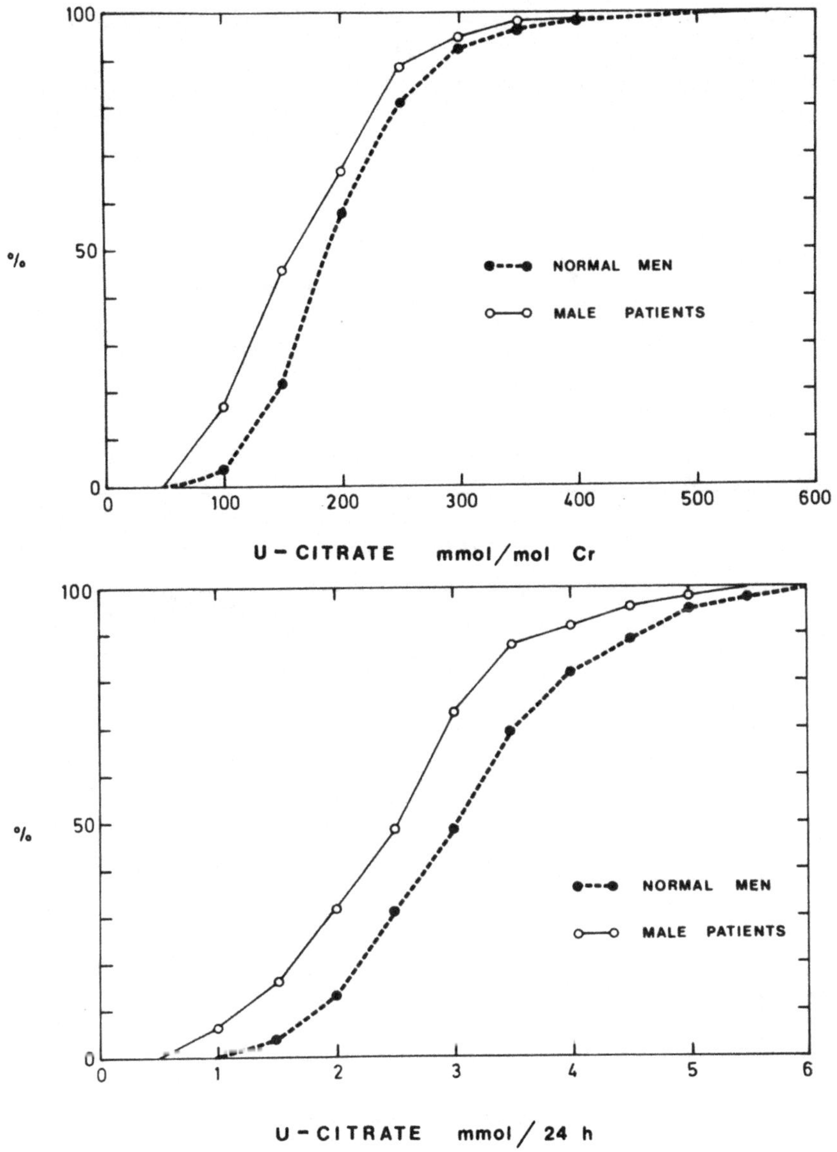

Figure 2. Cumulative frequency distribution curves for citrate/creatinine quotients (top) and urinary citrate excretion (bottom) per 24 hours in male patients and and normal men.

The cumulative frequency distribution curves for urinary citrate/creatinine quotients in normal men and male patients with calcium oxalate stone disease (Figure 2) disclose a mean excretion for normal men of 201 ± 89 mmol/mol (± SD) and for male patients 176 ± 67 mmol/mol. The difference is statistically significant ($p < 0.05$).

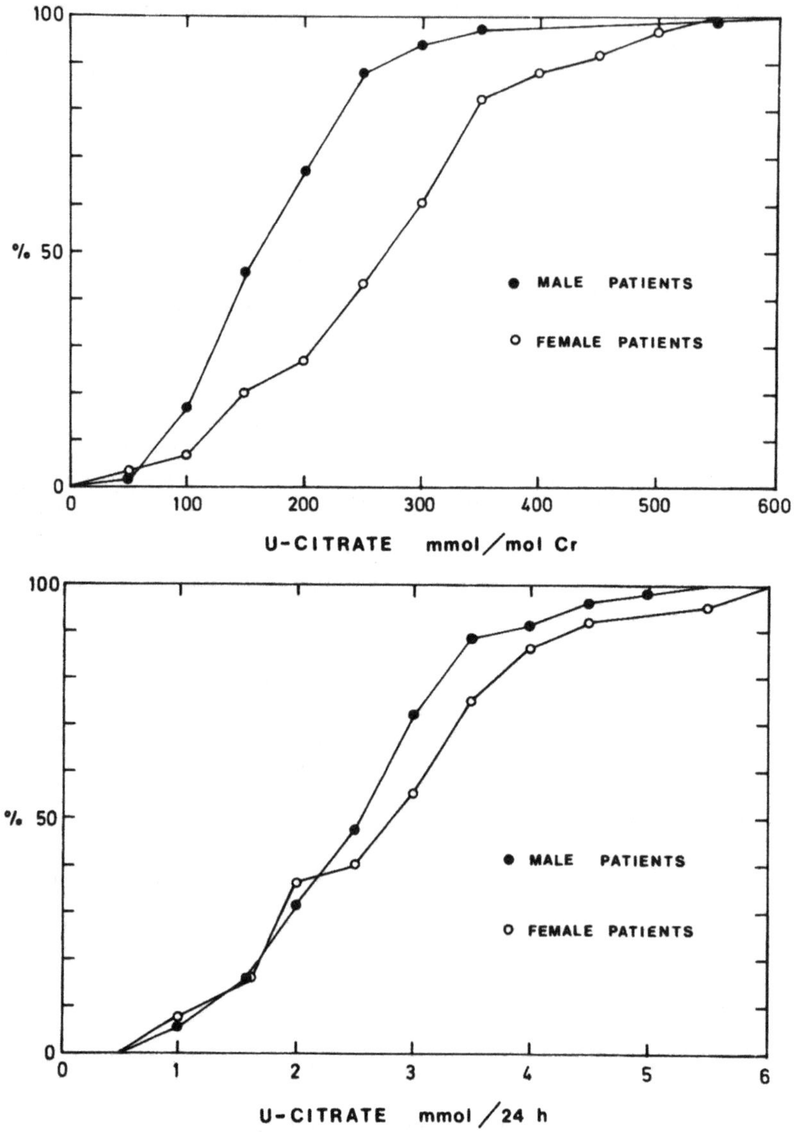

Figure 3. Cumulative frequency distribution curves for citrate/creatinine quotient (top) and urinary citrate excretion per 24 hours (bottom) in male and female patients with urolithiasis.

Cumulative frequency distribution curves for urinary citrate excretion during 24 hours in male and female patients with calcium oxalate stone disease are demonstrated in Figure 3. Mean citrate excretion was 2.48 ± 0.99 mmol (± SD) and 2.73 ± 1.30 mmol per day

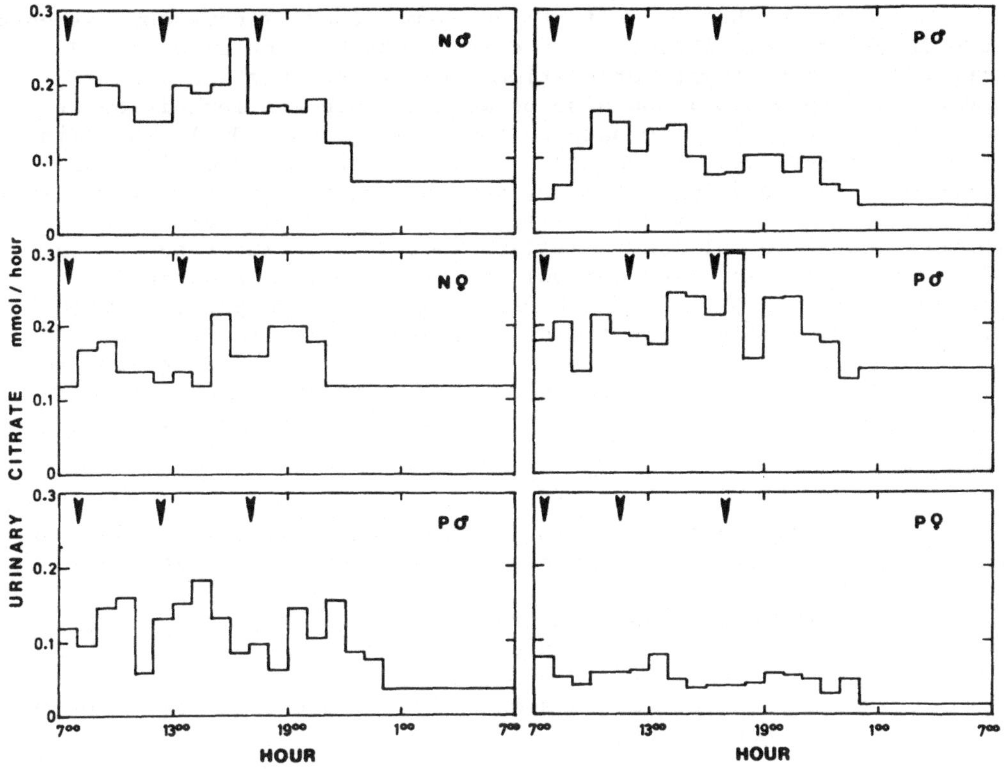

Figure 4. The diurnal variation of urinary citrate in 2 normal subjects and 4 patients with urolithiasis. The meals are indicated by arrows.

respectively. Although there was a slightly higher value in women, this difference did not reach the level of statistical significance.

When the citrate/creatinine quotient was considered the means for male patients were 267 ± 121 mmol/mol (± SD) and for female patients 176 ± 89 mmol/mol. This difference is highly significant ($p < 0.001$).

In a group comprising 30 normal men and 30 normal women, with the same age distribution the citrate excretion during 24 hours was 2.86 ± 0.94 (mean ± SD) mmol and 3.27 ± 0.73 mmol respectively, ($p < 0.05$). The citrate/creatinine quotient was in women 316 ± 108 and in men 207 ± 73 mmol/mol ($p < 0.001$).

Correlations between citrate and some other urinary constituents were investigated. There was no correlation between calcium and citrate. A significant correlation was obtained between magnesium and citrate ($p < 0.05$) and also between citrate and inhibition of calcium oxalate crystal growth in normal men ($p < 0.005$). No significant correlations were recorded between citrate and oxalate or between citrate and inhibition of calcium oxalate crystal growth in male patients. These results were obtained from 113 male stone formers and 32 normal men. Similar findings were recorded for women. All values were expressed per mol of creatinine. The diurnal urinary excretion of citrate in normal subjects and patients with urolithiasis varied during the day (Figure 4). There are meal related peaks of citrate excretion which might be important in protecting the urinary tract from crystallization during periods with an increased load of crystallization promoting substances.

CONCLUSIONS

1. Citrate appears to have a significant inhibiting effect on calcium oxalate crystal growth even at very low concentrations.

2. Urinary excretion of citrate was significantly lower in male patients with calcium oxalate stone disease than in normal men.

3. Women excreted larger amounts of citrate than men at least in the group of normal subjects.

4. No significant correlation was obtained between calcium and citrate, but weak correlations were recorded between magnesium and citrate. Furthermore a correlation was found between citrate and the inhibition index in normal subjects.

5. Urinary excretion of citrate varied during the day with meal-related peaks.

From these results it is evident that determination of citrate might be of value in the biochemical investigation and followup of patients with calcium oxalate stone disease.

REFERENCES

1. P. O. Schwille, D. Scholz, M. Paulus, W. Engelhardt, and A. Sigel, Invest. Urol. 16:457 (1979).
2. B. W. Greenbaum and N. Pace, Micro. Chem. J. 15:673 (1970).
3. W. G. Robertson, M. Peacock, and B. E. C. Nordin, Clin. Chim. Acta. 43:31 (1973).

MAGNESIUM EXCRETION IN URINE ON CONDITION OF INDIVIDUAL AS WELL AS STANDARD DIET IN HEALTHY CONTROLS AND CALCIUM OXALATE STONE FORMERS

D. Bach, A. Hesse, A. Strenge, and W. Vahlensieck

Urolithiasis Research, Department of Urology,
University Hospital
Bonn, West Germany

With our investigations we tried to answer the following questions:

1. Is there any subnormal excretion of magnesium (Mg) in calcium (Ca) oxalate stone-formers?

2. Do calcium oxalate stone-formers and healthy controls show any difference in their Mg excretion on condition of standard diet as well as of individual diet?

3. Is the Ca/Mg ratio qualified for estimating any risk of stone formation?

MATERIAL AND METHODS

In 33 calcium oxalate stone formers and 16 healthy controls as out-patients we analyzed the 24 h urine for Mg and Ca on one day individual diet. Sixty-seven calcium oxalate stone formers and 18 healthy controls were investigated as in-patients for 10 days on standard diet. Daily Mg and Ca intake was kept at 390 mg and 880 mg respectively. Liquid intake was maintained at 2400 ml/day. Twenty-four hour urines were collected daily and analyzed for Mg and Ca and other lithogenic and inhibiting substances. Ca and Mg were measured by atom absorption spectrophotometry (AAS).

The normal values we achieved from previous investigations with normal subjects in a steady state on a standard diet using five consecutive 24 h urines for the calculation of the mean value of urinary constituents, was as follows:

normal range for urinary Mg: 2.83 ± 0.70 mM

normal range for urinary Ca: 2.80 ± 1.05 mM

RESULTS

Urinary Mg while on a standard diet is shown in Table 1. The Mg excretion and concentration by calcium oxalate stone-formers and healthy controls on a standard diet are only slightly different and within the normal range. Table 1 also shows that Mg excretion by calcium oxalate-formers equals that of healthy controls on individual diet and is within the normal range. The mean concentration is greater in healthy controls, the difference, however, is not significant. When administering a standard diet it was observed that males, whether healthy or stone formers, show a higher Mg excretion and concentration than do females. (See Figures 1 and 2) Division of the mean of the daily Ca excretion and the mean of the daily Mg excretion results in the Ca/Mg ratio. Compared to the Ca/Mg ratio of healthy controls this value was found to be elevated in calcium oxalate stone formers both on individual diet and standard diet. See Table 1.

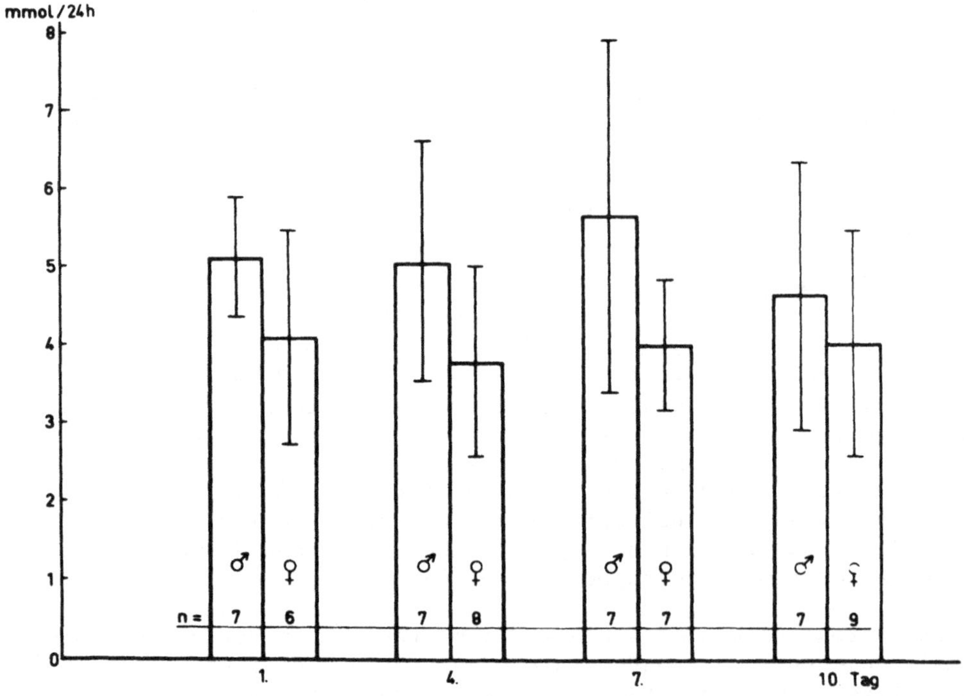

Figure 1. Mg excretion in 24 h urine on standard diet in male and female controls.

Table 1. Urinary Magnesium and Calcium[1]

	Standard diet				Individual diet			
	Controls (n=16)		Stone formers (n=67)		Controls (n=18)		Stone formers (n=33)	
	mmol/24 h	mmol/1	mmol/24 h	mmol/1	mmol/24 h	mmol/1	mmol/24 h	mmol/1
Ca	3.60±1.78	2.30±1.05	4.83±2.03	3.39±1.50	4.09±1.81	2.84±1.61	5.14±2.71	2.79±1.97
Mg	4.33±1.01	2.83±0.70	4.20±1.44	2.98±1.25	4.67±1.57	3.22±1.11	4.85±1.53	2.65±1.67
Ca/Mg	0.83		1.15		0.88		1.06	

1: Excretion and concentration of Ca and Mg (mean value ± SD) and the Ca/Mg ratio in healthy controls and Ca-oxalate stone formers on standard diet and individual diet. (Mean values on standard diet: Mean values of day 6 and 10 after reaching the steady state; Mean values on individual diet: Mean values of only one day)

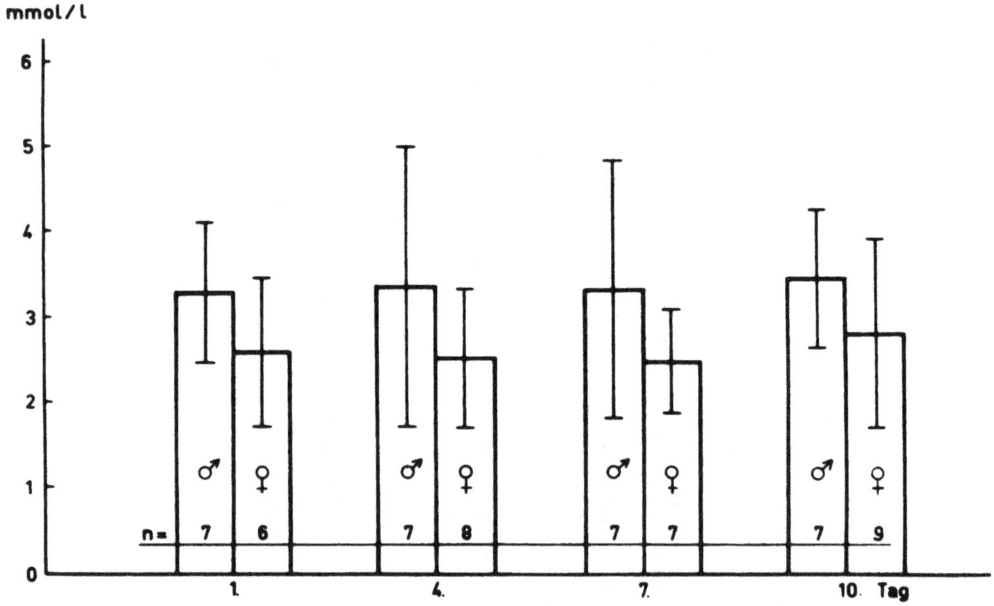

Figure 2. Mg concentration in 24 h urine on standard diet in male and female controls.

DISCUSSION

During the last years investigations of urinary Mg excretion by calcium oxalate stone formers values were both lower and greater than healthy controls[1,2,3]. Inasmuch as these results show great fluctuations, and the 24 h urines are usually not collected under standardized conditions, comparison between normal and stone formers is generally not useful. With our investigations on a standardized food regimen, unknown dietary factors to a large extent can be excluded. After 5 - 7 days an approximate "steady state" is reached, after which the excretion and concentration of lithogenic substances changes only slightly. On this standard diet we found that the excretion and concentration of Mg is not different in calcium oxalate stone formers compared to healthy controls, and thus hypoabsorption of Mg can be excluded in calcium oxalate stone formers. Investigations of 24 h urine collected at home while on an individual diet does not reveal any differences in the excretion and concentration of Mg between stone formers and controls. Thus insufficient dietary Mg was excluded in the stone-formers we investigated. However, this does not preclude that in the individual cases Mg deficiency caused by intestinal and pancreatic diseases or resections of parts of the intestine may be factors favoring stone formation.

Whether the difference in the Mg excretion found between male and female is significant as to the calcium oxalate stone formation, further investigations will have to show. In our opinion the elevation of the Ca/Mg ratio stone formers is due to a higher elevation of urinary Ca in stone formers. This we find confirmed by our investigations about hyperabsorption of Ca in stone formers.

The uncritical application of the Ca/Mg ratio for evaluation of risk of stone formation during prophylaxis seems questionable to us. Elevation of the value without exact knowledge about the single components may mislead to a diagnosis of hypomagnesiuria, while the actual cause is an elevated Ca excretion. When considering the mechanism by which Mg is thought to inhibit stone formers the mean daily concentration must be observed, since it is concentration not twenty-four hour excretion that will decide if crystallization might occur.

REFERENCES

1. B. Terhorst and D. Jonas, in:"Pathogenese und Klinik der Harnsteine II," W. Vahlensieck and G. Gasser, eds., Fortschr. Urol. Nephr. Steinkopff, Darmstadt (1974).
2. V. Revusova, in:"Urolithiasis Research," H. Fleisch, W. G. Robertson, L. H. Smith, and W. Vahlensieck, ed., Plenum Press, New York/London (1976).
3. A. Hesse, W. Berg, H.-J. Schneider, and E. Hienzsch, in:"Pathogenese und Klinik der Harnsteine V," G. Gasser and W. Vahlensieck, ed., Fortschr. Urol. Nephr. Steinkopff, Darmstadt (1977).

ACKNOWLEDGMENT

We want to thank Mr. cand. med. W. Dewes, Inst. Physiol. Chem. Bonn University (Director: Prof. Dr. F. Zilliken) for doing the statistical calculations.

CIRCADIAN EXCRETION OF URIC ACID ON CONDITION OF STANDARD DIET AFTER PURINE LOAD IN CALCIUM OXALATE STONE-FORMERS AND HEALTHY CONTROLS

W. Schneeberger[1], D. Bach[2], A. Hesse[2],
W. Dewes[3], and W. Vahlensieck[2]
1 Hospital for Rehabilitation, Bornheim-Merten,
2 Section for Urolithiasis Research, Department of Urology,
University Hospital, 3 Institute for Physiological
Chemistry of the Bonn University, Bonn, West Germany

Protein-rich nutrition after World War II shows a correlation with an increase of urolithiasis. Considerable significance is seen in the elevation of uric acid in serum and the increased excretion of uric acid in urine. Therefore, we studied the metabolism of uric acid in healthy controls and calcium oxalate stone-formers before and after an oral load with purines.

METHOD

Seventy calcium oxalate stone-formers and 27 healthy controls participated in the modified uric acid loading test by Ohlenschläger and Ulbrich (Fa. Fresenius, Bad Homburg, West Germany). Two grams of purines (980 mg adenine and 980 mg guanine) were given orally to all stone-formers and healthy controls and uric acid was measured one day prior to and two days following the test. The test was performed on days 11 and 12 on a standard diet. The 24 h urine was collected from all 70 stone-formers and 27 healthy controls and the uric acid excretion was measured one day prior to and two days after the purine load. In addition, 19 stone-formers and 11 controls collected the urine in 3 h fractions to determine uric acid content.

RESULTS

On the first and second day following the purine load uric acid was elevated above normal in the serum of stone-formers. In healthy controls the uric acid in serum also increased on the first day post load. However, the concentration stayed within the normal range and had returned to the pre-load values on the second day (Figure 1). Excretion of uric acid after the purine load in the two groups was

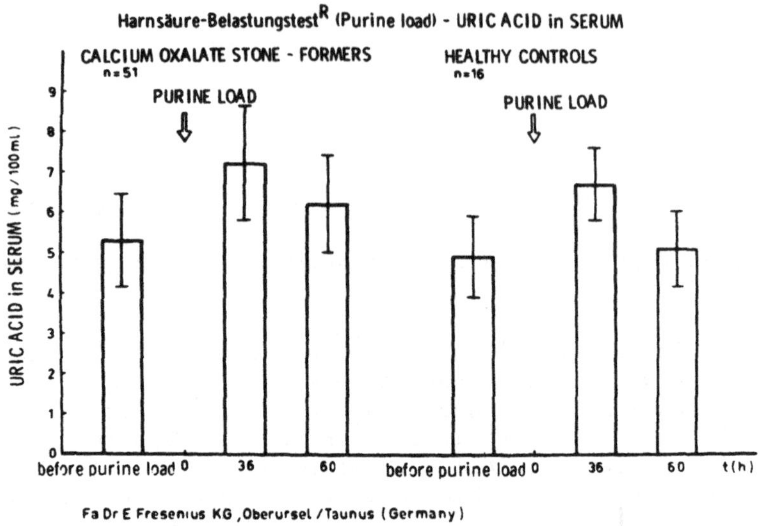

Figure 1. Serum concentration of uric acid (mg/100 ml) before and after purine load in 51 calcium-oxalate-stone-formers (left) and 16 healthy controls (right) after 10 days on standard diet.

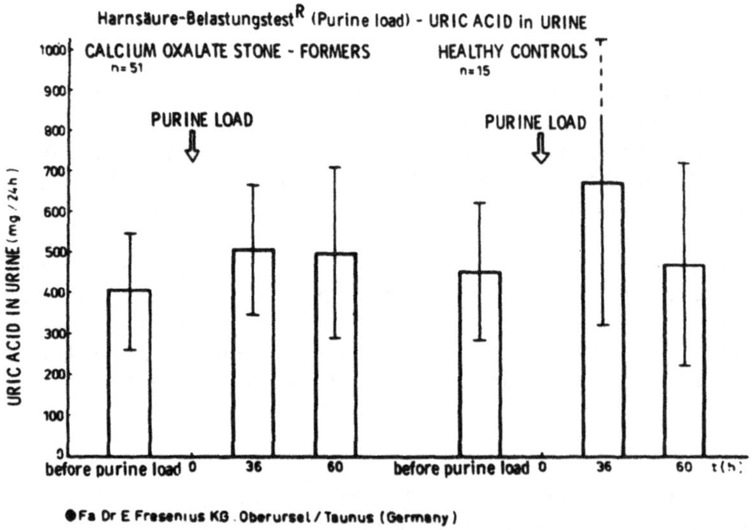

Figure 2. Urine concentration of uric acid (mg/24 h) before and after purine load in 51 calcium-oxalate-stone-formers (left) and 15 healthy controls (right) after 10 days on standard diet.

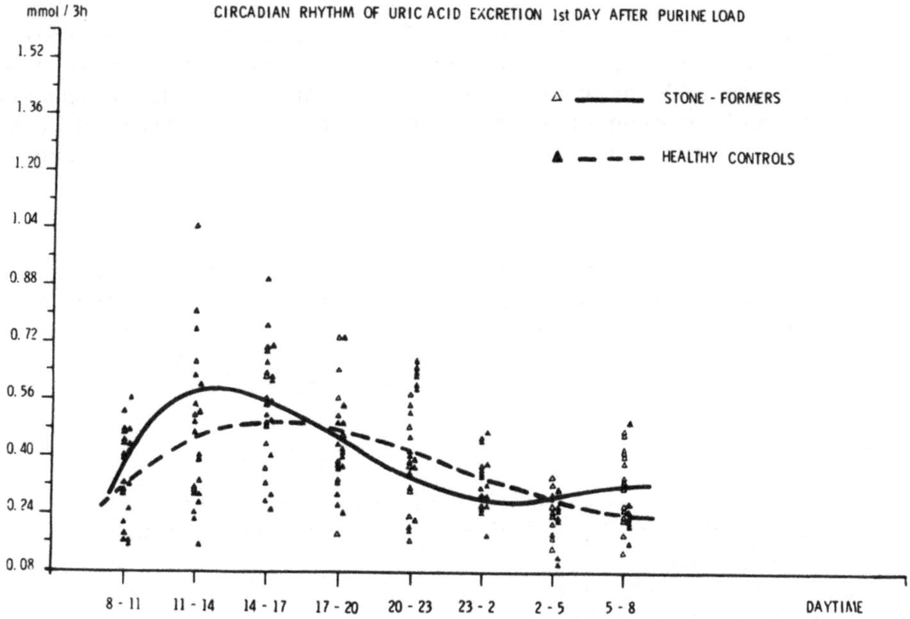

Figure 3. Circadian rhythm of uric acid (mmol/3 h) in 19 calcium-oxalate stone-formers and 11 healthy controls at the first day after purine-load on condition of a standard diet.

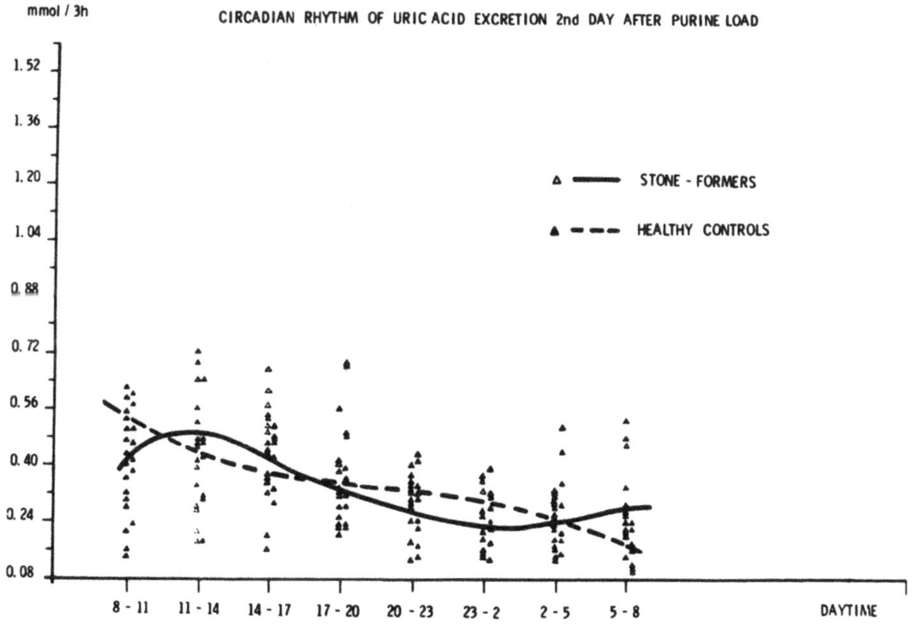

Figure 4. Circadian rhythm of uric acid (mmol/3 h) in 19 calcium-oxalate stone-formers and 11 healthy controls at the second day after purine load on condition of a standard diet.

increased equally, however, in stone-formers this increase remained unchanged for a longer period (Figure 2). The circadian excretion in stone-formers and controls resembled a sinusoid curve and showed in the calcium oxalate stone-formers in the first hours after the purine load a higher "peak" than in the healthy controls (Figures 3 and 4).

DISCUSSION

Following purine load calcium oxalate stone-formers have a protracted hyperuricemia and hyperuricosuria. This test enables us to diagnose a latent metabolic disorder of uric acid in calcium oxalate stone-formers. Those patients who show pathological values in this test can be specifically treated with Allopurinol.

REFERENCES

1. D. Bach, M. Rohde, W. Schneeberger, W. Hamm, W. Dewes, W. Vahlensieck, and F. Zilliken, Fortschr. Urol. Nephrol. 11:274 (1978).
2. D. Bach, W. Schneeberger, A. Hesse, and W. Vahlensieck, Therapiewoche 29:1482 (1979).
3. G. Ohlenschläger and H. Ulbrich, Therapiewoche 26:1254 (1976).
4. W. Schneeberger, D. Bach, W. Vahlensieck, and A. Hesse, Fortschr. Urol. Nephrol. 14:411 (1979).

HYPOPHOSPHATEMIA IN RECURRENT RENAL STONE FORMERS - CONSEQUENCE OF ARTERIAL HYPERTENSION?

W. Tschöpe, E. Ritz, and H. Wesch

Medizinische Universitat-Klinik, Sektion Nephrologie und Deutsches Krebsforschungszentrum, Abteilung für Nuklearmedizin, D-6900 Heidelberg, FRG

Fasting hypophosphatemia is commonly found in recurrent renal stone formers (calcium oxalate and/or -phosphate) with absorptive hypercalciuria[1,2]. However, not all authors were able to demonstrate lower plasma phosphorus levels in recurrent renal stone formers as compared with matched control individuals[3,4]. Hypophosphatemia is of interest in view of some recent proposals which try to link plasma phosphate and intestinal hyperabsorption of calcium in the pathogenesis of the hypercalciuria of recurrent renal stone formers via increased circulating levels of $1,25(OH)_2$ vitamin D[5].

In the present investigation, urinary calcium excretion and plasma phosphate were studied in a random sample of the general population and in recurrent renal stone formers (RSF). Some of the factors which correlated with fasting plasma phosphate levels were defined. It was concluded that arterial hypertension is one important factor which contributes to fasting hypophosphatemia.

PATIENTS AND METHODS

Male individuals (age 19-41 years) were randomly selected from the files of the city registration office with the aid of computer generated random numbers. Of the contacted individuals, 51% complied and participated in the study. The study was carried out in random sequence throughout the year. On the morning after the urine collection period, blood was drawn for serum chemistry (SMA-12-Technicon Autoanalyser, 25(OH)D[6], iPTH[7]). Individuals with serum creatinine >1.4 mg/dl with a GFR <80 ml/1.73 m^2 x min and fasting glucose >110 mg/dl were excluded. In addition, the same measurements were carried out at the same time of the year in 84 unselected male patients (age 19-55 years) with recurrent renal stone formation (RSF).

Metabolic causes of RSF other than hypercalciuria were excluded by appropriate studies. Eighty-four patients were compared with 238 controls. The results were analysed by U-test, Kruskal-Wallis-test, and multiple linear regression analysis.

RESULTS

Twenty-four hour UV_{Ca} was significantly higher ($p < 0.01$) in RSF (7 ± 3.15 mmoles/24 h; $\bar{x} \pm SD$) than in controls (CO) (5.5 ± 2.6). RSF and CO did not differ with respect to iPTH and urinary cAMP (RSF 255 ± 140 x 10^{-6} moles cAMP/mol creatinine; CO 276 ± 76). Fasting plasma phosphate levels were significantly lower ($p < 0.05$) in RSF (0.94 ± 0.18 mmol/l) than in CO (0.99 ± 0.16 mmol/l). TMP/GFR was similarly lower in RSF (2.32 ± 0.6 mg/dl; CO 2.54 ± 0.55 mg/dl; $p < 0.05$) (Table 1). However, a difference of plasma phosphate or TMP/GFR was no longer demonstrable if stone formers and controls were strictly age matched (RSF 1.01 ± 0.16 mmol/l; CO 0.99 ± 0.16). Similarly, no difference of plasma Pi or TMP/GFR was demonstrable if normotensive controls were compared with normotensive age matched stone formers.

Table 1. Physical and chemical parameters of the normal population, recurrent renal stone formers and age-matched recurrent renal stone formers. For better comparison, only $\bar{x}$ is given.

		CONTROLS (n = 238)	PATIENTS (n = 84)	AGE-MATCHED PAT (n = 42)
AGE	(years)	30,5	35,5 ★	30,6
WEIGHT	(kg)	75,5	76,5	74,5
RR syst.	(mmHg)	133	138 ★	134
RR diast.	(mmHg)	86	90 ★	88
CALCIUM	(mmol/l)	2,36	2,38	2,41
TMPi/GFR	(mg/dl)	2,54	2,32 ★	2,57
iPTH	(pmol/l)	30,3	19	20
25(OH)D	(nmol/l)	132	111	99
VOLUME	(ml/24h)	1394	1987 ★	1938
UV_{Ca}	(mmol/24h)	5,5	7 ★	6,4 ★
UV_{Na}	(mmol/24h)	207	225	207
Ca/Cr	(mol/mol)	0,34	0,44 ★	0,39 ★
cAMP	(µmol/mol Cr)	276	255	258

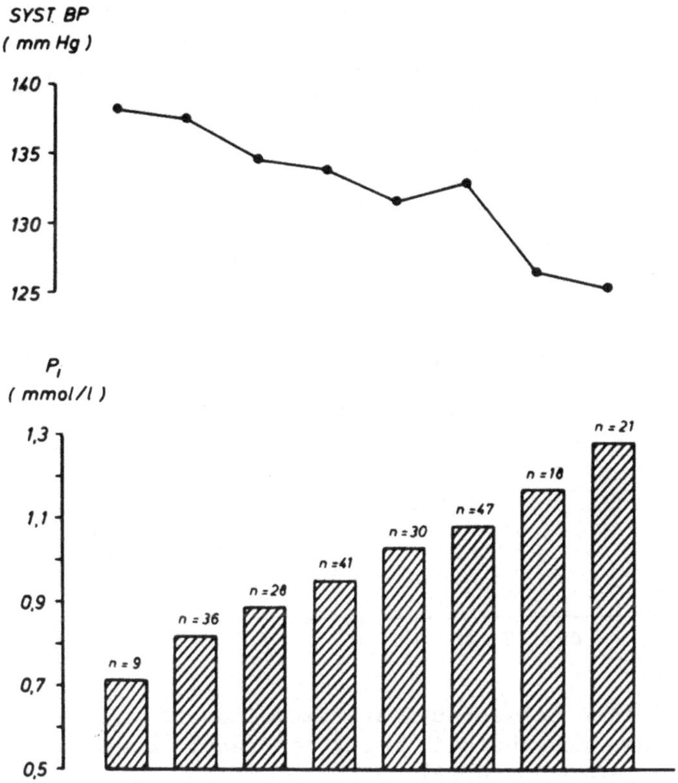

Figure 1. The relation between systolic blood pressure and fasting plasma phosphate in the normal male population (n = 238).

Both in RSF and in control individuals, a significant correlation was found between age and plasma phosphate (RSF: r = -0.4; CO: r = -0.26) and between systolic blood pressure and plasma phosphate (RSF: r = 0.27; CO: r = 0.23) (Figure 1).

UV_{Ca} correlated with plasma phosphate in RSF (r = -0.3) but not in controls (Figure 2).

DISCUSSION

The present study confirms the correlation between plasma phosphate and calcium excretion in recurrent renal stone formers. However, the study fails to show fasting hypophosphatemia in stone formers, if the effects of age and blood pressure on plasma phosphate are taken into account by appropriate selection of controls. The dependence of plasma phosphate on age or blood pressure is in agreement with previous reports in literature[8,9,10]. Ljunghall[8]

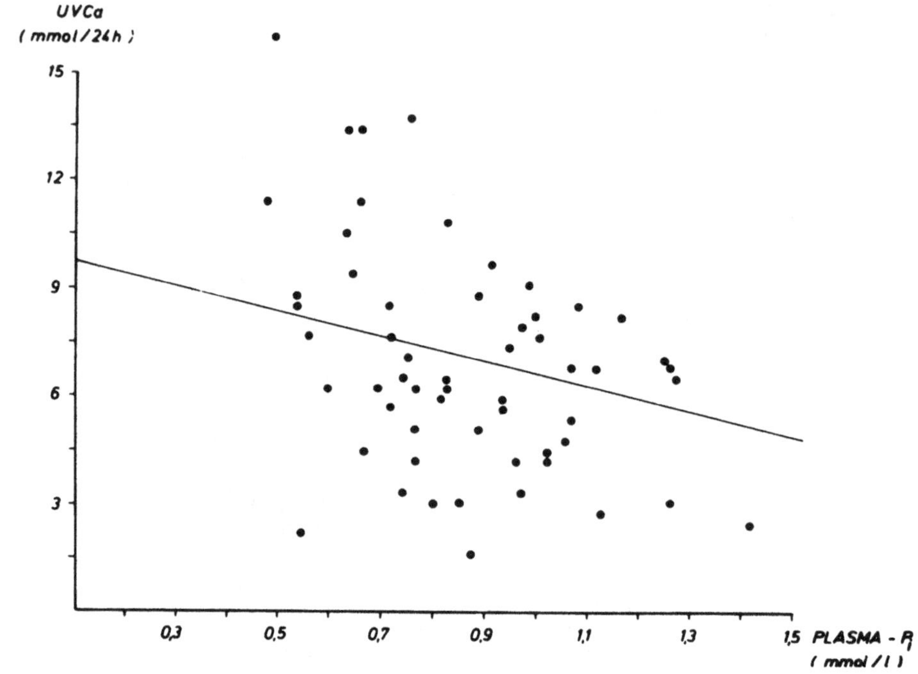

Figure 2. Relation between urinary excretion of calcium and fasting plasma phosphate in recurrent renal stone formers ($r = -0.3$; $p < 0.05$).

observed an inverse correlation between blood pressure and fasting plasma phosphate in a random population sample of non-stone forming probands comprising 2000 individuals. Furthermore, Heidland et al.[9] observed increased fractional phosphate clearance in individuals with various forms of hypertension. The reason for such hyperphosphaturia in hypertensive individuals is unknown and both peritubular passive forces and hormonal signals may play a role.

It remains unknown whether the rise in the urinary excretion of calcium and the fall in plasma phosphate with age, as found in the present study, result from the age-dependent decrease of GFR, the higher prevalence of hypertension, or from other factors.

It is of note, that in RSF, plasma phosphate was unrelated to PTH of cAMP.

We are aware of the fact that this study has cross-sectional character and does not prove or disprove causal relationships. However, the study documents the dependence of plasma Pi on blood pressure and age and suggests that control of these variables is mandatory in studies designed to analyze interdependence of plasma phosphate and urinary excretion of calcium.

REFERENCES

1. P. H. Hennemann, A. P. Forbes, P. H. Benedict, and H. R. Dudley, N. Engl. J. Med. 259:802 (1958).
2. F. H. Shen, D. J. Baylink, R. L. Nielsen, D. J. Sherrard, J. L. Ivey, and M. R. Haussler, J. Lab. Clin. Med. 90:955 (1977).
3. D. E. Barilla, J. E. Zerwekh, and C. Y. C. Pak, Min. Elect. Metab. 2:202 (1979).
4. Schonau, and F. Joergensen, Scand. J. Urol. Nephrol. 9:243 (1975).
5. R. W. Gray, D. R. Wilz, A. E. Caldas, and J. Lemann, Jr., J. Clin. Endocrin. Metab. 45:299 (1977).
6. R. E. Belsey, H. S. DeLuca, and J. T. Potts, J. Clin. Endocrin. Metab. 38:1046 (1974).
7. R. Bouillon, P. Konincks, and P. de Moor, in:"Radioimmunoassay and Related Procedures in Medicine," International Atomic Energy Agency, Vienna (1974).
8. S. Ljunghall, and H. Hedstrand, Br. Med. J. 1:553 (1977).
9. A. Heidland, H. Hennemann, R. Hensler, E. Heidbreder, and D. Gekle, Klin. Wschr. 49:1121 (1971).
10. E. Farnsworth, J. Clin. Invest. 25:897 (1946).

RELATIONSHIP OF URINARY CALCIUM TO SODIUM EXCRETION IN CALCAREOUS RENAL STONEFORMERS: EFFECT OF FUROSEMIDE

R. A. L. Sutton and V. R. Walker

Clinical Investigation Unit, Shaughnessy Hospital and Department of Medicine, University of British Columbia, Vancouver, British Columbia, Canada

There is normally a linear relationship between the fractional urinary excretion of sodium and calcium, both in man and experimental animals[1]. However, in identifying and classifying hypercalciuria in stone patients, the excretion of sodium has commonly been ignored[2].

In the present study, we have examined the relationship between sodium and calcium excretion in "fasting" urine and in 24-hour urine collections in normal subjects and in idiopathic calcium stoneformers. We have also investigated changes in urinary sodium and calcium excretion in the same subjects in response to furosemide (which inhibits the renal tubular reabsorption of both ions) in order to determine whether the response in normal subjects differ from those in stoneformers.

METHODS

Studies were carried out in 36 patients (45 ± 14 years, [mean ± S.D.]; 23M/13F) with idiopathic calcareous nephrolithiasis and in 20 healthy normal subjects (45 ± 11 years; 15M/5F). All individuals were placed on a low calcium diet (less than 400 mg calcium per day) with no salt restriction for one week prior to fasting urine collections and administration of furosemide.

A two-hour (0700 - 0900 hours) and a four-hour (0900 - 1300 hours) urine collection were then made following a 13-hour overnight fast. On a subsequent day, these two fasting urine collections were repeated with the additional administration of furosemide (60 mg p.o.) in a single dose between the two urine collections (0900 hours).

The increments in sodium and calcium excretion in response to furosemide were calculated as the difference between the ion/creatinine ratio before and after furosemide. To allow for circadian changes in ion excretions, the difference between the ion/creatinine ratios in the corresponding urines on the control day was subtracted from that on the diuretic day to give the net increment in ion excretion in response to furosemide.

Twenty-four hour urine collections were made on a separate occasion in 31 of 36 stoneformers and in 16 of the 20 normal subjects. These collections were made with all subjects on a free diet.

Urinary calcium was measured by atomic absorption spectrophotometry and sodium by emission flame photometry. Creatinine was estimated as the alkaline picrate.

RESULTS

Table 1 shows the sodium and calcium excretions expressed as the ion/creatinine ratios in normal subjects and stoneformers during a 2-hour period following an overnight fast, and in a 24-hour urine collection while the subjects ate a free diet.

Table 1

Fasting 2-hour	Normals	Stoneformers	P
n	20	36	
Na/creatinine	0.088 ± 0.009	0.075 ± 0.006	n.s.
Ca/creatinine	0.069 ± 0.011	0.124 ± 0.011	$p < 0.001$
Correlation of Ca/creatinine (y) vs Na/creatinine (x)	n.s.	$y = 0.052 + 0.964x$ $r = 0.53$, $p < 0.001$	
Non-fasting 24-hour			
n	16	31	
Na/creatinine	0.098 ± 0.010	0.102 ± 0.007	n.s.
Ca/creatinine	0.110 ± 0.014	0.168 ± 0.015	$p < 0.01$
Correlation of Ca/creatinine (y) vs Na/creatinine (x)	n.s.	$y = 0.078 + 0.878x$ $r = 0.43$, $p < 0.025$	

n.s. = not significant ($p > 0.05$)

In both collection periods, mean Na/creatinine ratios are not significantly different while mean Ca/creatinine ratios are significantly greater in the stoneformers than in the normal controls. The relationship between sodium and calcium excretions was examined in the normal subjects and the stoneformers in both the fasting state and in the 24-hour urine (Table 1). In the normal subjects no significant correlation was observed between the excretions of these ions in either collection period. In the stoneformers, however, a significant correlation was observed both in the fasting state (Figure 1: $p < 0.001$) and in the 24-hour urine ($p < 0.025$).

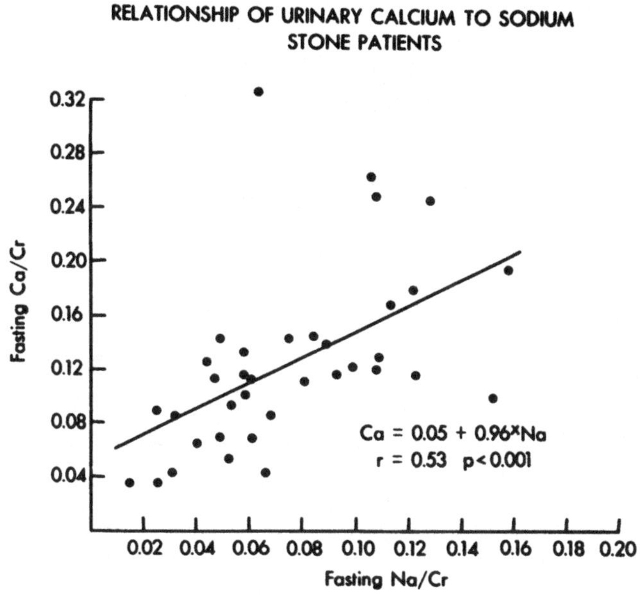

Figure 1

Table II shows the mean net increments in ion excretions in both groups of subjects in the four-hour period following the administration of furosemide, calculated as described above. Although the mean increment in sodium excretion was lower, and the mean increment in calcium excretion was higher in the stoneformers than in the normal controls, these differences were not statistically significant.

Figure 2 shows the relationship between the increments in sodium and calcium excretion following furosemide in normal subjects and stoneformers.

Table 2. Increments in Sodium and Calcium Excretion in Normal Subjects and Stoneformers in Response to Furosemide

	Normals	Stoneformers	p
n	15	36	
ΔNa/creatinine (mEq/mg)	0.523 ± 0.035	0.465 ± 0.026	n.s.
ΔCa/creatinine (mg/mg)	0.282 ± 0.035	0.340 ± 0.019	n.s.
Correlation of ΔCa/creatinine (y) vs ΔNa/creatinine (x)	y=0.072 + 0.402x x=0.66 p <0.01	y=0.171 + 0.365x r=0.48 p <0.005	

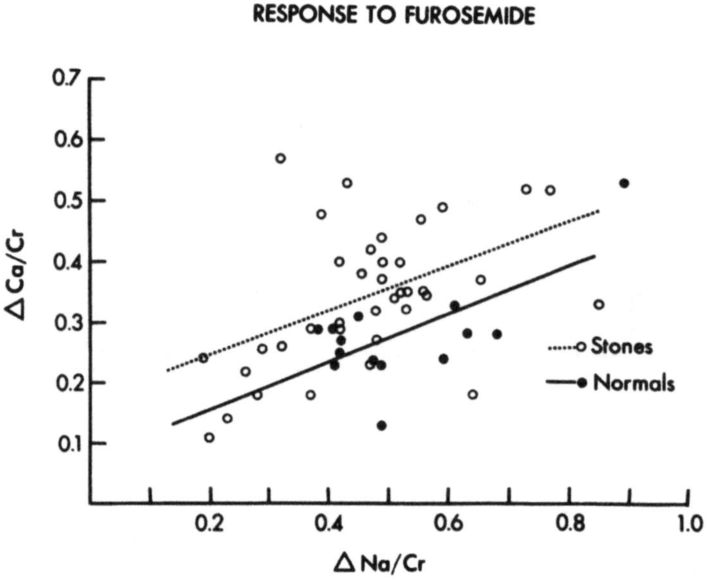

Figure 2

As shown in Table 2, there was a significant positive correlation between the increments in sodium and calcium excretion in both groups. Comparison of the two regressions shown in Figure 2 shows that the intercepts are significantly different ($p < 0.01$), whereas the slopes are not different ($p > 0.05$). Thus, in response to furosemide, for a given increment in sodium excretion, the stoneformers show a significantly greater increment in calcium excretion than the normals.

DISCUSSION

We have observed a significant positive correlation between calcium and sodium excretions in the urine of stoneformers, both in the fasting state and in a 24-hour urine collected while maintained on a free diet. Such a correlation was not observed in the normal subjects. These data suggest that sodium excretion (and therefore presumably dietary sodium intake) may be a determinant both of 24-hour urinary calcium excretion and of "fasting" calcium excretion in patients with calcium stones. It may be important to take account of urinary sodium excretion when defining both idiopathic hypercalciuria and "fasting" hypercalciuria.

We have previously examined the responses of normal subjects and calcium stoneformers to the diuretic agents hydrochlorothiazide and acetazolamide[3]. These data were interpreted as being consistent with the presence of a proximal tubular defect in fluid and ion reabsorption in the calcium stoneformers, associated with compensatory distal reabsorption of the delivered fluid and sodium but not calcium.

In the present study, in response to furosemide the mean increment in sodium excretion was not significantly different in the stoneformers from that in the normal subjects. However, for a given increment in sodium excretion in response to furosemide, the increment in calcium excretion was greater in stone patients than in normal subjects. Since furosemide causes a parallel inhibition of sodium and calcium reabsorption in the ascending limb of Henle's loop, prior to the distal tubule[4], this observation is consistent with a reduction in the capacity of the distal tubule to reabsorb delivered calcium in the stoneformers, which may also be associated with a compensatory increase in the capacity of this segment to reabsorb delivered sodium in the stoneformers.

REFERENCES

1. M. Walser, in:"Renal Pharmacology," Appleton-Century-Crofts, New York, (1971).
2. C. Y. C. Pak, R. Kaplan, H. Bone, J. Townsend, and O. Waters, N. Engl. J. Med. 292:497 (1975).
3. R. A. L. Sutton, and V. R. Walker, N. Engl. J. Med. 302:709 (1980).
4. B. R. Edwards, P. G. Baer, R. A. L. Sutton, and J. H. Dirks, J. Clin. Invest. 52:2418 (1973).

THE CLINICAL IMPORTANCE OF RENAL TUBULAR ACIDOSIS IN RECURRENT RENAL STONE FORMERS

U. Backman, B. G. Danielson, B. Fellström, G. Johansson,
S. Ljunghall, and B. Wikström
Department of Internal Medicine
University Hospital
S-750 14 Uppsala, Sweden

The incidence of renal tubular dysfunction, especially renal tubular acidosis (RTA) has usually been reported to be low among recurrent renal stone formers[1]. We have found, when the acidification capacity was routinely investigated in recurrent stone formers, that a large number of patients (20%) had defective urinary acidification[2] of which 95% had the incomplete form of the defect. A further analysis of the clinical and biochemical findings will be presented.

MATERIALS AND METHODS

Six hundred twelve recurrent renal stone formers were investigated according to our standard program for recurrent stone formers, including electrolytes in serum and urine, citrate, beta-2-microglobulin and cAMP in urine only. The renal acidification capacity was investigated by a short ammonium chloride test[3].

RESULTS

Two defects of the renal acidification capacity were diagnosed, namely the distal tubular acidosis (dRTA) and the proximal tubular acidosis (pRTA). All patients but five had the incomplete form, four patients had a complete dRTA and one patient complete pRTA. More females than males had the distal defect whereas among patients with pRTA there were more males. A family history of stones was more common in patients with RTA than among idiopathic stone formers.

The most pronounced biochemical finding was a low urinary excretion of citrate, the lowest excretion noted in patients with dRTA (Table 1). The urinary excretion of calcium was of the same

Table 1. Laboratory Characteristics of Patients with RTA

	n	U-Ca mmol/24h	U-citrate mmol/24h	U-cAMP µmol/g creat	Tubular Proteinuria (B_2-m > 370 µg/24h urine)
dRTA	45	8.1±3.8	1.5±1.1	3.9±1.0	(44%)
pRTA	67	7.1±3.1	2.2±1.1	4.3±1.5	(24%)
Controls		5.6±2.2	3.3±1.3	3.0±1.2	-

The clinical picture was more severe in patients with RTA than in patients with idiopathic stones with more operations and a higher stone frequency, twice as high as in the idiopathic stone formers (Table 2).

Table 2. Clinical Findings in Patients with RTA

	n	M	F	Age	Age of Onset	Heredity For Stones	n of Patients Operated
dRTA	45	18	27	39	28	(60%)	(69%)
pRTA	67	38	29	40	27	(35%)	(59%)

order as in our idiopathic stone formers and in the groups as a whole no evidence of secondary hyperparathyroidism was noted.

THERAPY

Most of the patients received prophylactic treatment, sodium bicarbonate or bendroflumethiazide. Patients with the complete form of the defect and those with low normal values of serum bicarbonate usually were given sodium bicarbonate. The treatment yielded an increased excretion of citrate in the bicarbonate-treated group and a reduced calcium excretion in all patients. During treatment there appeared to be fewer stone attacks and operations.

DISCUSSION

The present study revealed a rather severe stone disease in patients with renal acidification defects. Such a clinical picture has been described in patients with the complete form of RTA, but in our study most patients had the milder, incomplete form of the defect but nevertheless a severe stone disease. Although most patients had multiple stones in their kidneys, nephrocalcinosis was uncommon, thus these patients were different from patients with the complete form of RTA.

The more severe stone disease seen in our patients may in part be explained by more pronounced biochemical abnormalities than seen in idiopathic stone formers. It is well known that the urinary excretion of citrate is low in complete forms of RTA. It has been suggested that the low excretion is related to the degree of acidosis and normalized by correction of the acid-base status[4]. However, we found very low excretions of citrate also in our patients with the incomplete form of RTA, some patients having no measurable excretion at all in spite of a fairy normal acid-base status. Some patients with the complete form had a rather "normal" calcium excretion whereas some patients with the incomplete form had a rather high excretion. There was no evidence of renal hypercalciuria, which might have been suspected in this group of patients with tubular dysfunctions. Among our idiopathic stone formers about 30% had a positive family history of stone disease[5] whereas heredity was twice as common in patients with RTA when only first degree relatives were considered. However, we do not yet know the mode of inheritance in these cases but transmission of RTA as an autosomal dominant trait has been suggested[4]. Another possibility could be an over-representation in some families of some biochemical abnormality, which may lead to RTA[6].

Although RTA has been regarded to be uncommon in recurrent stone formers, a more thorough investigation of the acidification capacity will show a rather high incidence of the incomplete form of RTA. This diagnosis made only by an acid-loading test, seems important, since it appears to be associated with a more severe stone disease.

REFERENCES

1. F. L. Coe, NEJM 291:1344 (1974).
2. U. Backman, B. G. Danielson, G. Johansson, S. Ljunghall, and B. Wikström, Nephron 25:96 (1980).
3. U. Backman, B. G. Danielson, and M. Sohtell, Scand. J. Urol. Nephrol. Suppl. 35:33 (1976).
4. A. Sebastian, E. McSherry, and R. C. Morris, Jr., in:"The Kidney," Brenner and Rector, eds., Saunders, Philadelphia (1976).
5. B. Wikström, U. Backman, B. G. Danielson, B. Fellström, G. Johansson, and S. Ljunghall, (submitted for publication).
6. V. M. Buckalew, M. L. Purvis, M. G. Shulman, C. N. Herndon, and D. Rudman, Medicine 53:229 (1974).

EXPERIENCE WITH THE SHORT AMMONIUM CHLORIDE TEST

B. G. Danielson, U. Backman, B. Fellström, G. Johansson,
S. Ljunghall, and B. Wikström
Department of Internal Medicine
University Hospital
S-750 14 Uppsala, Sweden

INTRODUCTION

Since renal tubular acidosis is often complicated by stone formation, it seemed justified to investigate a stone forming population in order to study the incidence of renal acidification defects. For this purpose it was necessary to develop a clinically useful method and to standardize the ammonium chloride test.

MATERIALS AND METHODS

Ammonium chloride was given in an oral dose of 17.5 g to all patients except to children, where the dose was reduced in relation to body weight. The ammonium chloride was given as whole tablets, crushed tablets, capsules or in solution. Capsules were found to be absorbed very slowly. Ammonium chloride solution has an awful taste and was found impossible to use. Crushed tablets were found to be the most convenient way to administer the ammonium chloride, because rapid absorption was achieved without too many side effects, especially when given together with a small breakfast.

The degree of metabolic acidosis in each subject was measured in arterialized capillary blood samples using a blood gas analyser (Radiometer, Copenhagen, Denmark). Hourly urine samples were collected during 3-5 hours and analyzed for pH, titratable acid (TA), ammonium ions[1] and phosphate. Urinary pH was measured immediately after voiding. The urinary parameters were related to the degree of metabolic acidosis achieved by the ammonium chloride loading.

PATIENTS AND CONTROLS

From the investigation of 47 apparently healthy persons (age 20 to 45 years) recruited from the medical staff, the medical students as well as from a health survey reference values were obtained.

Five hundred eighty-six consecutive stone formers at the stone clinic were investigated using the standardized ammonium chloride test.

BICARBONATE LOADING TEST

To evaluate tubular reabsorption of bicarbonate some patients were investigated by a bicarbonate-loading test[2]. Bicarbonate was given intravenously in a continuous infusion following an induction of acidosis with ammonium chloride the previous day. The glomerular filtration rate was measured by inulin. Arterialized capillary samples were taken for analysis of acid-base status. Urine samples for measurements of pH and PCO_2 were taken under anaerobic conditions. The urinary bicarbonate was calculated from the Henderson-Hasselbach equation.

Four patients with normal acidification of the urine as well as five patients with a proximal renal tubular acidosis diagnosed by an ammonium chloride test were investigated.

RESULTS

From the investigation of the apparently healthy persons reference values were calculated for the urinary parameters in relation to the degree of metabolic acidosis obtained as illustrated in Figure 1. The critical level of acidosis appeared to lie around a base excess of -6 mmol/l, below which all subjects could acidify the urine to a pH below 5.0.

The frame of reference was used in the investigation of the stone formers. The distal type of RTA could be clearly distinguished by the inability of acidifying the urine to a value of 5.0 or below, as illustrated in Figure 1. The vast majority of the distal defects belonged to the incomplete type of the renal tubular acidosis (depicted as 2 in Figure 1).

The proximal type of RTA characterized by an increased urinary bicarbonate due to a defective bicarbonate reabsorption in the proximal tubules could also be distinguished by the test. The proximal RTA picture was characterized by an acidification of the urine to a pH below 5.0 but not until a low serum bicarbonate was present as illustrated in Figure 2. Most patients with the proximal defect had the incomplete type of the syndrome (depicted as 4 in Figure 2).

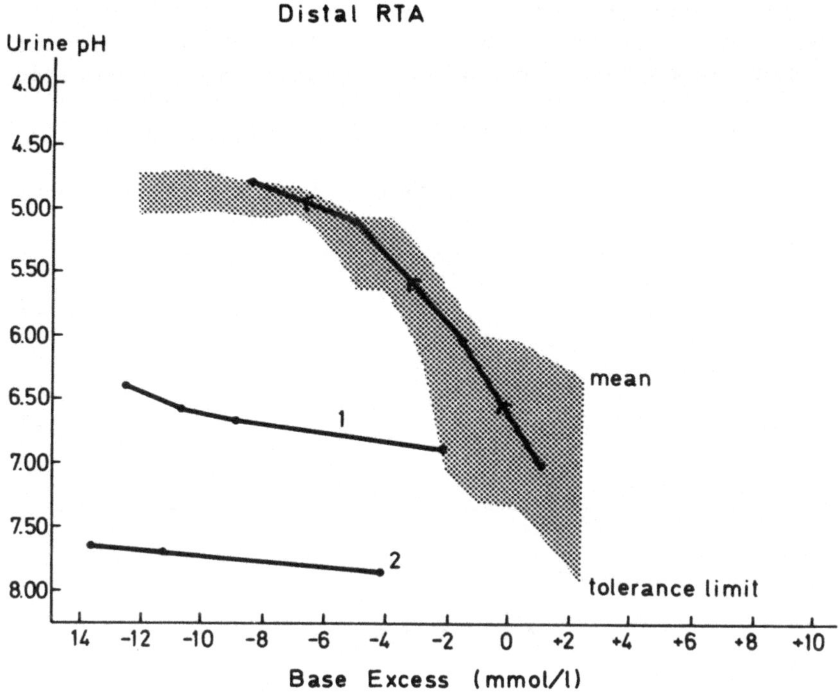

Figure 1. The urinary pH related to the metabolic acidosis in one control and in two patients with distal tubular acidosis of the incomplete type (1) and the complete type (2). The shaded area represents the frame of reference obtained from apparently healthy controls.

The patients with proximal RTA diagnosed by the ammonium chloride test were found to have a significantly lower bicarbonate threshold and an increased fractional bicarbonate excretion compared to the patients with normal acidification of the urine (Figure 3).

In patients with hyperuricosuria or gout the ammonium chloride test also showed a characteristic picture with a very low urinary pH at all levels of metabolic acidosis associated with normal TA but with a reduced ammonium ion concentration indicating an impaired renal ammonium production.

The number of patients found to have an impairment of the renal acidification are summarized in Table 1. Only four patients of 45 with a distal defect were found to have the complete form which is in accordance with previous findings in other stone populations.

The majority of affected patients were females. Only one patient of 66 with a proximal defect was found to have the complete form. Slightly more males than females were found to have proximal defects.

Table 1. Impairment of Renal Acidification

	Number of Patients	Males/Females	
	586		
Distal RTA	45	18	27
Complete	4		
Incomplete	41		
Proximal RTA	67	38	29
Complete	1		
Incomplete	66		

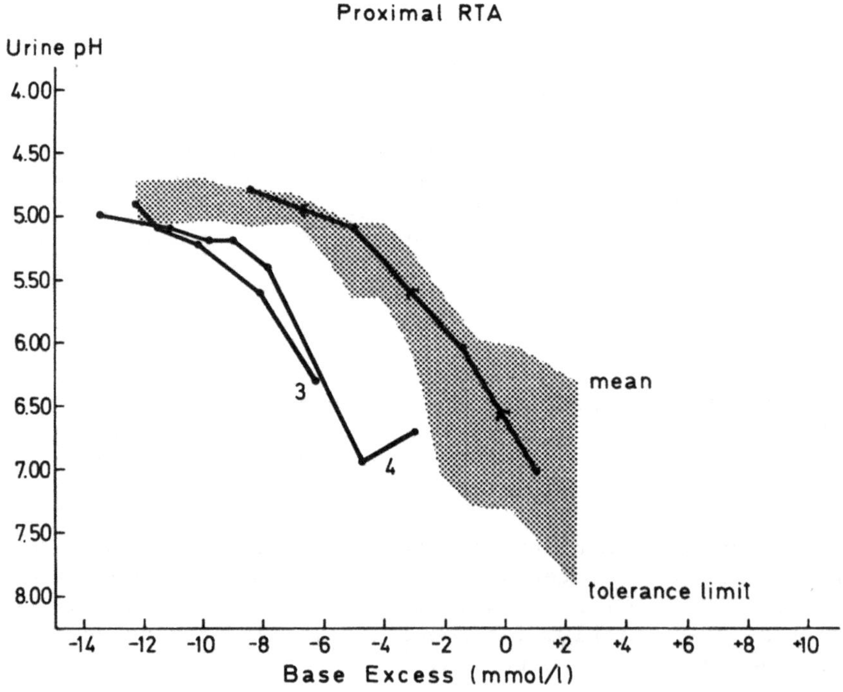

Figure 2. The urinary pH related to the metabolic acidosis in two patients with the proximal tubular acidosis of the complete type (3) and the incomplete type (4).

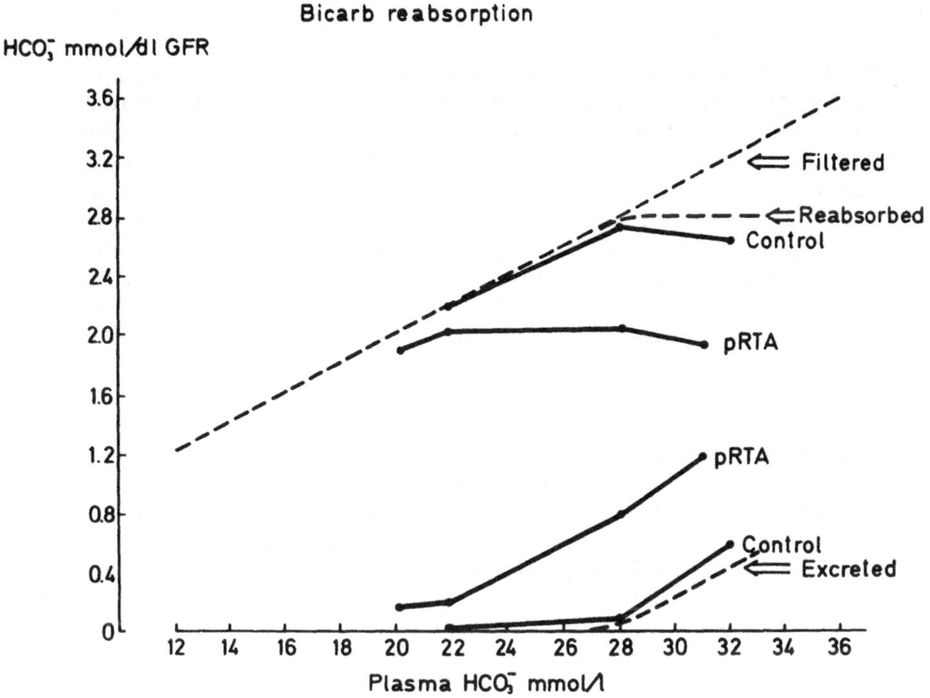

Figure 3. The relationship between plasma concentration, renal reabsorption and urinary excretion of bicarbonate in one control and in one patient with the incomplete proximal RTA. The dashed lines represent the filtered, the reabsorbed and the excreted bicarbonate in normal subjects.

DISCUSSION

Recent studies[3-5] have indicated that kidney stone formers may have tubular defects which may play a role for the stone formation. About 20% of the stone formers were found to have acidification defects. The majority of the affected patients were found to have the incomplete type of renal tubular acidosis. Since patients with RTA, both the complete and incomplete form seem to have a more severe stone disease than idiopathic stone formers the ammonium chloride test seems to be of value in clinical practice especially in the diagnosis of incomplete forms of renal tubular acidosis which otherwise will be overlooked.

SUMMARY

Using a standardized short ammonium chloride test it was possible to differentiate between patients with acidification defects of distal and proximal type. Twenty percent of the stone formers were found to have defects, the majority of which belonged to the incomplete type of RTA. Patients with hyperuricosuria had also characteristic acidification pattern. Since patients with RTA, both the complete and incomplete type, seem to have more severe stone disease than idiopathic stone formers the test seems to be of value in clinical practice especially in the diagnosis of incomplete forms of RTA which otherwise will be overlooked.

REFERENCES

1. K. Jørgensen, Scand. J. Clin. Lab. Invest. 9:287 (1957).
2. U. Backman, Scand. J. Urol. Nephrol. Suppl. 35 (1976).
3. S. Ljunghall, Scand. J. Urol. Nephrol. Suppl. 41 (1977).
4. U. Backman, B. G. Danielson, G. Johansson, S. Ljunghall, and B. Wikström, Nephron 25:96 (1980).
5. U. Backman, Eur. Urol. 4:50 (1978).

URINARY EXCRETION OF AMINO ACIDS BY SUBJECTS WITH RENAL CALCULI

William C. Thomas, Jr., Marjorie H. Malagodi, and Owen M. Rennert*
Research Service, Veterans Administration Medical Center, and College of Medicine, University of Florida, Gainesville, Florida; *Children's Memorial Hospital, University of Oklahoma, Oklahoma City, Oklahoma 73190

Idiopathic calcareous calculi remains a disorder of unknown cause, or causes. However, this affliction occurs predominantly in nonblack men, is affected by undefined geographic or climatic factors, and may be influenced by dietary habits[1]. In addition, the familial occurrence of idiopathic calculi has suggested that hereditary factors may exist that increase susceptability to this disorder[2]. Searching for a possible index of renal tubular dysfunction, McGeown[3] investigated the amino acid excretion of 110 patients with calcareous calculi. She reported that, except for 30 patients with some increase in urinary cystine, the amino acid excretion was reduced in the calculous patients as compared with the amino acid excretion of normal subjects. Of these 110 patients, twenty-three had hyperparathyroidism and the mean excretion of amino acid nitrogen was less in these than in the group as a whole. Subsequently, Hurn and associates[4] reported the urinary amino acid values of 15 patients with calcareous calculi, but they found a reduced excretion only in those patients with impaired renal function.

The present investigation was undertaken to determine whether the urinary excretion of amino acids by normal subjects differed from excretion of these acids by several subgroups of patients with calcareous calculi.

METHODS

All subjects were hospitalized in the Clinical Research Center and fed diets that were free of dairy products and provided 1 gm of protein per kilogram of body weight. On the day after admission a 24 hour collection of urine was obtained from each patient. During the collection period, specimens were refrigerated and aliquots of the 24 hour volume were immediately frozen until analyzed. Creatinine was determined on each collection by a modification of the method of Jaffe[5]. Quantitative analysis of urine aliquots for free amino acids was determined with a Durrum V500 amino acid analyzer using orthophathalic dicarboxaldehyde as the reacting reagent. With this reagent cystine and proline are not detected and the values for serine are increased by the inclusion of asparagine and glutamine. The results have been expressed as micromoles excreted per 24 hour.

RESULTS AND DISCUSSION

The mean urinary excretion of 18 amino acids by 8 healthy men, twenty-six patients (21 men and 5 women) with idiopathic renal calculi, 11 patients (6 men and 5 women) with medullary sponge kidneys, and 14 patients (all women) with hyperparathyroidism (subsequently proved by operation) are depicted in Table 1. Taurine, histidine, and glycine were the predominant amino acids in urine of normal subjects and those with calcareous calculi or hyperparathyroidism, and there was a reduced excretion of these 3 amino acids by the calculous patients. In the normocalcemic patients the decrease in urinary taurine, histidine, and glycine was sufficient to account for the observed reduction in the total of amino acids excreted per 24 hours.

It is evident from Table 1 that there was a similar pattern, both quantitatively and qualitatively, in the excretion of amino acids by the normal subjects and those with idiopathic calculi or medullary sponge kidneys. The amounts of these amino acids do not differ markedly from the values reported by Soupart[6] and others[7], except they found that either histidine or glycine was the most abundant of the urinary amino acids in their normal subjects. Taurine was the amino acid excreted in highest mean amounts by all of our groups except those with hyperparathyroidism. We attribute this increased taurine excretion as probably a consequence of a high dietary intake of meat before hospitalization[8].

The reduction in amino acid excretion by the patients with hyperparathyroidism is striking and probably does indicate an alteration in proximal tubular flux of amino acids in this disorder. These observations confirm those previously reported by McGeown[3]. The large amount of glycine excreted by these patients with hyperparathyroidism is probably because they were all women. Soupart[6] observed the increased excretion of glycine by women, and in our subjects women regularly excreted the greatest amount of glycine, independent of their type of stone disease. In contrast to the

Table 1. Urinary Amino Acids in Normal and Calculous Subjects (μmol/24 hr, mean values)

Amino Acids	Normals (N=8)	Idiopathic Stones (N=26)	Medullary Sponge (N=11)	Hyperpara-thyroidism (N=14)
Taurine	1152	911	1000	416
Histidine	1147	741	658	461
Glycine	984	904	877	715
Serine	584	379	361	191
Aspartic acid	306	308	289	81
Alanine	229	194	229	107
Threonine	138	145	178	68
Tryptophan	-	146	119	49
Lysine	118	223	105	116
Tyrosine	100	82	79	32
Phenylalanine	59	43	36	19
Ornithine	-	41	27	28
Valine	46	35	35	18
Glutamic acid	38	47	45	37
Arginine	33	29	32	20
Leucine	28	25	22	13
Isoleucine	14	11	-	9
Methionine	-	-	3	3
Total	4976	4264	4095	2383

N = number of subjects in each category.

findings of McGeown[3] and Soupart[6], but consistent with the observations of others[7,9], small amounts of glutamic acid were detected in all urine specimens.

These observations on normal subjects and patients with stone-forming diatheses do not provide evidence for a distinctive pattern of altered amino acid excretion by those with normocalcemic calculous disease. Both McGeown[3] and Resnick and associates[10] have indicated that there is some increase in urinary cystine in a number of patients with calcareous calculi, but unfortunately, we were not able to quantitate the excretion of this amino acid. A qualitative test for cystine in all of our patients revealed only that a trace amount was regularly present. In patients with hyperparathyroidism, however, a reduction in free amino acid excretion appears to be a distinctive and consistent finding.

REFERENCES

1. J. S. Joly, in:"Stone and Calculous Disease of the Urinary Organs," C. V. Mosby Co., St. Louis, (1940).
2. M. Resnick, D. B. Pridgen, and H. O. Goodman, N. Engl. J. Med. 278:1313 (1968).
3. M. G. McGeown, Clin. Sci. 18:185 (1959).
4. B. A. L. Hurn, R. G. Huntsman, H. Lehmann, J. Liddell, and A. B. Roos, Clin. Sci. 22:195 (1962).
5. D. L. Stevens, and L. T. Scaggs, Tech. Bull. Regist. Med. Technol. 30:207 (1960).
6. P. Soupart, Clin. Chim. Acta. 4:265 (1959).
7. D. C. Cusworth, and C. E. Dent, Biochem. J. 74:550 (1960).
8. J. G. Jacobsen, and L. H. Smith, Jr., Physiol. Rev. 48:424 (1968).
9. J. A. Young, and B. S. Freedman, Clin. Chem. 17:245 (1971).
10. M. I. Resnick, H. O. Goodman, and W. H. Boyce, J. Urol. 122:52 (1979).

ACKNOWLEDGMENT

This study was supported in part by the Medical Research Service, Veterans Administration and by NIH SCOR Grant AM 20586 and Clinical Research Center Grant RR 82, College of Medicine, University of Florida.

EXCRETION OF THE CA-BINDING AMINO ACID,

γ-CARBOXYGLUTAMATE, IN STONE-FORMERS

J. Joost, S. Silbernagl, and E. Jarosch

Departments of Urology, Physiology and Pediatrics
University of Innsbruck
Innsbruck, Austria

In recent years, there has been increasing interest in a particular Ca-binding amino acid, γ-carboxyglutamate (Gla), with regard to its role in many calcium-dependent physiological processes. This substance appears to be involved in hemostasis, bone calcification and ectopic mineralization. Research concerning the possible role in urinary Ca stone-formation is just beginning.

In 1974 a system for the metabolic control of Ca-binding was described involving certain blood clotting factors[1]. It was shown that the vitamin K-dependent structures in prothrombin are Gla residues. These are formed by carboxylation of glutamic acid in a post-translational step requiring vitamin K and bicarbonate (Figure 1). Gla residues act as Ca-binding sites and are essential for the activation of hemostasis. Gla is also present in a bone protein called osteocalcin[2], which may play an important role in bone calcification. In 1976 Gla was identified in the renal tissue of chicken, rat and rabbit[3]. Most of the renal Gla has been found in the cortex.

Lian[4] was the first to analyze kidney stone matrix for its content of Gla. She reported the presence of this amino acid in the EDTA-soluble, non-dialyzable proteins of Ca-containing calculi. Stones composed of struvite, uric acid and cystine do not contain Gla.

How much Gla is excreted in human urine? Gla was analyzed using an amino acid analyzer after special preparation of the urine[5]. Standards were made up using recrystallized, synthetic L-Gla[6]. Gla was measured in 10 healthy adult males and 25 Ca stone-formers (Figure 2). The latter all had a previous metabolic check-up and

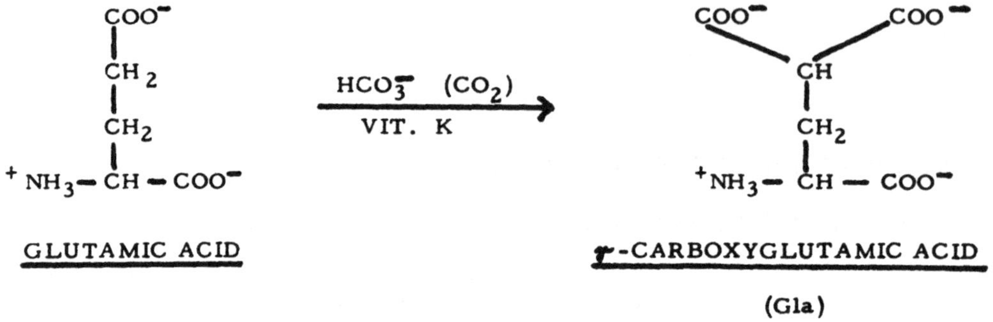

Figure 1.

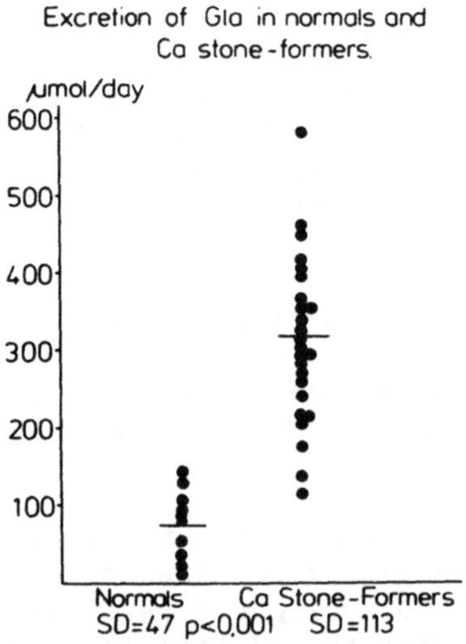

Figure 2.

were classified into groups defined as normocalciuric, absorptive and renal hypercalciuric as well as patients with primary hyperparathyroidism. In these stone-formers we found a significantly increased excretion of Gla per day with $\bar{x}$ = 307 µmol compared to $\bar{x}$ = 76 in normal subjects. No difference could be seen between the various normo- and hypercalciuric groups of stone-formers. Up to this time we have only measured Gla in 5 patients with uric acid stones. The mean value of 83 µmol/l was only slightly higher than that in normals with $\bar{x}$ = 63 (Figure 3). The Gla values of 4 cystinuric patients were in the normal range.

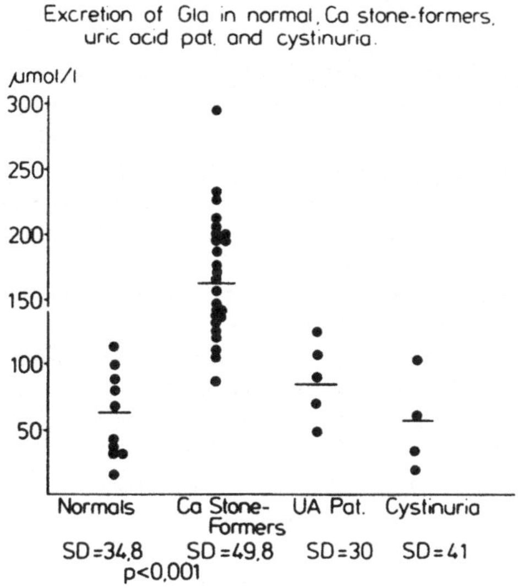

Figure 3.

We studied the possible influence of a low calcium diet on Gla excretion in 12 Ca stone-formers (Figure 4). The diet contained 400 mg Ca/day and was given for 5 days. Although there seems to be a trend downwards in Gla excretion, there is no statistically significant change. The same is true for the excretion of Gla on high Ca-diet (2 g/day) and in the fasting state (Figure 5).

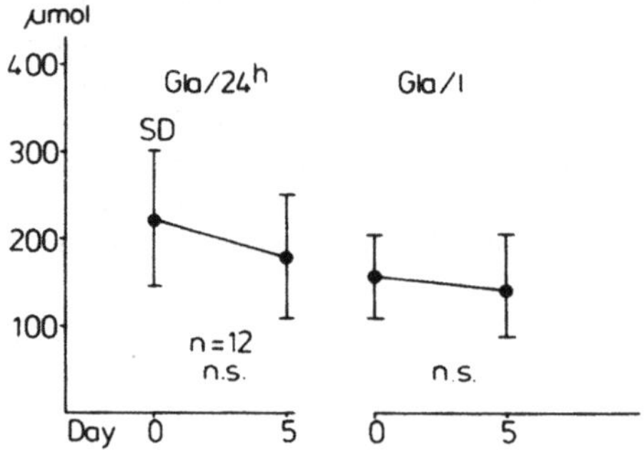

Figure 4.

In 15 Ca stone-formers (Table 1) Gla was analyzed simultaneously with serum parathyroid hormone and urinary oxalic acid, cAMP, pH and uric acid. The only significant correlation which could be found was with uric acid. This is surprising because the renal handling of Gla is quite different from uric acid. At the moment we have no plausible explanation for this correlation.

As already indicated the carboxylation system for glutamic acid seems to be dependent on vitamin K. This mechanism is predominantly true for the liver and is clinically used in anticoagulant therapy with vitamin K-antagonists. We therefore measured urinary Gla before and during anticoagulant medication with dicumarol (Sintrom^R) in 5 normal subjects (Figure 6). We could find only a slight, but not significant, increase on the 4th day of medication. Serial Gla determinations in one subject showed a significant increase on the 6th day with values returning to normal on the 10th

Table 1.

Relationships between urine Gla and plasma and urine biochemistry in Ca stone-formers.

	Number	Correlation	Significance	Gla
Parathyroid hormone ng/l	15	-0,08	n.s.	μmol/24h
Oxalic acid mg/24h	15	+0,24	n.s.	μmol/24h
Calcium g/24h	15	+0,48	n.s.	μmol/24h
Ca/creat. mg/mg	15	+0,37	n.s.	μmol/mg creat.
cAMP/creat. μmol/g creat.	15	-0,10	n.s.	μmol/mg creat.
pH	15	+0,15	n.s.	μmol/24h
Uric acid g/24	15	+0,77	p<0,01	μmol/24h

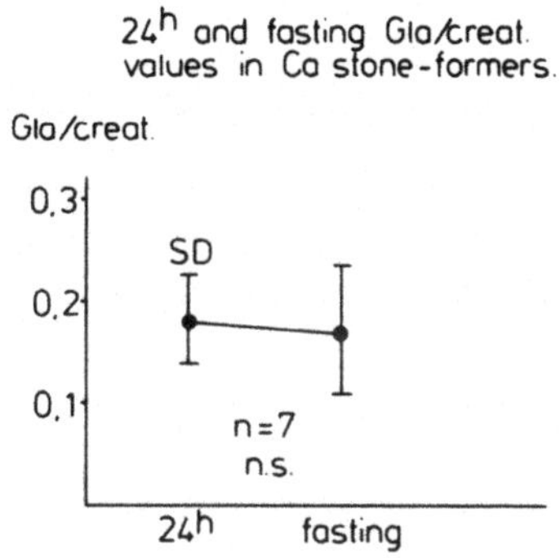

Figure 5.

day. Possible explanations for this lack of response to anticoagulants in our measurements might be: Firstly, that medication has been too short, although this seems unlikely because prothrombin has a half-life of only 60 hours. Secondly, urinary Gla might also be derived predominantly from extrahepatic origins such as bone, kidney etc. The rate of turnover and the contribution of possible breakdown of Gla-containing proteins from these sources are not clear.

Nothing is known about the possible role of Gla in renal calculi. Research has been done predominantly in the field of blood coagulation. Here Gla may be involved in the formation of metal-dependent intermolecular bridges between proteins or proteins and membranes[7]. In bone, Gla seems to interact with hydroxyapatite crystals[8]. These functions might also be related to Ca stone-formation. For us the first step to obtain more information about the raised excretion of Gla in Ca stone-formers and its possible role in kidney stones was to clarify the renal handling of this amino acid. So far plasma levels of Gla have not been measured because of its apparently low value. In that Gla has a low blood level, the relatively high urinary excretion might be due to a very low tubular reabsorption of this amino acid. If Gla should be absent or extremely low in plasma, urinary Gla must be of renal origin and/or secreted transcellularly in the tubule.

To elucidate the renal handling of Gla we infused this amino acid into rats and measured the clearance rate. In these preliminary studies Gla was analyzed by an ultra-micro ion-exchange chromatography with a sensitivity less than 1 pmol/amino acid. In the rat Gla blood levels were raised to 40 μmol/l. Clearance data from this experiment showed a fractional excretion of 50% of GFR. This corresponds to the renal handling of substances, as for instance urea, with no secretion and only passive reabsorption. In

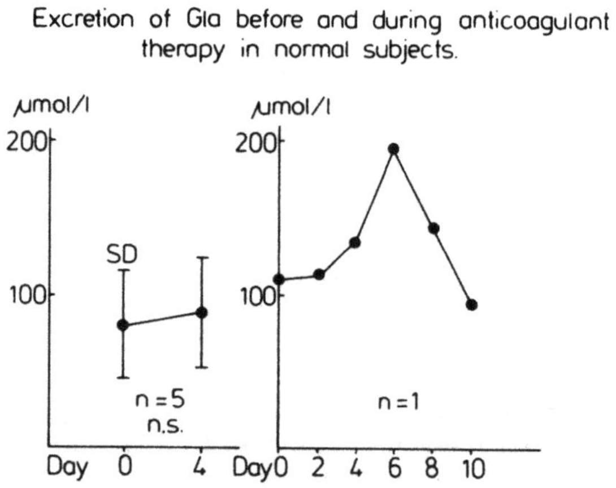

Figure 6.

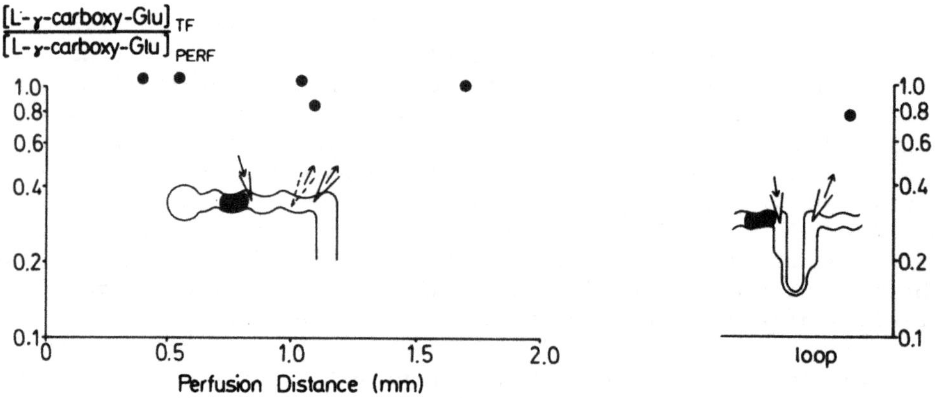

Figure 7.

one human subject examined an endogenous Gla plasma level of 1.15 μmol/l was found with a urinary concentration of 27 μmol/l. Assuming a normal GFR of 120 ml/min, the fractional excretion of Gla was 31%. Due to the fact that only one patient has been studied so far, the difference between a fractional excretion of 31% in the human compared with 50% in the rat does not seem to be significant.

To further clarify the reabsorption site of this amino acid single proximal convolutions of the rat were continuously microperfused with a solution of 0.5 mmol/l L-Gla and radioactive labelled Insulin (Figure 7). Volume reabsorption was excluded by an equilibrium solution. In the perfused section of the proximal tubule with a maximum length of 1.8 mm only a low (if any) reabsorption of Gla could be found. The loop (section between the last superficial loop of the proximal convolution and the first superficial loop of the distal convoluted tubule) showed a reabsorption of 25%. Considering the whole length of the proximal convolution to be 6 mm (whereas only 1.8 mm were perfused) and the loop together, these might fully account for the total kidney reabsorption of 50%. In addition, we may underestimate tubular reabsorption of Gla with our microperfusion experiments. Under free flow conditions the normal water reabsorption increases intratubular solute concentration and therefore enhances the reabsorption process.

SUMMARY

The Ca-binding amino acid, γ-carboxyglutamate, has been found in Ca-containing kidney stones. The urinary excretion was found to be 2-3 times higher in Ca-stone-formers than in normal subjects, uric acid and cystinuric patients. No correlations could be found with Ca, cAMP, parathyroid hormone, oxalic acid and urinary pH. The reason for the positive correlation between Gla and uric acid excretion is unclear. Anticoagulant medication showed no reduction of Gla in urine.

From our preliminary data on the renal handling of Gla, no secretion process could be demonstrated. Plasma concentrations of free Gla in man amounted to about 1 μmol/l. About one half of the glomerular load of Gla is reabsorbed, the other half is excreted. Our microperfusion experiments showed that Gla is most likely reabsorbed in the loop of Henle, mainly in the pars recta of the proximal tubule.

REFERENCES

1. J. P. Stenflo, P. Fernlund, W. Egan, and P. Roepstorff, Proc. Natl. Acad. Sci. 71:2730 (1974).
2. P. V. Hauschka, J. B. Lian, and P. M. Gallop, Proc. Natl. Acad. Sci. 72:3925 (1975).

3. P. V. Hauschka, P. A. Friedmann, H. P. Traverso, and P. M. Gallop, Biochem. Biophys. Res. Commun. 71:1207 (1976).
4. J. B. Lian, E. L. Prien, Jr., M. J. Glimcher, and P. M. Gallop, J. Clin. Invest. 59:1151 (1977).
5. J. Joost, E. Jarosch, G. Egger, and G. Hohlbrugger, in: "International Urinary Stone Conference," J. G. Brockis, ed., PSG Publishing Company, New York (1980).
6. W. Marki, M. Oppliger, P. Thanei, and R. Schwyzer, Helv. Chim. Acta. 60:798 (1977).
7. R. Sperling, B. C. Furie, M. Blumenstein, B. Keyt, and B. Furie, J. Biol. Chem. 253:3898 (1978).
8. J. P. Poser and P. A. Price, J. Biol. Chem. 254:431 (1979).

RENAL STONE FORMATION IN PRIMARY HYPERPARATHYROIDISM - ROLE OF TUBULAR DYSFUNCTION

S. Ljunghall, B. G. Danielson, G. Johansson, L. Wibell

Department of Internal Medicine, University Hospital

S-750 14 Uppsala, Sweden

The formation of calcium stones is perhaps the best recognized feature of primary hyperparathyroidism (HPT). Its frequency in different clinical series varies from 25% - 50%, the lowest figure being obtained in the most recent studies, where HPT was detected fortuitously during health screening studies. The mechanism for the markedly increased propensity for stones in HPT are not entirely clarified. For obvious reasons most interest has been directed to investigations of calcium metabolism but although HPT patients with stones have a higher mean urinary calcium than the stone-free individuals[1], hypercalciuria alone can not explain why some, but not all, HPT patients form stones.

Parathyroid hormone (PTH) promotes bicarbonate excretion by interfering with its reabsorption in the proximal tubules and excess secretion of PTH can therefore give rise to a picture of proximal renal tubular acidosis (RTA)[2]. It has also been claimed that a selective urinary excretion of low molecular weight (LMW) proteins ("tubular proteinuria") can be present in HPT and be reversible during the months following parathyroidectomy. Among consecutive normocalcemic, euparathyroid, patients with recurrent renal stones we[3] have previously found evidence of tubular dysfunction in more than 20%. Most of these had incomplete types of RTA but also tubular proteinuria was a common finding.

In the present study we have applied these tests to tubular function in a series of patients in order to evaluate the frequency of tubular dysfunctions and its relationship to stone formation in HPT.

PATIENTS AND METHODS

Altogether 64 patients (13 males, 51 females) with a mean age of 62 years (range 25-81 years) were studied. They were consecutively admitted cases of hypercalcemia who subsequently were proven to have HPT after neck exploration. Pre-operative evaluation was performed shortly before surgery whereas the post-operative studies were carried out not earlier than three months after the operation.

The urinary excretion of β_2-microglobulin was determined as an index of LMW-proteinuria by a radioimmunoassay technique (Phadebas, Pharmacia, Uppsala) in 2 h specimens obtained in the morning both before and after an intravenous calcium infusion test. The 24 h citrate excretion was measured by a citrate lyase method (normal range 1-5 mmol/24h). In 24 of the patients an ammonium chloride loading test was performed[3].

RESULTS

Out of the 64 patients in this study 29 had a history of stones. The stone-forming patients had a higher mean urinary calcium than the stone-free cases but there were no other differences in the serum or urinary electrolytes (see Table 1). In all the patients a pre-operatively raised serum concentration of PTH was normalized post-operatively and urinary calcium also decreased in every patient.

The urinary citrate excretion was of the same magnitude in the two groups of patients. A slight reduction was evident during the first postoperative period. The urinary excretion of β_2-microglobulin was raised in 12 patients (4 with stones). The excretion was not affected by calcium infusion and a raised output persisted also after parathyroid surgery.

Among the 24 patients, where the renal acidifying capacity was studied all had a normal basal acid-base status. During ammonium chloride loading one of them could not produce an acid urine despite systemic acidosis (distal RTA). One of the others had increased losses of bicarbonate and thus presented a picture of proximal RTA. The defective acidifying capacity persisted postoperatively.

DISCUSSION

In this series of consecutive patients with surgically proven HPT impaired acidifying capacity was a rare finding, and in the two cases where an incomplete defect was found it persisted also after correction of parathyroid hyperfunction. Although exogenous PTH will cause bicarbonate wasting and induce acidosis, it appears that in patients with mild-to-moderate HPT effects on the acidifying ability will not explain the increased propensity for stone formation.

Table 1. Laboratory Findings (mean values ± S.D.) in Patients with Primary Hyperparathyroidism

	Stone formers	Stone free
Males/females	7/22	6/29
Serum calcium (mmol/l)		
before op	2.88±0.15	2.82±0.16
after op	2.34±0.10a)	2.33±0.09a)
Serum alkaline phosphatase		
before op	3.8 ±1.1	4.1 ±1.8
after op	3.1 ±1.0	3.1 ±1.4
Serum PTH (μg/l) (normal range 0.22-0.50)		
before op	0.80±0.61	0.70±0.62
after op	0.41±0.04	0.41±0.05
Urinary calcium (mmol/24 h)		
before op	9.5 ±5.2b)	6.9 ±3.0
after op	4.2 ±2.1a)	3.5 ±1.9a)
Urinary magnesium (mmol/24h)		
before op	4.4 ±2.1	3.7 ±1.6
after op	3.7 ±1.8	3.2 ±1.0
Urinary urate (mmol/24 h)		
before op	3.3 ±1.4	2.7 ±0.5
after op	2.1 ±0.7a)	2.4 ±1.1
Ammonium chloride loading		
normal	10	12
tubular acidosis	1	1
Urinary citrate (mmol/24 h)		
before op	3.4 ±1.7	3.8 ±2.3
after op	2.5 ±1.1	2.2 ±1.5

a) $p < 0.05$ compared to pre-treatment values.
b) $p < 0.05$ compared to the stone-free group.

Increased excretion of β_2-microglobulin was more common and could be demonstrated in 20% of all HPT patients. In accordance with previous experience[4] this raised excretion persisted after parathyroidectomy and, although urinary proteins might be involved in the stone-forming process, excess excretion of tubular proteins was not a particular feature of the stone-forming HPT patients.

Urinary calcium was significantly higher in stone forming individuals. A recent study[1] has shown that in HPT there is a close relationship between the serum levels of $1,25(OH)_2D$, intestinal calcium absorption and calcium excretion. Thus hyperabsorbing patients with HPT will have an inappropriate hypercalciuria in relation to their serum calcium levels (which are not higher than in those with normal urinary calcium). The pattern is thus similar to that found in normocalcemic absorptive hypercalciuria although at a higher level of parathyroid function.

It has been reported[5] that, in some patients with HPT, operation will not correct their hypercalciuria and that post-operatively raised levels of parathyroid hormone can be found. These patients were believed to suffer from a primary renal defect in calcium reabsorption which lead to parathyroid stimulation. None of our patients failed to reduce both serum PTH concentrations and urinary calcium after successful parathyroid surgery. Although it is an intriguing concept that renal hypercalciuria in some cases could lead to an autonomous parathyroid hyperfunction, our experience from this series of consecutive cases indicates that such an event is not common in the development of HPT.

CONCLUSIONS

Patients with HPT and stones do not have an increased frequency of tubular defects compared with normocalcemic euparathyroid stone formers. Tubular dysfunction does not appear to be of importance for the increased propensity to form stones since it is not more common in stone-forming than stone-free patients with HPT and not reversed after correction of parathyroid hyperfunction.

REFERENCES

1. A. E. Broadus, R. L. Horst, R. Lang, E. T. Littledike, and H. Rasmussen, New Engl. J. Med. 302:421 (1980).
2. F. P. Muldowney, D. V. Carroll, J. F. Donohoe, and R. Freany, Quart. J. Med. 160:487 (1971).
3. U. Backman, B. G. Danielson, G. Johansson, S. Ljunghall, and B. Wikström, Nephron 25:96 (1980).
4. L. Wibell, P. A. Dahlberg, and F. A. Karlsson, Acta. Med. Scand. 206:507 (1979).
5. P. Bordier, A. Ryckewaert, J. Gueris, and H. Rasmussen, Am. J. Med. 63:398 (1977).

SHORT AMMONIUM CHLORIDE LOADING TEST FOR EVALUATION OF HYPERPARATHYROIDISM

Peter Alken

Department of Urology, University of Mainz

West Germany

The dilemma in the diagnosis of hyperparathyroidism (HPT) is reflected by three factors: Hypercalcemia is still regarded as the most important diagnostic sign, but unless multiple determinations of serum calcium are done, the so-called borderline cases will be missed. Tests that readily identify HPT combine either simple performance, widespread use and low accuracy (C_p, TRP, PEI, T_MP/GFR)[1] or sophisticated methods, limited use and high accuracy (PTH, Ca^{+++}, c-AMP). Consequently, some authors perform neck explorations to cure patients with recurrent nephrolithiasis who do not fulfill the diagnostic criteria of HPT. However, the stone recurrence rate may then reach 75%[2,3]. In this situation, to complete the diagnostic puzzle of hyperparathyroidism additional information is valuable.

PATIENTS AND METHODS

Twenty-five patients with recurrent calcium nephrolithiasis were evaluated metabolically during a 4-day test. Previously recorded values of serum calcium were elevated in 5 (Group A) and normal in 20 (Group B). The two patient groups did not differ significantly in age, sex, weight, height or C_{Cr}, which was normal in all cases.

One week prior to and during the test, 250 mg Ca/day was given, except for an additional 2 g calcium on day 2 and 1 g calcium on day 3. On day 4, 165 mg NH_4Cl per kg as crushed tablets was given at breakfast[4]. Fasting blood samples were drawn each day for the determination of calcium, phosphate and creatinine. On day 1, a 24-hour urine was collected for the calculation of C_{Cr}, C_p, TRP and PEI. Hourly portions of urine were collected during 7 hours after NH_4Cl

loading for the determination of calcium. Student's t-test was used for statistical analysis.

RESULTS

Table 1: Oral NH_4Cl loading induced a variable degree of hypercalciuria in all patients. This was most pronounced in Group A patients, who showed higher peak values of calcium excretion and a more persistent hypercalciuria.

Table 1. Calcium excretion profiles after NH_4Cl loading in 25 stone patients.

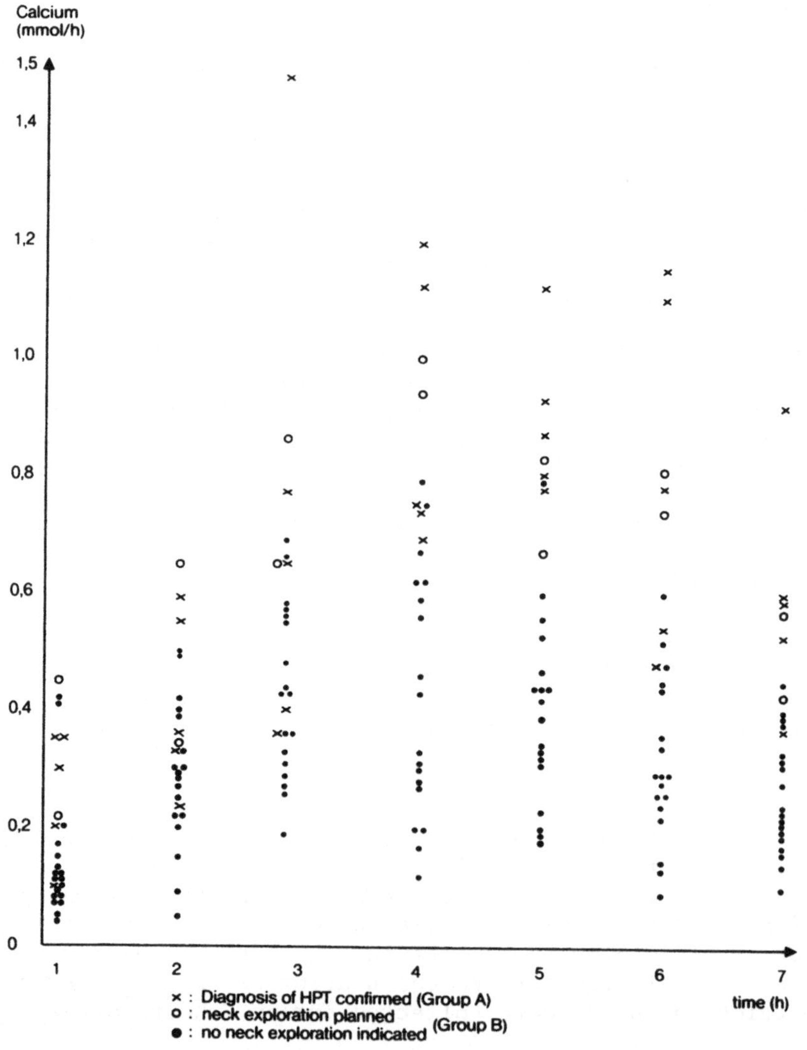

Table 2. Peak values of calcium excretion (mmol Ca/h; Group A: x = 1.056; s = 0.237. Group B: x = 0.570; s = 0.219. A vs B: $p < 0.001$). Total calcium excretion (mmol/7 h; Group A: x = 4.542; s = 1.258; Group B: x = 2.541; s = 0.981; A vs B: $p < 0.001$). Mean values of serum calcium determinations (mmol/l; Group A: x = 2.74; s = 0.205; Group B x = 2.50; s = 0.114; A vs B: $p < 0.001$). Symbols as in Table 1.

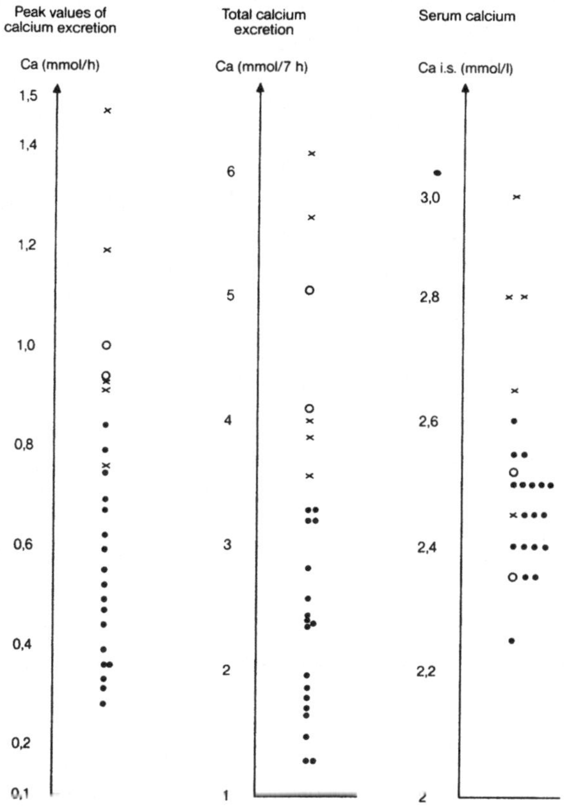

Table 2: Peak values of calcium excretion, the total amount of calcium excreted during the 7-hour period, and the mean values of four serum calcium determinations showed statistically significant higher values for Group A patients. Noteworthy are the entirely normal values of serum calcium of one Group A patient during the 4-day test, and the only slightly elevated values of another patient in whom 9 consecutive determinations during the 7 months preceding the test showed only two pathological values (2,53/2,23/2,35/2,4/2, 3/2,4/2,5/2,7/2,7 Ca i.s. mmol/l).

Table 3. C_p, TRP and PEI; A vs B: n.s.
Symbols as in Table 1.

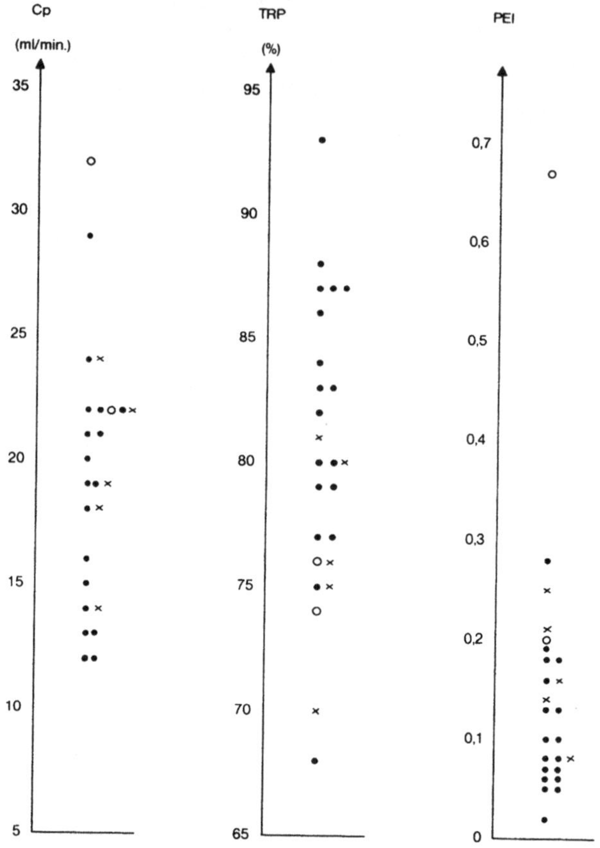

Table 3: Values of C_p, TRP or PEI were pathological in all Group A patients, but statistical analysis revealed no significant difference from Group B patients.

All Group A patients had parathyroid adenoma removed at neck exploration.

DISCUSSION

Coe et al.[5] found no hypercalciuria after short NH_4Cl loading in normal persons. The present series reveals a variable degree of hypercalciuria in stone patients, being most pronounced in HPT. Although the diagnostic set-up is not comparable to Coe's, control studies with NH_4Cl loading in 4 patients showing no or only slight hypercalciuria after parathyroidectomy seem to substantiate this difference. Further studies are needed to disclose the mechanism leading to hypercalciuria and may eventually allow an additional subgrouping of stone patients regarding renal or absorptive hypercalciuria. At present, the concomitant recording of urinary pH and calcium excretion after NH_4Cl loading offers information on HPT and RTA in stone patients with a negligible enlargement of the diagnostic set-up.

REFERENCES

1. U. Binswanger and J. A. Fischer, in:"Klinik der Inneren Sekretion," A. Labhart, ed., Springer, Berlin, New York, Heidelberg (1979).
2. H. Johansson, L. Thoren, I. Werner, and L. Grimelius, Surgery 77:691 (1975).
3. J. M. P. Siminovitch, R. E. James, C. B. Esselstyn, R. A. Staffron, and L. H. Banowsky, J. Urol. 123:335 (1980).
4. U. Backman, Scand. J. Urol. Nephrol. Suppl. 35 (1976).
5. F. L. Coe, J. J. Firpo, D. L. Hollandsworth, L. Segil, J. M. Canterburry, and E. Reiss, Kid. Int. 8:262 (1975).

SATURATION OF URINE IN PRIMARY HYPERPARATHYROIDISM:

ITS ROLE IN RENAL STONE FORMATION

A. Rapado, J. M. Castrillo, and M. Diaz-Curiel

Metabolic Unit, Fundacion Jimenez Diaz and Facultad de Medicine of Universidad Autonoma
Madrid, Spain

Renal lithiasis is a common clinical finding in primary hyperparathyroidism although its incidence seems to have been decreasing in recent years[1]. The incidence ranges from 36% to 76% (mean 55%)[2]. The incidence of stone-formation was 66% in 159 cases studied in our Foundation over the past 24 years, compared with a 2.7% incidence of hyperparathyroidism in 3,158 cases with renal lithiasis studied over the last 10 years[3].

The physicochemical basis for renal stone formation in hyperparathyroidism is the increase of solutes in the urine of these patients (mainly calcium and phosphate) together with a tendency for urinary pH to become alkaline. These changes result in an increase in the saturation of urine with calcium phosphates[4,5] as well as in the typical composition of the stones in these patients[6].

We have studied different indices of urinary saturation in a series of patients with primary hyperparathyroidism, before and after undergoing parathyroidectomy, in order to assess the effect of this procedure on the possible recurrence of lithiasis[7-9].

MATERIAL AND METHODS

Twenty-eight patients (23 females and 5 males) with primary hyperparathyroidism proven by surgery, were studied. Their ages ranged from 16 to 63 years (mean: 45). In 25 cases the surgical finding was an adenoma and 3 patients had parathyroid hyperplasia. Renal stones were found in 21 patients, of whom 14 did not have a recurrence of stone formation after parathyroidectomy and 5 showed clinical improvement with a reduction in stone incidence rate. In 2 cases renal stone formation remained clinically active. One of these two patients presented with recurrent urinary infection and the other had hypercalciuria which persisted after the operation. Clinical activity was determinated by the number of stones formed.

In every case the index of relative supersaturation with calcium oxalate, uric acid, brushite, and octacalcium phosphate was estimated from Marshall's nomograms[10] in 24 h urines collected prior to and at least 6 months after the operation. Urinary calcium was measured by atomic absorption spectrophotometry, uric acid by Caraway's method and the pH by means of the glass electrode following techniques already described[11]. Statistical analysis was carried out using the paired t-test.

RESULTS

Table 1 shows the values of the indices studied before and after parathyroidectomy in 28 patients, of whom 21 had renal lithiasis. The overall results did not reveal any significant differences between the cases with renal stones and the group of hyperparathyroid patients as a whole.

Table 1. Relative Urinary Supersaturation in 28 Cases of Primary Hyperparathyroidism
(R.L.=21 cases with associated renal lithiasis) (mean values ± S.E.M.)

		Preoperative	Postoperative	P
Calcium Oxalate	Total	0.836 ± 0.035	0.801 ± 0.048	n.s.
	R.L.	0.844 ± 0.037	0.808 ± 0.051	n.s.
Brushite	Total	0.511 ± 0.078	-0.043 ± 0.125	<0.001
	R.L.	0.600 ± 0.086	-0.058 ± 0.147	<0.001
Octacalcium Phosphate	Total	0.328 ± 0.119	-0.448 ± 0.151	<0.001
	R.L.	0.506 ± 0.115	-0.420 ± 0.171	<0.001
Uric Acid	Total	-1.023 ± 0.260	-0.133 ± 0.230	<0.001
	R.L.	-1.409 ± 0.281	-0.287 ± 0.287	<0.001

Calcium oxalate supersaturation did not change significantly, the mean value being in the metastable zone in all cases. Both the brushite and the octacalcium phosphate indices were significantly reduced, their mean values moving from the metastable to the undersaturated zone. The relative saturation of uric acid rose significantly but it always remained within the undersaturated zone.

DISCUSSION

Our results suggest that the supersaturation of urine with calcium phosphates plays a role in the genesis of the renal stone formation in hyperparathyroidism. The clinical importance observed after the parathyroidectomy in the cases with renal lithiasis was in agreement with reports of other authors[7,8].

We believe that the reduction in the urinary excretion of calcium, phosphate and bicarbonate[12], resulting from the normalization of parathyroid function, causes the significant fall in the saturation of urine with calcium phosphate from the metastable region to the region of undersaturation. This confirms Pak's findings[13].

With regard to calcium oxalate about whose significance in the renal stone formation of the hyperparathyroidism there is much controversy[14], parathyroidectomy did not seem to yield significant changes. However, we must point out that the mean value of the relative supersaturation index for calcium oxalate in our cases of hyperparathyroidism is higher than that in the general stone-forming population as reported by Nordin[15].

Hyperuricosuria has been recently suggested to increase the risk of calcium stone formation[16]. In our cases this parameter appeared to be irrelevant, clinically and physicochemically, in spite of a significant increase in urinary saturation with uric acid and parathyroidectomy.

In summary, our studies show that the physicochemical basis for renal stone formation in primary hyperparathyroidism depends, at least in part, on the supersaturation of urine with brushite and octacalcium phosphate. These findings confirm the importance of parathyroidectomy in the treatment of renal lithiasis associated with hyperparathyroidism.

REFERENCES

1. H. Heath, S. F. Hodgson, and M. A. Kennedy, New Engl. J. Med. 302:189 (1980).
2. A. Rapado and J. M. Castrillo, in:"Problemas Actuales de Urologia," L. Cifuentes Delatte, C. Alferez, E. Garcia de la Pena y R. Vela, eds., Salvat, Barcelona (1977).
3. A. Rapado, A. Mancha, J. M. Castrillo, M. L. Traba, M. Santos, and L. Cifuentes-Delatte, in:"Urolithiasis Research," H. Fleisch, W. G. Robertson, L. H. Smith, and W. Vahlensieck, eds., Plenum Press, New York (1976).
4. W. G. Robertson, in:"Calcium, Phosphate, and Magnesium Metabolism," B. E. C. Nordin, ed., Churchill Livingstone, Edinburgh (1976).

5. L. H. Smith, C. J. Van Den Berg, D. M. Wilson, D. A. Scholz, and D. C. Purnell, Kid. Int. 12:461 (1977).
6. L. Cifuentes-Delatte, A. Rapado, M. Santos, M. L. Traba, and J. M. Castrillo, Rev. Clin. Esp. 138:305 (1975).
7. M. G. McGeown, Lancet 1:586 (1961).
8. A. R. Harrison and G. A. Rose, in:"Urinary Calculi: Recent Advances in Aetiology, Structure and Treatment," L. Cifuentes-Delatte, A. Rapado, and A. Hodgkinson, eds., S. Karger, Basel (1973).
9. J. W. Muir and L. R. I. Baker, Br. Med. J. 3:738 (1978).
10. R. W. Marshall and W. G. Robertson, Clin. Chim. Acta. 72:253 (1976).
11. A. Rapado, M. L. Traba, J. M. Castrillo, A. Mancha, M. Santos, and L. Cifuentes-Delatte, in:"Problemas Actuales de Urologia," L. Cifuentes-Delatte, C. Alferez, E. Garcia de la Pena, and R. Vela, eds., Salvat, Barcelona (1977).
12. F. P. Muldowney, D. V. Carroll, J. F. Donohoe, and R. Freaney, Quart. J. Med. 160:487 (1971).
13. C. Y. C. Pak, in:"Calcium Urolithiasis," H. Fleisch, W. G. Robertson, L. H. Smith, and W. Vahlensieck, eds., Plenum Press, New York (1976).
14. C. Y. C. Pak and K. Holt, Metabolism 25:665 (1976).
15. B. E. C. Nordin, in:"Calcium, Phosphate, and Magnesium Metabolism," B. E. C. Nordin, ed., Churchill Livingstone, Edinburgh (1976).
16. F. L. Coe, in:"Nephrolithiasis: Pathogenesis and Treatment," Year Book, Chicago (1978).

CLINICAL DISORDERS

MEDULLARY SPONGE KIDNEY (TUBULAR ECTASIA) IN CALCIUM UROLITHIASIS

E. R. Yendt, S. Jarzylo, W. A. Finnis, and M. Cohanim

Departments of Medicine and Radiology, Kingston General Hospital and Queen's University, Kingston, Ontario, Canada

The project described in this presentation has been in progress for the past five years and has two main objectives. The first is to define the incidence of medullary sponge kidney in patients with calcium stones and the second is to attempt to determine the relationship between the milder degrees of the condition frequently encountered in our study and stone formation. During the course of our study, we have obtained all available intravenous urograms performed on our patients and reviewed them jointly with our radiologist colleague (S.J.) for evidence of tubular ectasia, a term which we prefer to "medullary sponge kidney" which we consider to be inappropriate for the milder degrees of the disorder. When the quality of the available x-rays was considered to be inadequate, infusion nephrotomography has, when feasible, been performed in an attempt to obtain better quality films.

The diagnosis of tubular ectasia was based on the demonstration in the intravenous urogram of ectatic tubules in three or more renal papillae. A diagnosis of tubular ectasia was not made when ectatic tubules were present in only one or two renal papillae because it is difficult to be certain that urographic abnormalities of such minimal degree actually are ectatic tubules. Moreover we found that the incidence of lesions interpreted as ectatic tubules in only one or two papillae was approximately the same (6 – 8%) in patients with stones as in those without. Although papillary blushing is considered by some authorities to be indicative of a minor degree of tubular ectasia[1], we did not diagnose tubular ectasia in our study when this was the sole radiographic abnormality.

During the past eleven years, we have investigated 1035 patients with calcium urolithiasis. Tubular ectasia was present in 132 patients, an incidence of 13% whereas in 214 patients without stones, the incidence was only 2%. However, in the last 400 patients, tubular ectasia has been diagnosed in 82 patients, an incidence of 21 % and in the last 200 patients the incidence of tubular ectasia was 23%. This is a much higher incidence of this disorder than has previously been reported. The higher incidence of tubular ectasia found by us is partially explained by the fact that we have looked very hard for these lesions, which many radiologists either fail to recognize or fail to report. Moreover we have found that the quality of the intravenous urograms performed in most stone patients is totally inadequate for the detection of minor degrees of tubular ectasia and whenever possible we have attempted to obtain an x-ray examination of higher quality.

We have used a grading system for the quality of intravenous urogram ranging through grade I (poor), grade II (fair), grade III (good), and grade IV (excellent). In our experience the quality of the intravenous urogram must be either good or excellent before the diagnosis of tubular ectasia can be ruled out with reasonable certainty. To qualify as a good or excellent examination, an intravenous urogram must clearly outline most calyceal fornices, detail must not be obscured by overlying bowel contents and ureteral obstruction must not be present. The majority of excretory urograms performed on patients referred to us are either poor or fair in quality. In our last 25 patients a total of 53 intravenous urograms have been performed, of which only three were classified as good, the remainder being poor or fair. We have encountered numerous cases in which a milder degree of tubular ectasia was not evident in the intravenous urograms which accompanied the patient which were only fair or poor in quality, but was readily apparent when better quality films were obtained.

For various reasons, however, it has not always been possible to obtain an intravenous urogram of adequate quality in our patients. It may not be ethically acceptable to repeat the examination and to expose the patient to additional radiation if the purpose of the exercise is largely academic. Some patients may be reluctant to undergo another x-ray procedure when one has been performed in the recent past; others may have developed a sensitivity to the contrast medium. Even when we do repeat the examination utilizing high dose infusion nephrotomography and an x-ray machine with a small focal spot, the quality of the films is occasionally still inadequate for our purposes. The result is that an intravenous urogram of satisfactory quality is available in only about one half our patients at the conclusion of our investigations. When this is taken into consideration, the incidence of tubular ectasia may be considerably higher than even our figures would indicate.

Of the 132 patients with tubular ectasia, 81 were males and 51 were females. Eighty-seven were normocalciuric and 35 were hypercalciuric (24 hour urinary calcium exceeding 375 mg per day in males and 300 mg per day in females on unrestricted diets). However in the patients thus classified as being normocalciuric, urinary calcium was significantly higher than normal.

Although the relationship between the classical form of medullary sponge kidney and renal stone formation is generally recognized, the significance of the milder cases of tubular ectasia identified in our study remains to be established. We have been attempting to identify differences between patients with calcium stones associated with tubular ectasia and those without tubular ectasia on the assumption that the demonstration of such differences would increase the likelihood of a relationship between tubular ectasia and stone formation. I should now like to review briefly the progress made along these lines to date.

The major clinical difference noted in our patients with tubular ectasia relates to the number of renal stones in situ at the time of referral to us. Fifty of 76 patients (66%) with tubular ectasia had stones in situ including 6 with widespread nephrocalcinosis whereas of 38 patients without tubular ectasia only 15 (39%) had stones in situ and none of these had nephrocalcinosis. In the patients with tubular ectasia, the calcifications were often thought to be situated with the substance of a renal papilla rather than in the collecting system. Excluding the patients with nephrocalcinosis, the mean number of stones in situ was 3.0 per patient in the patients with tubular ectasia but only 1.0 per patient in those without tubular ectasia. We have found that thiazides prevent further stone formation equally well in patients with tubular ectasia as in those without[2].

The first distinct biochemical difference noted in these patients with tubular ectasia was that in 10 patients the serum ultrafiltrable calcium levels were slightly below the normal range - an abnormality which we have not encountered in stone patients without tubular ectasia (Figure 1). Serum ultrafiltrable calcium has been measured routinely in our research laboratory for the past 12 years by a modification of the method of Toribara et al.[3]. We have established a narrow normal range of 5.15 - 5.85 mg % for this method which has been much more useful in detecting minimal degrees of hypocalcemia or hypercalcemia than the total serum calcium, even when the latter is corrected for alterations in serum protein levels. Following treatment with thiazides, serum ultrafiltrable calcium levels in these patients rose to the mid-normal range. (Figure 1) We then compared the mean serum ultrafiltrable calcium level in three groups of patients - calcium stone patients with tubular ectasia, calcium stone patients without tubular ectasia and patients with stones (Figure 2). This analysis was confined to male patients since the number of female patients was initially not sufficient for

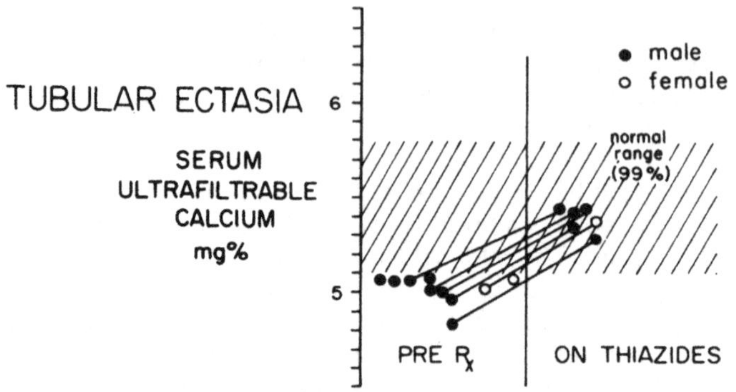

Figure 1. Serum ultrafiltrable calcium levels were slightly below the normal range in 10 patients with tubular ectasia but rise to normal during thiazide therapy. Each symbol represents the value for serum ultrafiltrable calcium of an individual patient. This abnormality has not been encountered in other groups of stone patients.

a meaningful analysis. The number of patients with calcium stones who did not have tubular ectasia was relatively small because patients were placed in this category only when a negative intravenous urogram was of good or excellent quality. The mean serum ultrafiltrable calcium is identical in patients with uric acid stones 5.46 ± .04 mg% (mean ± SE) and those with calcium stones who do not have tubular ectasia (5.46 ± .03 mg%) but is reduced in patients with calcium stones who do have tubular ectasia (5.41 ± .02 mg%). (In 33 patients who were considered to have ectatic tubules in only one or two renal papillae the serum ultrafiltrable calcium

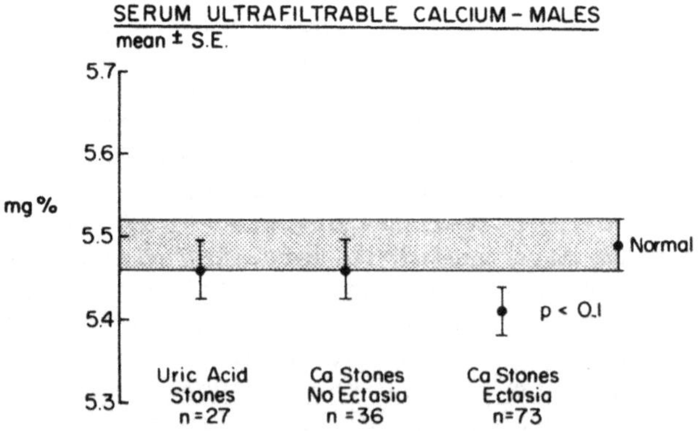

Figure 2. Mean serum ultrafiltrable calcium level - males (± standard error) is reduced in patients with calcium stones who have tubular ecstasia but the difference falls just short of statistical significance.

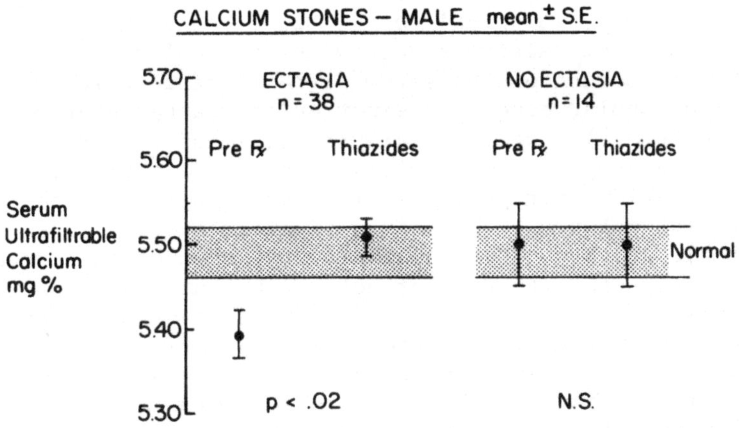

Figure 3. A statistically significant rise in the mean serum ultrafiltrable calcium level occurs in patients with calcium stones after one year or more of thiazide therapy but there is no significant change during thiazide therapy in patients who do not have tubular ectasia.

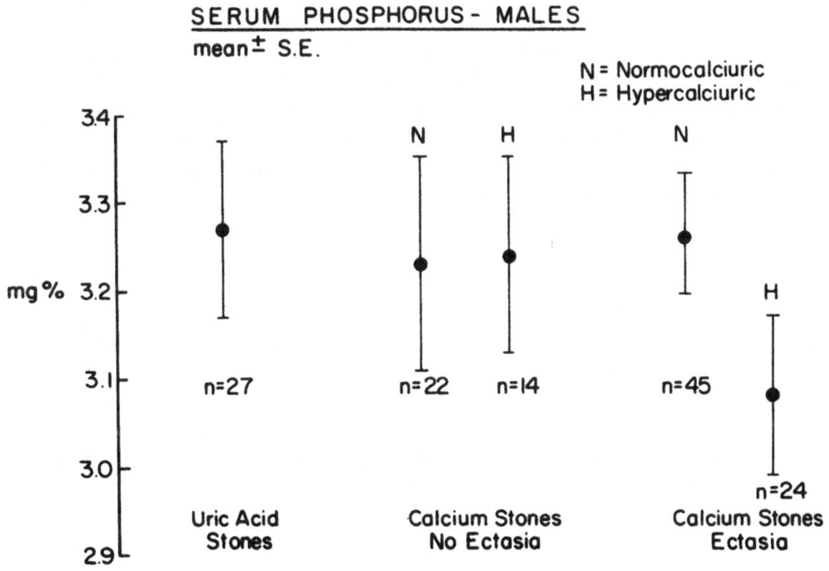

Figure 4. Mean fasting a.m. serum inorganic phosphorus levels in various groups of stone patients – males (mean ± standard error). The only group of patients with reduced serum phosphorus is the hypercalciuric patients with tubular ecstasia but the difference is not statistically significant.

was 5.46 ± 0.03 mg%, identical to the value found in patients with uric acid stones and calcium stones without tubular ectasia). Although the reduction of the serum ultrafiltrable calcium in patients with tubular ectasia has not quite reached statistical significance ($p<0.1$) a statistically significant difference does emerge when one compares serum ultrafiltrable calcium levels before and during thiazide therapy in calcium stone patients with and without tubular ectasia. There is a significant rise in serum ultrafiltrable calcium after thiazides have been administered for one year in patients with tubular ectasia but not in those without tubular ectasia. (Figure 3). The mean fasting serum inorganic phosphorus level was virtually identical in male patients with uric acid stones, normocalciuric and hypercalciuric patients with calcium stones who did not have tubular ectasia and normocalciuric patients with tubular ectasia. The only group of patients with a reduction in the mean serum phosphorus level were the hypercalciuric patients with tubular ectasia but the difference is not statistically significant (Figure 4).

We are obviously interested in the possibility that the tendency towards hypocalcemia seen in patients with tubular ectasia leads to secondary hyperparathyroidism which is reversible during thiazide therapy. Although we find elevated serum PTH levels in approximately 25% of our patients with tubular ectasia we as yet have insufficient longitudinal data to accurately assess the effects of thiazide therapy. Moreover we have insufficient data in patients who do not have tubular ectasia to assess whether or not secondary hyperparathyroidism is limited to patients with tubular ectasia. The vagaries of the PTH assay complicates this aspect of our studies and we are now measuring urine cyclic AMP in our patients in an effort to resolve this question.

Four of our patients (all female) with tubular ectasia have had overt hyperparathyroidism corrected by surgical removal of parathyroid adenomas. The association between medullary sponge kidney and hyperparathyroidism has also been reported in the literature in at least 14 patients[4,5]. We have investigated two additional patients with normal total serum calcium but with intermittent elevation of the serum ultrafiltrable calcium both before and during thiazide therapy; these patients have not been operated on but may be further examples of the same association. It is tempting to speculate that a renal calcium leak is associated with tubular ectasia leading to secondary hyperparathyroidism and finally to tertiary hyperparathyroidism, a suggestion which has also been made in the literature[6]. There is however no real proof for this hypothesis at the present time.

When we examined the composition of the urine in hypercalciuric patients with calcium stones there appeared to be some very clear cut differences between patients with tubular ectasia and those with-

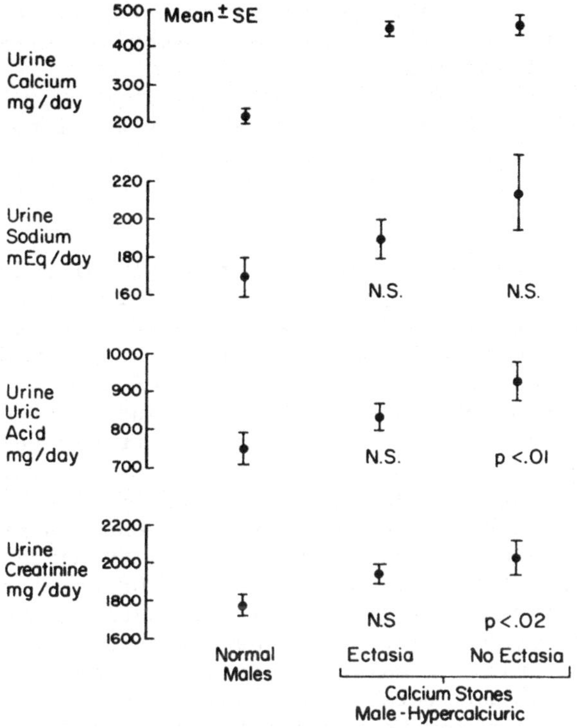

Figure 5. Mean (± standard error) 24 hour urinary calcium, sodium, uric acid and creatinine excretion in 18 normal male subjects, 26 hypercalciuric male calcium stone patients with tubular ectasia and 15 hypercalciuric male calcium stone patients who did not have tubular ectasia. Urinary creatinine and uric acid excretion is significantly higher than normal in the patients without tubular ectasia but not in the patients with tubular ectasia. The urine collections were made in out-patients on unrestricted diets.

out. In the patients who did not have tubular ectasia, daily urinary creatinine and uric acid excretion was significantly higher than in normal male subjects but this was not found in patients with tubular ectasia (Figure 5). Data for urinary phosphorus excretion (not included in Figure 5) are similar to those obtained for uric acid - these being significantly higher than normal urine phosphorus in hypercalciuric patients who do not have tubular ectasia. Urinary sodium was also higher in the patients without tubular ectasia although this difference ($p<0.1$) has not quite reached statistical significance. Urinary calcium excretion was similar in the two groups of patients. One possible interpretation of these findings is that body size and diet may be important factors contributing to hypercalciuria in patients who do not have tubular ectasia but are relatively unimportant in patients with tubular ectasia who have a renal tubular calcium leak.

Diminished renal concentrating ability and impaired urinary acidification have been reported in patients with medullary sponge kidney[1] but these aspects of renal function have not been investigated in our studies.

In summary, we have found a surprisingly high incidence of tubular ectasia of 23% in patients with calcium stones whereas in 214 non stone patients the incidence was only 2%. We have also found that the quality of the intravenous urogram performed in most stone patients is not adequate for the demonstration of these lesions and when this is taken into consideration the incidence of the disorder may be considerably higher. Serum ultrafiltrable calcium levels tend to be lower in patients with tubular ectasia than in other groups of stone patients and undergo a significant rise to normal during thiazide therapy whereas no significant change in serum ultrafiltrable calcium levels occurs during thiazide therapy in patients who do not have tubular ectasia. Urinary creatinine, uric acid, and phosphorus excretion is significantly higher than normal in hypercalciuric patients who do not have tubular ectasia but not in patients with tubular ectasia. These data strongly suggest that calcium and phosphorus metabolism is different in patients with tubular ectasia than in those without ectasia and that the pathogenesis of both the hypercalciuria and the stone formation may be different in these two groups of patients. Although we do not regard our data as conclusive, we do believe that they are sufficiently suggestive to warrant a careful search for tubular ectasia in patients with calcium stones and that patients with this abnormality should be examined as a separate group in studies related to the pathogenesis of calcium stones and/or hypercalciuria.

REFERENCES

1. J. J. Kniper, K. D. Gardner, Jr., ed., John Wiley and Sons, New York (1976).
2. E. R. Yendt and M. Cohanim, Kid. Int. 13:397 (1978).
3. T. Y. Toribara, A. R. Terepka, and P. A. Davey, J. Clin. Invest. 36:78 (1957).
4. D. S. Rao, B. Frame, M. A. Block, and A. M. Parfitt, JAMA 238:1912 (1977).
5. O. L. Tiktinsky and V. V. Nekachalov, Eur. Urol. 4:330 (1978).
6. P. Bordier, A. Ryckewart, J. Gueris, and H. Rasmussen, Am. J. Med. 63:398 (1977).

ACKNOWLEDGMENTS

This work was supported by grants from the Medical Research Council of Canada (MT 681).

CLINICAL AND LABORATORY FINDINGS IN PATIENTS WITH MEDULLARY SPONGE KIDNEY

U. Backman, B. G. Danielson, B. Fellström,
G. Johansson, S. Ljunghall, and B. Wikström
Department of Internal Medicine
University Hospital
S-750 14 Uppsala, Sweden

Structural abnormalities of the urinary tract are usually thought to predispose to renal stone formation. Medullary sponge kidney is probably a congenital abnormality. Because of such structural abnormalities, a higher incidence of tubular dysfunction may be anticipated. However, a broad investigation of renal tubular function has not been performed in larger series. The renal acidification capacity has only been investigated in a few patients and found to be defective in some of these[1]. In some cases the diagnosis of renal tubular acidosis (RTA) might have been overlooked[2,3]. It seems important to diagnose the acidification defect since it seems to be associated with a more severe stone disease[4].

Other factors which have been regarded to be of importance for stone formation in patients with medullary sponge kidney is hypercalciuria. Renal hypercalciuria and primary hyperparathyroidism have both been discussed[1,5].

In the present study, the clinical picture in medullary sponge kidney was related to the presence of metabolic abnormalities with special attention paid to parathyroid and renal tubular function.

MATERIAL

Among 612 recurrent stone formers medullary sponge kidney was diagnosed from the typical findings on pyelography in 14 men (mean age 46 years, range 23-72 years) and 8 women (mean age 38 years, range 26-59 years). The age of onset was 30 years. In 15 patients the typical radiological findings were seen in both kidneys, in 5 patients in one kidney and in 2 patients only one part of one kidney was affected. Three patients had been operated for stones, one of them twice. In two cases a resection of the diseased part had been performed. The mean stone episode rate was 0.6 stones/year. A positive family history of stone disease was seen in 8 patients. Urinary tract infections were uncommon and seen sporadically in 3 patients.

Out of the 22 patients, 14 (9 men and 5 women) went through a more detailed investigation. All patients were investigated as outpatients without dietary restrictions.

METHODS

All patients were investigated according to our standard program for stone formers[6]. Serum and urinary electrolytes were measured by atomic absorption. Parathyroid hormone concentrations (PTH) were determined by a commercial method (Medicinsk Laboratorium, Copenhagen). The urinary excretion of cyclic AMP (cAMP) was measured with a radioimmunoassay technique which gives a normal range of 0.2-0.6 μmol/mmol creatinine[7]. The fasting urinary calcium was determined after an overnight fast as described by Pak et al[8]. The renal threshold of phosphate (TmP/GFR) was determined in the same samples[9]. The renal acidification capacity was investigated by a short ammonium chloride test[10]. The subjects were given 17 g ammonium chloride whereafter the acid-base status and the urinary acidification (pH, titratable acid and ammonium ions) were followed each hour. Tubular proteinuria was estimated by investigating the 24 h urinary excretion of β_2-microglobulin which was measured by a radioimmunoassay technique (Phadebas, AB Pharmacia, Diagnostics, Uppsala, Sweden). Reference values are 30 - 370 μg/24 h. Urinary citrate output was analyzed by an enzyme method (citrate lyase), with a normal value of 3.2 ± 1.2 mmol/24 h.

RESULTS

One patient had a reduced GFR (20 ml/min) possibly due to dysplasia of the kidneys, judged from pyelography. In all the others serum creatinine and creatinine clearance were within the normal range. One patient had hypercalcemia and neck exploration revealed a parathyroid adenoma. All the other patients had normal serum values for calcium, magnesium and urate (Table 1). The urinary excretions of calcium, magnesium and urate were within the same range as for idiopathic stone formers. (Table 1).

Fasting urinary calcium excretion was also within normal limits in all patients and the excretion was inversely related to cyclic AMP in a similar way as previously found in control subjects (Figure 1). The patient with renal failure had a raised serum PTH and a low urinary cAMP whereas there was no consistent evidence of parathyroid hyperfunction in the others.

Table 1. Serum and Urinary Data for Calcium, Magnesium and Urate in Patients with Medullary Sponge Kidney Disease, Idiopathic Stone Disease and Controls

	Medullary sponge kidney disease (n = 22)	Idiopathic stone formers (n = 70)	Controls (n = 58)
Serum calcium (mmol/l)	2.44 ± 0.13	2.41 ± 0.07	2.41 ± 0.08
Urinary calcium (mmol/24h)	7.8 ± 4.0	6.9 ± 2.6	5.0 ± 2.2
Serum magnesium (mmol/l)	0.82 ± 0.07	0.83 ± 0.07	0.83 ± 0.05
Urinary magnesium (mmol/24h)	5.0 ± 2.1	4.1 ± 1.2	4.4 ± 1.3
Serum urate (mmol/l)	330 ± 88	270 ± 74	305 ± 52
Urinary urate (mmol/24h)	2.4 ± 0.71	3.1 ± 0.9	3.2 ± 1.0

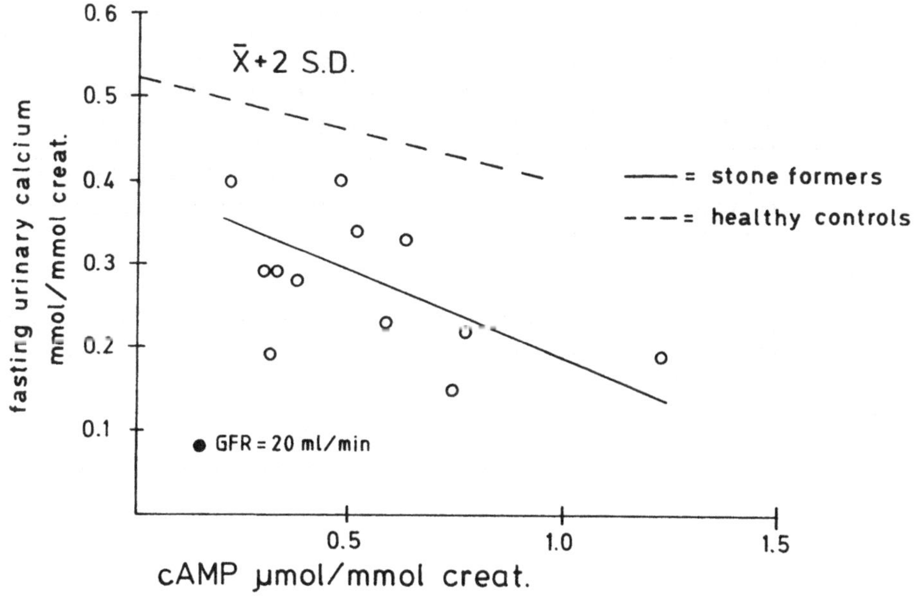

Figure 1. The relationship between the urinary excretion of calcium and cyclic AMP (cAMP) after an overnight fast in 14 patients with MSK. The regression line for recurrent stone formers is indicated together with the mean +2SD obtained from healthy controls.

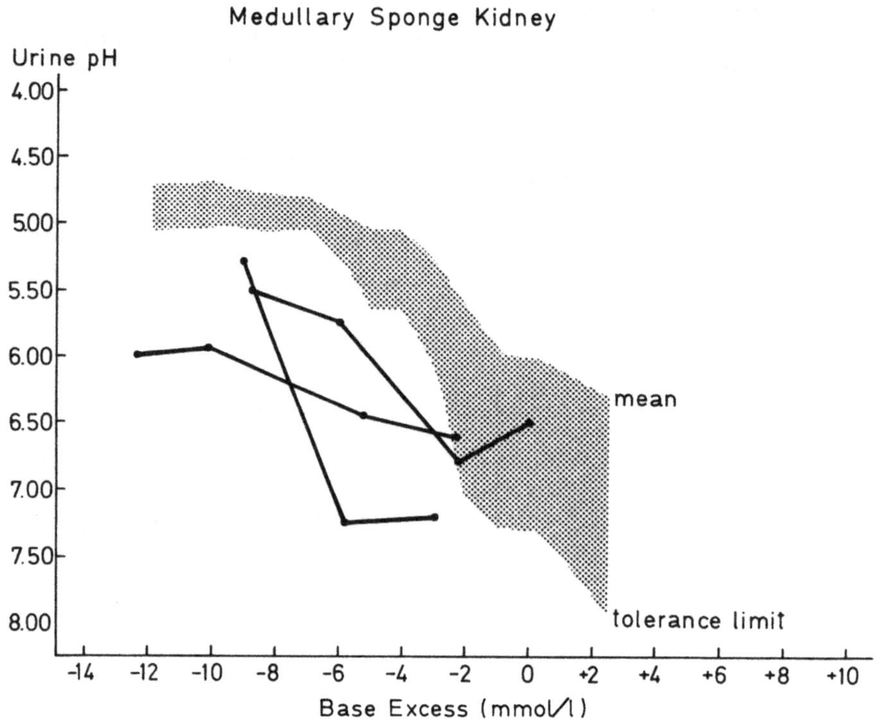

Figure 2. Three patients with defective urinary acidification compared to a frame of reference obtained from persons with normal acidification (shaded area). The two patients with the lowest urinary pH of 6.0 and 5.5 respectively were judged to have a distal defect; the third with a pH of 5.25 probably had a mixed defect with loss of bicarbonate.

Incomplete forms of renal tubular acidosis (RTA) were diagnosed in 3 patients (Figure 2). Two of these patients had only one kidney affected.

The urinary excretion of citrate was low, when compared to other stone formers. In spite of a usually normal acidification capacity the excretion was of the same order as in our patients with distal tubular acidosis (Figure 3).

The urinary excretion of β_2-microglobulin was increased in two patients with one of whom was the one with low GFR (Figure 4). The frequency of tubular proteinuria corresponds to that found in our idiopathic stone formers. The renal threshold phosphate concentration (TmP/GFR) was normal in all patients. Serum phosphate was raised only in the patient with renal failure.

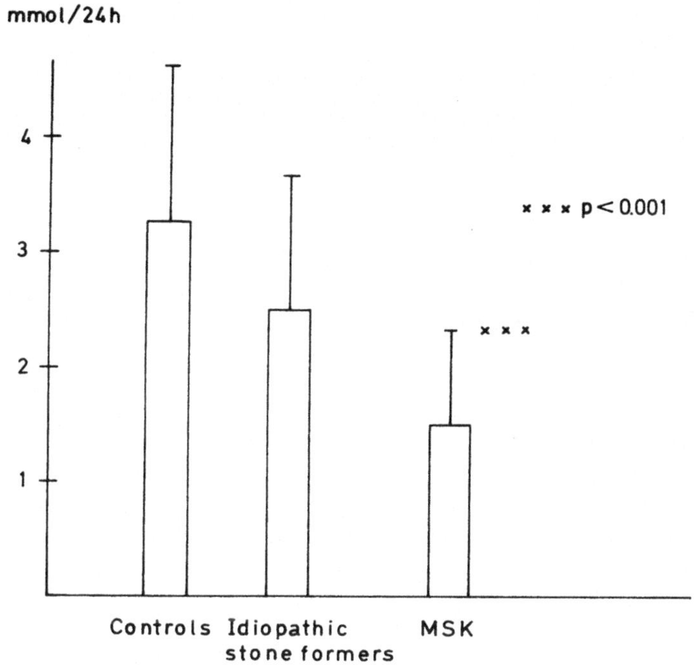

Figure 3. The urinary excretion of citrate in patients with MSK compared to the excretion in idiopathic stone formers and controls.

DISCUSSION

The incidence of medullary sponge kidney in our stone material of 612 recurrent stone formers was 3.5% which is about the same as found in other large series of consecutive stone formers[11,12]. Although the diagnostic criteria described in 1948 by Cacchi and Ricci [13] make sponge kidney as a discrete disease entity, its relationship to other cystic processes in the kidney sometimes seems hazy. As in other series in most of our patients (68%) both kidneys were affected[14].

Some authors have pointed to a moderate degree of ectasia of the collecting ducts which has been considered to be a normal variant[15]. The clinical importance of these changes has been discussed and considered by some to be slight[15] and often diagnosed by chance as the patients seldom exhibit symptoms whereas others classify them in the same group as medullary sponge kidney[5].

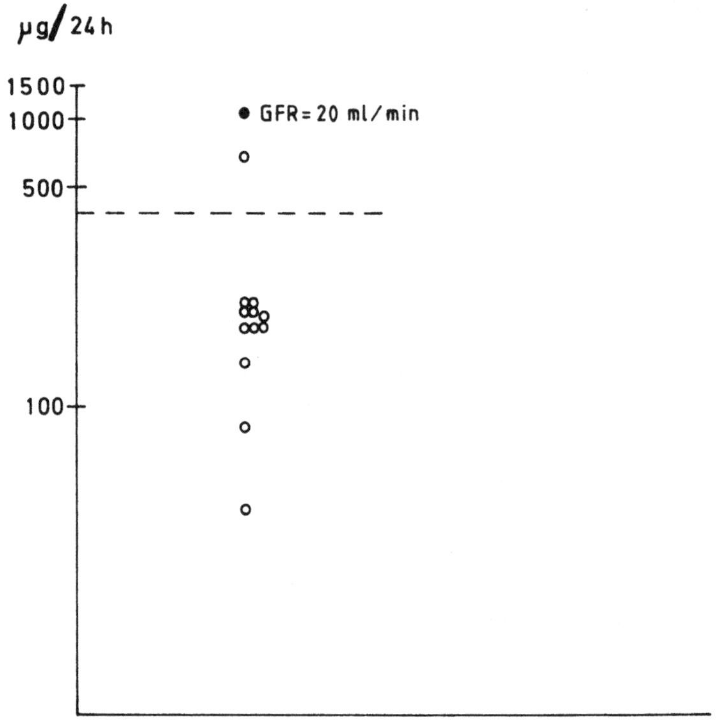

Figure 4. The urinary excretion of β_2-microglobulin in patients with MSK. The upper normal limit is indicated (dashed line).

Medullary sponge kidney is usually considered to be a benign disease as regards glomerular filtration rate. When renal failure has developed, it has usually been contributed to chronic pyelonephritis[2] but glomerulopathy has also been suggested[16]. The reason in our patient was obscure.

Some authors suggest that hyperparathyroidism can induce renal lesions indistinguishable from medullary sponge kidney[1]. Several cases are reported in the literature with both diagnoses[1,17,18] and some authors conclude that the association between the two diseases is greater than could be explained by chance only[1,18]. We also had one patient where it was difficult to differentiate between the two diagnoses. Other authors explain the coexistence by the development of secondary hyperparathyroidism due to hypercalciuria[5]. The treatment in these cases would then be directed to the treatment of hypercalciuria.

Except for the case with renal failure there was in the others no evidence of secondary hyperparathyroidism, furthermore, the inverse relationship between the fasting urinary calcium and cAMP was the same as for our controls and idiopathic stone formers, suggesting a picture of absorptive hypercalciuria[19].

Although there was no evidence of renal hypercalciuria, a higher incidence of tubular dysfunction in patients with structural abnormalities of the distal part of the nephron might be anticipated. The most constant finding in other studies was a reduced concentration capacity[2,20]. Renal acidification capacity has only rarely been studied. In the large material of Ekström et al.[2], at least one patient had an incipient acidosis suggesting an acidification defect as the glomerular filtration rate was normal. In the described cases and in our three patients with renal tubular acidosis glomerular filtration rate was normal. The acidification defect could therefore not be caused by renal insufficiency[14]. Probably the defect was of importance for the stone formation as all these patients had an early onset of stone disease. An early onset was a typical feature also in our other stone formers with renal tubular acidosis[4]. Thus, acidification defects should be suspected above all in young patients, as symptoms of medullary sponge kidney usually appear in the middle age[2,14].

The incidence of renal tubular acidosis in our patients with medullary sponge kidney was the same as in our recurrent stone formers. Disturbances of the proximal tubules were not clearly diagnosed in our series, neither proximal acidification defects nor tubular proteinuria being found.

One outstanding biochemical feature in our patients was a low urinary excretion of citrate. Hypocitraturia is a typical finding in patients with complete forms of renal tubular acidosis[21] but we found it also in our patients with the incomplete form[22]. The citrate excretion in all our patients with medullary sponge kidney was of the same order as in the distal type of RTA although most of them had normal acidification.

Patients with medullary sponge kidney had a clinical picture similar to that of other stone formers with a stone episode rate of 0.6 stones/year. They did not exhibit an increased frequency of infection or stone operations[6].

In conclusion, in spite of the structural abnormalities of the distal part of the nephron, patients with medullary sponge kidney did not have defective tubular function more often than our recurrent stone formers. Nor was there any evidence of renal hypercalciuria. The severity of the stone disease was not related to the tubular defects. As a group, patients with medullary sponge kidney should be investigated and treated according to the principles for other recurrent stone formers.

REFERENCES

1. R. C. Morris, H. Yamauchi, A. J. Palubinskas, and J. Howenstone, JAMA 28:883 (1965).
2. E. Ekström, E. Engfeldt, C. Lagergren, and N. Lindvall, in: "Medullary Sponge Kidney," Almkvist and Wiksell, Stockholm (1959).
3. F. Schabel, M. Fink, and J. Glatzl, Pädiatrie und Pädologie 11:417 (1976).
4. U. Backman, B. G. Danielson, G. Johansson, S. Ljunghall, and B. Wikström, Nephron 25:96 (1980).
5. E. R. Yendt and M. Cohanim, Kid. Int. 13:397 (1978).
6. B. Wikström, U. Backman, B. G. Danielson, B. Fellström, G. Johansson, and S. Ljunghall, (submitted for publication)
7. O. Wålinder, S. Ljunghall, and L. Wibell, Scand. J. Urol. Nephrol. 12:67 (1978).
8. C. Y. C. Pak, M. Ohata, E. C. Lawrency, and W. Snyder, J. Clin. Invest. 54:387 (1974).
9. R. J. Walton and O. L. M. Bijvoet, Lancet II:309 (1975).
10. U. Backman, B. G. Danielson, and M. Sohtell, Scand. J. Urol. Nephrol. Suppl. 35:33 (1976).
11. G. F. Mayall, Clin. Radiol. 21:171 (1970).
12. J. N. Lavan, F. C. Neale, and S. Posen, Med. J. Aust. 2:1049 (1971).
13. R. Cacchi and V. Ricci, Att. Ital. Urol. 5:59 (1948).
14. H. M. Spence and R. Singleton, J. Urol. 107:176 (1972).
15. A. J. Palubinskas, Radiology 81:963 (1963).
16. H. M. Levitt, R. McCoy, and B. F. Fetter, J. Urol. 112:710 (1974).
17. F. J. Stella, S. G. Massry, and C. R. Kleeman, Nephron 10:332 (1973).
18. M. D. H. Gremillon, M. J. W. Kee, and C. D. A. Mcintosh, JAMA 237:799 (1977).
19. S. Ljunghall, U. Backman, B. G. Danielson, G. Johansson, B. Jung, R. Källsen, L. Wibell, and O. Wålinder, Scand. J. Nephrol. Suppl. 41:77 (1977).
20. P. O. Granberg, C. Lagergren, and N. O. Theve, Scand. J. Urol. 5:177 (1971).
21. A. Sebastian, E. McSherry, and R. C. Morris, Jr., in:"The Kidney," Brenner and Rector, eds., Saunders, Philadelphia, (1976).
22. B. Wikstrom, U. Backman, B. G. Danielson, B. Fellstrom, G. Johansson, and S. Ljunghall, in:"Proceedings Fourth International Urolithiasis Research Symposium," L. H. Smith, B. Finlayson, and W. G. Robertson, eds., Plenum Press, New York.

HEREDITARY HYPERURICOSURIC UROLITHIASIS

O. Sperling

Department of Clinical Biochemistry, Beilinson Medical Center, Petah-Tikva, and Department of Chemical Pathology Tel Aviv University Medical School, Tel Hashomer, Israel

Hyperuricosuria is a major factor in uric acid stone formation. As a hereditary condition it is very rare, reflecting either purine overproduction (metabolic uricosuria) or renal uricosuria.

HEREDITARY METABOLIC HYPERURICOSURIC UROLITHIASIS

Uric acid lithiasis due to inborn errors of metabolism associated with excessive purine production has been established in 2 enzyme abnormalities: deficiency of hypoxanthine-guanine phosphoribosyltransferase (HGPRT)[1] and superactivity of phosphoribosylpyrophosphate (PRPP) synthetase[2-4]. Both are inherited by an X-linked pattern and are characterized by excessive purine production and recurrent (malignant) juvenile uric acid lithiasis.

HGPRT Deficiency

HGPRT deficiency was first discovered in the rare pediatric, X-linked neurological Lesch-Nyhan syndrome[1], in which uric acid lithiasis appears at a very young age. Partial HGPRT deficiency (0.01 to 17% of normal HGPRT activity) also causes purine overproduction and uric acid stones and occurs in 1 to 2% of patients with metabolic gout[5,6]. HGPRT deficiency, by decreased salvage nucleotide synthesis, causes accumulation of substrate PRPP and presumably a lowered nucleotide concentration. Each leads to accelerated purine synthesis *de novo* through activation of glutamine PRPP amidotransferase, catalyzing the first committed and rate limiting step in the pathway of purine synthesis.

PRPP Synthetase Superactivity

PRPP synthetase superactivity as a cause of purine overproduction was found in a family with gout and malignant uric acid lithiasis[2,7]. PRPP synthetase was found to be mutationally altered in its allosteric site, as reflected in feedback resistance to physiological inhibitors. Additional superactive mutants of PRPP synthetase were reported, including a mutant enzyme with increased specific activity[3] and one with higher affinity for the substrate ribose-5-phosphate[4], but are very rare among the gouty population. The purine overproduction in all PRPP synthetase mutants is caused by the increased production of substrate PRPP. The pattern of inheritance of the PRPP synthetase abnormality has been shown to be X-linked[8].

Unconfirmed Enzyme Abnormalities

Two additional enzyme abnormalities are considered to cause uric acid overproduction, superactivity of glutathione reductase[9] and deficiency of glucose-6-phosphatase (glycogen storage disease type 1)[10]. The mechanism of purine overproduction is held to be accelerated activity of the pentose phosphate pathway leading to increased ribose-5 phosphate availability and increased generation of PRPP. This mechanism, however, has yet not been conclusively established.

HEREDITARY RENAL HYPERURICOSURIC UROLITHIASIS

Hereditary hyperuricosuria may also occur in subjects with normal purine production, in the syndrome of renal hypouricemia[11]. Genetic renal hypouricemia is rare, appearing usually as one of the many manifestations of the Fanconi syndrome[12] or Wilson's disease[13]. When not associated with such broad tubulopathies, genetic renal hypouricemia may represent a defect in renal urate handling. This latter type has been shown to be frequently associated with mild uricosuria and urolithiasis[11]. Ten families are presently documented with hereditary renal hypouricemia of the isolated type[14-22], of which 7 are from Israel[16,18-22].

The most plausible model for renal urate handling in man consists of 4 components: glomerular filtration, pre-secretory tubular reabsorption, tubular secretion and post-secretory tubular reabsorption[16,23]. According to this model, almost all filtered urate is reabsorbed in the proximal tubule by a high-affinity-high-capacity transport mechanism; the amount of urate in urine derives almost exclusively from tubular secretion, occurring predominantly in the proximal tubule, which is balanced by reabsorption occurring either simultaneously or more distally (post-secretory reabsorption). The exact nature of the renal lesion causing the increased urate clearance has not yet been clarified. According to the above model increased urate clearance may result from defective tubular reabsorption, either at the presecretory or postsecretory sites or at both. To evaluate the defective site in the various patients with renal uricosuria, the PZA suppression test[24] and the probenecid test were applied. Based on the response of uric acid excretion in the various patients, 3 different types of tubular lesions were postulated[14-16,24,26-28].

CLINICAL SIGNIFICANCE

Hypouricemia has, as far as known, no clinical significance[11]. On the other hand, 4 out of the 8 propositi with inborn isolated renal hypouricemia[14,18,20] had urinary tract stones (2 uric acid stones, one a stone of unidentified composition). In the 2 patients with uric acid stones, the hypouricemia was associated with marked hyperuricosuria (24 h urinary uric acid > 1000 mg/day). Furthermore, moderate hyperuricosuria was present in 6 other hypouricemic propositi[11]. Thus, hyperuricosuria appears to be a common feature of isolated renal hypouricemia.

The mechanism of the hyperuricosuria in these subjects has not been finally clarified. It might reflect purine overproduction or diversion of intestinal urate elimination to urinary urate excretion. Since there is no evidence for purine overproduction[17,29], the hyperuricosuria in renal hypouricemia would appear to be "renal hyperuricosuria". Idiopathic hypercalciuria was found to be associated with renal hypouricemia in 4 of the propositi[14,16,20]. In 3, the hypercalciuria was proven to be of the absorptive type.

GENETIC ASPECTS

In 6 of the families both males and females were affected, compatible with autosomal inheritance, whereas in the other families this mode of transmission has not been excluded. In one family[16] the autosomal inheritance was proven to be recessive while in the others[14,20], autosomal recessive inheritance was compatible with the distribution. The results obtained with the pyrazinamide and probenecid tests in the various renal hypouricemic families reported indicate heterogeneity of the genetic abnormality in the tubular defect.

OTHER TYPES OF HEREDITARY RENAL HYPERURICEMIA

Theoretically, there may also be a high frequency of hyperuricosuria and urolithiasis in other types of hereditary renal hypouricemia, i.e. of the nonisolated type. However, no data are available to support this possibility.

REFERENCES

1. J. E. Seegmiller, F. M. Rosenbloom, and W. N. Kelley, Science 155:1682 (1867).
2. O. Sperling, P. Boer, S. Persky Brosh, E. Kanareck, and A. de Vries, Eur. J. Clin. Biol. Res. 17:703 (1972).
3. M. A. Becker, L. J. Meyer, A. W. Wood, and J. E. Seegmiller, Science 179:1123 (1973).
4. M. A. Becker and J. E. Seegmiller, Arthritis Rheum. 18:687 (1975).
5. T. F. Yu, M. E. Balis, T. A. Krenitsky, J. Dancis, D. N. Silvers, G. B. Elion, and A. B. Gutman, Ann. Int. Med. 76:255 (1972).
6. O. Sperling, M. Frank. R. Ophir, U. A. Liberman, A. Adam, and A. de Vries, Eur. J. Clin. Biol. Res. 16:147 (1971).
7. E. Zoref, A. de Vries, and O. Sperling, J. Clin. Invest. 56: 1093 (1975).
8. E. Zoref, A. de Vries, and O. Sperling, Human Heredity 27:73 (1977).
9. W. K. Long, Science 138:991 (1962).
10. W. N. Kelley, F. M. Rosenbloom, J. E. Seegmiller, and R. R. Howell, J. Pediatr. 72:488 (1968).
11. A. de Vries and O. Sperling, Biomed. 30:75 (1979).
12. I. A. Wallis and R. I. Eagle, Am. J. Med. 22:13 (1957).
13. C. Bishop, W. T. Zindhahl, and J. H. Talbott, Proc. Soc. Biol. Med. 86:440 (1954).
14. M. L. Greene, R. Marcus, G. D. Aurbach, E. S. Kazam, and J. E. Seegmiller, Am. J. Med. 53:361 (1972).
15. A. K. Khachadurian and M. J. Arslanian, Ann. Int. Med. 78:547 (1972).
16. O. Sperling, A. Weinberger, I. Oliver, U. A. Liberman, and A. de Vries, Ann. Int. Med. 80:482 (1974).
17. I. Akaika, T. Nishizawa, E. Yano, A. Takeuchi, Y. Nishida, T. Yoshimura, and Y. Horiuchi, Ann. Clin. Res. 7:318 (1975).
18. D. Benjamin, O. Sperling, A. Weinberger, J. Pinkhas, and A. de Vries, Nephron 18:220 (1977).
19. D. Benjamin, O. Sperling, A. Weinberger, and J. Pinkhas, Biomedicine 29:54 (1978).
20. M. Frank, M. Many, and O. Sperling, Br. J. Urol. 51:88 (1979).
21. R. Weitz and O. Sperling, J. Pediatr. (in press).
22. Garty and O. Sperling, (in preparation).
23. R. E. Rieselbach, Adv. Exp. Med. and Biol. 76B:1 (1977).
24. T. H. Steele and R. E. Rieselbach, Am. J. Med. 43:868 (1967).
25. A. B. Gutman and T. F. Yu, Am. J. Med. 23:600 (1957).
26. E. Praetorius and J. E. Kirk, J. Lab. Clin. Med. 35:865 (1950).
27. D. M. Wilson and N. P. Goldstein, Kid. Int. 4:331 (1973).
28. J. S. Bennett, J. Bond, I. Singer, and A. Gottlieb, Ann. Int. Med. 76:751 (1972).
29. K. Kawabe, T. Muruyama, and I. Akaoka, J. Urol. 116:690 (1976).

2,8-DIHYDROXYADENINURIA: OR WHEN IS A URIC ACID STONE NOT A URIC ACID STONE?

H. A. Simmonds*, K. J. Van Acker+, M. J. Dillon**,
T. M. Barratt**, C. F. Potter*, A. Sahota*, and
J. S. Cameron*
*Purine Laboratory, Guy's Hospital Medical School,
London Bridge, SE1 9RT, U.K.; +Department of Pediatrics,
University of Antwerp, Wilrijk, Belgium; **The Hospital
for Sick Children, Great Ormond Street, London, WC1N 3JH
U.K.

Purine nucleotides important for normal cellular metabolism are derived endogenously from de novo synthesis and also from recycling of pre-formed purines via the so-called salvage pathway (Figure 1). The latter pathway contains a number of enzymes, the absence of which can lead to disturbances of purine metabolism and also severe clinical symptoms[1]. An example is the deficiency of the salvage enzyme hypoxanthine-guanine phosphoribosyltransferase (HGPRT) which can lead either to the Lesch-Nyhan syndrome or X-linked gout[1].

Until recently little was known about the consequences for purine metabolism of a defect of the other salvage enzyme, adenine phosphoribosyltransferase (APRT). From 1968 onward a number of individuals had been identified with a decreased APRT activity in erythrocyte lysates during screening for HGPRT deficiency[2].

Disturbances of urate metabolism, sometimes accompanied by gout and/or stones, were noted in some of these heterozygotes. The fact that these characteristics were found with equal frequency in family members with normal APRT activity made a direct connection between APRT deficiency and abnormalities of urate metabolism unlikely.

Complete lack of the APRT enzyme was only recently recognized as a rare cause of supposedly "uric acid" stones in young children[3,4]. The stones are composed of 2,8-dihydroxyadenine (2,8-DHA), the extremely insoluble metabolite formed from adenine by xanthine oxidase (XO) via the 8-hydroxy intermediate in the absence of the APRT enzyme. The stones are radiolucent and indistinguishable from

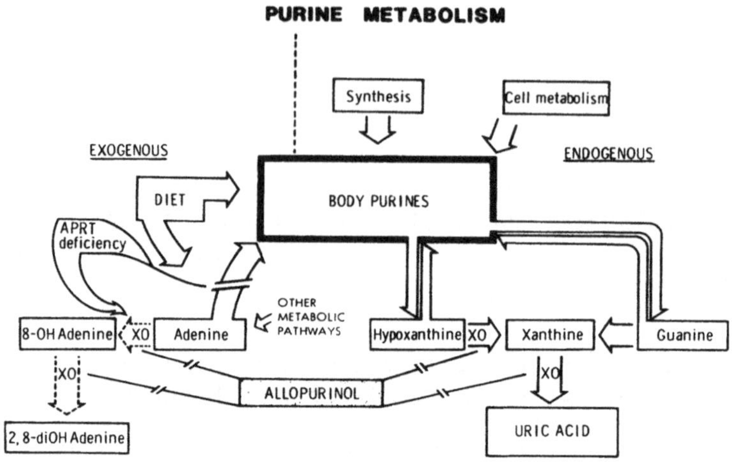

Figure 1. Pathways of purine metabolism.

those composed of uric acid when analysed by routine chemical techniques, hence their frequent confusion with the latter, and almost certain misdiagnosis in the past[4].

Since the first two homozygotes were identified independently in Paris and London, another five have been described by the same two groups[5-8]. Two of these homozygotes were asymptomatic and only identified during the course of the family studies[5-8], despite the excretion of comparable levels of 2,8-DHA. The presentation of a recent case in coma, with acute or chronic renal failure due to bilateral obstructive uropathy through 2,8-DHA stones, indicates the wide spectrum of severity which may be encountered (Dillon et al. - in preparation). The child has been left with severe renal impairment, which stresses the importance of recognition in all instances and early treatment of stone formers. The clinical symptoms are determined exclusively by the extreme insolubility of 2,8-DHA. There is a frequent history of the passage of gravel or small stones, sometimes from birth, accompanied by severe abdominal colic, dysuria and/or urinary tract infections[3-8].

Considerable data now exist from studies in the first four homozygotes and one large kindred[9], which confirm that the defect is inherited as an autosomal recessive trait (Figure 2).

Homozygotes show no evidence of immunodeficiency, are otherwise clinically normal and have no over-production or excretion of uric

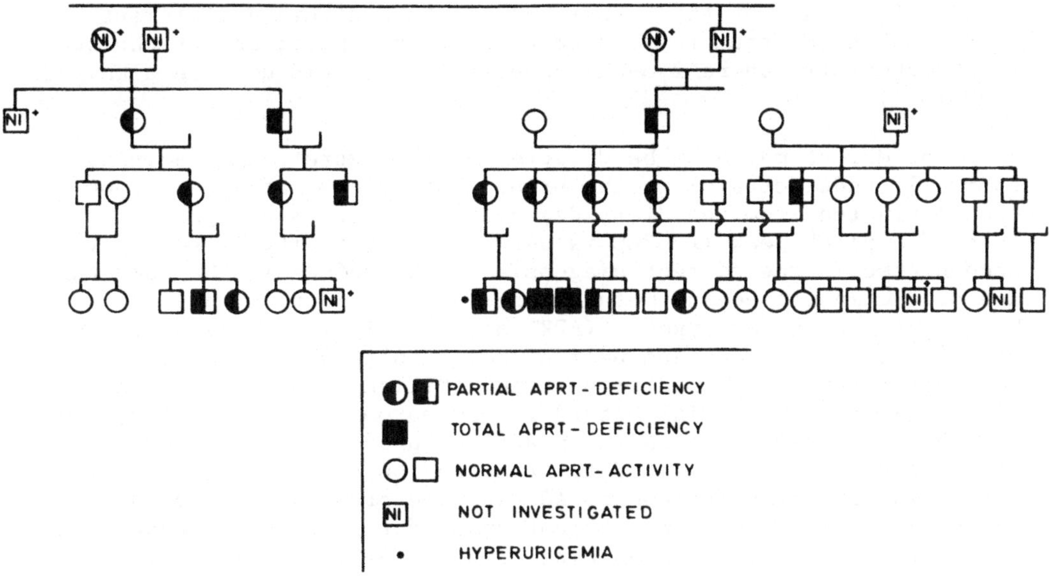

Figure 2. Pedigree of a family with APRT deficiency.

acid. Heterozygotes are indistinguishable from normal. This indicates that unlike the companion salvage enzyme HGPRT, APRT is apparently not involved in the over-all control of endogenous purine metabolism in man. However, the case presenting in uraemic coma demonstrates that APRT deficiency is a potentially fatal condition, and emphasizes the importance of identifying affected children.

In the first two cases the stones had been repeatedly reported as "uric acid"[3,4], because a similar chemical structure makes it impossible to distinguish between uric acid and its amino analogue, 2,8-DHA, by many of the tests used routinely in stone identification, namely, colorimetry, thermogravimetric analysis or the murexide test[7]. Some indication of the true composition of the stone is given by the appearance. Stones consisting of 2,8-DHA are generally friable and pale grey on crushing compared with uric acid which are usually hard, smooth, and pale yellow. Correct stone identification depends on the use of infra-red or mass spectrometry[7,8] which are not always available. Uric acid and 2,8-DHA may be distinguished by the action of uricase on the former but not the latter; a different ultra-violet spectrum in acid compared with alkali; or a technique of wet chemistry where 2,8-DHA appears in the acid not the alkaline fraction[7].

The defect may also be detected by the excretion of adenine (normally undetectable) in the urine, but unless caffeine compounds are eliminated from the diet, degradation products can produce a false "adenine" peak if HPLC is used[7]. Another pitfall recently encountered in the correct diagnosis of the defect is the fact that one of the most frequent methods used for the identification of homozygotes or heterozygotes (APRT activity in lysed erythrocytes) will produce erroneous and near normal results where the patient has recently received a blood transfusion (Dillon et al - in preparation). Another potential hazard for asymptomatic homozygotes, and possibly heterozygotes, is the practice in some countries of the addition of adenine to blood for transfusion to prolong its shelf-life. Massive transfusions of ACD-adenine preserved blood have produced renal failure in some patients, fatal in one instance. At post mortem, 2,8-dihydroxyadenine crystals were identified in the kidney[10].

The surgical renal biopsy findings in the female homozygote for APRT deficiency, who had permanent renal damage, are similar to the above report, and others of animal models of adenine toxicity[7]. Crystals were found obstructing the tubular lumens as well as in the interstitium, where some crystals had initiated a giant cell reaction. The picture was consistent with acute on chronic renal failure (Dillon et al. - in preparation).

The disorder, 2,8-dihydroxyadeninuria, is an example of the unusual situation where effective therapy was available prior to the recognition of the defect. The xanthine oxidase inhibitor, allopurinol, preferably without alkali, has been used successfully in all stone-formers to date.

The solubility of 2,8-DHA, unlike that of uric acid, is not altered within the physiological pH range and two studies have suggested that alkali may even have an adverse effect[5]. A dose of 10 mg/kg allopurinol has been effective in most cases, but this has had to be reduced to 5 mg/kg in the child who has suffered permanent renal damage. This is because oxipurinol, the active metabolite of allopurinol, is retained in renal failure and the dose must be reduced accordingly[11]; severe bone marrow depression has been noted in some instances. Where possible, plasma oxipurinol levels should be carefully monitored and maintained below 100 μmol/l.

Our young patient with severe renal impairment and APRT deficiency was from a commune and had been fed a macrobiotic diet rich in purines, indicating the importance of dietary purine restriction and the recognition of foods (such as "marmite" vegetable extract) which are rich in adenine and must be avoided. Although allopurinol appears to have an additional beneficial effect in reducing the absorption of dietary purine in some instances, it is ineffective in this regard in homozygotes (see Simmonds et al. this symposium). Thus, dietary restriction together with allopurinol will always be necessary.

Although dietary restriction is beneficial there is still a significant production of adenine from endogenous sources. Studies in homozygotes have indicated that there is no significant pathway for adenine production via purine metabolism[5], and the extent of production from the polyamine pathway (of which adenine is a by-product) is being explored. This is important because _in vitro_ studies have suggested that adenine itself is toxic to mammalian cells[12]. Because of the adenine accumulation induced by therapy, frequent clinical check-ups of allopurinol-treated homozygotes are therefore vital in order to determine the long term toxicity of adenine _in vivo_. Recent studies have shown that adenine is effectively secreted by the kidney[13] which should control adenine levels in body fluids.

Asymptomatic homozygote siblings are at present untreated and provide effective clinical controls, but must also be watched with care, for all the above reasons. Affected homozygotes have all been children to date, which raises the question of what changes might occur at puberty and, more specifically, where have all the affected adults gone?

SUMMARY

In summary, despite the apparent rarity of 2,8-dihydroxyadenine as a constituent of urinary stones, the severity of the clinical manifestations in some instances stresses the importance of subjecting all supposedly uric acid stones in children and young adults, to detailed analysis. The possibility that 2,8-DHA stones may be the cause of acute renal failure in young children should not be forgotten. In addition to the above pitfalls, the importance of dietary restriction and of allopurinol, preferably without alkali, in treatment, is underlined. The difficulty of diagnosis from APRT enzyme levels alone in transfused subjects is also emphasized.

REFERENCES

1. J. E. Seegmiller, in:"Urolithiasis Research," H. Fleisch, W. G. Robertson, L. H. Smith, and W. Vahlensieck, eds., Plenum Press, New York (1976).
2. W. N. Kelley, R. I. Levy, F. M. Rosenbloom, J. F. Henderson, and J. E. Seegmiller, J. Clin. Invest. 47:2281 (1963).

3. P. Cartier and M. Hamet, C. R. de Acad. Sci. (Paris) 297:883 (1974).
4. H. A. Simmonds, K. J. Van Acker, J. S. Cameron, and W. Snedden, in:"Urolithiasis Research," H. Fleisch, W. G. Robertson, L. H. Smith, and W. Vahlensieck, eds., Plenum Press, New York (1976).
5. K. J. Van Acker, H. A. Simmonds, C. F. Potter, and J. S. Cameron, New Engl. J. Med. 297:127 (1977).
6. T. M. Barratt, H. A. Simmonds, J. S. Cameron, C. F. Potter, G. A. Rose, D. G. Arkell, and D. I. Williams, Arch. Dis. Child. 54:25 (1979).
7. H. A. Simmonds, Clin. Nephrol. 12:195 (1979).
8. R. J. Reveillaud, M. Daudon, M. F. Protat, La Nouvelle Press Medicale 8:3965 (1979).
9. K. J. Van Acker, H. A. Simmonds, C. F. Potter, and A. Sahota, in:"Purine Metabolism in Man III," A. Rapado, R. W. E. Watts, and C. H. M. M. De Bruyn, Plenum Press, New York (1979).
10. J. S. Falk, G. T. O. Lindblad, B. J. M. Westman, Transfusion 12:376 (1972).
11. G. B. Elion, F. M. Benezra, T. D. Beardmore, and W. N. Kelley, in:"Purine Metabolism in Man III," A. Rapado, R. W. E. Watts, and C. J. M. M. De Bruyn, Plenum Press, New York (1979).
12. J. F. Henderson and F. W. Scott, Pharmac. Ther. 8:539 (1980).
13. A. Ericson, T. Groth, F. Niklasson, and C. H. De Verdier, Scand. J. Clin. Lab. Invest. 40:1 (1980).

RENAL CALCULI IN TRIAMTERENE USERS

Bruce Ettinger, Norman O. Oldroyd, and Fritz Sörgel

Department of Medicine, Kaiser-Permanente Medical Center, San Francisco, California; the Louis C. Herring Company, Orlando, Florida; and the University of California School of Pharmacy, San Francisco, California

Since we recognized the first case of triamterene nephrolithiasis[1], we have attempted to compile and investigate all similar cases. In the last 18 months, we found 436 additional cases among the 160,000 calculi (0.3%) submitted to the Louis C. Herring company and obtained clinical histories for one quarter of the cases. The purpose of this communication is to: 1) describe the appearance of triamterene in urinary calculi, 2) describe the chemical tests used to identify and quantitate these deposits, and 3) report the clinical findings of patients who have passed these stones.

Microscopic crystallographic analysis of calculi suggests the presence of triamterene and its metabolites, the combination of which we will denote "triamterene" for this study. We did not see visible crystals of this material but learned to recognize the typical patterns of "triamterene" deposition. The "triamterene" may appear as the central nucleus, an amorphous deposit around which calcium oxalate or uric acid is deposited. "Triamterene" may add to the size of nucleated stones by being laid down in lamina or intercrystalline patches, or it may form encrustations on the outside of stones.

Those "triamterene" stones which contain no other material known to form calculi appear mustard to gold-colored and usually show con centric lamellae formed over an amorphous nucleus. They are sometimes colored various shades of brown by incorporation of urinary pigments and occasionally have a hyaline appearance when the "triamterene" is in a matrix of mucoprotein. "Triamterene" deposits may be mistaken for amorphous salts of uric acid, protein, or microcrystalline apatite which is stained by urinary pigments.

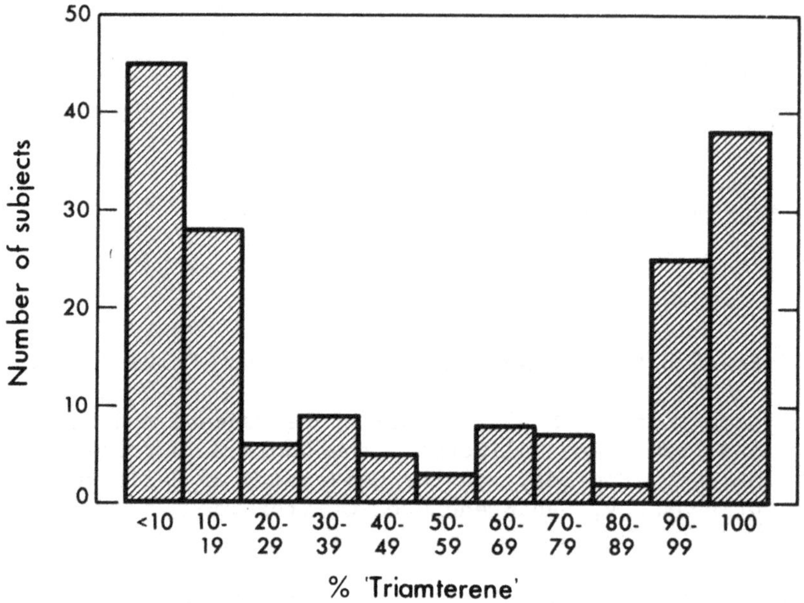

Figure 1. Crystallographic estimates of "triamterene" content in patients with renal calculi.

Estimates of the percentage composition based on crystallographic analysis appear in Figure 1. Of these calculi, 36% were entirely or nearly all "triamterene," whereas 48% showed minor amounts of "triamterene" (<20%) with major amounts of calcium oxalate monohydrate, calcium oxalate dihydrate, or uric acid. In no case did "triamterene" appear admixed with magnesium ammonium phosphate, carbonate apatite, or brushite.

Identification of "triamterene" by a simple chemical spot test aided in the analysis. Material suspected of being "triamterene" was exposed to long-wave ultraviolet light after being dissolved in 8% lactic acid or 3% ammoniacal n-butanol. A characteristic intense blue fluorescence was noted even when minute quantities were present.

Because the fluorescent test was not entirely specific, we performed subsequent analyses by infrared spectroscopy and thin-layer chromatography. We pulverized the calculous material, dissolved it in 8% lactic acid, extracted the "triamterene" with 5 to 10 ml of methanol, and applied 0.3 ml of the extract to a silica gel-G, thin-layer plate. The solvent system used in developing the plates was n-butanol, ammonia, chloroform, and methanol in a ratio of 50:15:15:15[2]. Fluorescent densitometry allowed us to quantitate triamterene and its two major metabolites (parahydroxy triamterene and parahydroxy triamterene sulfate), which were present in the calculi in a fairly consistent pattern (Table 1).

Table 1. Quantitation of Triamterene and its Metabolites ("Triamterene") in Ten Calculi

Total "Triamterene"		TLC Analysis of Metabolites		
Crystallographic Estimate (%)	TLC Analysis (%)	Triamterene (%)	Parahydroxy Triamterene Sulfate (%)	Parahydroxy Triamterene (%)
100	74.6	69	24	7
90	55.6	72	15	13
100	47.9	39	50	11
92	36.3	43	46	11
100	34.9	67	27	6
100	29.5	38	43	19
100	27.5	40	43	18
100	26.1	47	34	19
90	26.0	27	50	23
100	20.4	39	50	11
Mean97.2	37.9	48	38	14

TLC = thin-layer chromatography

Triamterene is rapidly metabolized to parahydroxy triamterene, then to parahydroxy triamterene sulfate (Figure 2)[3,4]. The urinary excretion of the latter compound is nearly complete in eight hours. During this time, the ratio of parahydroxy triamterene sulfate to triamterene is between 4 and 10 to 1. The sulfate metabolits and the native triamterene found in our stone material were often present in nearly equal amounts, with triamterene predominating occasionally. Very little parahydroxy triamterene was found in the calculi. Triamterene and its metabolites accounted for 20% to 75% of the weight of those stones which were shown to be free of the usual substances known to form calculi (Table 1). There appears to be an unusually large component of protein matrix in these stones when compared to the 2% to 3% of calcium oxalate stones and the 9% to 11% of cystine stones reported by Boyce[5].

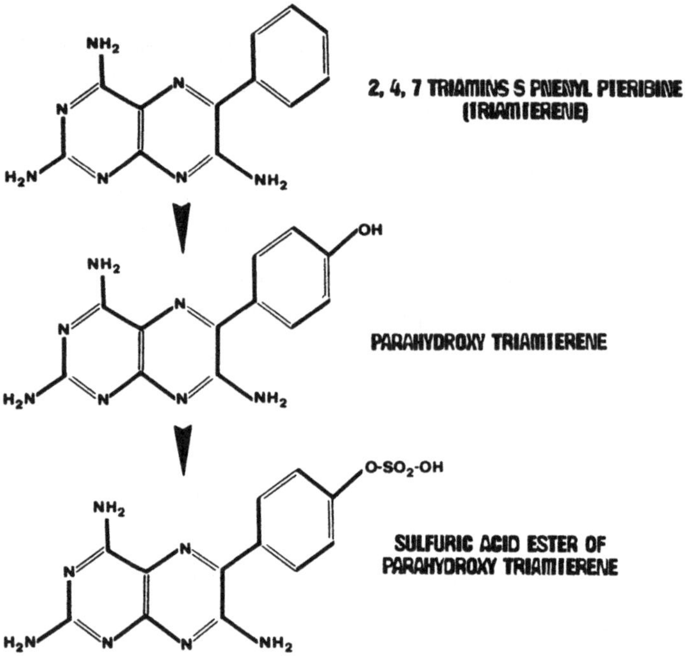

Figure 2. Chemical steps in triamterene metabolism.

Clinical histories confirmed the use of triamterene by all patients, and 97% used Dyazide®, a mixture of triamterene and hydrochlorothiazide. The vast majority of patients had used Dyazide for several years, but a few had begun taking Dyazide only a few months prior to stone passage. Most patients were taking Dyazide at the time of stone passage, but a few had discontinued the use of triamterene as much as one to two years prior to the passage of their stones.

For the purpose of this analysis, we divided the triamterene stone patients into two groups, those forming largely triamterene stones (> 80% by crystallographic analysis and denoted "high-T") and

---

®Dyazide: Smith, Kline & French, Philadelphia, Pennsylvania.

those with only a small percentage of triamterene in their calculi (< 20% and denoted "low-T"). Two other comparison groups were drawn from the clinic population at Kaiser-Permanente Medical Center, San Francisco, California. We reviewed the medical records of 100 consecutive stone-free Dyazide users and 100 consecutive patients who had passed calcium oxalate stones, verified by crystallographic analysis. Table 2 summarizes the clinical data for these four groups. The male-to-female ratio among the stone-free Dyazide users was nearly equal and a similar ratio existed among patients with triamterene stones. The calcium oxalate stone group showed the expected male predominance. Stone-free Dyazide users and triamterene stone formers were older, by an average 15 years, than the patients suffering from simple stones. Recurrent calculous disease was present in half the patients with calcium stones and in a similar proportion of patients with "low-T" stones, whereas only 29% of those patients with "high-T" stones had had previous stone events. Spontaneous passage of "high-T" stones was common, because these calculi were smaller and more friable. The mean weight of the "high-T" stones was 8.8 mg and 77% were passed spontaneously, whereas the mean weight of the "low-T" stones was 71.6 mg and 54% were passed without surgical intervention. Simple calcium oxalate stones had a mean weight of 23 mg and were passed spontaneously in 88% of the cases. Perhaps the addition of "triamterene" to calcium stones augmented their size enough to make passage difficult.

Table 2. Clinical Characteristics of Subjects with "Triamterene" (T) Stones

	Patients with Triamterene Stones		Control Groups	
	"Low-T"	"High-T"	Stone-Free Dyazide Users	Patients with Simple Calcium Stones
Male:Female ratio	1:2	1:5	1:1	5.9
Age (yr):				
Male	57.6	60.3	58.5	46.7
Female	57.2	55.1	59.0	43.2
Previous Calculi (%)	53	29	4	48
Spontaneous Passage (%)	54	77	-	88

Table 3. Drug Histories of Subjects with "Triamterene" (T) Stones

	Patients with Triamterene Stones			
	"Low-T"	"High-T"	Stone-Free Dyazide Users	Patients with Simple Calcium Stones
Mean daily Dyazide dose (no. capsules)	1.7	2.2	1.6	-
Daily dose > 2 capsules (%)	7	17	8	-
Regular use of other drugs (%):				
any	75	83	68	15
propanolol	22	40	18	2
alpha-methyldopa	22	18	16	1
allopurinol	6	12	3	4
hydralazine	6	12	3	0

Hypertension was the indication for Dyazide use in 86% of stone-forming patients and 90% of the control group. Table 3 summarizes the drug histories for the four groups. The mean dose of Dyazide was 28% higher in those patients with "high-T" stones and their use of propranolol, allopurinol, and hydralazine hydrochloride was twice as great as in "low-T" stone-formers. The "high-T" stone-formers were more likely to use multiple drugs than the stone-free Dyazide group or the "low-T" group. Of the "high-T" stone subjects, 11% used four Dyazide capsules (or their equivalent) daily, whereas none of the "low-T" stone group used these high dosages.

On the basis of their higher Dyazide dosage and multiple drug therapies, we suspect that patients with triamterene stones have more severe hypertension than the stone-free Dyazide users. On the other hand, we found numerous examples of triamterene stone formation in subjects who took Dyazide once a day.

Dyazide, the most commonly administered form of triamterene, is widely used: we estimate that three million people in the United States use Dyazide. Our sample of stones received at the Louis C. Herring company represents one fifth of the kidney stones passed in the United States[6]. We did not seek triamterene exhaustively in our sample but performed the chemical analyses only if obvious deposits of triamterene were seen microscopically. We can project, conservatively, that 1,450 stones containing some triamterene are being passed each year in the nation. These 1,450 stone events, occurring among three million people exposed to triamterene, result in an annual triamterene stone incidence of 0.5 per 1,000 persons taking Dyazide. We do not know the incidence of non-triamterene stones among these Dyazide users. The annual age-/sex-specific incidence of renal calculi expected for Dyazide users is approximately 1.3 to 1.6 per 1,000[6,7].

Only a few months' exposure to the usual doses of the drug is necessary. One third of these stones are all or nearly all triamterene. They occur in older patients, 71% of whom have had no previous stone history. Larger than usual dosage contributes to one sixth of the cases, and multiple drug use is twice as common in stone-formers. We have demonstrated that triamterene contributes to the growth of urinary calculi and we suspect these larger calculi result in an increased need for surgery.

Our studies do not show whether Dyazide contributes to a higher incidence of renal calculi. It is possible that a reduction in the rate of urolithiasis brought about by Dyazide's thiazide component may offset the lithogenic effects of triamterene. Until the risk of renal calculi among Dyazide users is known, it would be prudent to exercise caution in prescribing this drug to patients with a history of renal calculi.

REFERENCES

1. B. Ettinger, E. Weil, N. S. Mandel, and S. Darling, Ann. Int. Med. 91:745 (1979).
2. B. Grebian, H. E. Geissler, and E. Mutschler, Arzneim.-Forsch. 26:2125 (1976).
3. B. Grebian, H. E. Geissler, and H. Knauf, Arzneim.-Forsch. 28:1420 (1978).
4. K. Lehman, Arzneim.-Forsch. 15:812 (1965).
5. W. H. Boyce, Am. J. Med. 45:673 (1968).
6. R. Sierakowski, B. Finlayson, R. R. Landes, C. D. Finlayson, N. Sierakowski, Invest. Urol. 15:438 (1978).
7. C. M. Johnson, D. M. Wilson, W. M. O'Fallon, R. S. Malek, and L. T. Kurland, Kid. Int. 16:624 (1979).

CYSTINE STONE - THERAPY WITH ALPHA-MERCAPTO-PROPIONYLGLYCINE - TEN YEARS OF EXPERIENCE WITH FORTY-TWO PATIENTS

Richard E. Hautmann

Department of Urology, Faculty of Medicine, Rheinisch-Westfälische Technische Hochschule
Aachen, West Germany

INTRODUCTION

The aim of management in cystinuria is simply to keep the urinary cystine concentration less than supersaturation and, thus, to prevent cystine precipitation and subsequent stone formation. This goal may be achieved by reducing the volume of cystine excreted into the urine[1-4], increasing the volume of urine in which the cystine is dissolved[5,6], or increasing the solubility of cystine in the urine[7] (Table 1). However, in clinical experience with cystinuria treatment, results continue to be poor. The most promising form of therapy at present is changing cystine to a chemically more soluble form. Until now, reliance has been placed primarily on D-penicillamine[8]. However the drug has serious side effects that limit its application. Alpha-mercapto-propionylglycine (MPG) is a newly developed drug, promising higher effectiveness and lack of toxic side effects[9].

PRINCIPLE

D-penicillamine, as well as n-acetyl-DL-penicillamine[10], acetylcysteine[11] and the newly developed drug alpha-mercapto-propionylglycine[9] (MPG) are mercaptans or thiols. Their mechanism of action is based on the thiol disulfide exchange reaction (Figure 1). It is known that thiols dissociate like acids to yield active anions that undergo exchange reactions with disulfides. With a suitable water soluble thiol it is possible to transform the less soluble L-cystine into a water soluble disulfide derivate[12,13].

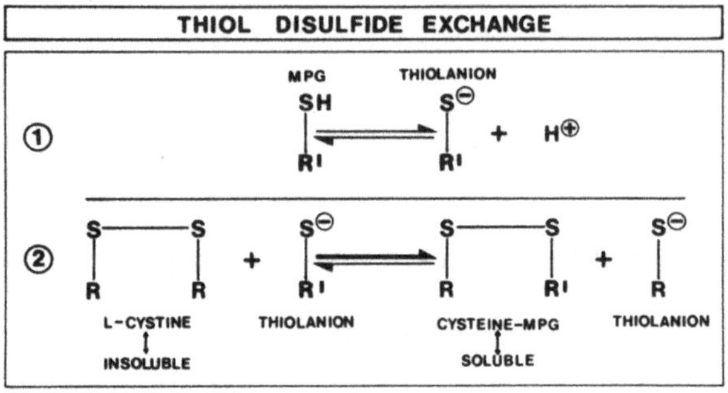

Figure 1

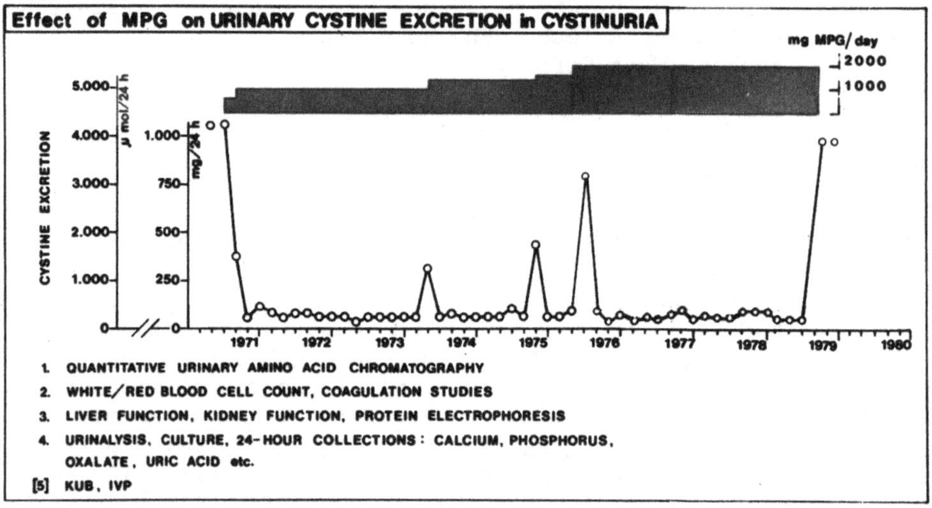

Figure 2

Table 1. Treatment of Cystinuria

TREATMENT OF CYSTINURIA

		Drawbacks
1. CYSTINE EXCRETION ↓	LOW PROTEIN DIET	growing child
2. URINE VOLUME ↑	FLUID INTAKE 4-7 liters / day bedtime, 2.00 a.m. acetazolamide	hypertension cardiovascular disease renal insufficiency
3. CYSTINE SOLUBILITY ↑	ALKALINIZATION above pH 7.5 bicarbonate (10-30gm day) citrate	phosphate precipitation hypercalcaemia edema alkalosis
4. CHANGING CYSTINE TO A CHEMICALLY MORE SOLUBLE FORM	D-penicillamine N-acetyl-DL-penicillamine acetyl-cysteine α-mercapto propionyl glycine (MPG)	side effects

MATERIAL AND METHODS

From 1970 to 1980, 17 female and 25 male cystinuric patients with a mean age of 37 years have been treated with MPG. The diagnosis of cystinuria depended upon the infra-red analysis of the multiple passed or removed urinary tract stones and the quantitative urinary amino acid chromatography in these patients. The daily dose of MPG varied between 600 and 2,000 mg (Figure 2). The dose of MPG required was adjusted to the urinary cystine level, which should be less than 100 mg per day if calculi are to be prevented. Hydration was maintained not by reference to fluid intake but rather by insistence on an output of 2,000 cc per day or more in instances of severe cystinuria. The urinary pH was maintained at approximately 6.8 to 7.0. The patients were monitored by a series of routine tests: 1) quantitative urinary amino acid chromatography (every other month), 2) KUB every year; excretory urography only when stones are present, 3) serum studies (complete liver function, coagulation studies, renal function and protein electrophoresis), 4) urine studies (urinalysis, pH, culture, 24-hour collections for creatinine, calcium, phosphorus, uric acid and so forth), and 5) white and red blood cell counts and platelets.

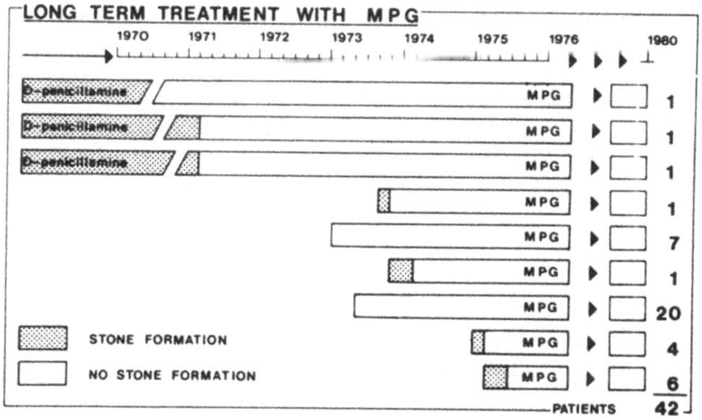

Figure 3

Table 2.

SIDE EFFECTS

D-penicillamine	MPG
1. GRANULOCYTOPENIA	1. SOFT FAECES (31/42)
2. THROMBOCYTOSIS	2. SKIN RASH (9/42)
3. EOSINOPHILIA	3. FEVER (3/42)
4. PROTEINURIA (NEPHROTIC SYNDROME)	4. CHANGED SLEEPING RHYTHM (1/42)
5. GLOMERULONEPHRITIS	5. LOSS OF EFFECTIVENESS SLIGHT (27/42) COMPLETE (1/42)
6. MACULAR RASH	
7. EPIDERMOLYSIS BULLOSA	
8. RETINAL HAEMORRHAGES	
9. LOSS OF TASTE	
10. ANTIPYRIDOXINE EFFECT	
11. SERUM SICKNESS (?) RASH, FEVER, ARTHRALGIA LYMPHADENOPATHY	
12. IMPAIRED WOUND HEALING	
50 percent — WITHDRAWAL	0 percent

Table 3.

COMPARISON : D-penicillamine – MPG

		D-penicillamine	MPG
USE AND DOSE			
ADMINISTRATION	:	ORALLY, PERMANENT	
DAILY DOSAGE grm. divided aliquots	:	1.0 -3.0	0.5 - 2
MONITORING OF EFFICACY	:	CYSTINE LEVEL: LESS THAN 100 mg/day	
ADJUNCTIVE THERAPY	:	MODERATE DIURESIS ALKALINIZATION pH 6.5 PYRIDOXINE	
EFFICIENCY			
STONE DISSOLUTION IN VITRO	:	++	+++
IN VIVO	:	++	+++
STONE PREVENTION	:	++	+++
DRAWBACKS			
SIDE EFFECTS	:	+++	(+)
LOSS OF EFFECTIVENESS	:	?	+

RESULTS

Figure 3: 1) There was no recurrent stone formation except at the immediate onset of the MPG therapy when 14 of the 42 patients continued to pass small calculi. However, in these patients this must be attributed to their failure to follow the MPG regimen appropriately in the early days of the therapy. 2) The routinely performed tests were normal through the years, and there were no major side effects (Table 2). 3) Unfortunately, the continued use of MPG during this 10-year period resulted in a slight loss of effectiveness in 27 out of the 42 patients (Table 2). In these patients the dosage had to be increased stepwise from 600 to 2,000 mg per day. The exact dosage was dictated by the urinary excretion of cystine which should be less than 100 mg per day if calculi are to be prevented. 4) After a stepwise dose increase to finally 2,500 mg per day after a treatment period of 9 years, the cystine excretion in only one patient showed no further response and, thus, this patient is the only treatment failure (Figure 2).

CONCLUSIONS

Because of its high effectiveness and its lack of toxicity MPG currently should be the treatment of choice in cystinuric stone-forming patients (Table 3).

REFERENCES

1. C. E. Dent, and B. Senior, Brit. J. Urol. 27:317 (1955).
2. D. R. Smith, F. O. Kolb, and H. A. Harper, J. Urol. 81:61 (1959).
3. M. Lotz, J. T. Potts, Jr., J. M. Holland, W. S. Kiser, and F. C. Bartter, J. Urol. 95:257 (1966).
4. F. O. Kolb, J. M. Earli, and H. A. Harper, Metabolism 16:378 (1967).
5. S. R. Weinberg, and P. A. Tabenkin, Arch. Intern. Med. 90:850 (1952).
6. C. E. Dent, M. Friedman, H. Gree, and L. C. A. Watson, Brit. Med. J. 1:403 (1965).
7. S. Z. Freed, J. Urol. 113:96 (1975).
8. J. C. Crawhall, E. F. Scowen, and R. W. Watts, Brit. Med. J. 1:588 (1963).
9. R. Hautmann, B. Terhorst, H. W. Stuhlsatz, and W. Lutzeyer, J. Urol. 117:628 (1977).
10. G. S. Stokes, J. T. Potts, Jr., M. Lotz, and F. C. Bartter, Clin. Sci. 35:467 (1968).
11. W. P. Mulvaney, T. Quilter, and A. Mortera, J. Urol. 114:107 (1975).
12. A. P. Ryle, and F. Sanger, Biochem. J. 60:535 (1955).
13. A. Phil, L. Eldjarn, and K. F. Nakken, Acta. Chem. Scand. 12:1357 (1958).

ACKNOWLEDGMENT

This work was generously supported by the MARTIN-BRINKMANN-FOUNDATION, Bremen, West Germany.

THE NATURAL HISTORY OF CYSTINURIA: A 15 YEAR FOLLOW-UP IN 106 PATIENTS

F. Linari, M. Marangella, B. Fruttero, and M. Bruno

Division Nefrologia Emodialisi, Ospital Mauriziano
Umberto I
Turin, Italy

From 1963 through 1979 we saw 106 patients with cystinuria: 62 had recurrent stone disease and 44 were stone free. Three of the stone-forming patients had the "pure" form of cystinuria[1,2], and 59 had the classic form. They came from 35 families and we were able to study 18 families. In all cases the diagnosis was made by chemical analysis and/or I.R. spectrography, and/or x-ray diffraction of the stone, and by urinary aminoacid patterns (ion exchange column, lithium buffer[3]).

The frequency distribution of cystinuria in the patients without lithiasis showed a grossly bimodal behavior with two subgroups, the former with a small increase in cystine, the latter with higher levels. This distribution probably reflects a genetic heterogeneity of cystinuria: the first group may correspond to heterozygous genotype III, the second to heterozygous genotype II, according to Rosenberg[4]. Urinary levels of cystine, arginine, lysine and ornithine in the two subgroups are reported in Table 1. Cystinuria levels range within narrow values in each family, except in two out of 15 in which both subjects with low and high levels were present. This suggests the transmission of two different alleli and the presence of double heterozygotes among the stone-formers of these families.

Sixty-two out of 106 cystinuric patients (Table 2) were affected by recurrent cystine urolithiasis. The frequency distribution of the onset age of lithiasis is shown in Figure 1.

Up to the first observation, a cumulative number of 593 calculi in 618 years had been formed by these patients. The lithiasis was monolateral in 22.6%, bilateral in 77.4%. Eighty-five surgical procedures were carried out in 53 patients: 23 ureterolithotomies,

Table 1. Daily Excretion of Cystine, Arginine, Lysine, Ornithine in Heterozygotes Cystinurics Type II and III Compared to Controls (μmol/24 h, mean ± SD)

Group	Cyst	ARG	LYS	ORN
Type III Heterozygotes	227.9± 77.7$^{\zeta}$	127.5±73.0^{+}	1240.8±519$^{\zeta}$	136.7± 76.5$^{\zeta}$
Type II Heterozygotes	951.5±236.6$^{\zeta}$	893.0±1456*	2389.7±1687.6$^{\Delta}$	535.2±827.0$^{\Delta}$
Controls	35.6± 6.6	59.9± 5.8	555.8± 500	17.0± 5.2

* $p < 0.05$; + $p < 0.01$; Δ $p < 0.005$; ζ $p < 0.001$

Table 2. Clinical-Epidemiological Features in 62 Cystinuric Stone Formers

	m	SD
Age (last observation)	32.7	13.7
Age (first stone episode)	17.2	10.1
Follow-up (years)	14.9	11.31
Stone episodes/pt./yr.	1.22	1.00
Stone surgery/pt./yr.	0.311	0.491

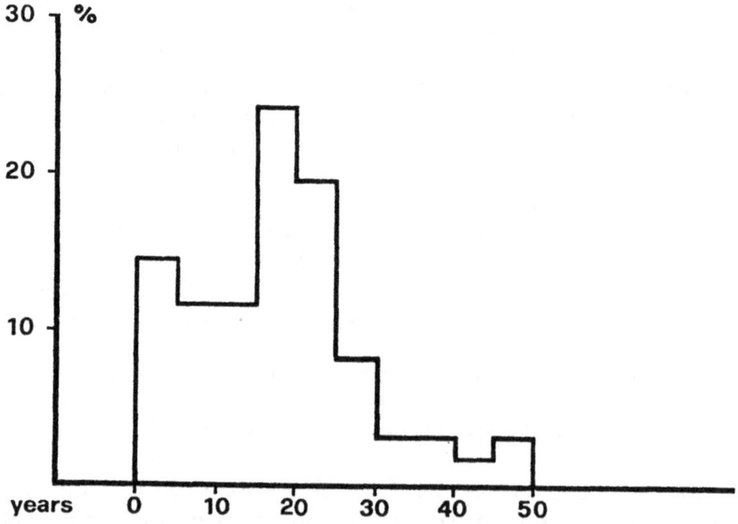

Figure 1. Frequency distribution of the onset age of stone disease.

Table 3. Biochemical Pretreatment Parameters of 46 Classic Cystinurics (mean ± SD)

	Cystinic Lithiasis	Controls	P
GFR (ml/min/1.73 m^2)	101.3± 21.6	115.9±16.9	<0.05
Urinary CYS (μmol/24 h)	2630.5± 964.0	35.6± 6.6	<0.001
Urinary ARG (μmol/24 h)	2348.5±1572.6	59.9± 4.8	<0.001
Urinary LYS (μmol/24 h)	2727 ±1577	555.8± 500	<0.001
Urinary ORN (μmol/24 h)	1851 ±1048.4	17.0± 5.2	<0.001
Plasma CYS (μmol/l)	23.2± 15.15	29.3± 2.3	N.S.
Total Plasma AA. (μmol/l)	2545 ±340.3	2106 ± 260.2	N.S.
Calciuria (mg/24 h)	167.8± 96.1	139.5± 51.4	N.S.
T_mPO_4/GFR (mg%)	3.41± 0.58	3.03± 0.65	N.S.

Table 4. Dibasic Aminoacids Excretion in Three "Pure" Cystinurics

	Pure Cystinuria	Controls	P
Cystine	4394.3 ± 889.51	35.6 ± 6.6	0.001
Arginine	51.3 ± 7.53	59.9 ± 4.8	N.S.
Lysine	205.5 ± 126.7	555.8 ± 500.0	N.S.
Ornithine	16.4 ± 1.41	17.0 ± 5.2	N.S.

fifty-six pyelolithotomies, 6 nephrectomies. Tables 3 and 4 show the main pre-treatment biochemical parameters of classic and pure cystinuric patients, respectively.

The management of cystine stone disease was performed by increasing urine volume and by decreasing cystine excretion with sulphydrilant drugs. Alkali administration was used only when drugs had to be withdrawn because of side-effects and when a stone-dissolution attempt was decided.

Table 5. Mean Follow-up Before and After Pharmacological Treatment in 49 Patients

Drug	No	Follow-up B. Treatment		Follow-up A. Treatment	
Thiola	22	7.3	8.5	2.56	1.6
D-Pen	13	11.3	9.9	2.9	1.97
Thiola + D-Pen	14	14.0	12.1	9.1	2.7
Total	49	507.5		220.0	

Table 6. Clinical Parameters Before and After D-Penicillamine in 27 Patients

	Before		After		P
Mean Follow-Up (Years)	12.80	11.03	3.42	2.1	
Stone Episodes/ Pt/Year	1.18	0.94	0.21	0.29	0.001+
Operations/Year	0.115		0.01		0.011o
Stone Size Reduction or Dissolution	---		6		
Urinary Tract Infection	55.5%		25.9%		N.S.o

+ Student T-test for paired data; o q (x^2)

Table 7. Biochemical Data Before and After D-Penicillamine

	Before		After		P
Urinary Cystine	2545.5	843.8	787.1	319.9	0.001+
Urinary Arg+Lys+Orn	6280.7	3504.9	6388	3116.7	N.S.
Plasma Cystine	32.8	25.5	34.23	24.2	N.S.

+ Student T-test for paired data.

Forty-nine of the stone forming patients were treated with D-Penicillamine or 2-Mercaptopropionyl-glycine (2MPG) or both, for an average period of 4.43 ± 3.60 years per patient (altogether 220 years, Table 5).

We treated 27 patients (20 males and 7 females) with D-Penicillamine. Patients' ages ranged from 16 to 67 years. Treatment was carried out for an average period of 3.42 years per patient, with initial doses of 1 - 2 g/day and average maintenance doses of 0.95 ± 0.35 g/day, rechecked within 6 months. A clinical and biochemical improvement was achieved as shown in Tables 6 and 7, and Figure 2.

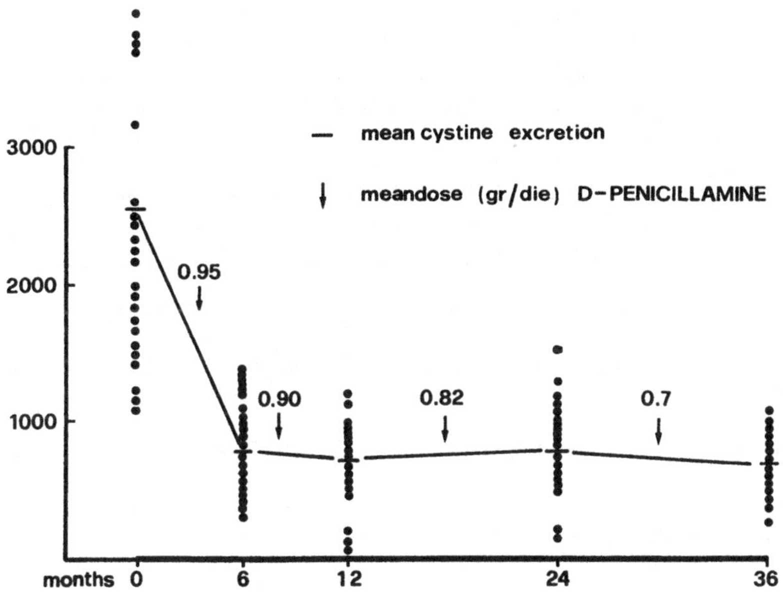

Figure 2. Daily excretion of cystine (μmol/24 h) under D-Penicillamine.

Thirty-six patients, 22 males and 14 females, were treated with 2MPG. Patients' ages ranged from 9 to 67 years. Treatment was carried on with initial doses of 1 - 2 g/day for about 6 - 20 days and was first reduced to lower doses of 1.64 ± 0.46 g/day, on the average, within 6 months, and later on, to maintenance doses of about 1 g/day. In no case was it necessary to give more than 2 g/day of 2 MPG to lower urinary cystine under 900 μmol/24 h. Clinical and biochemical results are reported in Tables 8 and 9. Figure 3 shows the trend of cystinuria related to the mean 2MPG doses used throughout each period.

Table 8. Clinical Parameters Before and After 2MPG in 36 Patients

	Before	After	P
Mean Follow-Up (Years)	10.17 ± 10.33	3.53 ± 2.19	
Stone Episodes/ Pt/Yr	1.19 ± 0.88	0.21 ± 0.33	0.001++
Operations/Yr	0.117	0	0.0005+
Stone Dissolution or Reduction		6	
Urinary Tract Infection	28.9%	25%	N.S.+

++ Student T-test for paired data; + q (x^2)

Table 9. Biochemical Data Before and After 2MPG

	Before	After	P+
Urinary Cystine (μmol/24 h)	2455.3 ± 935.6	958.8 ± 494.8	0.001
Urinary Arg+Lys+Orn (μmol/24 h)	7583.3 ± 3100.2	6966.9 ± 3081.2	N.S.
Plasma Cystine (μmol/l)	20.03± 10.01	17.73± 5.41	N.S.

+ Student T-test for paired data

The results achieved with 2MPG and D-Penicillamine have been compared both by matching data from the 22 patients who underwent 2MPG only, with the data from the 13 patients under D-Penicillamine only, and by evaluating the clinical course in those patients (14) who were given first D-Penicillamine and later 2MPG. No significant differences could be pointed out relative to the main clinical parameters (Figures 4 and 5). Side effects are fairly frequent (Table 10), but promptly disappear with treatment withdrawal and usually don't reappear when the drug is restored. Differences

Table 10. Side-Effects Under D-Penicillamine and 2MPG

	D-Penicillamine	2 - MPG	P+
Skin Rash	11.1%	8.3%	N.S.
Fever	7.4%	2.8%	N.S.
Joint Pain	3.7	--	N.S.
Proteinuria (> 1 gr/24 h)	3.7	--	N.S.
Gastroenterology Problems	22.2	8.3	N.S.

+ P (x^2)

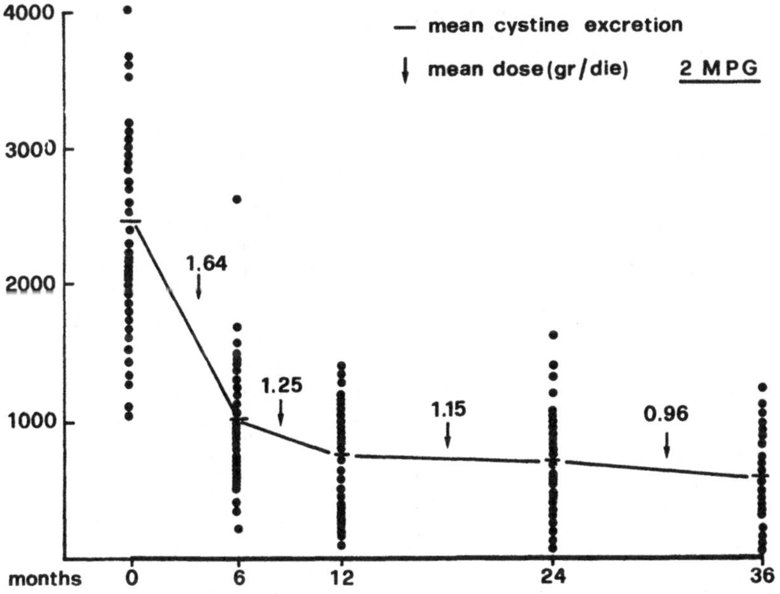

Figure 3. Daily excretion of cystine µmol/24 h under 2MPG.

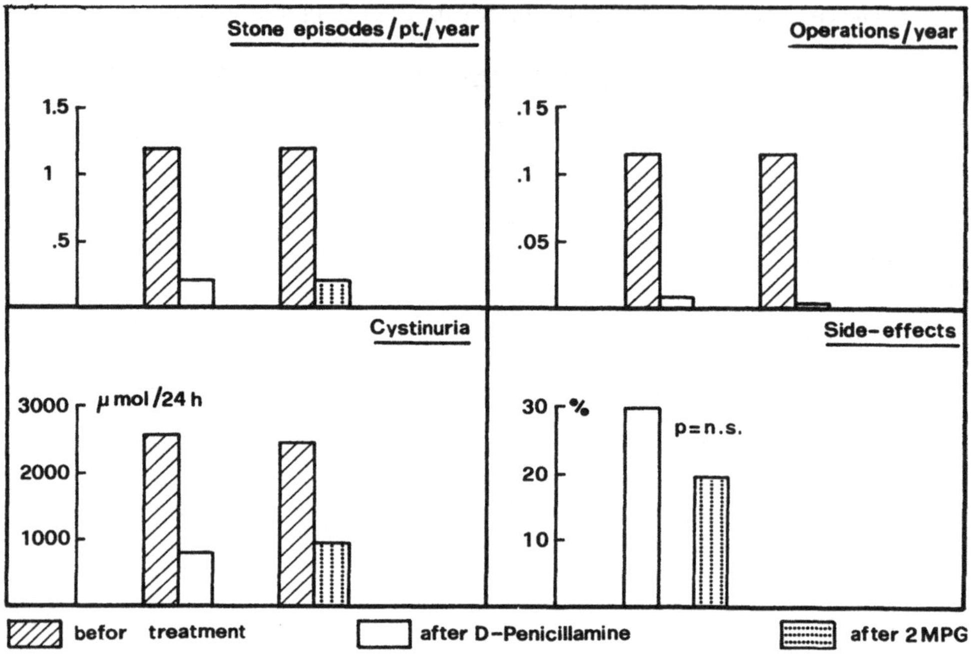

Figure 4. Comparison between the effects observed in patients who received D-Penicillamine or 2MPG only.

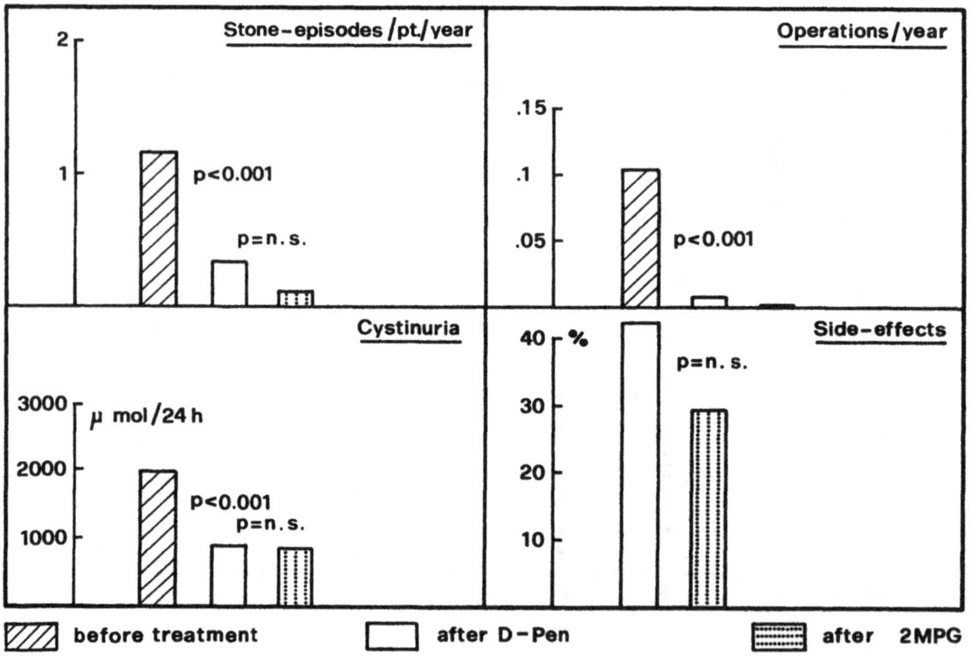

Figure 5. Comparison between D-Penicillamine and 2MPG effects in 14 patients who received both drugs.

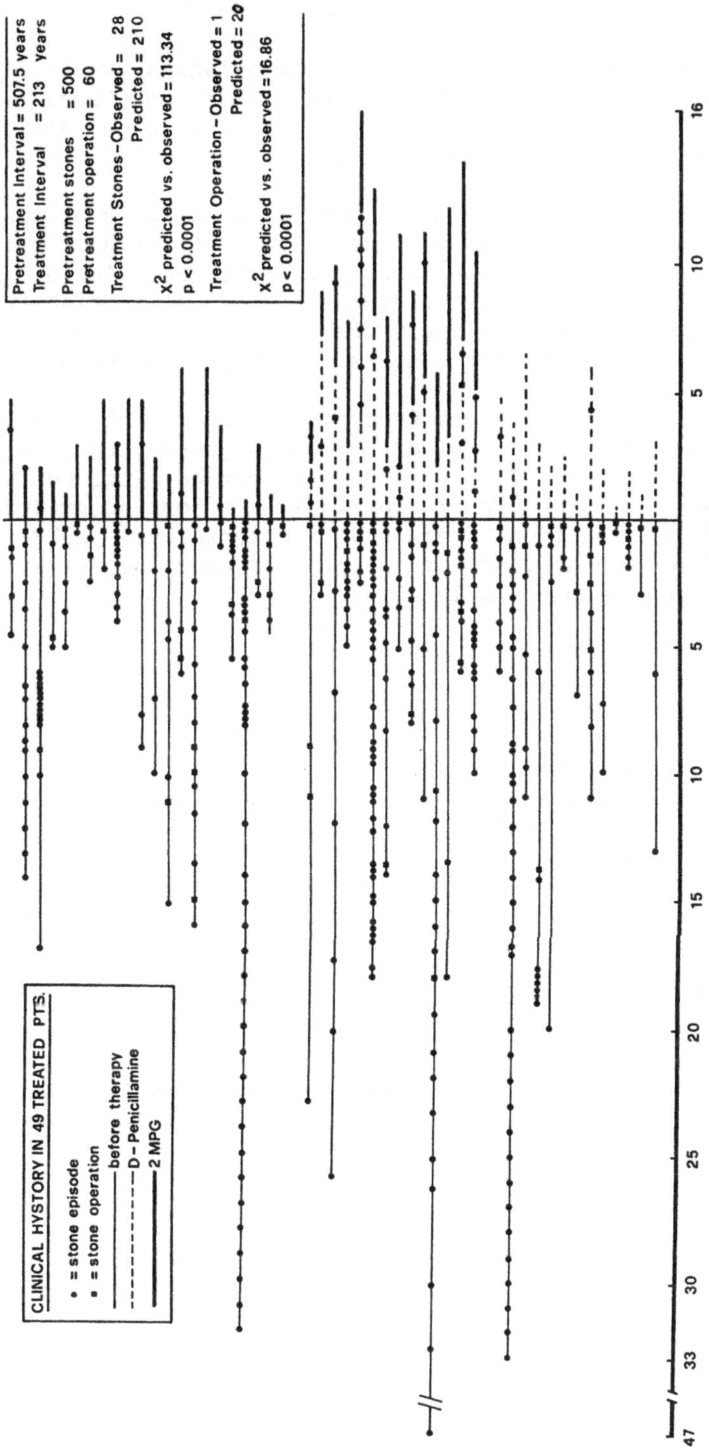
CLINICAL HYSTORY IN 49 TREATED PTS.
• = stone episode
▪ = stone operation
before therapy
D - Penicillamine
2 MPG
Pretreatment Interval = 507.5 years
Treatment Interval = 213 years
Pretreatment stones = 500
Pretreatment operation = 60
Treatment Stones - Observed = 28
Predicted = 210
X2 predicted vs. observed = 113.34
p < 0.0001
Treatment Operation - Observed = 1
Predicted = 20
X2 predicted vs. observed = 16.86
p < 0.0001
YEARS
16
10
5
5
10
15
20
25
30
33
47

Figure 6.

between the two drugs are not significant but D-Penicillamine side-effects tend to be more frequent and more important.

We checked regularly some humoral immunological tests in all the patients under 2MPG: no significant abnormality was found concerning the complement components, circulating immunocomplexes, anti2MPG antibodies or autoantibody production.

There appears to be no doubt about the usefulness of the pharmacological management of patients with cystinuria in preventing stone recurrencies[5]. As shown in Figure 6 the reduction of stone-episodes and of stone surgery obtained under treatment is striking. The efficacy of treatment is indirectly confirmed by those patients who, after treatment interruption, had a prompt relapse of lithiasis.

In conclusion, the history of cystine stone disease is positively influenced by therapy and it gives a good prognosis, when suitably treated. A follow-up of 14.9 ± 11.3 years per patient, on the average, shows a favorable evolution in most of our 62 patients: 68% have normal renal function; frequency of chronic pyelonephritis is fairly low; only two patients are at present under hemodialysis because of renal failure (Table 11).

Table 11. To Date Clinical Situation in 62 Cystinuric Patients

Stone Episodes/Pt	10.21
Chronic Pyelonephritis	12 (19.4%)
Uninephrectomy	6 (9.7%)
Hemodialysis	2 (3.22%)
Normal Renal Function	42 (67.7%)

REFERENCES

1. J. Brodehl, K. Gelissen, and S. Kiwalewsky, Klin. Wschr. 45:38 (1967).
2. F. Ramos, F. Vivanco, L. Cifuentes-Delatte, and A. Rapado, in:"Urinary Calculi," L. Cifuentes-Delatte, A. Rapado, and A. Hodgkinson, eds., Karger, Basel (1973).
3. A. Mondino, G. Bongiovanni, S. Fumero, and L. Rossi, J. Chromatogr. 74:255 (1972).
4. L. E. Rosenberg, Science 154:1341 (1966).
5. P. J. Dahlberg, C. J. Van Den Berg, S. B. Kurtz, D. M. Wilson, and L. H. Smith, Mayo Clinic Proc. 52:533 (1977).

GLUTAMINE THERAPY OF CYSTINURIA

C. J. Van Den Berg, D. M. Wilson, L. H. Smith, and
J. D. Jones
Mayo Clinic

Rochester, Minnesota

Cystinuria is an inherited disorder characterized by abnormalities in the transport of cystine, lysine, ornithine, arginine, and possibly cysteine in both the intestinal tract and renal tubule. Clinically this is important only because of the insolubility of cystine in the urine with resultant cystine calculus formation.

A review of the management of 89 cases of homozygotes at the Mayo Clinic (1) showed that the current management of stones in these patients is still not satisfactory. Medical treatment includes increasing the solubility of cystine by increasing urine volume and the use of d-penicillamine. Treatment with urine alkalinization and increased oral fluids alone is frequently associated with continued stone formation and the addition of d-penicillamine has been very helpful in this situation. Unfortunately, d-penicillamine is not an innocuous drug and in the study cited, there were 23 drug complications in 21 of 43 patients treated. These included 12 patients with rash, fever and lymphadenopathy, four with high-grade proteinuria, one with granulocytopenia and six with taste abnormalities.

A recent report by Miyagi et al.[2] suggested that glutamine (a non-toxic amino acid) caused a marked fall in the urinary excretion of cystine in one patient with Type II cystinuria (those with markedly decreased gut transport of cystine and increased urinary excretion of lysine and cystine in heterozygote relatives)[3]. In this patient, intravenous infusion of glutamine decreased the urinary cystine excretion by 45% and oral L-glutamine (2.1 - 8 gm daily) decreased the urinary excretion of cystine from 2555 mg to 240 mg by the third day. Serum glutamine was not measured in the patient studied, however, increased by 40 - 170 μM in one normal control given 8 gm of glutamine. In addition, the urinary pH increased during glutamine administration. While the increase in urine pH was similar to that expected in normal people loaded with oral glutamine[4], the mechanism whereby glutamine decreased the urinary excretion of cystine was not clear.

To substantiate this potentially important therapy and to further elucidate a mechanism of action for glutamine in patients with cystinuria, we studied five patients with homozygous cystinuria of undetermined type. All patients had a history of known cystine calculi but were stone-free at the time of the study. All patients discontinued oral alkali and d-penicillamine for at least one week prior to the study. All patients had normal liver function tests and there was no history or data suggesting intestinal malabsorption or any disorder of acid base or ammonia metabolism. All patients were studied for seven days--three control days and four on 700 mg oral L-glutamine powder q 8 hours. We measured: (1) urinary excretion, fractional excretion (FE) and blood levels of cystine, ornithine, arginine and lysine, (2) systemic pH and renal excretion of ammonia, titratable acidity (TA), HCO_3^-, total acid excretion (TAE) and citrate excretion. Freshly voided urine samples were checked for the presence of cystine crystalluria by scanning electron microscopy.

Patients were admitted to the Clinical Study Unit on a controlled diet of their usual fare. Control data from 24 hour urines were averaged from day one and two. GFR (inulin clearance), fractional excretion (% of filtered load excreted) of amino acids, uric acid, PO_4, NH_4^+, TA and HCO_3^- were determined on day 3. Glutamine was started on day 4 and the 24 hour urine data were again averaged from days 6 and 7 (there was no difference between them)--FE studies as on day 3 were analyzed on day 6.

There were no significant changes in any of the parameters studied (Table 1). We saw no rise in serum glutamine or any other serum amino acid 2 hours after the 700 mg dose of glutamine. There was also no change in the total excretion of FE or ornithine, arginine or lysine. Urine crystal studies revealed no change in cystine crystals which were seen in all patients before and during glutamine therapy. Data by Thier, et al (personal communication) using as much as 8 gm of oral glutamine daily in five patients, one of whom was a Type II cystinuric, also showed no changes in the urinary excretion of cystine. The reason for this difference in response from the patient of Miyagi, et al. is not clear, but if glutamine has any role in the treatment of these patients, the type of patient or therapeutic key remains to be elucidated.

Table 1.

Patient #	Pre Glutamine Cystine mg/24°	Post Glutamine Cystine mg/24°
1	1199	1097
2	825	1098
3	1073	1264
4	811	881
5	1190	1136
Mean	(1020)	(1095)

Mean Data	Pre-Drug	Post-Drug
Cystine mg/gm creat.	529	555
FE cystine	86	90
NH_3 mM/24 hours	31.3	31.8
TA mM/24 hours	18.2	19
HCO_3 mM/24 hours	12.3	17.1
TAE mM/24 hours	37.2	33.7
Uric acid (FE)	9.7	11.1
PO_4 (FE)	14.3	14.9
Serum cystine μM/dl	4.0	4.1
Serum glutamine μM/dl	67.4	63.6
GFR ml/min/1.73 sq. m.	97	98
Urine pH	6.36	6.52

REFERENCES

1. P. J. Dahlberg, C. J. Van Den Berg, S. B. Kurtz, D. M. Wilson, and L. H. Smith, Mayo Clinic Proc. 52:533 (1977).
2. K. Miyagi, S. Nakada, and D. Ohshiro, New Engl. J. Med. 301: 196 (1979).
3. S. O. Thier and S. Segal, in:"Metabolic Basis of Inherited Disease," J. B. Stanbury, ed., McGraw-Hill Co., New York (1972).
4. T. Welbourne, M. Weber, and N. Bank, J. Clin. Invest. 51:1852 (1972).

ACKNOWLEDGMENTS

This investigation was supported by AM 20605 and RR 585 grants from the National Institutes of Health.

URINARY STONE FORMATION IN BOWEL DISEASE

M. Peacock, C. P. Bambach*, W. G. Robertson,
J. E. Aaron, and G. L. Hill*
M.R.C. Mineral Metabolism Unit and *Department of
Surgery, The General Infirmary
Leeds LS1 3EX, U.K.

Urinary stone formation is now a well recognized sequela of bowel disease[1,2]. It occurs in patients with inflammatory bowel disease and in patients with an ileostomy or a bowel resection, particularly of the small bowel. The formation of urinary stones, however, seems to be related more to surgical treatment than to the underlying bowel disease or to its medical management. The prevalence of stone disease in patients following bowel surgery is between 5 and 15% and both uric acid[3] and calcium oxalate[4] stones may be formed.

Although urinary stone formation is a common complication of bowel surgery, patients with this type of stone disease only account for a small proportion of the total population of uric acid and calcium oxalate stone-formers[5]. Nevertheless, the understanding of the etiological factors involved in this type of stone formation is important not only for the management of patients requiring bowel surgery but also for the appreciation of the role of diet, digestion and bowel function on urinary stone formation in general.

In this study we examine whether stone formation in bowel disease can be accounted for by changes in the urinary risk factors which we have previously defined in relation to idiopathic stone disease[6].

PATIENTS AND METHODS

Patients

The prevalence of urinary stone disease in patients who had undergone bowel surgery in the Department of Surgery at the Leeds

General Infirmary from 1960 to 1975 was established by postal questionnaire. The patients formed three groups according to the type of surgical operation. The first (ileostomy group, IL), had undergone a proctocolectomy and ileostomy and had less than 10 cm of small bowel resected. The second (ileostomy with small bowel resection group, IL BR) were similar to the first but had between 20 cm and 300 cm of small bowel resected. The third (small bowel resection group, BR) did not have an ileostomy but had between 20 cm and 300 cm of small bowel resected. Twenty-seven of the ileostomy group, 17 of the ileostomy and small bowel resection group and 17 of the small bowel resection group agreed to have further investigations.

Materials and Methods

A 24-hour urine was collected from each patient on a free diet and analyzed for volume, pH, calcium, oxalate, uric acid and glycosaminoglycans inhibitor (GAGS)[6].

Fasting blood and an iliac bone biopsy were taken from 24 patients with over 20 cm of small bowel resected with or without an ileostomy. Osteomalacia and osteoporosis were diagnosed using histomorphometric criteria as previously described[7]. Plasma 25 hydroxy vitamin D (25OHD) was measured by competitive binding assay[8].

Calculations and Statistical Analysis

The significance of the differences between groups was assessed using Student's t-test or the Wilcoxon sum of rank test. Relative supersaturation indices for uric acid and calcium oxalate were obtained from nomograms[9] and the relative probability of calcium and uric acid stone formation (P_{SF}) was calculated as previously described[6].

RESULTS

The prevalence of urinary stone disease in our patients assessed by postal questionnaire was 12.4% (Table 1). The ileostomy with small bowel resection group (IL BR) had a prevalence of 23%, the ileostomy group (IL) had a prevalence of 11.8% and the small bowel resection group (BR) of 8%.

The 24-hour excretions of the urinary risk factors for calcium oxalate and uric acid stone are shown in Figure 1. As compared to normal subjects the IL and IL BR group had a significant reduction in volume, pH and glycosaminoglycans inhibitor. IL BR group had also a significant reduction in urine calcium. BR group had a significant increase in oxalate but a significant reduction in calcium. The 24-hour urine concentrations of the urinary risk factors are shown in

Table 1. Prevalence of Urinary Stone Formation in Patients with Bowel Disease: Leeds

	TOTAL	STONE	PERCENT
ILEOSTOMY (IL)	170	20	12
ILEOSTOMY + S.B.RESECTION (ILBR)	30	7	23
S.B.RESECTION (BR)	50	4	8

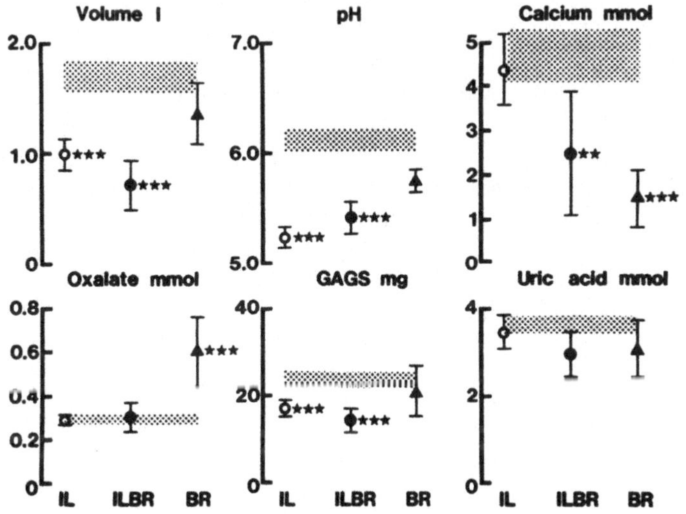

Figure 1. Mean (±2SE) 24-hour excretions of the urinary stone risk factors in patients with bowel disease: IL = ileostomy; IL BR = ileostomy with a small bowel resection greater than 30 cm; BR = small bowel resection greater than 30 cm with no ileostomy; the shaded area represents the mean ±2SE in 85 normal subjects, apart from uric acid which was in 15 normal subjects (*P =<0.05, **P<0.01, ***P<0.001).

Figure 2. All three groups had a significant increase in oxalate concentration. Groups IL and IL BR had a significant increase in uric acid concentration. Group IL had a significant increase and group BR a significant decrease in calcium concentration. Figures 3 and 4 show that all three groups had a significantly increased probability of forming both calcium oxalate and uric acid stones as compared to normal subjects. The risk was greatest in group IL BR and least in group BR.

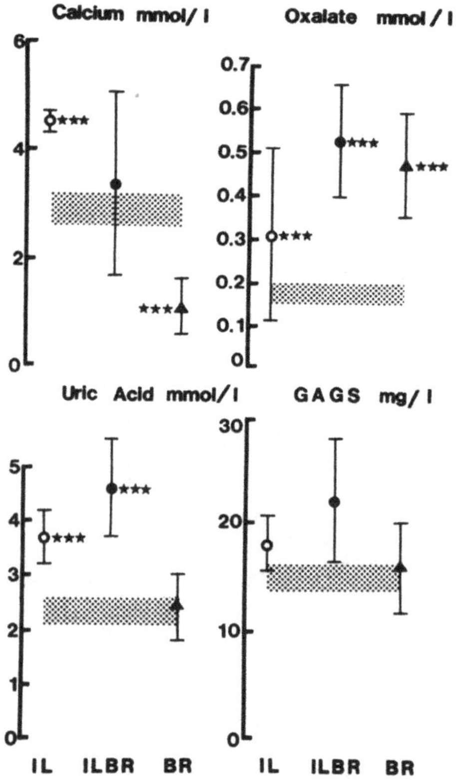

Figure 2. Mean (±2 SE) 24-hour urine concentrations of the urinary stone risk factors in patients with bowel disease (see Figure 1 for details).

Over 30% of patients with small bowel resection, with or without an ileostomy, had histological evidence of osteomalacia (Figure 5). This was associated with low plasma 25OHD concentrations, although many patients without osteomalacia also had low concentrations. The osteomalacic patients had a significantly lower calcium excretion, a similar oxalate excretion and higher supersaturation values for calcium oxalate as compared with the non-osteomalacic patients (Figure 6).

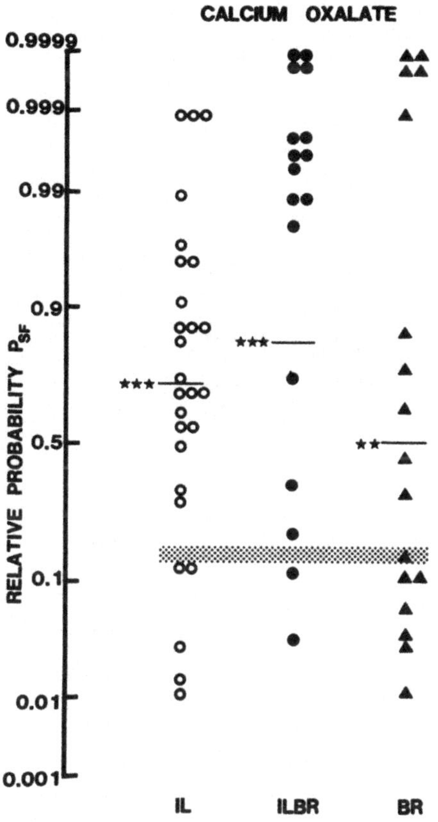

Figure 3. The relative probability of forming calcium oxalate stones (P_{SF}) in patients with bowel disease as compared with normal subjects (see Figure 1 for details).

The osteomalacic patients treated with vitamin D showed a rise in 24-hour urine calcium and oxalate excretion and a rise in calcium oxalate supersaturation (Figure 7).

DISCUSSION

The overall prevalence of urinary stone disease of over 12% in our patients is in general agreement with published figures. The highest prevalence was found in ileostomy patients with a significant length of small bowel resected and the lowest in patients who had

had a resection of small bowel but had no ileostomy (Table 1). The differences in urinary stone prevalence between the three groups were reflected in the differences in calculated probability of stone formation from the 24-hour urine biochemistry (Figures 5 and 6).

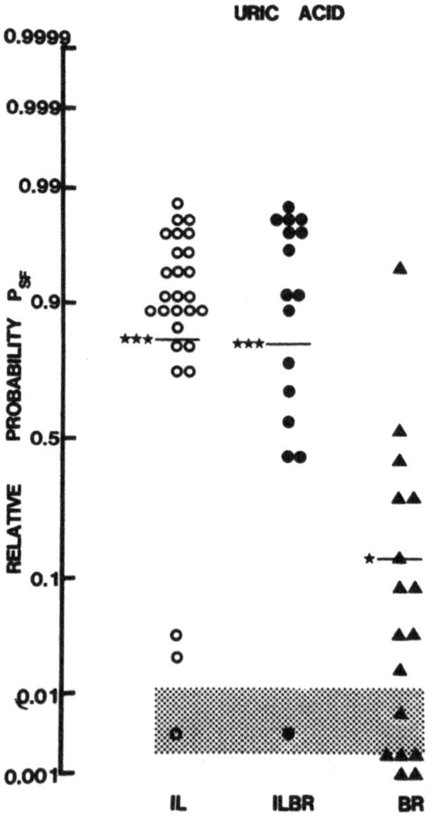

Figure 4. The relative probability of forming uric acid stones (P_{SF}) in patients with bowel disease as compared with normal subjects (see Figure 1 for details).

Patients with an ileostomy have an increased risk of forming both uric acid and calcium oxalate stones mainly because of a low urine volume and pH. These urinary changes reflect the great difficulty ileostomy patients have of conserving water and base in the absence of colonic function. In the ileostomy patients with small bowel resection the urine volumes are even lower and despite having a very low urine calcium excretion still have an increased risk of forming calcium oxalate stones. In patients with small bowel resection and no ileostomy the urine volume and pH are low

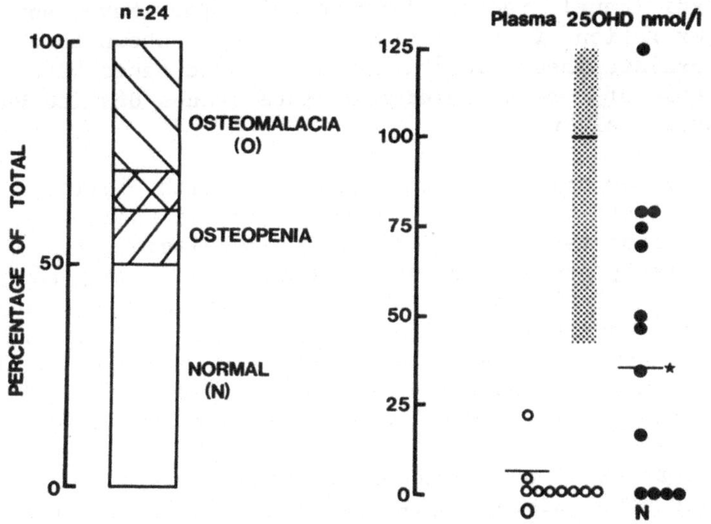

Figure 5. The percentage of iliac crest bone biopsies with osteomalacia, osteopenia or normal histology in patients with small bowel resection (left hand panel) and the plasma 25 hydroxy vitamin D concentrations in patients with osteomalacia (o) and in patients with normal bone histology (N) (right hand panel) (Normal Mean and Range (±2SD) is shown in shaded area).

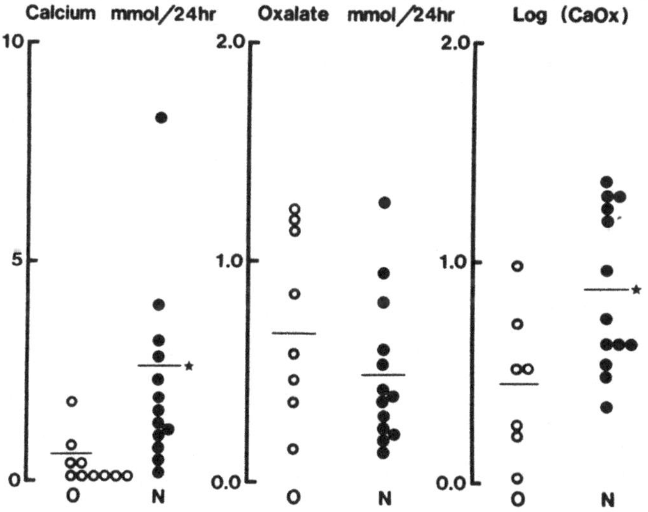

Figure 6. 24-hour calcium, oxalate and relative supersaturation of calcium oxalate (log CaOx) in osteomalacia (o) and non-osteomalacic (N) patients with small bowel resection.

but not significantly reduced from normal. They have, however, an increased excretion of oxalate, which has been shown to be due to increased oxalate absorption[10], and as a consequence have an increased risk of forming calcium oxalate stones despite having a very low urine calcium.

The very low urine calcium in patients with small bowel resection reflects calcium malabsorption and is associated with a high incidence of vitamin D deficient osteomalacia. This low urine calcium partially protects these patients from forming calcium oxalate stones. Treatment of osteomalacia in these patients with vitamin D increases the risk of forming calcium stones. The true prevalence of stone in small bowel resection is probably, therefore, higher than the one we have reported in this series and will depend to some extent on the vitamin D status of this population.

The formation of uric acid and calcium oxalate stones in patients with bowel disease agrees with our hypothesis that stone formation can be accounted for and predicted by a limited number of urinary risk factors[6]. Furthermore it illustrates that dietary and digestive factors have substantial effects on the urinary risk factors and are probably also acting in idiopathic stone disease, although less dramatically, as we have discussed elsewhere[11,12].

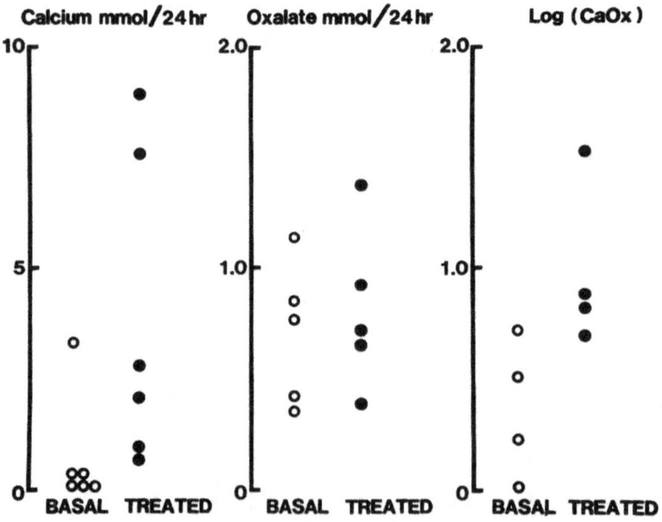

Figure 7. 24-hour calcium, oxalate and relative supersaturation of calcium oxalate in untreated (basal) and vitamin D treated bowel patients with osteomalacia.

SUMMARY

1. The prevalence of urinary stone disease was established by postal questionnaire in 250 patients who had undergone bowel surgery. They formed three groups according to the type of surgery which had been performed: an ileostomy group with less than 10 cm of small bowel resected(IL); an ileostomy group with between 20 and 300 cm of small bowel resected (II BR) and a small bowel resection group with between 20 and 300 cm of small bowel resected but without an ileostomy (BR). The overall prevalence was over 12.4%, the prevalence in group IL was 11.8%, in group IL BR 23.3% and in group BR 8%.

2. The risk of forming uric acid and calcium oxalate stone as compared to normal subjects was calculated from the biochemistry of a 24-hour urine collection in 61 unselected patients. All three groups had a significantly increased risk of forming both types of stone which correlated with the prevalence of stone in the three groups. In groups IL and IL BR the main risk factors were a low urine volume and pH; and in group BR a high urine oxalate.

3. Over 30% of patients with small bowel resection, with or without an ileostomy, had vitamin D deficient osteomalacia and a significantly lower urine calcium than the non-osteomalacic patients which decreased their risk of forming calcium oxalate stones. Treatment with vitamin D increased the urine calcium and increased the risk of forming stones.

4. Urinary stone formation in bowel disease can be accounted for and predicted by changes in the urinary risk factors for calcium oxalate and uric acid stones.

REFERENCES

1. J. J. Deren, J. G. Porush, M. F. Levitt, M. T. Khilnani, Ann. Int. Med. 56:843 (1962).
2. E. A. Gelzayd, R. I. Breuer, and J. B. Kirsner, Am. J. Dig. Dis. 13:1027 (1968).
3. R. C. Bennett and R. P. Jepson, Aust. NZ. J. Surg. 36:153 (1966).
4. L. H. Smith, H. Fromm, and A. F. Hofmann, N. Eng. J. Med. 286: 1371 (1972).
5. M. Peacock and W. G. Robertson, in:"Urinary Calculous Disease," J. E. A. Wickham, ed., Churchill Livingstone, London (1979).
6. W. G. Robertson, M. Peacock, P. J. Heyburn, D. H. Marshall, and P. B. Clarke, Br. J. Urol. 50:449 (1978).
7. B. E. C. Nordin, M. Peacock, J. Aaron, R. G. Crilly, P. J. Heyburn, A. Horsman, and D. Marshall, Clin. Endocrin. Metab. 9:177 (1980).
8. J. F. Morris and M. Peacock, Clin. Chim. Acta. 72:383 (1976).

9. R. W. Marshall and W. G. Robertson, Clin. Chim. Acta. 72:253 (1976).
10. V. S. Chadwick, K. Modha, and R. H. Dowling, N. Eng. J. Med. 289:172 (1973).
11. W. G. Robertson, M. Peacock, P. J. Heyburn, F. A. Hanes, D. Ouimet, A. Rutherford, and V. J. Sergeant, in:"Proceedings Fourth International Urolithiasis Research Symposium," L. H. Smith, B. Finlayson, and W. G. Robertson, eds., Plenum Press, New York (in press).
12. W. G. Robertson, M. Peacock, D. Ouimet, P. J. Heyburn, and A. Rutherford, in:"Proceedings Fourth International Urolithiasis Research Symposium," L. H. Smith, B. Finlayson, and W. G. Robertson, eds., Plenum Press, New York (in press).

PREVALENCE OF NEPHROLITHIASIS IN MALABSORPTIVE SYNDROMES

K. Dharmsathaphorn, D. Freeman, H. J. Binder, and J. Dobbins
Department of Internal Medicine, Yale University School of Medicine
New Haven, Connecticut 06510

Patients with inflammatory bowel disease have an increased incidence of nephrolithiasis, especially after resection or bypass of part of the bowel[1]. Many of these stones are composed of calcium oxalate though uric acid stones appear to be more common after an ileostomy. Patients with ileal disease have increased absorption of dietary oxalate, with resultant hyperoxaluria, because of increased solubility of oxalate and increased permeability of the colon to oxalate[1]. Increased solubility is related to steatorrhea. Unabsorbed fatty acids bind to calcium preventing the formation of insoluble calcium oxalate, thus oxalate remains in solution available for absorption. Fatty acids (and bile acids) also increase the permeability of the colon to oxalate[2].

Several investigators have found a direct correlation between the degree of steatorrhea and urinary oxalate excretion[3-5]. In these studies hyperoxaluria has been observed in patients with steatorrhea of many different etiologies including chronic pancreatitis. In addition to hyperoxaluria, steatorrhea causes diarrhea, which may result in dehydration and metabolic acidosis[6]. Thus, one might expect to find a higher incidence of kidney stones in patients with steatorrhea of any cause. Therefore, we attempted to determine the prevalence of kidney stones in patients with steatorrhea and whether steatorrhea alone is a risk factor for nephrolithiasis.

We reviewed the available records of all adult patients who had a 72-hour fecal fat determination. Age, sex, diagnosis, presence of nephrolithiasis were recorded as well as the following laboratory data: urine specific gravity, serum uric acid, calcium, phosphorus, albumin, carotene, B_{12}, folate, iron, total iron binding capacity and red blood cell folate. Nephrolithiasis was considered present when there was radiologic or surgical evidence of a kidney stone or when the patient gave a history of passing a stone. Steatorrhea was defined as fecal fat excretion greater than 6 g/24 h, and diarrhea was defined as fecal weight greater than 225 g/24 h.

The patients were divided into two groups on the basis of fecal fat determination: patients with steatorrhea and those without steatorrhea. Clinical and laboratory data in the two groups were comparable except for the following: patients with steatorrhea had a greater stool weight, and lower serum calcium, albumin, and carotene. Twelve percent of the patients with steatorrhea had a history of nephrolithiasis, compared to 4% in the patients without steatorrhea ($p < 0.01$).

The prevalence of nephrolithiasis according to clinical diagnosis was 3.5% in patients with steatorrhea without ileal disease, 33% in patients with steatorrhea and ileal disease and 4% in patients with ileal disease without steatorrhea. Most of the patients with nephrolithiasis had both ileal disease and steatorrhea. Only a few patients with steatorrhea of other cause than ileal disease had a history of stone disease. Likewise, few patients with ileal disease but without steatorrhea had stones.

Utilizing simple odds ratios, we determined the association between nephrolithiasis and other clinical variables. Steatorrhea, male sex, diarrhea, ileal disease and age were associated with a significantly increased risk of nephrolithiasis. Ileal disease was not associated with nephrolithiasis in the patients without steatorrhea.

The association between nephrolithiasis and each of the above variables was then analyzed while controlling for the influence of the other variables. First, the partial associations were tested in order to determine whether there was any direct association between pairs of variables and whether the corresponding association depended on a third variable (confounding variable)[8]. This analysis revealed that the association between nephrolithiasis and steatorrhea was independent of age and diarrhea. We therefore focused on the association between nephrolithiasis, ileal disease and the degree of steatorrhea (Table 1). From this table we can conclude that the association between nephrolithiasis, ileal disease and steatorrhea depends upon the degree of steatorrhea. We noted no association between steatorrhea and nephrolithiasis in patients without ileal disease. Therefore, we conclude that the association between nephrolithiasis and steatorrhea depends on the presence of ileal disease. Conversely, the association between nephrolithiasis and ileal disease depends upon the presence of steatorrhea.

Table 1. Prevalence Rate of Nephrolithiasis
Percent

Stool fat g/day	Patients without ileal disease	Patients with ileal disease
<6	4	5
6-20	2.5	24
>20	8	51

These findings are in agreement with the current literature, i.e. there are no reports of an increased incidence of nephrolithiasis in pancreatic insufficiency, celiac disease, primary biliary cirrhosis or causes of steatorrhea other than ileal disease, despite the occurrence of hyperoxaluria in many of these patients. They also suggest that only those patients with ileal disease and steatorrhea will have an increased incidence of nephrolithiasis.

Stone analysis, when available, revealed that about half the stones were composed of calcium oxalate and half of uric acid. Steatorrhea and ileal disease thus appears to result in an increased incidence of uric acid stones as well as calcium oxalate stones. These findings are consistent with studies reporting an increased incidence of uric acid as well as calcium containing stones in patients with inflammatory bowel disease[9-10]. Uric acid metabolism has not been well investigated in patients with ileal disease, therefore we cannot draw firm conclusions about the mechanism of uric acid stone formation in these patients. Uric acid stones appear to be more common after an ileostomy and most of our patients with uric acid stones had an ileostomy. As previously stated, steatorrhea may cause dehydration and metabolic acidosis; factors which predispose to uric acid stone formation.

These results suggest that hyperoxaluria alone is not enough to increase the incidence of nephrolithiasis since most patients with steatorrhea have increased absorption of dietary oxalate and hyperoxaluria, assuming adequate dietary oxalate content. Smith et al. have recently reported that patients with ileal disease and nephrolithiasis have decreased Mg, K, sulfate and citrate in their urine[11]. These substances are important in that they increase the solubility of calcium oxalate in urine. Thus, the increased incidence of calcium oxalate stones in patients with ileal disease could be the result of increased oxalate in the urine relative to decreased solubilizing substances such as citrate, Mg, etc. These solubilizing substances are decreased in urine presumably because of malabsorption and diarrhea.

In summary, the increased incidence of nephrolithiasis depends upon the presence of both ileal disease and steatorrhea, and increases with the severity of steatorrhea. Both uric acid and calcium oxalate stones are associated with ileal disease and steatorrhea.

REFERENCES

1. J. W. Dobbins, J. Clin. Gastroenterol. 1:165 (1979)
2. J. W. Dobbins and H. J. Binder, Gastroenterology 70:1096 (1976).
3. E. Hylander, S. Jarnum, H. J. Jensen, and M. Thale, Scand. J. Gastroenterol. 13:577 (1978).
4. G. B. McDonald, D. L. Earnest, and W. H. Admirand, Gut 18:561 (1977).
5. H. Andersson and R. Gillberg, Lancet 2:677 (1977).
6. H. J. Binder, Gastroenterology 65:847 (1973).
7. W. G. Cochran, in:"Statistical Methods," 6th edition, State University Press, Ames, Iowa (1967).
8. Y. M. M. Bishop, S. E. Fienberg, and P. W. Holland, in:"Discrete Multivariate Analysis," MIT Press, Cambridge, Massachusetts (1975).
9. J. J. Deren, J. G. Porush, M. F. Levit, and M. G. Khilnani, Ann. Int. Med. 56:843 (1962).
10. E. A. Gelzayd, R. I. Breuer, and J. B. Kirsner, Am. J. Dig. Dis. 13:1027 (1968).
11. L. H. Smith, P. G. Werness, D. M. Wilson, and S. F. Phillips, (abstract) Clin. Res. 28:486A (1980).

THE INFLUENCE OF GASTROINTESTINAL ANATOMY ON OXALATE EXCRETION AND KIDNEY STONE INCIDENCE IN PATIENTS WITH ENTERIC HYPEROXALURIA

Björn Nordenvall, Lars Backman, and Lasse Larsson

Department of Surgery, Karolinska Institute at Danderyd Hospital, Stockholm, Sweden; Department of Clinical Chemistry, University Hospital, Linköping, Sweden

INTRODUCTION

Jejunoileal bypass operations result in malabsorption with diarrhea, especially during the first postoperative year. Hyperoxaluria and increased risk of forming renal calculi have been found in these patients[1,2].

We have in an earlier study found that the stone incidence varies in patients operated with different types of intestinal bypass[3]. The stone incidence was significantly higher after end-to-end jejunoileostomy (25 stone formers out of 82 patients) than after end-to-side anastomosis (7 out of 83, $p < 0.001$). The stone incidence seems to be even higher after biliointestinal shunt (5 out of 10). Increased absorption of dietary oxalate is thought to be the major cause of the hyperoxaluria[4]. This hyperabsorption is related to the degree of steatorrhea after intestinal resections[5].

The aim of the present study was to estimate the urinary excretion of oxalate, calcium, magnesium, and citrate. These parameters might give some information concerning the various risks of forming kidney stones after different types of operations or at different periods after surgery.

MATERIAL AND METHODS

We have studied thirty patients operated with intestinal bypass because of severe obesity one to seven years before the investigation. The patients had undergone three types of jejunoileostomy (group 1-3, Figure 1). There were ten patients in each group. Five patients in each group had had postoperative kidney stones.

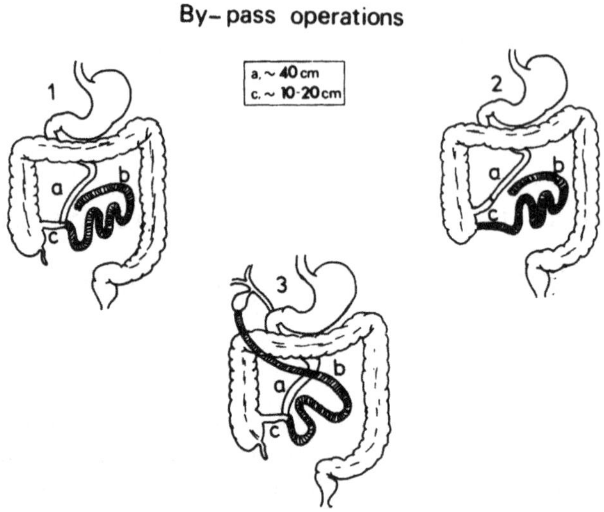

Figure 1. Three types of intestinal bypass for obesity (group 1-3). 1. End-to-side jejunoileostomy[6]. 2. End-to-end jejunoileostomy[7]. 3. Bilio-intestinal shunt[8].

The patients had their normal diet during the urine collection period of 3 days. Urinary oxalate was determined by a method described by Hodgkinson and Williams[9]. The upper reference limit was 400 µmol/24 h. Urinary calcium and magnesium were analyzed by atomic absorption technique[10,11]. The upper reference limit for the quotient calcium/magnesium was 2. Urinary citrate was determined according to Greenbaum[12]. The lower reference limit was 2 mmol/24 h.

Data are given as mean ± SEM. Unpaired data were compared by Wilcoxon's sum of ranks test.

RESULTS

Oxalate

The mean urinary oxalate excretion was 986 ± 49 µmol/24 h, with a range of 512 ± 1497 µmol/24 h. The excretion was significantly higher in group 3 (1178 ± 68) compared to group 1 (863 ± 58 $p < 0.01$) and group 2 (869 ± 65, $p < 0.05$, Figure 2).

No differences in oxalate excretion were found in patients with or without kidney stones (992 ± 72 and 948 ± 56) and there was no evidence of any decrease in oxalate excretion with time after operation (Figure 3).

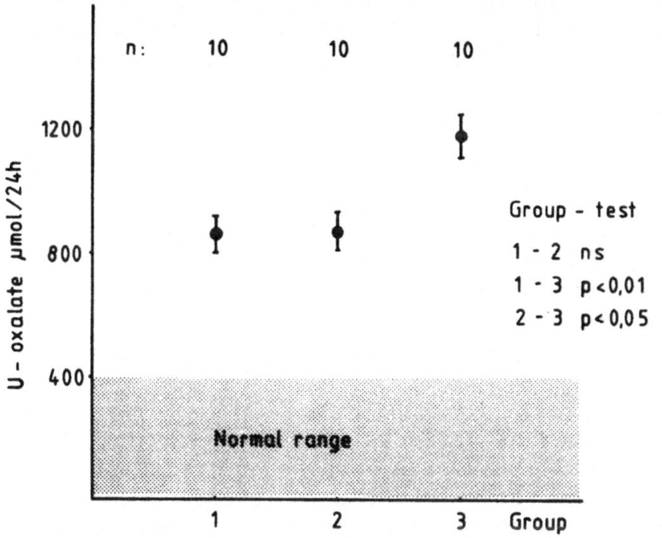

Figure 2. Mean urinary oxalate excretion after three types of intestinal bypass operations (group 1-3, see Figure 1).

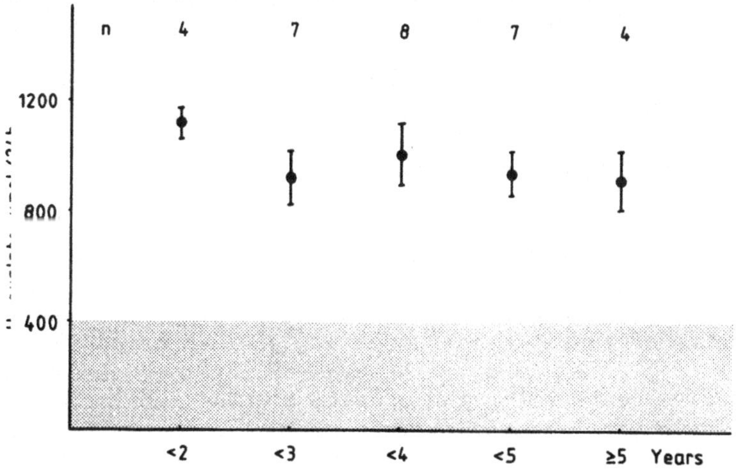

Figure 3. Urinary oxalate excretion after intestinal bypass operations. The influence of time after surgery.

Calcium and Magnesium

The mean excretion of calcium and magnesium were normal (3.4 ± 0.3 mmol/24 h and 2.1 ± 0.3 mmol/24 h). The mean quotient calcium/magnesium was higher than normal (2.5 ± 0.4). There were no differences between the patient groups 1-3 or between patients with or without stones.

Citrate

The mean excretion of citrate in the patients was lower than normal (1.7 ± 0.2 mmol/24 h). There were no differences in citrate excretion between the patient groups 1-3 or between the patients with or without stones.

DISCUSSION

A great number of patients throughout the world have been operated with small-intestinal bypass as treatment for massive obesity during the years 1954-1980. Several severe complications have appeared after this operation, one of the most frequent being kidney stones. Like other patients with intestinal disease and steatorrhea, hyperoxaluria is common.

It is to be expected that this hyperoxaluria would tend to decrease with time roughly parallel to the diminishing frequency of diarrhea, which is very prominent in the early postoperative period. This study has shown that the hyperoxaluria persisted unchanged one to seven years after intestinal bypass operations.

A significantly higher excretion of oxalate was found in patients with a bilio-intestinal shunt. One explanation could be that these patients had an increased degree of steatorrhea due to low bile concentration in the intestine in circuit.

The excretion of oxalate was the same in patients with end-to-side and end-to-end anastomosis in spite of the different stone incidence. Also, patients with postoperative kidney stones had the same degree of hyperoxaluria as those without. This indicates that the incidence of kidney stones does not seem to be correlated to the degree of hyperoxaluria. The hyperoxaluria persisted unchanged more than five years after the operation. The mean urinary quotient of Ca/Mg was higher and the citrate excretion lower than in the normal population. These factors increase the risk of forming renal calculi in the patients.

It seems likely that the risk of attaining kidney stones remains unchanged for indefinite time after small-intestinal bypass operation.

REFERENCES

1. S. Dickstein and B. Frame, Surg., Gyn. and Obst. 136:257 (1973).
2. J. P. O'Leary, W. C. Thomas, and E. R. Woodward, Am. J. Surg. 127:142 (1974).
3. L. Backman, B. Nordenvall, and D. Hallberg, Urol. Res. 7:189 (1979).
4. V. S. Chadwick, K. Modha, R. H. Dowling, NEJM 289:172 (1973).
5. D. L. Earnest, G. Johnson, H. E. Williams, and W. M. Admirand, Gastroenterology 66:1114 (1974).
6. J. M. Payne, and L. T. De Wind, Am. J. Surg. 118:141 (1969).
7. M. Buchwald, and R. L. Varco, Surgery 70:62 (1971).
8. D. Hallberg, and U. Holmgren, Acta Chirurgica Scand. 145:405 (1979).
9. A. Hodgkinson, and A. Williams, Clin. Chim. Acta. 36:127 (1972).
10. D. L. Trudeau, and E. F. Freier, Clin. Chem. 13:101 (1967).
11. J. L. Hansen, and E. F. Freier, Am. J. Med. Tech. 33:158 (1967).
12. B. W. Greenbaum, and N. Pace, Microchem. J. 15:673 (1970).

THERAPY FOR ENTERIC HYPEROXALURIA: A COMPARISON OF CALCIUM SUPPLEMENTATION AND URINARY ALKALINIZATION

John G. Gregory, Ki Y. Park, Robert Wilt, and Alex Feigl

Section of Urology, St. Louis University
School of Medicine
St. Louis, Missouri

Of the commonly considered factors causatively related to calcium oxalate stone formation; urinary pH, inhibitor factors, urinary volume, levels of calcium, oxalate, and uric acid, it appears at the present time that the level of urinary oxalate is the factor most significantly responsible for stone formation[1]. Such being the case, it is intuitively reasonable to consider with particular interest any patients having a predisposition toward the hyperoxaluric state. No large group of patients is better suited for such a study than are those who have enteric hyperoxaluria. Since 1972 we have had occasion to study 681 patients who have had a small bowel bypass procedure performed for reasons of morbid obesity.

Stone formation in this etiologically homogeneous group has been 16.4%. The majority of patients formed one or only an occasional stone. (Figure 1) Despite early concern, the stone morbidity in this group of patients has not been excessive[2], most of the stones passed spontaneously and only two of the patients we have followed were considered so severely jeopardized by stone formation so that the small bowel bypass procedure has been, by necessity, reversed. In the past several years the small bowel bypass procedure has fallen in popularity and as such the urgency to develop a method of therapeutic management for the enteric hyperoxaluric patient is less acute. Nevertheless we feel the enteric hyperoxaluric model is a good one against which therapeutics for more generalized types of oxalate stone disease can be tested, especially in light of evidence suggesting the presence of increased gastrointestinal oxalate absorption in some "idiopathic" stone formers[3].

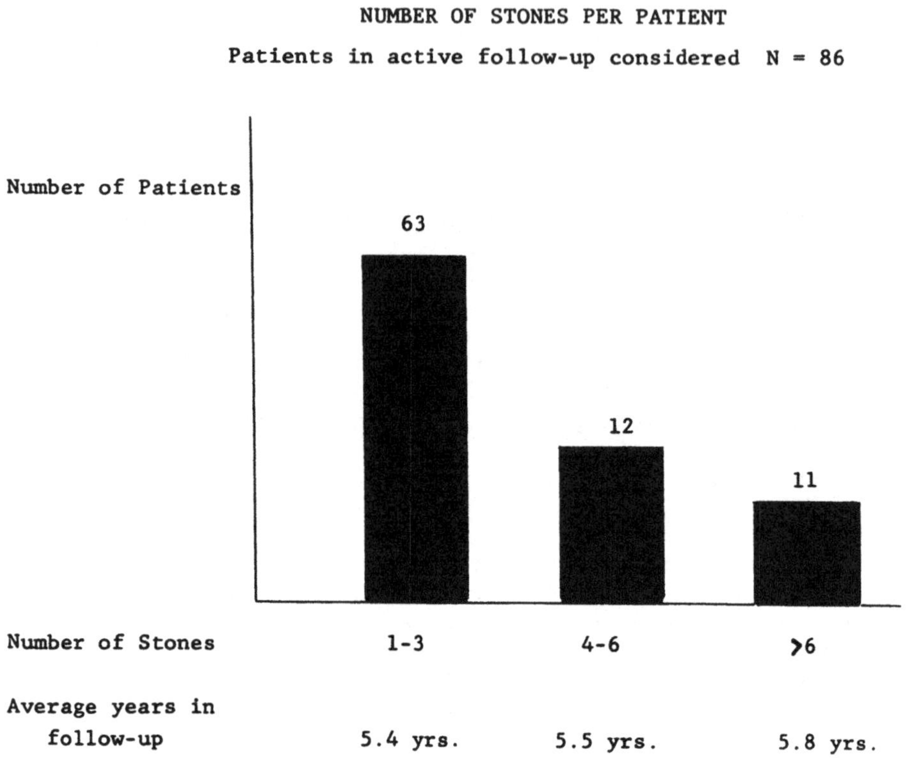

Fig. 1.

Small bowel bypass patients are uniformly hyperoxaluric. The urinary oxalate being of exogenous origin[4]. (Figure 2) The individual with the intact bowel absorbs less than 10% of the measured dietary oxalate whereas the individual with the shortened bowel can absorb up to 50% of the same oxalate[5], predominantly via the colon[6]. In addition to being hyperoxaluric the bowel shortened patient demonstrates hypocalciuria. It is thought that the steatorrhea that occurs following bypass causes a formation with the intragut calcium of an intralumenal soap, thus reducing the formation probability in the gut of insoluble calcium oxalate salt but allowing instead the free, highly soluble oxalate to be absorbed in large quantities across the gut lumen[7]. If this mechanism is correct it is certainly reasonable to employ oral calcium supplementation as a therapeutic modality hoping, by mass action, to overload the gastrointestinal tract with calcium and force the reaction toward the formation of insoluble calcium oxalate. In the small bowel bypass patient an inverse relationship has been demonstrated between dietary calcium and urinary oxalate.

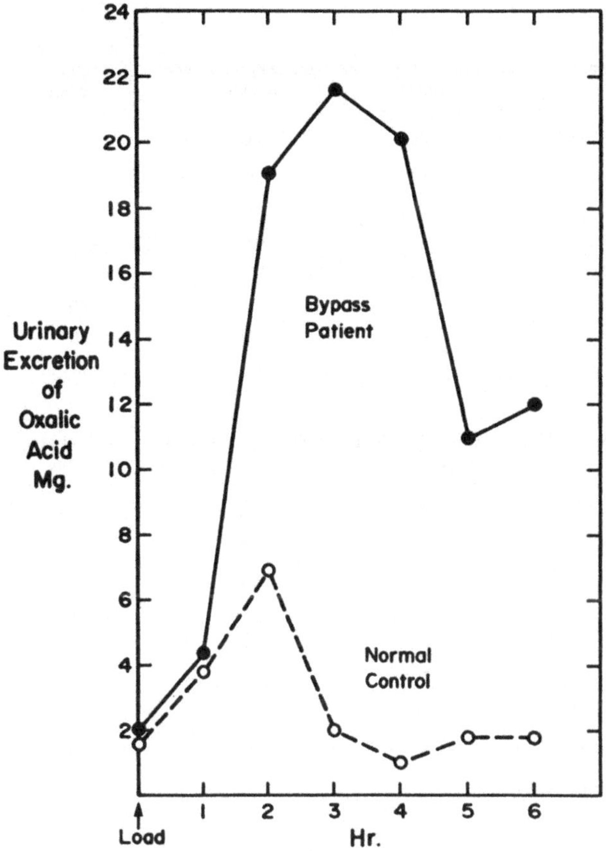

Fig. 2. The urinary excretion of oxalate following an oral load of 200 mg sodium oxalate in a normal individual and a small bowel bypass patient.

A second therapeutic approach to enteric hyperoxaluria was first encountered in our laboratory while developing methodology for oxalate quantitation[9]. In the course of preliminary experiments we noted that calcium oxalate precipitation occurred best at pH 5.0, and in fact at an alkaline pH calcium oxalate precipitation did not occur. This effect is shown in an acute dog experiment where the animal was infused with sodium oxalate resulting in time in an elevated urinary calcium oxalate ion product recorded as the negative log of the ion product and in an appreciable increase in urinary crystallization (Figure 3A). When the animal was alkalinized prior to oxalate infusion crystallization was suppressed until a much higher ion product, again recorded as the negative log (Figure 3B).

(a)

Urine Specimen	Urine pH	Urinary Calcium µg/ml	Urinary Oxalate µg/ml	Wt.of CaOx Crystals µg/ml	-log ion product
1	5.8	76	26	0	6.26
2	5.9	81	65	11	5.83
3	5.8	98	149	89	5.39
4	5.9	120	205	140	5.17
5	5.8	96	161	120	5.37
6	5.9	128	278	200	5.01
7	5.8	88	406	250	5.00

(b)

Urine Specimen	Urine pH	Urinary Calcium µg/ml	Urinary Oxalate µg/ml	Crystals µg/ml	-log ion product
1	8	116	39	0	5.90
2	7.8	88	72	0	5.75
3	8	94	124	0	5.49
4	8	96	161	14	5.37
5	7.9	100	256	33	5.50
6	8	70	431	49	5.08
7	8.1	72	491	77	5.01

Fig. 3. Awake Animals

3(a). infused with sodium oxalate
3(b). alkalinized with sodium bicarbonate prior to infusion with sodium oxalate

Measurement made of urinary oxalate, calcium and crystal content.

In an attempt to analyze the effect of these two therapeutic modalities, calcium supplementation and alkalinization, we have clinically compared the effects in the same small bowel bypass patients of one week of no treatment control, one week of calcium carbonate therapy given as 2 grams of calcium carbonate powder 5 times a day and 1 week of sodium bicarbonate therapy, the bicarbonate given so that the patients maintained a urinary pH of 7.0 or greater as tested by the patient at each voiding. On the last day of the 7 day treatment schedule multiple urine collections were taken and analyzed for pH, total calcium, oxalate and crystal content (recorded as that percent of the total oxalate present in crystal form), and for an estimate of the urinary calcium oxalate concentration product ratio (CPR)[10]. Pak and co-workers[11] have shown a good correlation between the CPR and the more laborious method of determining activity product ratio, as long as close attention to technique is employed[12].

	Date	Urine Specimen	Time Voided	Volume Voided	pH	Microscopic Observation	Percent Crystals	Oxalate µg/ml	Calcium µg/ml	CPR	-log IP
Patient D.W.	12-6-79	1	7:00 am	105 cc	5.0	DB	7.0	155	32	5.2	5.86
		2	12:45 pm	150 cc	5.0	DB	2.0	128	22	4.1	6.10
		3	2:45 pm	170 cc	5.0	DB	2.0	166	20	3.9	6.03
Control		4	7:00 pm	180 cc	5.0	DB	2.0	125	18	3.6	6.20
Specimens		5	10:00 pm	90 cc	5.0	DB	3.0	288	16	4.4	5.89
	12-7-79	6	12:10 am	60 cc	5.5	DB	15.0	118	52	13.4	5.76
		7	3:30 am	75 cc	5.0	DB	17.0	186	66	17.0	5.46
		8	6:15 am	50 cc	5.2	DB	20.0	163	80	17.6	5.44
		9	8:45 am	95 cc	5.0	DB	7.0	136	32	4.8	5.91
		10	11:00 am	140 cc	6.0	DB	2.0	174	20	4.9	6.01
	12-14-79	1	3:30 am	50 cc	5.8	DB	25.0	126	160	10.3	5.25
		2	6:45 am	80 cc	5.5	DB	34.0	115	98	10.5	5.50
Specimens		3	8:30 am	105 cc	6.0	DB	50.0	162	88	13.5	5.40
following		4	11:15 am	70 cc	6.0	DB & Oct	52.0	149	108	11.1	5.35
calcium		5	1:00 pm	60 cc	5.8	DB	7.0	66	114	5.6	5.68
loading		6	2:00 pm	180 cc	5.0	DB	3.0	65	96	3.7	5.76
		7	3:45 pm	240 cc	5.0	DB	2.0	48	76	2.3	5.99
		8	6:00 pm	90 cc	5.0	DB	2.0	59	76	3.3	5.92
		9	10:30 pm	150 cc	5.0	DB	4.0	84	88	3.2	5.68
	12-15-79	10	2:00 am	150 cc	5.0	DB	5.0	73	72	3.1	5.83
	12-22-79	1	12:15 am	30 cc	7.8	x	0	107	60	1.5	5.74
		2	7:00 am	60 cc	8.0	x	0	118	52	1.6	5.76
		3	7:45 am	70 cc	8.0	x	0	161	48	1.4	5.66
Specimens		4	9:45 am	60 cc	7.9	x	0	107	48	.97	5.84
following		5	1:15 pm	60 cc	8.0	x	0	163	52	1.8	5.62
alkalinization		6	3:30 pm	210 cc	8.0	x	0	108	8	.8	6.61
		7	5:30 pm	30 cc	8.0	x	0	179	4	.65	6.69
		8	8:30 pm	80 cc	8.0	x	0	164	6	1.0	6.56
	12-23-79	9	12:20 am	120 cc	8.0	x	0	160	10	1.26	6.34
		10	5:50 am	150 cc	8.0	x	0	106	8	.83	6.61

DB = Dumbbell crystals (CaOx monohydrate)
Oct = Octahedral, dodecahedral and bipyramidal
CPR = Concentration product ratio [10]

Fig. 4. The urinary findings in a single small bowel bypass patient: on no medication, following calcium loading, and following alkalinization.

A typical patient is seen in Figure 4. On no therapy the patient shows the typical urine pattern of high oxalate, low calcium, acid pH and marked crystal formation. After 1 week of calcium therapy the pH and volume remained unchanged, urinary oxalate does decrease, but urinary calcium also increases, the crystal content increased in some specimens as does the CPR value. After 1 week of bicarbonate therapy the pH of the urine samples is increased, urinary volume remains the same as does the urinary oxalate content, urinary calcium decreases, urinary crystals are not seen and the CPR falls dramatically.

A summary of the comparative values found in 10 small bowel bypass stone forming patients (Figure 5) demonstrates the capability of urinary alkalinization to prevent calcium oxalate crystallization in this small group of patients.

	Normal Subjects (n=24)	Small bowel bypass stone former (n=30)	Small bowel bypass stone former with $CaCO_3$ (n=10)	Small bowel bypass stone former with alkalinization (n=10)
Urinary pH	5.8	5.0	6.1	7.8
Total Volume (ml/24 hr)	1,670	850	867	910
Calcium (µg/ml)	107 ± 18	75 ± 8	115 ± 10	45 ± 6
Oxalate (µg/ml)	22 ± 2	144 ± 7	85 ± 6	128 ± 5
Calcium Oxalate Crystal (µg/ml)	0	65.5	48	5.2
CPR*	2.94	11.5	9:5	2.85

*CPR = ratio of the concentration product of calcium and oxalate

Fig. 5. Effect of oral calcium and alkalinization upon urinary oxalate and calcium excretion in the small bowel bypass patients. The mean values are indicated.

Unfortunately, urinary alkalinization is not easily achieved in the small bowel bypass patient. Large amounts of alkali must be consumed to alkalinize most patients. Sodium bicarbonate is the least expensive and most readily available agent but cannot be used in hypertensive individuals, has an objectionable taste and causes

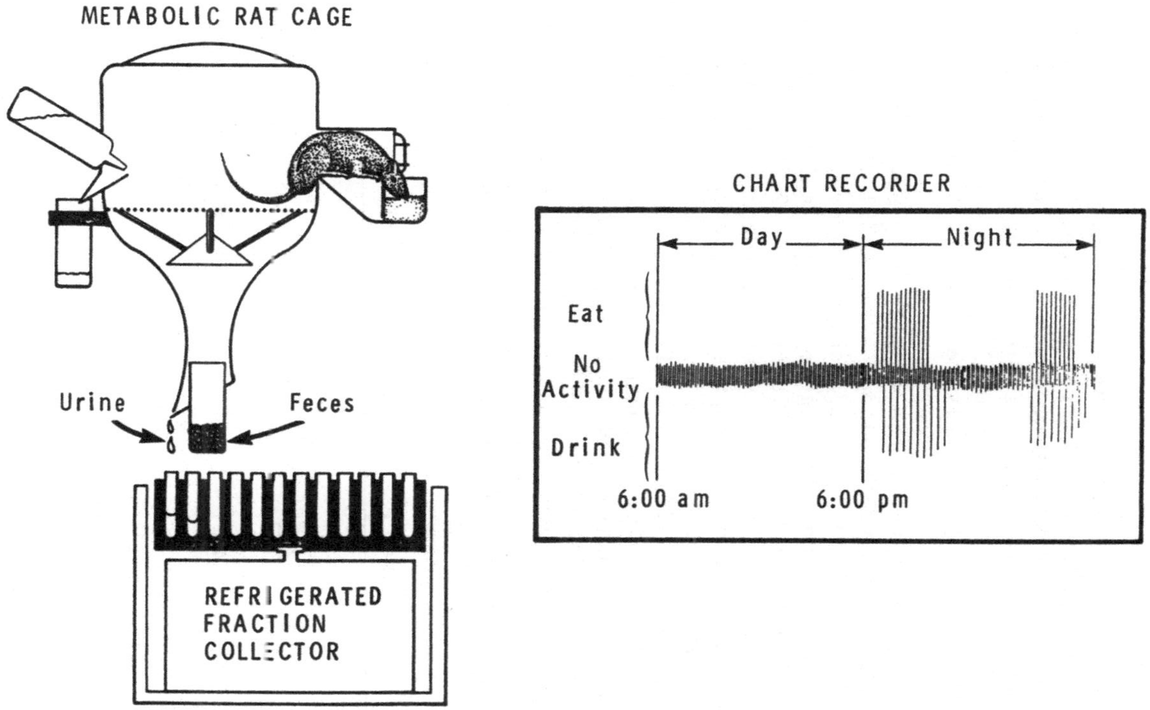

Fig. 6. Schematic of metabolic chamber with urine collection and intake monitors.

flatulence. Polycitra K (potassium citrate - Willen Co.) is not palatable, expensive and only available in liquid form. Citrolith (potassium and sodium citrate - Beach Co.) is palatable and is available in tablet form but must be taken in large quantities and is expensive.

Despite the practical difficulties associated with the alkalinization of bypass patients, the concept that a pH change can demonstrably effect crystallization and stone formation we felt warranted further consideration as did the fact that calcium ingestion may in addition to lowering oxalate act to elevate urinary calcium, an observation previously reported by Stauffer[13].

In an attempt to explore the relationship between calcium and oxalate absorption we have developed a rat model made hyperoxaluric by feeding a diet containing added sodium oxalate. The rat is maintained in a metabolic chamber (Figure 6) which allows separation of urine and feces with the urine aliquotted over 24 hours by a refrigerated fraction collector. Electrical contacts allow records to be made of actual drinking and feeding time and in turn an estimate of the amount of food and fluid consumed. Light and dark periods are controlled and the animals are undisturbed for 24 hours. At appropriate times individual animals are sacrificed and the kidneys analyzed for calcium and oxalate content. Individual animals are quite consistent in their eating and drinking patterns. (Figure 7) Intake predominantly occurs during active periods (in this experiment the 12 dark hours) with nearly simultaneous consumption of food and water occurring in most animals.

Collection Period	Day 1	Day 2	Day 3	Day 4
Active				
1st 6 hours	$\frac{2.8}{3.1}$	$\frac{2.1}{2.8}$	$\frac{3.1}{3}$	$\frac{2.8}{3}$
2nd 6 hours	$\frac{4.1}{3}$	$\frac{3.1}{3.1}$	$\frac{2.5}{2.8}$	$\frac{3.2}{3}$
Quiet				
1st 6 hours	$\frac{0}{.6}$	$\frac{0}{0}$	$\frac{.3}{.2}$	$\frac{0}{.1}$
2nd 6 hours	$\frac{2.1}{.5}$	$\frac{1.2}{.5}$	$\frac{1.0}{.2}$	$\frac{1.0}{.5}$

Fig. 7. Feeding time for normal 150 gram rat.

$$\frac{\text{eating min/hr}}{\text{drinking min/hr}}$$

	Day 1	Day 2	Day 3	Day 4
Food g / Water ml	25/43	25/40	23/41	24/39

Fig. 8. 24 hour intake of food and water for normal 150-gram rat.

	Urine μg/ml		Kidney mg/g	
DIET	Oxalate	Calcium	Oxalate	Calcium
Control	50	100	0.2	0.1
5% Sodium Oxalate	500	40	0.8	0.2
5% Sodium Oxalate 5% Calcium Chloride	100	100	0.2	0.2
5% Sodium Oxalate 5% Calcium Carbonate	100	75	0.2	0.1

Fig. 9. Urine and kidney levels of calcium and oxalate. Collections made after 10 days maintenance on the diet indicated. There are 3 animals in each group. Mean values are indicated.

The total amounts of food and water consumed are likewise quite consistent for the individual animal. (Figure 8)

After establishing normal values for individual animals we added five percent sodium oxalate to the diets of the animals and again after 4 days measured timed excretion levels of calcium and oxalate (Figure 9). The addition of sodium oxalate acted to increase the urinary oxalate and decrease the urinary calcium presumably by gut binding of calcium by oxalate. The tissue levels of oxalate did not appreciably change from those observed in normal animals. The animals were next given a combination of 5% sodium oxalate in their water and 5% calcium chloride in their food (Figure 9). This combination reduced the urinary oxalate to near normal levels and did not increase the tissue calcium oxalate levels. Animals given calcium carbonate behaved in a similar fashion but were noted to have a urinary pH one unit above the control level.

From an observation of the individual feeding records it is clear that the rat eats and drinks at the same time and in this experiment acts ideally to cause the presence in the GI tract of calcium and oxalate at identical points in time. To interfere with this sequence of events we next explored the possibility of an intermittent calcium oxalate diet. To do this we fed a rat sodium oxalate in a normal diet for 5 days and then discontinued the supplemental feedings and recorded the urinary oxalate values (Figure 10). It appeared that the urinary oxalate levels remained elevated after discontinuing oxalate supplementation, slowly lowering over the ensuing 48 hours.

Time Hours	Urinary Oxalate μg/ml
0- 6	300
6-12	200
12-18	120
18-24	100
24-30	110
30-36	75
36-42	85
42-48	50

Fig. 10. Urinary oxalate excretion of an animal on control diet following 5 days of 5% sodium oxalate added diet.

We next alternated supplemental calcium with supplemental oxalate feedings adding oxalate to the diet for 5 days then removing oxalate and adding calcium. Following several weeks of this alternating protocol considerable tissue levels of calcium oxalate were found (Figure 11).

Time on Diet Weeks	Diet	Kidney Assay Calcium mg/g	Kidney Assay Oxalate mg/g
5	5% NaOx 5.5% $CaCl_2$	.1	.240
4	5 days 5% NaOx alternate 5 days 5% $CaCo_3$	2.4	3.3
4	5 days 5% NaOx alternate 5 days 5.5% $CaCl_2$	4.1	9.8
5	5 days 5% NaOx alternate 5 days 5% $CaCo_3$	1.0	2.1
5	5 days 5% NaOx alternate 5 days 5.5% $CaCl_2$	4.4	9.6

Fig. 11. Renal tissue levels of calcium and oxalate following intermittent feeding of calcium and oxalate. Figures represent individual animals.

We feel these rat experiments are in accordance with our patient studies and support the idea that while calcium feeding can reduce urinary oxalate the calcium and oxalate must not be given intermittently for in such cases the effect will be opposite to that desired in terms of urinary oxalate and especially in terms of tissue calcium oxalate levels. In the enteric hyperoxaluric patient we wonder if it is ever possible, because of the continuous eating pattern these patients have, to cause the presence in the gut of calcium at each and every time the oxalate intake is high.

Alkalinization appears to be of some use as a method of defense against crystallization and stone formation as has been demonstrated by our patient trials and infused dog preparation. We feel it is this alkalinization effect that explains the relatively reduced tissue levels of calcium oxalate in those rats receiving the oxalate-

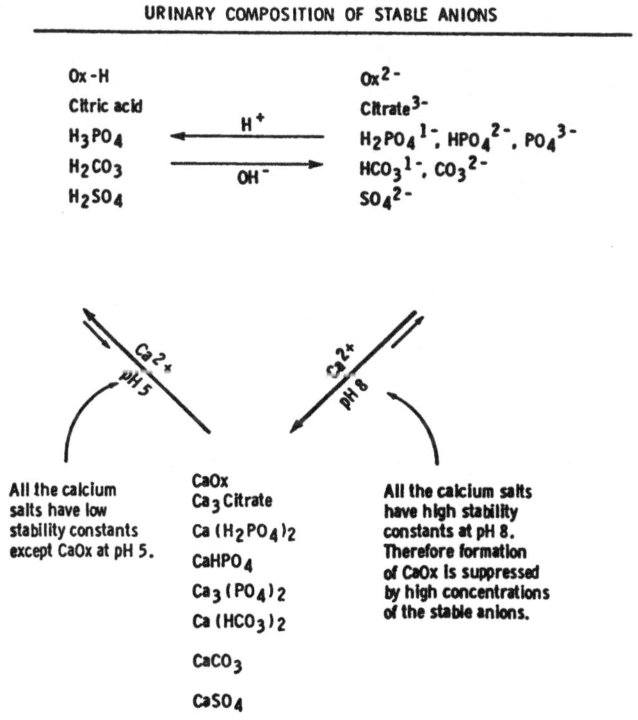

Fig. 12. Urinary composition of stable urines.

$CaCO_3$ alternating diet. The marked effect observed in urine we feel is due to a conversion at an alkaline pH of urinary acids to anionic forms and by the urinary clearance of a percentage of the administered salts as additional anions. These anions compete with oxalate for calcium and form stable soluble salts. Such does not occur at pH 5.0 because at this pH the predominantly stable salt of calcium is calcium oxalate (Figure 12).

From our studies to date we feel that we have demonstrated 1) the importance of analyzing individual events occurring in the kidney not a summary of a 24 hour average, 2) that the urine may be a poor mirror of events occurring in the kidney, 3) calcium therapy for hyperoxaluria will probably reduce urinary oxalate but may well, and especially if given intermittently, increase urinary calcium and the amount of renal calcium oxalate deposits, 4) alkalinization may well play a role as an alternative form of therapy for calcium oxalate stone disease.

REFERENCES

1. W. G. Robertson, M. Peacock, P. J. Heyburn, A. H. Marshall, and P. B. Clark, Br. J. Urol. 50:449 (1978).
2. J. G. Gregory, K. Y. Park, and H. W. Schoenberg, J. Urol. 117:631 (1977).
3. A. Hodgkinson, Clin. Sci. Mol. Med. 54:291 (1978).
4. V. S. Chadwick, K. Modha, and R. H. Dowling, N. Eng. J. Med. 289:172 (1973).
5. D. L. Earnest, G. Johnson, H. E. Williams, and W. H. Admerand, Gastroenterology 66:1114 (1974).
6. R. Modigliani, D. Labayle, C. Aymes, and R. Denvil, Scand. J. Gastroenterology 13:2 (1978).
7. D. L. Earnest, Trans. Assoc. Am. Phys. 88:224 (1975).
8. I. Hessov, C. N. Holm, and L. P. Hansen, Digestion 17:268 (1978).
9. K. Y. Park and J. G. Gregory, Clin. Chem. 26:1170 (1980).
10. C. Y. C. Pak and M. Ohata, Kid. Int. 7:154 (1975).
11. C. Y. C. Pak, Y. Hayashi, B. Finlayson, and S. Chu, J. Lab. Clin. Med. 89:891 (1977).
12. C. Y. C. Pak and S. Chu, Invest. Urol. 11:211 (1973).
13. J. Q. Stauffer, Am. J. Clin. Nutr. 30:64 (1977).

RETROSPECTIVE FOLLOW-UP OF PATIENTS WITH STRUVITE CALCULI

Robert R. Bruce and Donald P. Griffith

Department of Urology, Baylor College of Medicine,

Houston, Texas

The cause and effect relationship of urinary infection and urinary calculi is an ancient concept. Contemporary clinical and experimental investigations support the traditional belief that infection-induced calculi result primarily as a consequence of the hydrolysis of urea by the bacterial enzyme urease[1]. The accumulated information supports the widespread clinical experience that infection induces the formation of struvite and carbonate apatite calculi. The exact incidence of infection-induced calculi is unknown. Available data is collected largely from reference laboratories that analyze many calculi. Such data indicates that the incidence of struvite calculi is up to 20% of calculi analyzed[2]. This may be a falsely elevated figure, because most struvite calculi are removed surgically and sent for analysis whereas a high percentage of other types of stones, such as calcium oxalate, are passed spontaneously and may not be recovered by the patient or sent by the physician for analysis. Struvite stones comprise approximately 15% of the calculi analyzed at the Baylor-affiliated Urolithiasis Laboratory. Since 1973, 2066 struvite calculi have been analyzed. A questionnaire was devised to evaluate the clinical course of these patients retrospectively. These questionnaires were sent to the attending physician for completion. An attempt was made to design a form that could be filled out easily and quickly in order to obtain a good response rate. The main objectives of the study were to evaluate the incidence of recurrent infection, recurrent calculi, and the types of procedures performed for removing calculi. The format was constructed in such a manner that the information obtained could be easily electronically processed for tabulation and analysis. Approximately 600 questionnaires were returned, and of these 527 were adequate for analysis. Ninety-two percent of the stones were removed surgically. Follow-up ranged from 5-74 months with a mean of 14.5 months.

In this series 54% of the patients were female and 46% were male. Pre-treatment urine culture data was available on 74.5% of the patients. Proteus, Pseudomonas, and Klebsiella accounted for the majority of the infections. Approximately 10% of the patients were infected with more than one organism. 25.5% of the cases were uninfected or there was no data available. A recurrent infection was defined as infection at presentation and infection evident on evaluation 30 days or longer after initial treatment. Initial treatment usually consisted of surgical lithotomy and postoperative antimicrobial treatment. The stone recurrence rate for the entire group was 4.5%. One-hundred eight patients developed urinary infection after their initial treatment, the rate of recurrent infection being 20.4%. Of the 108 patients who had recurrent infection 24 patients or 22.5% developed recurrent calculi. The most common procedure performed was pyelolithotomy, which comprised 30% of the operations performed. Nephrolithotomy and ureterolithotomy had an equal incidence of 18%. 16.5% of the operations consisted of open or endoscopic removal of bladder calculi. 7.7% of the calculi were passed spontaneously. The total number of nephrectomies for the group was 55 or 10.4%. However, the nephrectomy rate for patients that developed recurrent calculi was 25%.

Several investigators have shown that urea-splitting organisms are the major, if not the only, bacteria that induce the formation of struvite calculi[3,4]. The bacterial species Proteus, Staphylococcus, Pseudomonas, and Klebsiella are most often associated with calculogenesis. This is consistent with our findings. Because E. coli is rarely if ever the cause of stone formation, the presence of cultures positive for E. coli probably represent secondary infections or concomittant infections with urea-splitting organisms. The vast majority of Proteus species have urea-splitting potential as compared to 63% for Klebsiella and 32% for Pseudomonas. The other organisms cultured and the negative cultures in our series may represent unusual organisms that elaborate urease or those that are difficult to culture by routine methods. Anerobic organisms and mycoplasma species may elaborate urease and could therefore induce formation of struvite stones in the presence of sterile aerobic urine cultures.

Boyce, Wickham and others have reported a rate of recurrent stone formation of 18% in large series[5,6]. The recurrence rate of 4.5% in our series is considerably lower but may reflect the fact that many of the patients in other series were selected from tertiary referral centers. Though the recurrence rate of 4.5% is not alarmingly high, the magnitude of morbidity can be significant. The chronicity and the progressive downhill course of some patients with recurrent stones and recalcitrant urinary infection has prompted some clinicians to refer to this condition as "stone cancer".

Effective treatment should be directed toward total removal of calculous material and urinary catheters plus total eradication of urinary infection. Long-term culture-specific antibiotic therapy that maintains sterile urine is an effective adjunctive measure that retards calculogenesis. When urinary infection persists despite antimicrobial treatment, recurrent calculogenesis is likely to develop. Adjunctive therapy with urease-inhibiting agents may be effective in patients whose urine cannot be sterilized with oral antimicrobial regimens. Additional clinical trials of culture-specific antimicrobial agents and urease-inhibiting drugs are warranted in the 20% of patients with persistent urea-splitting urinary infection.

In summary, the rate of recurrent infection is approximately twenty percent, and the rate of stone recurrence for patients followed for a mean period of 14.5 months was 4.5%. Recurrent infection-induced calculi should be viewed as a chronic illness with life-threatening potential, and these patients should be managed aggressively with antimicrobial and surgical therapy.

REFERENCES

1. D. P. Griffith and D. M. Musher, Invest. Urol. 11:228 (1973).
2. D. P. Griffith, in:"Nephrolithiasis - Pathogenesis and Treatment," F. L. Coe, ed., Year Book Medical Publishers (1978).
3. J. A. Anderson, Invest. Urol. 12:381 (1975).
4. D. P. Griffith and D. M. Musher, in:"Colloquium on Renal Lithiasis," B. Finlayson and W. C. Thomas, Jr., eds., University of Florida Press, Gainesville (1976).
5. J. A. Wickham, N. Coe, and J. P. Ward, J. Urol. 116:148 (1976).
6. W. H. Boyce and E. B. Elkins, J. Urol. 111:307 (1974).

INFECTED RENAL LITHIASIS: RESULTS OF LONG-TERM SURGICAL AND MEDICAL MANAGEMENT

J. W. Segura, S. B. Erickson, D. M. Wilson,
C. J. Van Den Berg, and L. H. Smith
Department of Urology and Nephrology, Mayo Clinic

Rochester, MN 55901

Patients with infection stones composed of struvite ($Mg-NH_4-PO_4$) and associated with infections with urease producing bacteria have been difficult to manage[1-10]. Recurrence of infection, regrowth of stones, and multiple surgical procedures have been common in many long-term studies and some workers have felt that surgery for infected stone was contraindicated because of the high recurrence rate. A long-term study was begun in 1966 to evaluate the effectiveness of a combined program of treatment of infected renal calculi by aggressive surgical removal of stones, careful diagnostic evaluation, and close medical follow-up. This paper concerns the results of this long-term study.

METHOD

Seventy-nine patients (29 men and 50 women) were studied. All had bacteriuria with urease producing bacteria and all had renal stones containing struvite and carbonate apatite. All patients had a complete metabolic work-up, an excretory urogram and microbiological studies of the urine.

RESULTS

The mean follow-up since the last surgical procedure was 6.1 years (range 2-13.3) and the mean time from the discovery of stones to the last operation for stone was 10 years (range 0-40 years), and the mean age at the time the stone was discovered was age 40.

One or more operations were done in 78 patients and over half of the patients had multiple surgical procedures. Urease producing bacteria were cultured from the stones in every case and the most common organisms cultured were Proteus species.

Table 1. Infected Renal Lithiasis
Associated Metabolic Renal Lithiasis

Idiopathic calcium urolithiasis (CaOx nidus)		
With hypercalciuria	yes	24 pt
	no	10
Primary hyperparathyroidism		5
Gout (uric acid nidus)		2
Immobilization		2
Type I RTA		2
Milk alkali syndrome		2
Cystinuria		1
Corticosteroid therapy		1
Total		49 pt (62% of 79)

Diagnostic evaluation revealed an associated metabolic abnormality predisposing to stone formation in 62% of the 79 patients (see Table 1). Structural abnormalities which would predispose to stone formation were noticed in 14% of the 79 patients (see Table 2). Thus, in over three-fourths of the patients a definable cause for the urolithiasis other than infection was discovered.

Table 2. Infected Renal Lithiasis
Structural Aberrations

Obstruction of ureter or ureteropelvic junction	3 pt
Ileal conduit	3
Medullary sponge kidney	1
Neurogenic bladder	1
Ureterovesical reflux	2
Congenital megaureters	1
Total	11 pt (14% of 79)

Renal function was decreased preoperatively in 23 of the 79 patients and was improved after surgery in 6, decreased in 7 and not changed in 66 (see Table 3). Long-term follow-up revealed that 91%

were free of recurrent infected stones, although in 15% new metabolic stones had formed. Recurrent infection occurred in one patient out of four, but in about half the patients there was no new stone or infection (see Table 4).

Table 3. Infected Renal Lithiasis
Renal Infection

Preoperative	
Creatinine clearance <60 ml/min	23 (29% of 79)
At latest follow-up	
Improved	6
No change	66
Decreased	7 (dialysis 1)

Table 4. Infected Renal Lithiasis
Long-Term Follow-Up

Finding	No.	%
Free of new stone and infection	40	51
Recurrent infection	20	25
Recurrent infected stone (retained stone material in 6)	7	9
Metabolic stone formed	12	15
Total	79	100

DISCUSSION

This study demonstrates the high morbidity and chronicity of infected renal lithiasis. By using a multidisciplinary approach that considers the infection, primary metabolic anatomic and functional disorders which may predispose to stone formation and emphasizing careful long-term follow-up, it is apparent that excellent results can be achieved.

The patients were treated preoperatively with 24 hours of bactericidal antibiotic therapy, usually Ampicillin, or, if necessary an aminoglycoside. Such bactericidal therapy was carried through surgery and the hospital period and the patients were discharged on a suppressive medication program, originally methenamine salts and NH_4Cl for urinary acidification. More recently a suppressive program utilizing trimethoprim and sulfamethoxazole has been used. The patients were seen initially at three months after surgery, then usually at three to six months and then afterward as necessary, but no less frequently than annually with continuing follow-up critical to successful management.

REFERENCES

1. J. T. Priestley and J. H. Dunn, J. Urol. 61:194 (1949).
2. J. C. A. Ruys and W. A. Moonen, Arch. Chir. Neerlandicum 20:7 (1968).
3. N. J. Nemoy and T. A. Stamey, JAMA 215:1470 (1971).
4. J. A. Libertino, H. R. Newman, B. Lytton, and R. M. Weiss, J. Urol. 105:753 (1971).
5. M. Singh, G. C. Tresidder, and J. Blandy, Br. J. Urol. 43:658 (1971).
6. M. Singh, R. Chapman, G. C. Tresidder, and J. Blandy, Br. J. Urol. 45:581 (1973).
7. W. H. Boyce and I. B. Elkins, J. Urol. 111:307 (1974).
8. L. H. Smith, in:"Renal Calculi," W. C. Thomas, Jr., ed., C. C. Thomas, Springfield, Illinois (1976).
9. D. P. Griffith, Kid. Int. 13:372 (1978).
10. S. N. Rous and W. R. Turner, J. Urol. 118:902 (1977).

ACKNOWLEDGMENT

This work was supported by grant number AM 20605 from the National Institutes of Health.

INFECTION-INDUCED STONES: STATUS OF CLINIC TRIALS WITH UROSTAT™ (ACETOHYDROXAMIC ACID)

Donald P. Griffith, Pat Moskowitz, and Stuart Feldman

Department of Urology, Baylor College of Medicine
Houston, Texas 77030

The cause and effect relationship between urinary infection and urinary stones has been since antiquity. Bladder stones that we now perceive as infection induced have been found in Egyptian mummies dating back to 5,000 B.C. Hippocrates recognized that putrifying loin abscesses were commonly associated with renal stones. Marcet (1817) suggested that the evolution of ammonia during putrification alkalinized urine and that such alkalinization was "unavoidably attended by the precipitation of phosphates contained in urine." Recent experimental and clinical investigations from a number of investigators have validated these historical concepts.

EXPERIMENTAL INVESTIGATIONS

Experimental investigations have shown that the bacterial enzyme - urease - is the primary biochemical inducer of struvite ($MgNH_4PO_4 \cdot 6H_2O$) and carbonate-apatite [$Ca_{10}(PO_4)_6CO_3$] stones. Both enzyme and substrate (urea) must be present for crystallization of struvite. The hydrolysis of urea (ureolysis) by urease generates high levels of urinary ammonia and alkalinity - events that bring about supersaturation of urine with respect to calcium phosphate and magnesium ammonium phosphate. Such supersaturation rapidly brings about crystallization of struvite and apatite. Urease inhibition prevents the biochemical changes and prevents crystallization and calculogenesis. The validity of the hypothesis has been confirmed *in vitro* and *in vivo* in a number of closely controlled investigations which have recently been summarized[1].

CLINICAL MANIFESTATIONS

Infection-induced urinary stones manifest clinically (a) as soft, mushy, poorly mineralized matrix concretions within the pyelocaliceal system, (b) as branched "staghorn" renal calculi that completely fill the pyelocaliceal system, and (c) as bladder stones. The bladder stones develop predominantly in patients who utilize indwelling catheters or intermittent self-catheterization.

The organic matrix that commonly occurs in association with these stones is poorly understood. Preliminary investigations[2] have shown that this matrix material contains large concentrations of glycoaminoglycans (GAG). It is probable that the alkalinity and ammonia generated from ureolysis cause chemical injury to the urothelium and that such an insult results in GAG production by mucosal or submucosal cells.

Infection-induced stones are not common but are life-threatening - particularly in patient populations who are "at risk" of chronic urinary tract infection. For example, only ten to fifteen percent of the urinary stones analyzed by commercial laboratories contain struvite. However, the actual incidence may be much less because struvite stones tend to be analyzed more frequently than metabolic stones. Struvite stones are usually removed surgically (and sent for analysis) whereas metabolic stones usually pass spontaneously (and may not be recovered or analyzed). On the other hand, chronic urinary infection, recurrent stones and progressive azotemia were the cause of death in almost 50% of the World War II and Korean conflict veterans with spinal cord injury who have been followed for twenty and fifteen years respectively[3].

Modern treatment consists of surgical removal of all calculous material and concomitant administration of antimicrobial agents to completely eliminate infection. If infection persists within tissues and/or if calculous material is left behind, then persistent infection is likely. Persistent urea-splitting infection places the patient in a "high risk" category for recurrent stone formation. A recent literature review[4] suggests that urinary infection persisted in approximately 40% of patients treated in this conventional manner and that perhaps 60% of those at risk developed recurrent stones. A recent review of our own experience has shown that approximately 20% of patients treated in a conventional manner (surgery and antibiotics) harbor persistent infection; approximately 20% of those at risk (with infection) developed recurrent stones (mean follow-up = 14.5 months)[5].

HYDROXAMIC ACIDS

For the past nine years we have been studying the biochemical interactions of urease and hydroxamic acids. This work has recently been reviewed[1]. Most of the hydroxamic acids which are characterized by a

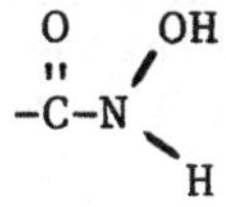

configuration are effective inhibitors of urease. When considered on the basis of structure, activity, and toxicity, acetohydroxamic acid (AHA) appears to offer the greatest pharmacologic promise.

Pharmacokinetic and preliminary clinical trials of the clinical use of AHA have been reported[6-8]. These studies showed that AHA is rapidly and completely absorbed from the gastrointestinal tract; peak blood levels occur in approximately one-half hour. Approximately 40-60% of an oral dose is excreted unchanged in urine. The percentage of unaltered AHA that is recovered in urine is higher (and the half-life is longer) in patients taking high doses as compared to low doses. This finding indicates that AHA is partially metabolized and that as the metabolic pathway becomes saturated a larger percentage of unaltered AHA is excreted in urine. Unpublished ^{14}C-AHA studies have shown that 25-30% of AHA is metabolized to CO_2 and excreted via the lungs[9]. Approximately 10% is excreted in the urine as acetamide. The half-life (which is 5-10 hours in volunteers with normal renal function) is prolonged in patients with renal insufficiency.

Patients must concentrate their urine to a reasonable extent to develop therapeutic concentrations of AHA (in urine). Though urease inhibition has been reported with concentrations as low as 8 mcg/ml[10], we have strived to obtain urinary AHA concentrations as high as possible to give the highest probability of efficacy.

CLINICAL TRIALS OF AHA

Seventy-six (76) patients ranging in age from 3-86 years have been treated with AHA for three months or longer. This population is derived from a larger population of 124 potential candidates. Reasons for failure of 48 patients to participate include: (a) advanced azotemia, (b) cured with conventional therapy, (c) advanced co-existent disease, (d) patients' disinterest, (e) absence of a documented urea-splitting urinary infection, (f) patients' concern for side effects (i.e., headaches, rash) during the first week of treatment, and (g) logistical and/or expense problems.

Of the 76 patients 31 (41%) had an anatomically functional urinary tract; the other 45 (59%) had some form of urinary diversion (i.e., intestinal conduit, Foley catheter, nephrostomy tube, etc.). Thirty-seven (49%) of the seventy-six patients were either paraplegic or quadriplegic.

Forty-six (46) of the patients had undergone ninety-seven surgical lithotomy procedures (average = 2.1 procedures/patient) prior to beginning treatment. After initiating treatment 25 patients underwent 38 surgical procedures for removal of stones. Three of these 38 procedures were performed to remove new/or larger stones that developed during AHA treatment. The other 35 procedures were performed to remove stones that were present prior to treatment with AHA.

Forty-three (43%) percent of the 76 patients had laboratory evidence of renal insufficiency prior to beginning treatment. Patients with a serum creatinine greater than 2.5 mg/dl were treated infrequently and patients with a serum creatinine greater than 3.0 mg/dl were not offered treatment.

All candidates were offered treatment with AHA. Patients with serum creatinine less than 2.5 mg/dl were/are offered treatment at the following oral dose: for greater than 70 kg body weight (BW) - one (1) 250 mg dose four times per day at 6-hour intervals; for 50-70 kg BW - one (1) 250 mg dose three times per day at 8-hour intervals; and for less than 50 kg BW - one (1) 250 mg dose two times per day at 12-hour intervals. Adult patients with serum creatinine of 2.5 -3.0 mg/dl were offered treatment with one (1) 250 mg dose two times per day at 12-hour intervals regardless of body weight.

This clinical trial was initiated in 1974 and was terminated in November, 1979. Patients were treated for 3-60 months (mean = 17.2 months for a total inclusive treatment period of 1,309 patient moths).

SIDE EFFECTS/TOXICITIES

Treatment was interrupted for one week or longer on 66 occasions for an accrued time of 52 patient months. Thus, net treatment time for all 76 patients was 1,257 patient months. The cause for these temporary interruptions is listed in Table 1.

A higher percentage of patients reported mild, tolerable side effects that were usually transient. Such side effects include:

Headaches - 75% of patients reported mild headaches during the first week of treatment. Simple analgesics usually gave relief.

GI Upset - 50% of patients reported a change in bowel habits - usually mild. Diarrhea/constipation was noted with approximately equal frequency. Symptoms occurred at all times during treatment.

Tremulousness/Weakness - 4% of patients reported a diminished sense of well-being, weakness and/or tremulousness.

Flushing Sensation with Alcohol - 8% of patients reported a warm, erythematous flushing sensation following ingestion of alcoholic beverages. The sensation characteristically persists for 30 minutes and disappears spontaneously.

Table 1. Temporary Treatment Interruptions

	Instance	%
Surgical Procedures	19	27
Toxic Reactions		
Mild anemia	12	17
Severe anemia	2	3
Phlebitis	9*	13
Pulmonary emboli	1*	1.4
Side Effects		
Headache	8*	11
Rash	2	3
GI upset	4*	6
Tremulousness	3*	4
Logistical/Social	7	10
	70	

*4 patients had more than one reaction/side effect. Percentages are based on 70 causes for interruption of treatment.

Forty-eight (48) of the 76 patients were on treatment with AHA when this uncontrolled trial was formally terminated in November, 1979. The reasons for termination are detailed below:

	No. of Patients	%
Completion of Study	48	63
Early Termination/Voluntary		
Toxic Reactions/Side Effects	7xx	9xx
Anemia (1)		
Phlebitis (5)		
Rash (1)		
Loss of Candidacy	21	28
Sterile Urine Postop (8)		
Secondary Medical Problems (2)		
Death (1)		
Azotemia (1)		
Compliance (9)		
	76	100

[xx]These patients were also reported as having temporary interruptions in treatment. These patients elected not to resume treatment.

Signs and symptoms invariably returned to normal following cessation of treatment with AHA.

Blood transfusions were given to only one (1) patient to treat his anemia. This severe reaction occurred in a patient with azotemia during the early phases of the investigation.

Anticoagulants were utilized in five (5) patients whose treatment was terminated because of phlebitis. Two (2) of these five had been treated with anticoagulants for phlebitis months to years before being treated with AHA.

One patient (#76) expired suddenly while on treatment. An autopsy demonstrated an acute myocardial infarction and severe occlusive coronary artery disease. There was no evidence of thromboembolism.

SCREENING BLOOD TESTS

Screening blood tests were analyzed pretreatment and at three-month intervals during treatment. The blood test data may be summarized as follows:

Renal Function (Blood urea nitrogen and creatinine) - The study population contained a large number of patients with mild to modest impairment in renal function. BUN and creatinine levels were not significantly altered during treatment.

Hematological Function [Hemoglobin (Hgb), Hematocrit (Hct), White Blood Count (WBC), Reticulocyte Count (Retic)] - The hematological status of the entire population is in the low normal range prior to treatment. A hemolytic anemia was detected in 14 patients. In two (2) patients the anemia was severe enough to require hospitalization. One patient was given blood transfusions. Erythrocyte fragility tests, Coombs' tests, and incubated fragility tests were performed on several patients at the time of their hemolytic reaction. These tests were normal. The reticulocyte count was invariably elevated in patients who showed evidence of hemolysis (i.e., a falling Hbg and Hct). A mild elevation in reticulocytes occurred in 33% of patients. Treatment was not altered because of the mild reticulocytosis. Significant alterations in the white blood cell (WBC) counts were not observed. Even patients who had severe hemolysis had little change in the WBC count. No change was noted in the morphological character of platelets; platelet counts were not performed.

Iron (Fe) - Serum Fe was commonly in the low normal or below normal range prior to treatment. This finding probably results from their chronic urinary infection and chronic renal disease.

We perceived no significant changes in these parameters as a group phenomena. However, we developed the clinical impression that patients who took oral iron (to treat a pre-existent anemia) concomitantly with AHA may have had incomplete intestinal absorption of both drugs.

Liver Function (Albumin, SGOT, Total Bilirubin, Alkaline Phosphatase) - We perceived no appreciable change in liver function studies. Bilirubin levels became mildly and transiently elevated in the two patients who had the most severe hemolytic anemia.

Electrolytes (Ca, Phosphorus, Na, K, Cl) - We perceived no appreciable change in these parameters.

Serum Glucose, Cholesterol, Triglycerides, Total Lipids, and Uric Acid - We perceived no significant change in these parameters.

URINARY CHEMISTRIES

Urinary chemistries have been reported previously[4,7,8]. Urinary alkalinity and NH_3 were reduced in virtually every patient studied.

Figure 1 characterizes the urinary ammonia and pH levels in a patient with congenital paraplegia (meningomyelocele) treated with two different doses of AHA. Note that neither dose completely normalized his urinary pH and ammonia levels. However, the patient commented upon the improved clarity (loss of turbidity) and diminished ammoniacal odor of his urine.

Figure 2 details the changes in urinary ammonia and alkalinity in patients with 1.0 gm/day of AHA for two weeks or longer.

RADIOGRAPHIC DATA

Documentation of the therapeutic efficacy of AHA as determined by radiographic changes in stone size/number is exceedingly difficult owing to the absence of a suitable control population, interruptions in treatment and incompletely documented patient compliance. In a sub-set study wherein patients were used as their own historical controls treatment with AHA significantly retarded stone growth[8].

Anecdotal observations include the following: (a) Rapid stone growth/recurrence has occurred in 5 patients since cessation of AHA (November 1979) and randomization into a double-blind protocol (April 1980). None of these patients had had stone growth during the preceding 12-36 months during which time they were on treatment with AHA. (b) Stone growth/recurrence occurred during temporary interruptions in AHA treatment in three patients who had temporary interruptions in treatment because of side

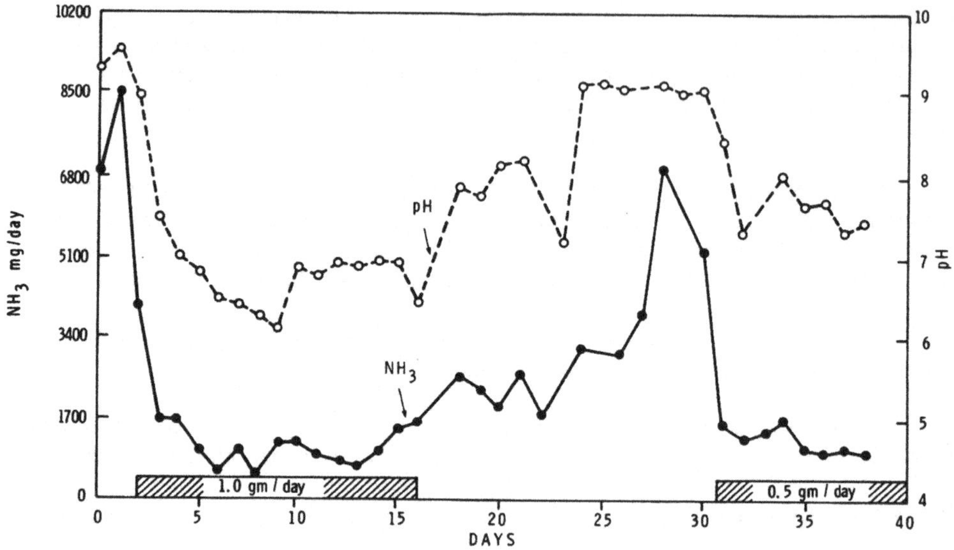

Fig. 1. Urine pH and ammonia in D.C., a 21-year-old paraplegic with an ileal conduit, chronic <u>Proteus</u> urinary infection and bilateral staghorn renal calculi treated with 2 doses of acetohydroxamic acid. Urinary pH and ammonia were reduced but not normalized (normal pH < 6.5; ammonia < 800 mg/day).

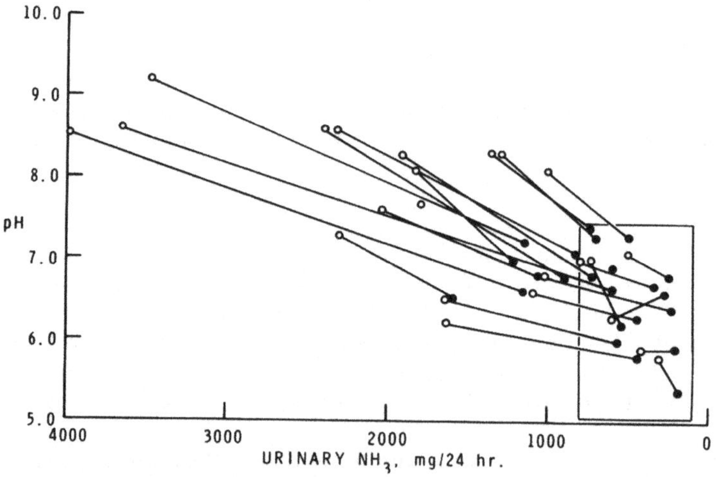

Fig. 2. Changes in urinary pH and ammonia induced in 23 patients during long-term treatment with acetohydroxamic acid (AHA), 500 mg per os twice daily. Open circles denote <u>Proteus</u>-infected patients on no treatment; closed circles denote <u>Proteus</u>-infected patients on AHA; rectangle enclosure means values ± SD of patient controls (N=20) with sterile urine.

effects or toxic reactions. Similar events probably occurred in two other patients but are incompletely documented. (c) Stone dissolution has been a rare occurrence (3-4 kidneys). (d) Most patients note that their urine becomes less cloudy and less ammoniacal during treatment. Virtually all patients note a recurrence of turbidity and ammoniacal odor when treatment is interrupted. (e) Several patients have noted less inflammation/excoriation about the stomas of their ileal conduits while on treatment.

SUMMARY AND CONCLUSIONS

There is an abundant amount of experimental and clinical data to support the contention that the bacterial enzyme urease is the primary biochemical mediator of infection-induced stones composed of struvite and carbonate-apatite. Peroral treatment with AHA at doses of approximately 15 mg/kg/day (i.e., 1.0 gm/day in divided doses) effectively reduces urinary alkalinity and ammoniuria in patients with recalcitrant urea-splitting bacteriuria who have sufficient renal function to concentrate the drug in their urine. Such treatment reduces the turbidity and ammoniacal odor of urine.

Dissolution of stones has occurred infrequently. The therapeutic efficacy of AHA and probably any other urease inhibitor will likely result from its ability to retard or prevent stone growth or recurrence in patients whose urea-splitting urinary infection cannot be eliminated with conventional therapy. Such an effect, however, is incompletely documented.

Treatment with AHA does not replace conventional treatment. Surgical candidates with potentially curable stone disease should be offered curative procedures. Patients who harbor persistent urea-splitting bacteriuria or who are poor surgical candidates will probably benefit from long-term adjunctive chemotherapy with AHA.

Side effects and toxicities that result from AHA are dose-related and apparently reversible. A lesser incidence of side effects is likely with a smaller dose which may be equally as effective as the large doses used in this trial. We are convinced that the hemolytic anemia is AHA induced but are less certain about the phlebitis. The phlebitis that we have encountered may be an endemic problem in the study population.

Multi-center clinical trials are warranted.

REFERENCES

1. D. P. Griffith, R. R. Bruce, and W. N. Fishbein, in: "Nephrolithiasis," F. L. Coe, B. M. Brenner, and J. H. Stein,

eds., Churchill Livingstone, New York, p. 231 (1980).
2. C. Sato, Personal communication.
3. J. Donnelly, R. H. Hackler, and R. C. Brents, J. Urol. 108: 558 (1972).
4. D. P. Griffith, Kid. Int. 13:372 (1978).
5. R. Bruce and D. P. Griffith, in:"Proceedings of the IV International Symposium on Urolithiasis Research," (in press).

ACKNOWLEDGMENT

Supported in part by grants from the NIH R01 AM20159, the RSA (NIHR) 13-P-59243/6, the Veterans Administration, and the Baylor Urolithiasis Laboratory.

UREASE INHIBITORS IN THE TREATMENT OF INFECTION INDUCED STONES: SOME CHEMICAL, PHARMACOLOGIC AND CLINICAL CONSIDERATIONS

William N. Fishbein

Biochemistry Division, Armed Forces Institute of Pathology, Washington, D.C. 20306

Urease, the most potent of all amidases, is widely distributed in bacteria, plants, and invertebrates, although absent from the tissues of vertebrates[1]. It is at present the only example known of a nickel metalloenzyme[2,3], and its activity persists over a wide range of H+, urea, ammonia, and bicarbonate concentrations. When present in bacteria invading the urinary tract, it faces an environment peculiarly suited to elicit damage to the host. The potential amounts of ammonia and bicarbonate in urinary urea are, respectively, about 25x and 180x their usual levels in urine, and the hydrolysis constant of ammonium carbonate is about pH 9. Significant ureolysis will therefore result in (1) marked increase in urinary ammonia, (2) dramatic increase in urinary bicarbonate, (3) increase in urine pH leading to the appearance of carbonate and some ammonia vapor. These three factors comprise a vicious circle abetting cell damage and stone formation. They can be aborted, indirectly by bacteriostasis, and/or directly, by inhibiting urease.

The primary hydroxamic acids (HA) are all potent inhibitors of urease, by virtue of both the similarity of their structure (R-CO-NHOH) to the amide groups of urea, which permits access to the active site, and their chelate properties, which results in binding to the nickel atoms, and inhibition of the enzyme[4,5]. The long-chain aliphatic hydroxamates, although potent in vitro inhibitors and patentable, are poorly absorbed and not excreted in the urine[6] and are, moreover, ineffective[7] at pH < 7. The 1-4 carbon hydroxamates were synthesized in our laboratory[8] and studied in mice to compare their disposition, toxicity, and inhibitory potency. All were rapidly absorbed and rapidly, though incompletely, excreted in the urine[9].

Table 1. Acute toxicity of short-chain aliphatic hydroxamates in CAF-1 mice. All deaths occurred within 24 hours; survivors recovered in one day and remained well 3 months later.

Hydroxamate	Route	Dosage Levels	Total Mice	m moles/kg LD_{50}	m moles/kg 95% Cl	g/kg LD_{50}	g/kg 95% Cl
Aceto-	po	5	50	63.2	60.5-69.2	4.74	4.54-5.19
	sc	5	50	32.4	22.8-41.0	2.43	1.71-3.08
	ip	4	100	35.5	33.7-37.3	2.66	2.53-2.80
Formo-	ip	5	50	12.4	10.0-15.6	0.75	0.61-0.95
Propiono-	ip	5	50	22.6	21.1-24.2	2.01	1.87-2.16
Isobutyro-	ip	6	60	38.0	36.5-39.5	3.91	3.76-4.07

The 1-carbon compound (FormoHA) was the most toxic (Table 1), and the least completely excreted in urine (24%), although it provided the most complete shortterm blockade of ^{14}C-urea hydrolysis [10]. On the chronic toxicity tests it was fatal in 14 days at 0.32 g/kg/day with pronounced leukopenia, rather than anemia, which predominated with the other compounds (Table 2). The 2-carbon compound (AcetoHAHA) was nearly as potent an inhibitor[11], but was much less toxic (LD_{50} = 2.7 g/kg) and was the most completely excreted in urine (65%). On chronic toxicity tests it was fatal in 13 days at 1 g/kg/day with anemia too pronounced to be explained solely by erythropoietic blockade. It was innocuous for 100 days, however at 0.5 g/kg/day. The complete disposition of this compound was ascertained using 1-^{14}C-AHA. It was absorbed and excreted about half as fast as urea, and was distributed throughout total body water. About 20% was reduced to acetamide and excreted in the urine and 15% was hydrolyzed to acetate and/or carbonate[12]. The 3-carbon compound (PropionoHA) had inhibitory properties and acute and chronic toxicities similar to AHA. It was less completely excreted in urine, however (35%), and was the only homolog that failed to show prolonged urease inhibition 16-22 hrs after a single dose (Table 3). It is also the only homolog that has been shown to be non-teratogenic[13,14]. The 4-carbon compound (IsobutyroHA) was as toxic as AHA, but only 2/3 as potent a urease inhibitor. Its excretion pattern[9] and chronic toxicity (Table 2) were similar to PropionoHA.

These considerations would favor the selection of AcetoHA or PropionoHA, for the clinical therapy of urinary tract infection with ureolytic bacteria. Only the former has been evaluated for toxicity in man, where single large doses (9-10g) were administered to patients with terminal hepatic coma (Table 4). Modest declines in hemoglobin and platelet counts were statistically significant, suggesting that hematopoietic suppression and probably some hemolysis is likely to represent an early manifestation of toxicity, as it does for the related compound, hydroxyurea (aminohydroxamate)[15]. AcetoHA was shown to be effective in reducing blood ammonia levels in patients with hepatic decompensation[16,17]. It was also used to slow down the rate of ureolysis in sheep on urea-supplemented diets, and thereby more than doubled their nitrogen retention[18]. Much more information on the therapeutic potential (and toxicity) of this compound has recently become available as a result of the diligent studies of Griffith, et al.[19].

Table 2. Chronic toxicity of short-chain aliphatic hydroxamates in CAF-1 mice. In several cases the red cell decline is too abrupt to result from etythropoietic blockade alone.

Hydroxamate	Daily Dose g/kg/sc	Total Days	Deaths	Day of Death	Survivors:% Initial Value Day	WBC	RBC	Weight
Aceto-	0.25	88	0/10		(52)	81	96	90
	0.5	63	0/10		(30)		78	95
	0.5	100	0/10					110
	1.0	13	10/10	8-13	(5)	46	44	88
					(10)	35	17	68
Formo-	0.2	42	1/10	22				97
	0.2	110	2/10	11				112
	0.32	14	10/10	5-14	(7)	36	66	78
Propiono-	0.2	42	0/10					105
	0.8	44	10/10	17-44	(17)	95	26	97
					(38)	45	12	83
Isobutyro-	0.15	42	0/10					96
	0.6	42	2/10	20-26				86
	1.8	9	10/10	2-9	(3)	93	33	92
					(7)	68	11	74

Table 3. Inhibition of hydrolysis of labelled urea (given sc) in mice at times noted after ip injection of several hydroxamic acids. Mean ± SE are shown. Labelled urea was injected at 0 hours and again at 16 hours. Adapted from[10]. Amino-hydroxamate = hydroxyurea.

	% Inhibition of ^{14}C-Urea Hydrolysis				
	3.33 mm/kg	13.33 mm/kg (6.72 mm/kg for Formo-)			
Hydroxamate	0-2 Hrs	0-2 Hrs	2-4 Hrs	4-6 Hrs	16-22 Hrs
Formo-	67 ± 5	76 ± 5	51 ± 3	49 ± 10	24 ± 2
Aceto-	61 ± 10	90 ± 2	69 ± 4	65 ± 6	31 ± 3
Propiono-	54 ± 4	85 ± 3	63 ± 8	44 ± 12	-8 ± 10
Isobutyro-	40 ± 11	70 ± 2	64 ± 6	43 ± 11	18 ± 6
Amino-	17 ± 9				
None	0 ± 7				

Table 4. Hematologic effects of single large oral doses of acetohydroxamate (150 mg/kg body weight) in patients with hepatic decompensation. Hemograms were done on the day of treatment and two days later. Several patients had poor renal function, and two developed nausea from the drug. Although small, the fall in hemoglobin, and especially in platelet count, was significant on a paired-trial basis.

		g% Hb			WBC ($x10^3$)			Platelets ($x10^3$)		
Patient	Trial	Before	After	Change	Before	After	Change	Before	After	Change
1	1	11.8	11.2	-0.6	10.2	7.8	-2.4	205	174	-31
	2	10.5	11.4	+0.9	7.2	5.4	-1.8	218	172	-46
	3	12.6	9.9	-2.7	7.6	10.4	+2.8	166	146	-20
2	4	12.1	9.6	-2.5	12.9	11.1	-1.8	---	137	---
	5	7.9	8.3	+0.4	---	14.1	---	117	52	-65
3	6	12.4	10.4	-2.0	6.8	8.6	+1.8	172	154	-18
	7	10.6	---	---	13.1	10.5	-2.6	264	188	-76
4	8	8.3	8.9	+0.6	---	11.9	---	122	102	-20
5	9	9.0	8.4	-0.6	3.0	4.5	+1.5	44	43	-1
6	10	12.5	10.0	-2.5	6.2	2.5	-3.7	---	49	---
	Mean	10.77	9.79	-1.00	8.38	8.68	-0.78	163.5	121.7	-34.6
	SD	1.81	1.12	1.45	3.47	3.64	0.24	68.7	56.0	25.7
	P		>.10	<.10		>.10	>.10		>.10	<.01
	Declines/Total:			6/9			5/8			8/8

REFERENCES

1. A. M. Delluva, K. Markley, and R. E. Davies, Biochim. Biophys. Acta. 151:646 (1968).
2. N. E. Dixon, C. Gazzola, R. L. Blakelay, and B. Zerner, J. Am. Chem. Soc. 97:4131 (1975).
3. W. N. Fishbein, M. J. Smith, K. Nagarajan, and W. Scurzi, Fed. Proc. (USA) 35:1680 (1976).
4. K. Nagarajan and W. N. Fishbein, Fed. Proc. (USA) 36:700 (1977).
5. N. E. Dixon, C. Gazzola, J. J. Watters, R. L. Blakeley, and B. Zerner, J. Am. Chem. Soc. 97:4130 (1975).
6. K. Kobashi, S. Takebe, and J. Hase, Yakugaku Zasshi, 93:1564 (1973).
7. K. Shimbayashi, Y. Cbara, T. Yonemura, N. Deguchi, and M. Nakanashi, Jap. J. Vet. Sci. 35:327 (1973).
8. W. N. Fishbein, J. Daly, and C. L. Streeter, Anal. Biochem. 28: 13 (1969).
9. W. N. Fishbein and C. L. Streeter, J. Pharm. Exp. Therap. 174:239 (1970).
10. W. N. Fishbein and J. E. Daly, Proc. Soc. Exp. Biol. Med. 134: 1083 (1970).
11. W. N. Fishbein, Biochem. Med. 1:111 (1967).
12. W. N. Fishbein, C. L. Streeter and J. Daly, J. Pharm. Exp. Therap. 186:173 (1973).
13. S. Chaube and M. L. Murphy, Cancer Res. 26:1448 (1966).
14. T. von Kreybig, R. Preussmann and W. Schmidt, Arzneimittel-Forsch 18:645 (1968).
15. W. N. Fishbein, Johns Hopkins Med. J. 121:1 (1967).
16. W. N. Fishbein, P. P. Carbone, and H. D. Hochstein, Nature 208:46 (1965).
17. W. H. J. Summerskill, F. Thorsell, J. Feinberg, and J. S. Aldrete, Gastroenterology 54:20 (1968).
18. C. L. Streeter, R. R. Oltjen, L. L. Slyter and W. N. Fishbein, J. Anim. Sci. 29:88 (1969).
19. D. P. Griffith, in:"Proceedings Fourth International Urolithiasis Research Symposium," L. H. Smith, B. Finlayson, and W. G. Robertson, ed., Plenum Press, New York (in press).

ACKNOWLEDGMENT

This investigation was supported in part by Grant AM 10960 from the National Institutes of Health under the auspices of Universities Associated for Research and Education in Pathology, Inc. The opinions or assertions contained herein are the private views of the authors and are not to be construed as official or as reflecting the views of the Department of the Army or the Department of Defense. In conducting the research described in this report, the investigators adhered to the "Guide for Laboratory Animal Facilities and Care," as promulgated by the Committee on the Guide for Laboratory Animal Facilities and Care of the Institute of Laboratory Animal Resources, National Academy of Sciences-National Research Council.

COMPLICATIONS AND MANAGEMENT OF "NEGLECTED" RENAL STONES

S. M. Singh, S. N. Wadhwa, P. Trehan, N. P. Gupta,
R. Yadav, and K. K. Malhotra
Departments of Urology and Nephrology,
All India Institute of Medical Sciences
New Delhi, India

In developed countries, with better facilities for medical and surgical treatment of urolithiasis, calculi usually are not "neglected" although even from affluent countries, there are reports of patients in whom surgery was advised, but they have failed to take advantage of it. This study of 50 patients with renal/ureteric stone "neglected" by the patients so far as orthodox treatment is concerned have been collected from the records of patients admitted to the Institute Hospital during the period from January 1, 1979, to March 31, 1980. The reason for neglect has been most often patient fear of and unwillingness to undergo surgery, but to nearly an equal extent it has been due to claims by practitioners of "folk lore" medicine or rival system of medicine that they had some medicine to dissolve the stone. Ninety percent of the stones have contained calcium and 10% contained uric acid. There have been no cystine stones in this group.

The age distribution ranged from 1 to 70 years with the majority of the patients in the third, fourth and fifth decades. Thirty-seven were males and 13 were females.

The minimum duration of symptoms was 1 year and the maximum 36 years as is shown in Table 1.

The symptoms and signs at the time of admission are given in Table 2. One or more of the symptoms and signs of chronic renal failure were present in most patients. Many patients had more than one symptom and/or sign.

The complications in the series are given in Table 3.

Table 1. Total Duration of Symptoms

Duration of Symptoms	No. of Patients
1 to 2 years	2
3 to 4 years	9
5 to 6 years	10
7 to 8 years	7
9 to 10 years	6
11 to 15 years	4
16 to 20 years	6
21 to 30 years	6
Over 30 years	2
Total	50

Table 2. Symptoms and Signs at Admission

Symptoms	No. of Patients
Flank pain	48
Frequency and dysuria	25
Nausea and vomiting	24
Hematuria	16
Intermittent fever	13
Stone passage	11
History of Hypertension	9
Anuria	10
Oliguria	7
Signs	
Anemia	32
Renal angle tenderness	12
Hypertension	20
Kidney mass	4
Fluid overload	8
Dehydration	6

Many of the patients had undergone treatment by more than one system of medicine and where it was thought that allopathic treatment had also been ill-advised or inaccurate these patients are also included in the group. Also included are patients who had one operation and were advised further surgery either on the same kidney or for a stone on the other side. The advice was not heeded, and lead to complications and therefore these patients have also been included in this group as indicated in Table IV.

Table 3. Complications of Renal Stones

Complication	No. of Patients
Anemia	32
Hydronephrosis	27
Chronic pyelonephritis	24
Urinary infection	23
Chronic renal failure	22
Hypertension	20
Pyonephrosis	16
Non-functioning kidney	8
Fluid overload	8
Acute renal failure	7
Perinephric abscess	3

Table 4. Treatment Received Before Admission

Type of Treatment	No. of Patients
Allopathic treatment	9
Homeopathic and Ayurvedic treatment	28
Operated and neglected	5
No treatment	8

Investigations - Certain biochemical studies were done in all patients, and details are given in Table 5.

Table 5. Most of Investigations and Biochemical Studies were done in all Patients

Serum Calcium Levels

Serum levels	No. of Patients
<10 mg%	19
10 to 11 mg%	23
11 to 11.5 mg%	6
11.5 to 12 mg%	1
12 to 13.0 mg%	1
Mean serum calcium 12.6	

Urinary Calcium in 24 hours

Urine levels	No. of Patients
<100 mg	6
101 to 200 mg	39
201 to 300 mg	4
301 to 350 mg	-
350 to 400 mg	-
>400 mg	1

Serum Uric Acid Levels

Serum levels	No. of Patients
2 to 4 mg%	6
4 to 6 mg%	15
6 to 8 mg%	14
8 to 10 mg%	8
>10 mg%	7

Urinary Uric Acid in 24 hours

<100 mg	2
101 to 200 mg	15
201 to 300 mg	24
301 to 400 mg	5
401 to 500 mg	2
>500 mg	2

MANAGEMENT

The management of each patient has had to be individualized. Patients admitted with renal failure, acute and/or chronic, have needed: 1) Initial workup to determine size and distribution of stone, and biochemical status; 2) correction of fluid balance; 3) hemodialysis or peritoneal dialysis as indicated before appropriate surgery could be performed. (Table 6)

Table 6. Dialysis

Hemodialysis	
Pre-operative	16
Post-operative	5
Peritoneal	
Pre-operative	8
Post-operative	0

Listed below are the types of operations performed (Table 7) and complications of surgery (Table 8).

Table 7.

	No. of Patients
Bilateral Operation (renal/ureteric stones)	10
Unilateral Operation (renal/ureteric stones)	36
Permanent nephrostomy	2
Conservative medical treatment	2

Table 8. Various Operations Performed

Extended pyelolithotomy	27
Pyelolithotomy	21
Nephrostomy	10
Pyelonephrolithotomy	6
Lower polar nephrectomy	5
Nephrectomy	4
Ureterolithotomy	9
Basketing	2

Many patients had more than 1 operation.

Table 9. Operative and Post-Operative Complications

Hemorrhage	3
Infection	12
Wound dehiscence	2
Retained calculi	5
Ureteric colic	2
Fistula	1

TREATMENT

Ureteric Stones

Patients with obstructive uropathy without renal failure due to ureteral stones have done well with simple ureterolithotomy. Hydronephrosis has disappeared and kidney function has returned to normal.

Kidney Stones

Problems in the surgical management of "neglected" kidney stones have been posed by many factors: a) Multiplicity of stones; b) adhesions of the kidney to the perirenal fat and fascia making surgery difficult and hazardous; c) renal failure; d) presence sometimes of only one functioning kidney.

Principles of renal calculus surgery were strictly observed for removal of calculi as popularized by Gilvernet[1] and Boyce[2]. Following surgery efforts have been made to sterilize the urine with appropriate antibiotics. Depending upon the chemical composition of the stone, appropriate dietetic and medical therapy has been given.

RESULTS OF TREATMENT

Results of treatment are shown in Table 10.

Table 10. Results

Relief of symptoms	41/50	82%
Improvement in renal function.*	23/29	79.9%
Improvement in hypertension	14/20	80%
No improvement	3/50	6%
Died within 4 weeks of surgery	3/50	6%

*Sixteen of 22 patients with chronic renal failure s-abilized their serum creatinine between 2 and 3.2 mg/dl. Renal function was normal in all seven patients with acute renal failure.

DISCUSSION

This series shows that the results of neglect in the treatment of renal stones can be disastrous even in this Institute where the type of treatment now being offered has improved greatly from that of 20 years ago with hemodialysis and peritoneal dialysis being more readily available. However, the morbidity and mortality is far higher than where renal stones are treated on time. From this paper we conclude that renal stones demand expert medical and surgical treatment in both developed and under-developed countries.

REFERENCES

1. J. Gilvernet, Urol. Internat. 20:255 (1965).
2. W. H. Boyce, in:"Renal Calculi Urologic Surgery," second edition, Harper & Row Publishers, Inc., New York (1975).

FIELD PREVENTIVE PROGRAM OF BLADDER STONE DISEASE IN THAILAND

A. Valyasevi, S. Dhanamitta, and S. Watthana-Kasetr

Faculty of Medicine, Ramathibodi Hospital, Mahidol University, Rama VI Road, Bangkok 4, Thailand

Previous investigations in Thailand have revealed several etiological factors involved in the pathogenesis of bladder stone formation[1,2]: (a) a low dietary phosphate intake; (b) a consumption of high oxalate-containing vegetables; (c) a high urinary ammonia and uric acid excretion; and (d) a reduced urine volume from some degree of dehydration. These factors lead to heavy oxalate and urate crystalluria and crystal clumping which may eventually form the nuclei of stones.

In 1974, a field trial was started in Ubol Province, Northeast Thailand (endemic stone area). The aims were to test the effectiveness of oral inorganic phosphate supplementation (60 mg P/kg body weight/day) for: (a) protection against calcium oxalate crystalluria; (b) prevention of the occurrence of presumptive and/or positive stone symptoms*, and (c) reduction in the incidence of overt stone disease.

METHODS

The study took place in 9 villages of the Pibul district. The occurrence of presumptive and positive stone symptoms among the preschool children living in these villages was 17% at the time of the survey in 1973. The high prevalence in this area made it suitable for the study.

*Presumptive symptoms include dysuria, cloudy urine and hematuria. Positive systoms include passing gravel or tiny stones and stone operation.

Detailed description of the study designs, selection of subjects and field procedures have been previously reported[3]. The study was started in June 1974 covering 1062 pre-school children with negative stone history; among these, 451 subjects received placebo and 611 received oral orthophosphate supplementation* in the amount to supply approximately 60 mg per kg body weight per day.

Routine examination of random morning samples were performed on all subjects every two to three months. Qualitative tests for protein, sugar and pH were evaluated by using Combistix.(R) A microscopic examination was made for cellular debris and crystals. Crystalluria and clumping of crystals were scored by type, size and number. Special examination of urine was performed where a stone episode was suspected during the 24 hours over which the urine sample was collected. Microscopic examination and chemical analyses were also performed in these samples.

During febrile or diarrheal episodes, random urine samples were collected and examined. If heavy crystalluria and/or clumping were found, 24 h urine samples were collected and analyzed.

RESULTS AND DISCUSSION

The results presented here cover a 5 year period from June 1974 to May 1979. The total number of subjects with negative stone history was 1062 and the dropout rate less than 10%.

Effectiveness of the Oral Orthophosphate Supplementation

1. Protection against calcium oxalate crystalluria. The total number of subjects who have completed the 5-year study were 180 (94 males and 86 females). More male subjects have calcium oxalate crystalluria and clumping than females. In the males receiving the placebo a significantly higher percentage had crystalluria involving 8 of the 11 cases of crystalluria reported. Comparison of the occurrence of crystalluria and clumping, between the two sexes showed that a higher percentage occurred in males.

Since calcium oxalate crystalluria and clumping are more common in males than females, the effects of phosphate were analyzed separately for the two sexes. Comparison of crystalluria and clumping in males were made in two ways: (a) as percent of individuals with crystalluria after receiving phosphate supplementation for 3 years (the number of subjects is maximum), and (b) as number of

* The phosphate was prepared as a solution of Na_2HPO_4 (88.015 g) and KH_2PO_4 (13.609 g) with a pH of approximately 7.0.

occurrences of crystalluria and clumping after receiving the supplementation for 5 years. There was significantly less crystalluria (with or without clumps) in the phosphate-supplemented group compared with the placebo group ($0.05 > p > 0.025$).

The above findings confirm our previous short-term study[4,5] that oral orthophosphate supplementation can significantly reduce calcium oxalate crystalluria and clumping.

2. Reduction in the occurrence of presumptive stone symptoms. There were 174 subjects in the placebo group and 159 in the phosphate-supplemented group studied for 5 years. The number of subjects who presented the presumptive stone symptoms were approximately the same (22 in placebo and 21 in the phosphate-supplemented group). However, the children in the placebo group presented more frequent episodes of symptoms with longer duration compared with the phosphate-supplemented group ($0.05 > p > 0.01$). This suggests that phosphate supplementation reduces the severity of presumptive stone symptoms.

3. Reduction in the incidence of overt stone disease. During the 5 years of the study, 5 subjects in the placebo group developed positive stone disease compared with 3 subjects in the phosphate-supplemented group. Furthermore, the positive stone symptoms in the placebo group (4 out of 5) had a long duration of the symptoms (31, 11, 6 and 56 days) preceeding the stone episodes; whereas, in the phosphate-supplemented group, the symptoms developed only 3 to 4 days before the stone episodes. It thus appears that the stone episodes were considerably less severe in the phosphate than the placebo group. Although the number of overt stone cases seemed small, the number of cases in the placebo group was close to that expected in the time period of study. Since the number in the phosphate group was less than expected, it showed an indication of possible effect of oral orthophosphate supplementation in the reduction in the incidence of overt stone disease.

Correlation Between the Occurrence of Diarrhea, Fever, and the Presumptive Symptoms of Bladder Stone Disease

It is anticipated that dehydration plays an important role in the occurrence of bladder stone disease in Thailand through diarrhea, vomiting and febrile episodes which frequently occur among village children. The possible correlation between the occurrence of diarrhea, fever and the presumptive stone symptoms has been evaluated in this study.

The evaluation was performed in all subjects receiving placebo during the 5 year study during which 387 subjects developed stone symptoms. There was a significant correlation between diarrhea and urinary symptoms (cloudy urine, hematuria and stone passed) in 169 boys ($0.5 > p > 0.01$). In females there was a correlation between dysuria and gravel in urine and fever and diarrhea ($0.05 > p > 0.01$). It is possible that these urinary symptoms arose from urinary tract infection or dehydration. In our experience however, these symptoms are more indicative of bladder stone disease than any other disease.

CONCLUSIONS

A field preventive program for bladder stone disease was carried out in Northeast Thailand covering approximately 1200 preschool children over a 5 year period. Oral orthophosphate supplementation (60 mg P/kg body weight/day) was found to (a) decrease the occurrence of oxalate crystalluria and clumping; (b) reduce the severity and duration of presumptive stone symptoms, and (c) reduce the occurrence of overt stone disease. No untoward effects of the phosphate supplementation were demonstrated. We suggest that oral orthophosphate supplementation be considered for the prevention of idiopathic bladder stone disease.

REFERENCES

1. A. Valyasevi and S. Dhanamitta, in:"Idiopathic Urinary Bladder Stone Disease," R. Van Reen, ed., Fogarty International Center Proceedings No. 37, DHEW Publication No. (NIH) 77-1068 (1977).
2. S. Dhanamitta, A. Valyasevi, and B. Susilavorn, in:"Idiopathic Urinary Bladder Stone Disease," R. Van Reen, ed., Fogarty International Center Proceedings No. 37, DHEW Publication No. (NIH) 77-1068 (1977).
3. A. Valyasevi, S. Dhanamitta, S. Watthana-Kasetr, and R. Van Reen, in:"Idiopathic Urinary Bladder Stone Disease," R. Van Reen, ed., Fogarty International Center Proceedings No. 37, DHEW Publication No. (NIH) 77-1068 (1977).
4. S. Dhanamitta, A. Valyasevi, and R. Van Reen, Am. J. Clin. Nutr. 20:1387 (1967).
5. A. Valyasevi, S. Dhanamitta, and R. Van Reen, Am. J. Clin. Nutr. 22:218 (1969).

ACKNOWLEDGMENT

This work was supported in part by the National Institutes of Health, U. S. Department of Health, Education and Welfare, Grant No. AM 13066-01-8.

TREATMENT

OBJECTIVE EVIDENCE FOR THE BENEFICIAL EFFECT OF A HIGH FLUID INTAKE IN THE MANAGEMENT OF NEPHROLITHIASIS

K. Sakhaee, J. E. Zerwekh, and C. Y. C. Pak

Section on Mineral Metabolism, Department of Internal Medicine, Southwestern Medical School, The University of Texas Health Science Center at Dallas, Dallas, Texas

The importance of oral fluid intake on the formation and prevention of renal stones has long been emphasized[1-5]. The nephrolithiasis occurring in hot climates has been attributed partly to the low urine output resulting from an excessive sweat loss and dehydration[2]. A recent study by Robertson identified a low urine volume as an important risk factor for nephrolithiasis[6]. Thus, it has been customary to recommend a high fluid intake in patients with renal stones to assure an adequate urine volume[3-5,7]. However, the physicochemical effects and the ability of this regimen to prevent stone-formation have not been shown.

Theoretically, a high fluid intake may inhibit stone-formation, since it will dilute urine, lower urinary concentration of stone-forming constituents, and reduce urinary saturation of stone salts[8]. However, this maneuver will also dilute urinary concentration of inhibitors[9], which normally retard crystallization of stone salts. Thus, it is theoretically possible that the decline in inhibitor activity may be sufficient to negate the "beneficial" effect of reduced saturation.

These circumstances led us to examine in detail the effect of urinary dilution on the crystallization of calcium (Ca) salts in urine. It will be shown that urinary dilution, achieved in vitro by addition of water to urine samples or in vivo by an increased fluid intake, reduced urinary state of saturation of brushite ($CaHPO \cdot 2H_2O$), Ca oxalate and monosodium urate. Moveover, the urinary limit of metastability of brushite did not change, and that of Ca oxalate significantly increased. This finding, which indicated a retardation of spontaneous nucleation of Ca oxalate, was unexpected from the dilution of inhibitor concentration.

MATERIALS AND METHODS

In Vitro Dilution

A 24-hour urine sample was obtained in an outpatient setting from each of 6 patients with Ca nephrolithiasis and 2 normal control subjects, while their fluid intake was deliberately limited in order to obtain urine volume of less than 1 liter/day. Each urine sample was divided into three equal portions. Appropriate amounts of distilled water was added to each portion to "artificially" produce urine volumes of 1.0, 1.5 and 2.0 liters/day. Crystallization studies[10] were performed in each diluted sample.

In Vivo Dilution

Four patients with nephrolithiasis and three normal control subjects participated in the study, after an informed written consent was obtained. They were maintained on a constant metabolic diet, with a daily composition of 400 mg Ca, 800 mg phosphorus (P) and 100 mEq sodium (Na) for 7 days. In one group (randomly chosen), the total fluid intake (including the amount contained in food) was kept at 1.8 liter/day during the first 4 days. On days 5, 6 and 7, the fluid intake was increased to 2.3, 2.8 and 3.3 liters/day respectively by an ingestion of appropriately larger amounts of distilled water. In the other group, the order of fluid intake was reversed; i.e. the total fluid intake was 3.3 liters/day during the first 4 days, and was reduced by 0.5 liter on each succeeding day by an appropriate reduction of distilled water intake. Urine was collected in 24-hour pools from days 4-7 for crystallization studies[10].

Crystallization Studies

Measures of crystallization included activity product ratio (APR) of brushite, Ca oxalate and monosodium urate, and formation product ratio (FPR) of brushite and Ca oxalate. They were determined by techniques described previously[10-12].

The APR represented the state of urinary saturation with respect to the solid phase[10,13]. The urine sample was incubated with an excess of the solid phase to steady-state. The ratio of activity products in the original sample and in the ambient fluid after incubation with the solid phase gave a quantitative measure of saturation with respect to that solid phase, where a value of 1 indicated saturation, greater than 1 supersaturation, and less than 1 undersaturation. The activity products of brushite, Ca oxalate and monosodium urate were calculated by the technique of Finlayson[13].

The FPR indicated the limit of metastability, or the minimum supersaturation required for spontaneous nucleation[10,12]. Strictly, it represented heterogeneous nucleation by naturally occurring nuclei. To samples rendered devoid of cellular debris and crystalline material by filtration (Millipore 0.22 micron), a solution of calcium chloride or sodium oxalate was added in increasingly large amounts, in order to cause precipitation of Ca phosphate or Ca oxalate respectively. The minimum APR which permitted precipitation at 3 hours represented the FPR.

Urinary Ca and magnesium (Mg) were analyzed by atomic absorption spectrophotometry, and Na by flame photometry. Urinary P was measured by the method of Fiske and Subbarow[14], uric acid by the enzymatic method[15], and oxalate by the technique of Hodgkinson and Williams[16]. Citrate was determined by the method of Beutler and Yeh [17], and pyrophosphate according to the method of Solomons and Styner[18].

The paired t-test was employed to test the significance of measures between various urine volumes.

RESULTS

Effect of In Vitro Dilution of Urine on Crystallization

When urine samples were diluted by an addition of water, urinary APR of brushite, Ca oxalate and monosodium urate decreased significantly (Table 1). Urine samples which were supersaturated to begin with (APR > 1), became less supersaturated with respect to Ca oxalate, and undersaturated (APR < 1) for brushite and monosodium urate, when urine volume was raised from 1 liter/day to 2 liters/day. The dilution of urine did not significantly alter the FPR of brushite (Table 1). However, the FPR of Ca oxalate rose significantly, i.e., a greater degree of supersaturation was required to initiate spontaneous nucleation.

Table 1. Effect of *In Vitro* Dilution of Urine (by Water Addition)

	Urine Volume (liter/day)		
	1	1.5	2.0
Activity Product Ratio			
Brushite	2.59±0.53	1.44±0.32**	0.83±0.18**
Monosodium Urate	1.50±0.53	1.33±0.35**	0.82±0.19**
Ca Oxalate	3.70±0.59	3.09±0.44*	2.60±0.47**
Formation Product Ratio			
Brushite	3.98±0.46	4.20±0.58	3.96±0.54
Ca Oxalate	11.92±2.40	14.98±2.54*	15.60±2.06*

Values are presented as mean ± SE. Significant difference from control (1 liter/day) is shown by * for p <0.05, ** for p <0.01.

Table 2. Effect of *In Vivo* Dilution of Urine on Urinary Chemistry and Crystallization

	Urine Volume (liters/day)			
	1.023	1.350	1.877	2.383
Ca, mg/day	148±17	160±22	150±16	149±19
Oxalate, mg/day	18.7±1.2	21.7±1.3	21.1±1.2	21.3±1.1
P, mg/day	576±21	591±29	600±50	615±21
Na, mEq/day	70±8	76±3	71±7	69±0
Uric Acid, mg/day	404±73	391±77	459±73	424±72
Citrate, mg/day	608±118	658±126	644±136	648±123
Magnesium, mg/day	101±4	96±4	91±5	87±5
Pyrophosphate, mg P/day	1.42±0.49	1.40±0.26	1.57±0.39	1.36±0.33
pH	5.88±0.11	5.78±0.11	5.84±0.11	5.71±0.11
Activity Product Ratio				
Brushite	2.59±0.24	1.89±0.31**	1.20±0.09†	0.99±0.13†
Monosodium Urate	1.58±0.43	0.91±0.24	0.59±0.10*	0.35±0.05**
Ca Oxalate	3.58±0.48	3.12±0.47	2.70±0.35**	2.11±0.34†
Formation Product Ratio				
Brushite	4.86±0.42	5.27±0.58	5.28±0.55	5.34±0.36
Ca Oxalate	11.52±0.51	13.52±1.21*	14.70±1.21**	15.33±1.94**

Values are presented as mean ± SE. Significant difference from control (1.023 liter/day) is shown by * for $p < 0.05$, ** for $p < 0.01$ and † for $p < 0.001$.

Effect of In Vivo Dilution

Mean urine volumes for the group were 1.023 ± 0.084 SE, 1.350 ± 0.108, 1.877 ± 0.072 and 2.383 ± 0.106 liters/day, corresponding to total fluid intakes of 1.8, 2.3, 2.8 and 3.3 liters/day, respectively.

With increasing urine volume, the urinary APR of Ca oxalate, brushite and monosodium urate progressively declined (Table 2). At the highest urine volume, urinary environment became less supersaturated with respect to Ca oxalate, saturated with brushite, and undersaturated with monosodium urate (APR < 1).

As in the *in vitro* dilution, the FPR of brushite did not change significantly when the urine volume rose with increased fluid ingestion (Table 2). However, the FPR of Ca oxalate significantly increased. The minimum supersaturation required for spontaneous nucleation of Ca oxalate was 11.52-fold with urine volume of 1.023 liter/day; it increased to 15.33-fold at urine volume of 2.383 liter/day. Thus, dilution of urine inhibited the nucleation of Ca oxalate.

In contrast, *in vivo* dilution of urine did not significantly alter urinary excretion of Ca, oxalate, P, Na, uric acid, citrate, Mg, pyrophosphate or pH ($p > 0.1$) (Table 2).

DISCUSSION

An important aspect of recent progress in urolithiasis research has concerned the disclosure that certain metabolic derangements may be associated with and play a pathogenetic role in renal stone-formation[19-21]. This appreciation has led to the introduction of new treatment programs, which are directed at ameliorating or correcting the underlying metabolic abnormalities[22]. The programs include thiazide[23], sodium cellulose phosphate[24], orthophosphate[25], and allopurinol[20]. The mode of action of these drugs, not only with respect to their physiological action but also with their effects on physical chemistry of stone-formation, is beginning to be delineated[22].

Unfortunately, the more conventional approach to management, such as oral fluid intake, has been neglected[3]. Although a high fluid intake has been generally recommended as an adjunct to treatment[3,4,8] the exact mode of action of urinary dilution on stone formation was not critically examined. Recent introduction of techniques for the assessment of crystallization of Ca salts in urine[10,12] allowed us to assess quantitatively the effects of urinary dilution.

Urinary dilution, achieved *in vitro* by addition of water to urine or *in vivo* by an ingestion of water, was shown to reduce urinary saturation of Ca phosphate (brushite), Ca oxalate and monosodium urate. This reduction occurred because of the decreased concentration of component ions and ensuing fall in ionic activities. Moreover, the dilution of urine significantly increased the limit of metastability[9,11] of Ca oxalate, though not that of brushite. Thus, a greater degree of supersaturation was required to elicit spontaneous nucleation of Ca oxalate.

The finding of a rise or no significant change in the limit of metastability with urinary dilution was unexpected, since the reduced concentration of urinary inhibitors[9] should also have occurred. If such inhibitors were the sole factors dictating the metastable limit, the minimum supersaturation required for spontaneous nucleation should have decreased upon urinary dilution. The results suggested the presence in urine of substances, which facilitate the spontaneous nucleation of Ca salts. The reduced concentration of such promoters[9,11] upon urinary dilution could then have increased the metastable limit. The chemical nature of promoters is not known; however, they must represent soluble material since studies of nucleation were performed in urine devoid of cellular debris and crystalline material. The preferential effect of urinary dilution on the limit of metastability of Ca oxalate rather than of brushite is unexplained.

The effects of *in vivo* dilution was qualitatively similar to that of *in vitro* dilution. An increased urinary output from water ingestion did not significantly modify the total urinary content of Ca, oxalate, P, Na, uric acid, citrate, magnesium, pyrophosphate or pH. We were unable to document a volume-dependent excretion of oxalate[26,27].

In summary, urinary dilution was found to reduce the propensity for the crystallization of Ca salts in urine by lowering the urinary saturation of brushite and Ca oxalate, and by increasing the minimum supersaturation required to elicit spontaneous nucleation of Ca oxalate. If the scheme involving etiological importance of monosodium urate in Ca urolithiasis proves to be valid[11,12,28], urinary dilution may also retard the crystallization of Ca salts by reducing the saturation and preventing the formation of the urate phase. These data provided objective evidence for the beneficial role of increased fluid intake in the management of urolithiasis. We would agree with Smith et al.[3] that a fluid intake sufficient to insure urine volume 2.5 l/day would be highly desirable.

REFERENCES

1. C. W. Vermeulen, E. S. Lyon, J. E. Ellis, and T. Borden, J. Urol. 97:573 (1967).
2. N. J. Blacklock, J. Roy. Naval Med. Serv. 51:99 (1965).

3. L. H. Smith, C. J. Van Den Berg, and D. M. Wilson, N. Engl. J. Med. 298:87 (1978).
4. A. E. Broadus and S. O. Thier, N. Engl. J. Med. 800:839 (1979).
5. W. G. Thompson, in:"Practical Dietetics," D. Appleton Co., New York, (1895).
6. W. G. Robertson, Intern. Urin. Stone Conf. 12 (1979).
7. B. E. C. Nordin, H. Barry, L. Bulusu, and R. Reed, in:"Urinary Calculi," L. Cifuentes Delatte, A. Rapado, and A. Hodgkinson, eds., S. Karger, Basel, (1973).
8. C. Y. C. Pak, in:"Calcium Urolithiasis: Pathogenesis, Diagnosis and Management," Plenum Press, New York (1978).
9. H. Fleisch, Kid. Int. 13:361 (1978).
10. C. Y. C. Pak and K. Holt, Metabolism 25:665 (1976).
11. C. Y. C. Pak, O. Waters, L. Arnold, K. Holt, C. Cox, and D. Barilla, J. Clin. Invest. 59:426 (1977).
12. C. Y. C. Pak, D. E. Barilla, K. Holt, L. Brinkley, R. Tolentino, and J. E. Zerwekh, Am. J. Med. 65:593 (1978).
13. C. Y. C. Pak, Y. Hayashi, B. Finlayson, and S. Chu, J. Lab. Clin. Med. 89:891 (1977).
14. C. H. Fiske and Y. Subbarow, J. Biol. Chem. 66:375 (1925).
15. L. Liddle, J. E. Seegmiller, and L. Laster, J. Lab. Clin. Med. 54:903 (1959).
16. A. Hodgkinson and A. Williams, Clin. Chim. Acta. 36:127 (1972).
17. E. Beutler and M. K. Y. Yeh, J. Lab. Clin. Med. 54:125 (1959).
18. C. C. Solomons and J. Styner, Calc. Tiss. Res. 3:318 (1969).
19. C. Y. C. Pak, in:"Urolithiasis Research," H. Fleisch, W. G. Robertson, L. H. Smith, and W. Vahlensieck, eds., Plenum Press, New York (1976).
20. F. L. Coe, Kid. Int. 13:418 (1978).
21. L. H. Smith, Urol. Clin. N. Amer. 1:241 (1974).
22. C. Y. C. Pak, in:"Fourth Workshop on Phosphorus," (in press).
23. E. R. Yendt and M. Cohanim, Kid. Int. 13:397 (1978).
24. C. Y. C. Pak, C. S. Delea, and F. C. Bartter, N. Engl. J. Med. 290:175 (1974).
25. W. C. Thomas, Kid. Int. 13:390 (1978).
26. P. M. Zarembski and A. Hodgkinson, Clin. Chim. Acta. 25:1 (1969).
27. D. G. Oreopoulos, H. Husdan, M. Leung, D. B. W. Reid, and A. Rapoport, Ann. Int. Med. 85:617 (1976).
28. W. G. Robertson, in:"Urolithiasis Research," H. Fleisch, W. G. Robertson, L. H. Smith, and W. Vahlensieck, eds., Plenum Press, New York (1976).

ACKNOWLEDGMENT

This work was supported by USPHS grants RO1-AM16061, P50-AM20543, and MO1-RR-00633.

REDUCTION OF URINARY OXALATE EXCRETION DURING CHRONIC THIAZIDE THERAPY

M. Cohanim and E. R. Yendt

Department of Medicine, Kingston General Hospital
and Queen's University,
Kingston, Ontario, Canada

Thiazide diuretics are effective in preventing calcific renal calculi[1,2]. Although the initial rationale for the use of these agents in stone prevention was based on their now well-known hypocalciuric action, it is possible that other thiazide-induced changes in the composition of the urine are of equal or greater importance.

Supersaturation of urine with calcium oxalate and deficiency of inhibitors of the growth and aggregation of calcium oxalate crystals appears to be of major importance in the pathogenesis of calcific calculi[3]. Changes in urinary oxalate concentration are relatively much more important than changes in urinary calcium in influencing the degree of calcium oxalate supersaturation[4]. Thus the effect of thiazides on the urinary excretion of oxalate must be clarified before the therapeutic efficacy of this agent can be fully explained.

SUBJECTS AND PROCEDURES

All patients underwent a complete stone investigation prior to thiazide therapy. Following the investigation, thiazide was administered in the form of hydrochlorothiazide, 50 mg twice daily in 31 patients and 25 mg twice daily in the remaining 18 patients. The patients were not hospitalized during the 24-h urine collection and were eating their usual diets. Dietary oxalate was not restricted during the treatment period and in many patients dietary oxalate was probably greater during thiazide therapy because of an increased intake of citrus fruit juices, which contain relatively large amounts of oxalate, to combat thiazide-induced hypokalemia.

Urinary oxalate excretion was measured by the method of Hallson and Rose[5], prior to thiazide therapy and at varying intervals throughout the course of treatment in 49 patients with recurrent calcific renal calculi.

Normal Subjects

Urine oxalate excretion measured in 27 non-hospitalized normal men and women eating their usual diets was 38.8 ± 10.3 mg/day (mean ± SD). In the 49 patients with calcific renal calculi urine oxalate was 45.9 ± 14.3 mg/day (mean ± SD).

Urolithiasis Patients During Thiazide Therapy

Urine oxalate excretion was measured in 20 patients during the first three months of thiazide therapy, in 14 patients after 6 months of thiazide therapy and in 13 patients after 6 to 12 months' therapy; the mean urine oxalate excretion did not differ significantly from pre-treatment values in any of these groups. (Table 1). In 32 patients, urine oxalate was measured on one or more occasions after thiazide therapy was continued for more than one year; in these patients the mean urine oxalate excretion after this period of treatment was significantly lower than pre-treatment values. (Table 1).

All pre-treatment values for urine oxalate determinations as well as all determinations made after one year or more of therapy are shown for the 24 males (Figure 1) and 8 females (Figure 2) comprising this group. It is noteworthy that the maximum reduction in urine oxalate excretion frequently did not occur until the second or third year of thiazide therapy.

DISCUSSION

We believe that the thiazide-induced reduction of urine oxalate excretion is related to reduced intestinal calcium absorption which has been demonstrated during chronic thiazide therapy. Although the acute effect of thiazides on intestinal calcium absorption is variable, there is fairly good evidence, that during long-term thiazide administration intestinal calcium is frequently diminished[1,6]. The similarity noted in the time pattern for the reduced urine oxalate excretion and the diminished intestinal calcium absorption during thiazide therapy is striking. It seems likely that reduced intestinal calcium absorption during long term thiazide therapy leads to greater precipitation of dietary oxalate as insoluble calcium oxalate in the intestinal lumen so that less oxalate is absorbed and excreted in the urine.

Table 1. Effect of Thiazide Therapy on Urinary Oxalate

Duration of Therapy	Number of Subjects	Urine Oxalate mg per day (mean ± SE)			Urine Oxalate mg % (mean ± SE)		
		Pre-Thiazide	On Thiazide	P	Pre-Thiazide	On Thiazide	P
3 months	20	41 ± 3.5	41 ± 3.5	N.S.	2.98 ± 0.28	2.87 ± 0.34	N.S.
6 months	14	48 ± 3.0	44 ± 4.0	N.S.	3.39 ± 0.30	2.64 ± 0.33	N.S.
6 - 12 months	13	47 ± 3.5	46 ± 3.5	N.S.	3.01 ± 0.17	2.48 ± 0.34	N.S.
12 - 48 months	32	46 ± 2.1	33 ± 1.9	<0.001	3.43 ± 0.26	2.04 ± 0.14	<0.001

N.S. - Not significant

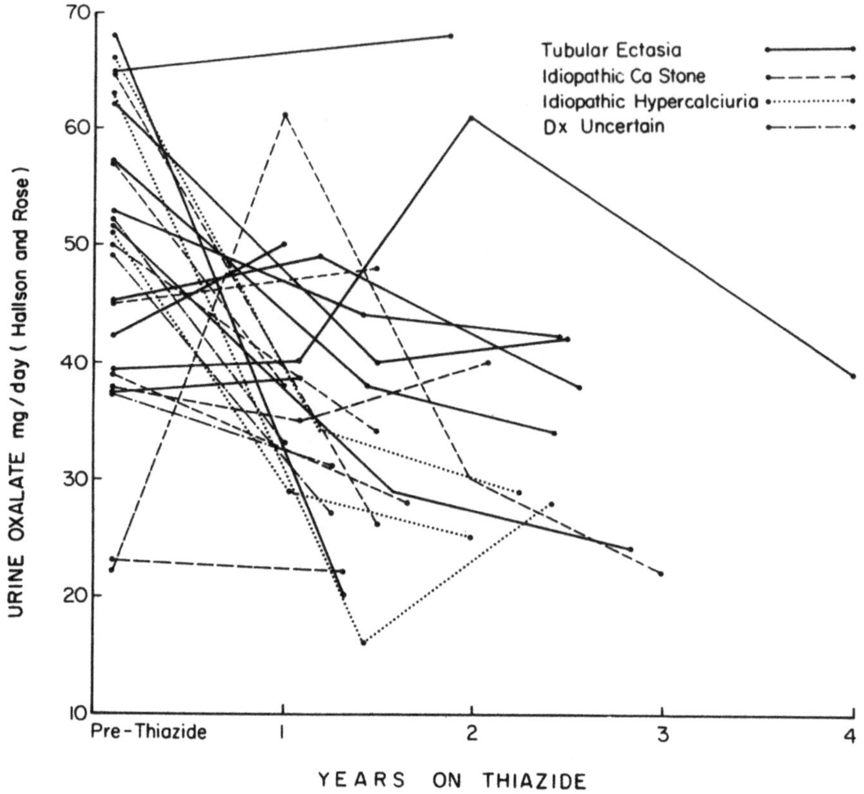

Figure 1.

The effect of thiazides on urine oxalate excretion is undoubtedly important insofar as renal calcific stone prevention is concerned and its potential importance is equal to or even greater than the hypocalciuric action. The observation is also of practical importance in therapy because it suggests that the drug may not exert its full therapeutic efficacy for at least one year after treatment is started. It also suggests that thiazide therapy may be effective in calcium urolithiasis when the hypocalciuric effect is relatively small.

REFERENCES

1. E. R. Yendt and M. Cohanim, Kid. Int. 13:397 (1978).
2. F. Backman, B. G. Danielson, G. Johansson, S. Ljunghall, and B. Wikstrom, Br. J. Urol. 51:175 (1979).

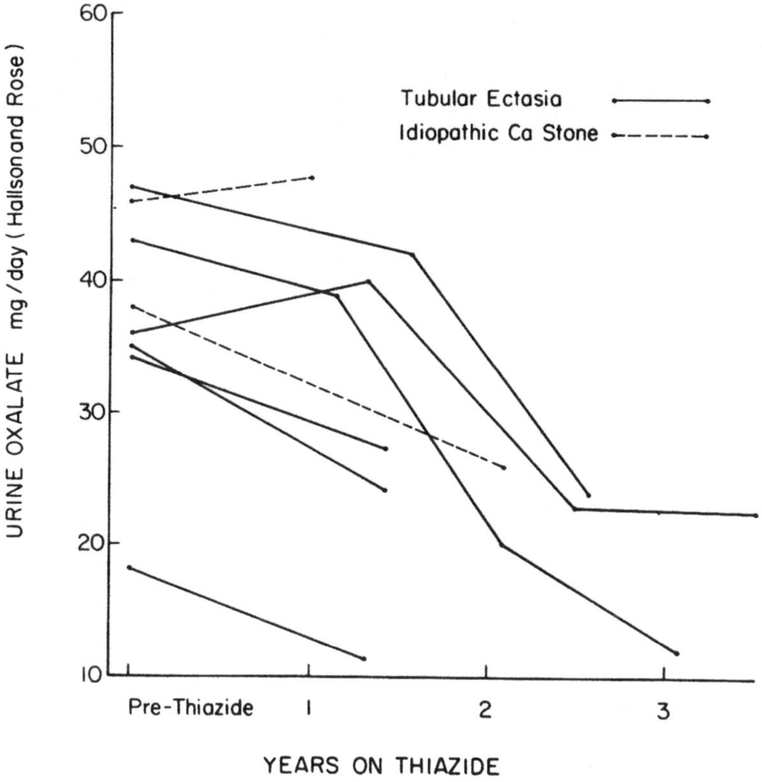

Figure 2.

3. W. G. Robertson, M. Peacock, R. W. Marshall, D. H. Marshall, and B. E. C. Nordin, New Engl. J. Med. 294:249 (1976).
4. W. G. Robertson, M. Peacock, and B. E. C. Nordin, in: "Urolithiasis, Physical Aspects," B. Finlayson, L. L. Hench and L. H. Smith, eds., National Academy of Sciences, Washington, D.C. (1972).
5. P. C. Hallson and G. A. Rose, Clin. Chim. Acta. 55:29 (1974).
6. U. Ehrig, J. E. Harrison, and D. R. Wilson, Metabolism 23:139 (1974).

ACKNOWLEDGMENT

This work was supported by Research Grant MT 681 from the Medical Research Council of Canada.

LONG-TERM TREATMENT WITH BENDROFLUMETHIAZIDE FOR PREVENTION OF RENAL STONES. CLINICAL EXPERIENCES.

S. Ljunghall, U. Backman, B. G. Danielson,
B. Fellström, G. Johansson, and B. Wikström
Department of Internal Medicine
University Hospital
S-750 14 Uppsala, Sweden

It has long been recognized that thiazides reduce the urinary calcium output and studies, where larger numbers of patients have been studied[1,2] have reported that during long-term follow-up most patients will be free of recurrences.

In this report we present our experience from long-term treatment with bendroflumethiazide in patients with recurrent calcium stones. The effects on the clinical course has been compared with the natural history of stone disease in a group of untreated stone patients.

PATIENTS AND CONTROLS

Since 1975 we have instituted treatment with bendroflumethiazide (2.5 mg twice daily with 0.57 g potassium chloride) in 168 patients (130 males and 38 females) with a mean age ± standard deviation of 43 ± 12 years. Prior to treatment they had on the average experienced renal stones for eight years with a mean stone episode rate of 0.8 stones/year. For comparison we have also followed a group of 43 patients with a mean age of 45 ± 11 years who did not receive any medical treatment. They had a history of stones for an average of seven years and during that time a mean stone episode rate of 0.5 stones/year. These patients received the same general advice about the necessity of a high fluid intake and were recommended to avoid excess calcium and oxalate intake[3].

All patients and controls were followed at regular intervals at our out-patient stone clinic.

RESULTS

Among the untreated controls there was an apparent reduction of the propensity to form stones. During follow-up for an average of three years the mean stone episode rate decreased from 0.5 to 0.3 stones/year, 55% of the patients experienced at least one recurrent stone.

During the same time seven of the patients treated with thiazide (10%) had formed any new stones. The mean stone episode rate had decreased to 0.08 stones/year.

The therapeutic failures could be explained by inadequate reduction of urinary calcium only in three cases. In these three individuals probably a habitual high sodium intake was of importance since urinary calcium decreased when sodium intake was reduced.

Mild side effects were not uncommon. Several young patients with a low blood pressure felt hypotensive symptoms during the first weeks of therapy. When treatment was instituted gradually such side effects were seldom incapacitating.

Asymptomatic hypokalemia occurred in two and symptomatic gout in one patient.

DISCUSSION

The difference between the patients treated with thiazide and the untreated patients as regards the natural history of stone disease seems so large that it could hardly have been caused by chance. Also in comparison with our experience from other forms of therapy thiazide appears to be the most effective way to prevent stone recurrences (Figure 1). However, it should be pointed out that this investigation, as all other studies on the effects of thiazide, was conducted as an open study. Until a well controlled double-blind trial has been carried out the definite role of thiazides for calcium stone prevention has not been definitely settled.

We instituted thiazides in consecutive numbers of idiopathic stone formers irrespective of the level of the urinary calcium output. The capacity to prevent stone formation was not restricted to the hypercalciuric patients. Also individuals with pre-treatment values clearly within the normal range generally displayed a reduction of their calcium excretion and absence of recurrences during follow-up.

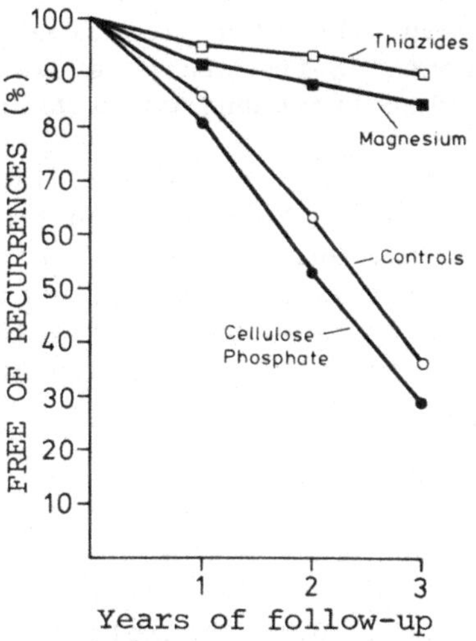

Figure 1. Effects of different modes of stone prevention among patients with recurrent formation of calcium-containing stones followed at our out-patient stone clinic.

If it is accepted that stone formation in most cases is the final result of an imbalance between supersaturation and inhibitory activity in the urine[4] any reduction of the urinary calcium should reduce the supersaturation of calcium salts and thereby the propensity to form stones. Our experience agrees with the view put forward by Yendt[1] that thiazides are effective also in normocalciuric individuals.

Possibly also effects other than the hypocalciuric response contributes to stone prophylaxis and explains why recurrences sometimes do not appear despite minimal reduction of urinary calcium. Among such effects are a decrease of urinary oxalate, increase of urinary magnesium and zinc[1,3].

Among our patients most cases of hypercalciuria are due to primary intestinal hyperabsorption of calcium[3] while in other reports higher frequencies of renal hypercalciuria have been reported. It is apparent from the present study that thiazides reduce not only renal but also absorptive hypercalciuria. Furthermore, we have found, in agreement with others[1], that during the long-term use of thiazides hyperabsorption is reduced together with hypercalciuria[5]. Although this particular point could be controversial[6], we do not believe that it is necessary to distinguish between renal and absorptive hypercalciuria before embarking on thiazide treatment.

During the five years we have used thiazides serious side effects have been uncommon, the main exception being a patient who developed symptoms of gout. Serum urate levels and clinical symptoms were reversed when treatment was withdrawn.

The continuing research in renal stone disease will probably provide us with a more detailed knowledge on the basic disturbances responsible for stone formation. Hopefully, also, possibilities to correct these abnormalities will arrive. Until this goal is achieved thiazides appear to be an acceptable substitute where stone recurrences are prevented in most consecutive stone patients with few and mild side effects.

REFERENCES

1. E. R. Yendt and M. Cohanim, Kid. Int. 13:387 (1978).
2. F. L. Coe, Ann. Int. Med. 87:404 (1977).
3. S. Ljunghall, U. Backman, B. G. Danielson, B. Fellström, G. Johansson, and B. Wikström, Scand. J. Urol. Nephrol. Suppl. 54 (in press).
4. W. G. Robertson, M. Peacock, P. J. Heyburn, D. H. Marshall, and B. E. C. Nordin, NEJM 294:249 (1976).
5. S. Ljunghall, U. Backman, B. G. Danielson, B. Fellström, G. Johansson, and B. Wikström, Scand. J. Urol. Nephrol. Suppl. 54 (in press).
6. J. Zerwekh, and C. Y. C. Pak, Metabolism 29:13 (1980).

LONG-TERM TREATMENT WITH BENDROFLUMETHIAZIDE FOR PREVENTION OF STONES. METABOLIC EFFECTS

S. Ljunghall, U. Backman, B. G. Danielson, B. Fellström,
G. Johansson, and B. Wikström
Department of Internal Medicine
University Hospital
S-750 14 Uppsala, Sweden

Since 1975 we have used thiazides for prevention of renal calcium stones. Our experience[1] confirms that of Yendt and Cohanim[2] that in most cases stone formation will virtually cease during several years of follow-up and that subjective side effects in general are mild.

However, considering that stone disease only rarely has a serious effect on a patient's everyday life, significant side effects are not acceptable. We have therefore, in this study, tried to evaluate some metabolic effects of long-term treatment with bendroflumethiazide (2.5 mg twice daily together with 0.57 g potassium chloride).

PATIENTS AND METHODS

Patients (130 males, 38 females) with recurrent formation of idiopathic calcium stones have been treated with thiazides for periods up to over four years.

Serum and urinary calcium and magnesium were measured by atomic absorption while urate was determined by a uricase method. In a group of 15 patients a more detailed study of calcium metabolism was performed both before and after three years' therapy. This study included longitudinal determinations of parathyroid hormone (PTH) and urinary cyclic AMP (cAMP), fasting urinary calcium and hydroxyproline and the 24-hour citrate excretion. At the end of this study (but not before) muscle biopsies were taken for determinations of magnesium and potassium[3] and the serum levels of zinc, copper and iron were analyzed. In ten of the patients the intestinal calcium absorption was measured with an isotope technique at the start of treatment and after three years.

RESULTS

The effect of long-term treatment with bendroflumethiazide on serum and urinary electrolytes are summarized in the Table.

Urinary calcium decreased during the first treatment month and remained on this lower level throughout follow-up. The reduction was not confined to those with pretreatment hypercalciuria but was evident over the whole range of values. Only in 7/168 individuals therapy failed to reduce the urinary calcium output. These non-responders had, during treatment, a higher excretion of sodium than the others. When sodium restriction was imposed urinary calcium decreased also in these cases.

When intestinal calcium absorption was measured before and after three years' treatment a mean reduction from 74% to 66% could be demonstrated. This reduction was correlated to the decrease of the calcium output.

The serum calcium concentrations increased slightly during the first months of therapy in most of the patients and remained slightly elevated during the first three years. This was evident although adjustments were made for alterations of the serum albumin content, which in the group as a whole remained unchanged at a level of 45 ± 2.5 g/l during the entire follow-up. Seventeen patients had at least one value above the upper limit of the normal range (2.60 mmol/l) but in ten of them this was only a transient elevation. Of the cases with repeatedly demonstrated hypercalcaemia most were evident already during the first month. When therapy was withdrawn in these patients all but two promptly normalized their serum calcium values. These two individuals had the most pronounced hypercalcaemia and also, in contrast to the others, simultaneously elevated levels of PTH. In one of them neck exploration was performed and displayed a typical parathyroid adenoma.

In the group of patients where parathyroid function was prospectively evaluated all determinations of PTH and cAMP were within the normal range and there were no changes during treatment.

Fasting urinary calcium was reduced but there were no consistent changes of the urinary hydroxyproline or citrate.

Initially, the urinary magnesium excretion increased but after the first year gradually returned to the pretreatment levels. The serum magnesium decreased during follow-up and six patients, all followed for more than three years, showed values below the lower limit of the normal range.

Table 1. Laboratory Effects (Mean Values ± S.D.) of Treatment With Bendroflumethiazide

Months of treatment	0	1	36
Number of patients	168	160	45
Serum values			
Calcium (mmol/l)	2.45± 0.06	2.51± 0.10***	2.49± 0.07*
Magnesium (mmol/l)	0.80± 0.05	0.79± 0.06	0.70± 0.06**
Phosphate (mmol/l)	0.97± 0.19	0.92± 0.19	0.94± 0.18
Potassium (mmol/l)	4.26± 0.29	3.87± 0.44***	3.84± 0.38***
Urate (μmol/l)	225 ±113	340 ±65***	347 ±57***
Alkaline Phosphatase (μkat/l)	2.96± 1.32	-	2.74± 0.83
PTH (μg/l)	0.37± 0.08	-	0.36± 0.08
Urine values			
Calcium (mmol/24h)	8.5 ± 2.4	4.7 ± 1.7***	5.3 ± 2.0***
Magnesium (mmol/24h)	4.5 ± 1.2	4.9 ± 1.3**	4.7 ± 1.2
Urate (mmol/24h)	3.4 ± 1.0	3.3 ± 0.7	3.1 ± 1.0
Citrate (mmol/24h)	2.7 ± 1.6	-	2.6 ± 1.5
Hydroxiproline (mg/mmol creat)	11.8 ± 3.7	-	10.7 ± 5.1
cAMP (mmol/mmol creat)	0.39± 0.15	0.47± 0.11	0.38± 0.07
Fasting urinary calcium (mmol/mmol creat)	0.37± 0.12	-	0.24± 0.11**
Volume (l/24h)	1.4 ± 0.4	1.4 ± 0.5	1.4 ± 0.4

*) $p < 0.05$; **) $p < 0.01$; ***) $p < 0.001$ compared to pretreatment values (paired t-test)

The muscle magnesium content, determined after three years' treatment were in all the investigated cases within the normal range with a mean value close to that of healthy stone-free individuals and untreated stone patients. The serum urate increased in every patient with an average of 90 µmol/l. This increase was unrelated to the pretreatment level. The urinary urate excretion was unchanged in the group as a whole.

DISCUSSION

Among most of our patients a sustained reduction of the urinary calcium excretion was achieved irrespective of the pretreatment level. Thus, also those with clearly normal values before therapy experienced a further reduction. Since they also appeared to benefit with respect to further stone formation our study supports the view proposed by Yendt[2] that thiazides could be used in stone patients regardless of the magnitude of the urinary calcium.

The cause of hypercalciuria in most of our patients[4] is intestinal calcium hyperabsorption and only rarely are any cases of resorptive or renal hypercalciuria documented. From our data it appears as if thiazides during long-term therapy causes a reduction of the raised intestinal calcium uptake and that during chronic use a new steady state is achieved where the reduced excretion is accounted for by a reduced uptake from the gut.

The findings of a slow but steady decline of the serum magnesium values suggest that during continued treatment magnesium deficiency could appear. The possibility of eventual magnesium deficiency should, therefore, be kept in mind and the necessity for regular magnesium supplements during thiazide treatment has not been ruled out. Theoretically they should further improve the stone-preventive effects of thiazides[3].

REFERENCES

1. S. Ljunghall, U. Backman, B. G. Danielson, B. Fellström, G. Johansson, and B. Wikström, Scand. J. Urol. Nephrol. Suppl. 54 (1980).
2. E. R. Yendt, and M. Cohanim, Kid. Int. 13:197 (1978).
3. G. Johansson, Scand. J. Urol. Nephrol. Suppl. 51 (1979).
4. S. Ljunghall, Scand. J. Urol. Nephrol. Suppl. 54 (1980).

EXPERIENCES WITH THIAZIDES IN A DOUBLE BLIND STUDY

D. Scholz, P. O. Schwille, and A. Sigel*

The Mineral Metabolism and Hormone Research Laboratory, Departments of Surgery and Urology*, University of Erlangen, Erlangen, West Germany

Thiazides are widely used in the prevention of calcific urinary calculi, as they reduce the urinary excretion of calcium and the stone recurrence rate[1]. In an attempt to separate specific from non-specific effects of thiazide treatment we undertook a double blind study using hydrochlorothiazide or placebo for over one year in patients with recurrent calcium lithiasis.

Patients with metabolically active calcium urolithiasis[2], but without primary hyperparathyroidism, were assigned in a random order: 25 (♂ = 14, ♀ = 11) in group A (= hydroclorothiazide^{+}) 26 (♂ = 17, ♀ = 9) in group B (= placebo^{+}). The mean age in group A was 46 years (29-63) and in group B 41 years (20-64). Both groups were comparable regarding weight and stone forming rate. Two tablets per day were taken (25 mg thiazide/tablet in group A). When serum potassium fell below 3.0 mval/l during treatment, potassium was substituted orally. Before and after 3 and 12 months of treatment the following clinical examinations were performed: on day 1 a 24 h urine was collected (except after 3 months) at home without dietary prescriptions, especially no salt restriction; on day 2, after an overnight fast of 12 - 15 hr, blood was taken between 8 a.m. and 9 a.m., and a fasting urine was collected over 2 h after drinking 600 ml of tap water. The last tablet was given on the evening of day 1.

All excretion rates of the 24 h urine were calculated for 1.73 m body surface. Results are indicated as means ($\bar{x}$) ± 1 standard error (SEM). To compare values before and during treatment, the X-test was used in cases of normal distribution, the t-test for paired data, otherwise the test of Wilcoxon and the test of Mann and Whitney were used. Normal values are indicated as median and interdecile range-80 (ID-80) for non-parametric distribution.

Table 1. Values in the 24 h urine of patients with recurrent calcium lithiasis before and after 12 months of treatment with thiazide (= A) or placebo (= B). Normal values are indicated as median with the respective interdecile range 80, patient values as means ± 1 standard error; n = number of observations. Creat. = creatinine, for other abbreviations see Methods section. [a]: $p < 0.05$; [b]: $p < 0.01$; [c]: $p < 0.001$ vs pretreatment values.

	Normal Values	Patients Pre-treatment A	n	B	n	After 12 months A	n	B	n
Volume; ml	1230; 760-1820	1820±136;	25	1891±166;	20	1820±166;	25	1658±142;	20
Calcium; mg	187; 98-276	249±20;	25	272± 32;	20	153±22;	25[c]	235±26;	20
Calcium; mmol/l	3.55; 1.50-6.00	3.84±0.36;	25	3.72±0.42;	20	2.28±0.29;	25[c]	3.85±0.53;	20
Magnesium; mg	108; 73-169	103±9;	25	102±9 ;	20	89±9 ;	25	85±5 ;	20[a]
Magnesium; mmol/l	3.37; 2.24-6.23	2.58±0.23;	25	2.43±0.18;	20	2.18±0.17;	25	2.26±0.15;	20
Sodium; mval	149; 76-209	197±15;	25	184±13;	19	173±14 ;	25	142±11;	19[a]
Potassium; mval	68; 44-93	61±5;	25	64±7;	19	60±5;	25	50±4;	19
Phosphate; mg	727; 516-983	784±70;	25	824±75;	19	737±46;	25	759±44;	19
Uric acid; mg	527; 308-763	641±45;	25	699±37;	19	593±50;	25	551±33;	19[b]
Oxalate; mg	32; 17-46	42±6;	16	47±6 ;	13	35±6 ;	16	22±6;	13[a]
Oxalate; mmol/l	0.29; 0.16-0.48	0.30±0.05;	16	0.31±0.05;	13	0.25±0.07;	16	0.20±0.05;	13
Citrate; mg	468; 273-715	345±74;	16	350±46;	16	332±70;	16	309±41;	16
RSP-CaOx	0.98; 0.85-1.20	0.96±0.07;	16	0.98±0.06;	13	0.71±0.08;	16[a]	0.71±0.08;	13[a]
RSP-CaP	0.41;-0.29-0.89	0.28±0.08;	25	0.40±0.09;	19	0.16±0.08;	25	0.27±0.12;	19
cAMP; μmol/g Creat.	2.82; 1.27-3.84	3.54±0.33;	15	3.07±0.40;	15	3.57±0.79;	15	2.76±0.25;	15

RSP = Relative supersaturation for calcium oxalate (CaOx) or calcium phosphate (CaP).

RESULTS

1. Serum and fasting urine before and during treatment: Total serum calcium and protein increased slightly in both groups after 12 months but the differences were not significant; ultrafiltrable and ionized calcium remained unchanged in group A with treatment. Serum potassium was down at 3 and 12 months ($p < 0.001$); serum urate was up at 3 and 12 months ($p < 0.001$). Serum phosphate was up in both groups after 12 months ($A = p < 0.05$; $B = p < 0.01$). Plasma PTH, glucose, triglycerides and alkaline phosphatase were the same in both groups and did not change with treatment. Urine pH, endogenous creatinine clearance and TM_{PO4} also did not change. The urinary excretion of calcium was decreased in both groups after 3 months of treatment (group $A = p < 0.001$; group $B = p < 0.05$) but in only group A after 12 months ($p < 0.01$). The urinary excretion of potassium was decreased in both groups ($A = p < 0.01$; $B = p < 0.05$) and the urinary excretion of uric acid and cAMP was decreased in group A ($p < 0.05$).

2. Results in 24 h urine collections: Before treatment and at 12 months of treatment 24 h urine collections were obtained and the results are presented in Table 1.

3. Other laboratory and clinical results: Systolic and diastolic blood pressure was lowered in group A during treatment. Bone mineral content measured by photon-absorptiometry in the distal radius of the non-dominant forearm was not affected by treatment in either group. Six patients in each group spontaneously passed stones during the follow-up period on treatment. This apparent lack of difference in response to treatment occurred in spite of the fact that there was a significant reduction in the urinary excretion of calcium in group A.

DISCUSSION

Our investigation proves that hydrochlorothiazide therapy in patients with recurrent calcium lithiasis causes a drastic and continuous reduction of calcium excretion in the urine under ambulatory treatment, and even with a lower dose than normally used and without salt restriction in the diet.

In contrast to the findings of others we do not find a thiazide induced change of urinary magnesium excretion. Apparent changes in urinary oxalate also occurred in the placebo group and may be caused by unspecific influences of treatment e.g. changed food intake or altered behavior by the patients. The daily urinary excretion of citrate was low before treatment and was not altered by thiazide as reported by others[3]. As small changes in urinary oxalate influence the activity product of CaOx in the same manner as great changes in urinary calcium[4], the RSP of CaOx decreased equally in both groups.

No side effects of thiazide therapy on the metabolism of glucose or fat were observed. The mild decrease of serum potassium in group A and the equal change of the urine values in both groups indicate that a depletion of whole body potassium was unlikely, when potassium was prescribed on the basis of serum potassium measurements. Although a mild hyperuricemia was found in group A, no clinical signs of gout were observed.

The relative low doses of thiazide used by us cannot be responsible for the stone recurrence rate, as calcium excretion was drastically reduced in the non-responders of group A, and recurrences were also reported for the daily dose of 2 x 50 mg[5]. Therefore, mechanisms other than elevated urinary calcium may be responsible for the new stone formation e.g. the decrease of magnesium or the increase of phosphate, uric acid and oxalate.

We conclude from these data, that the reduction of elevated urinary calcium alone does not prevent stone recurrence in all cases, but an exact interpretation of the number of non-responders to the drug in comparison with placebo treatment requires examination over a longer time period than one year. As thiazide therapy has the advantage of relative good compliance by the patients and low cost, preference should be given to this drug in the correction of urinary calcium excretion.

REFERENCES

1. E. R. Yendt, F. G. Guay, and D. A. Garcia, Can. Med. Assoc. J. 102:614 (1970).
2. L. H. Smith, Urol. Clin. N. Am. 1:241 (1974).
3. D. A. Garcia and E. R. Yendt, Can. Med. Assoc. J. 103:473 (1970).
4. W. G. Robertson and B. E. C. Nordin, in:"Renal Stone Research Symposium," A. Hodgkinson and B. E. C. Nordin, ed., Churchill, London (1969).
5. E. R. Yendt, R. J. A. Gagne, and M. Cohanim, Trans. Am. Clin. Climatol. Assoc. 77:96 (1965).

ACKNOWLEDGMENTS

We are grateful to K. Schwille, M. L. Rasenack, I. Goldberg, and B. Schreiber for technical assistance and secretarial help.

NEUTRAL POTASSIUM PHOSPHATE AND THIAZIDE: COMBINED TREATMENT IN RECURRENT STONE FORMERS

A. Scott Klein and Donald P. Griffith

Roy and Lillie Cullen Department of Urologic Research, Department of Urology, Baylor College of Medicine, Houston, Texas 77030

INTRODUCTION

Urinary calculous disease accounts for a large number of hospital admissions yearly and calcium oxalate is the most common stone found. Current theories of calculogenesis suggest that stones form as a consequence of two pathologic processes: (1) urinary solute supersaturation and (2) ineffective inhibition as shown by Robertson[1].

Thiazide diuretics have been shown by Yendt[2] to be effective in calcium oxalate (CaOx) stone management by: (1) reducing calciuria; (2) increasing urinary magnesium and zinc, and (3) possibly reducing oxaluria. However, thiazides also have the undesirable effects of: (1) reducing urinary citrate and (2) reducing body potassium stores.

Neutral potassium orthophosphate (K_2HPO_4 + KH_2PO_4) also have been shown by some[3] to be effective in the treatment of calcium stone disease. They exert their primary beneficial effect by increasing urinary inhibitor activity as a result of increasing urinary pyrophosphate; furthermore, they reduce calciuria, though to a lesser degree than seen with thiazides.

Combined thiazide and neutral K-phosphate therapy would have the potential additive effects of increasing urinary inhibitors and reducing urinary solute supersaturation. We reasoned that this form of therapy would be of benefit in refractory stone formers and that the potassium supplementation (14.25 mEq/capsule) would be sufficient to offset losses induced by the thiazide. Nephrocalcinosis, however, is a potentially serious side effect of combined treatment which may be induced or exacerbated by hypokalemia and alkalosis as shown by Holliday[4].

A report of patients on combined treatment is given and the results are reported.

MATERIAL AND METHODS

This is a retrospective analysis of 62 patients treated for periods up to three years. There were 53 males and 9 females with an average age of 40 years and a range of 13-61 years. This population had an average of 8.35 stone episodes per patient pretreatment and a mean treatment period of 1.5 years. Sixteen patients had more than 10 stone episodes pretreatment. Twelve patients in the group had continued to form stones on single drug treatment; eight were on thiazides, three on allopurinol, and one on magnesium oxide.

Stone episodes, defined as either spontaneous passage or surgical removal of urinary calculi, were determined before and during treatment. Radiographic studies consisted of renal tomograms or plain abdominal films. Serum and 24-hour urine chemistries were determined by standard laboratory methods. Patients were on an ad lib diet pretreatment. Modest restriction of dairy products and oxalate-rich foods was encouraged during treatment.

Our combined treatment program consisted of either hydrochlorothiazide, 50-100 mg per day, or chlorthalidone, 50-100 mg per day, and neutral k-phosphate in sufficient dosage to supply 1.5 gm of elemental phosphorus per day.

RESULTS

Stones were available for analysis from 35 patients. Thirty (86%) stones were predominantly calcium oxalate, 4 (11%) calcium phosphate and 1 (3%) uric acid.

Sequential radiographic studies were available in 56 patients. New stones formed during combined thiazide and phosphate therapy in two (2) patients (4%). An increase in size of pre-existing stones was identified in 7 (13%) patients; this included those forming new stones. No roentgenologic evidence of nephrocalcinosis was found in any of the patients studied.

Patient acceptance of the combined therapy was good. Two patients complained of diarrhea and indigestion from phosphate therapy, but this resolved by decreasing the daily dosage. Two patients developed symptomatic hypokalemia for which the thiazides were temporarily discontinued.

Table 1. Serum Changes at 1 and 3 Years on Thiazide and K-Phosphate

	PRETX	N	1 YEAR	P	PRETX	N	3 YEARS	P
Serum Calcium	9.7±.1	49	9.8±.07	NS	9.8±.13	15	9.7±.11	NS
Phosphorus	2.9±.08	49	3.0±.09	NS	3.1±.17	15	3.2±.15	NS
Creatinine	1.0±.03	49	1.1±.03	0.036	1.1±.06	15	1.1±.07	NS
Potassium	4.3±.06	49	3.8±.06	<0.001	4.3±.10	14	3.9±.12	0.02
Chloride	104±.4	49	101±.6	<0.001	103±.9	14	101± 1	0.06
CO_2	29±1.6	31	29±1.4	NS	28±.8	14	28±.8	NS

Table 2. Urine Changes at 1 and 3 Years on Thiazide and K-Phosphate

	PRETX	N	1 YEAR	P	PRETX	N	3 YEARS	P
Urine pH	6.0±.05	59	6.3±.05	<0.001	6.1±.11	14	6.3±.16	NS
Calcium	304± 18	62	158± 9	<0.001	295± 37	15	175± 25	0.002
Phosphorus	1039± 44	62	1642±72	<0.001	976±104	15	1574±170	0.005
Creatinine Clearance	132± 5	48	120± 3	0.018	123± 10	15	117± 11	NS
Calcium-Creatinine Ratio	0.156±.01	58	0.098±.01	<0.001	.161±.03	10	.120±.02	0.05

Serum studies are presented in Table 1. Serum calcium and phosphorus remained essentially unchanged over the three year period. Serum potassium showed a significant reduction of about 0.5 mEq per liter but remained within the normal range (5.0-3.5 mEq/l). The serum chloride also was reduced slightly; this reduction was not associated with an increased total CO_2. Although serum creatinine increased slightly at one year, the three-year data is unchanged from pretreatment. We did not feel this small one-year change was significant clinically.

Urine studies are presented in Table 2. Although the urine pH increased from 6.0 to 6.3 at one year and may reflect a mild alkalinizing effect of thiazides, the change at three years was not significant.

Significantly, there was a 48% and 41% reduction in 24-hour calcium excretion at one and three years respectively. Also, daily excretion of phosphorus increased by 58% and 61% at one and three years respectively. This increase in excreted phosphorus represents 40% of the daily dose administered.

The uncorrected creatinine clearance decreased slightly from 132 to 120 cc/minute at one year and an even smaller insignificant decrease from 123 to 117 cc/minute at three years.

The calcium-creatinine excretion ratio was significantly reduced at both the one- and three-year period. This reflects the previously mentioned reductions in calcium excretion.

A summary of the clinical course of patients is presented in Table 3. Column A shows an 86% overall reduction in predicted (83.4) vs actual (12) stone episodes with a highly significant chi-square value of 61.1. In those patients with serious stone disease (> 10 stone episodes pretreatment) shown in Column B, there was an 87.7% reduction in stone episodes (as compared with the predicted number of stones) with a chi-square of 25, also highly significant. Similar data in Column C for patients continuing to form stones on single drug programs showed a significant 82.5% reduction in stone episodes. Furthermore, patients with continued stone formation on thiazide-only treatment likewise had a significant reduction in stone episodes by 82%.

SUMMARY

The efficacy of combined thiazide and neutral K-phosphate therapy comes from several lines of evidence in our study. Only 2 (4%) patients formed new stones and only 7 (13%) patients had evidence of continued metabolically active stone disease during treatment. There was a significant reduction in stone episodes for the whole treatment group. In patients previously on single drug programs with continued stone formation, combined therapy resulted in a significant reduction in stone episodes. Likewise, the patients initially on thiazide-only treatment programs with continued active stone disease experienced similar reductions.

The safety of combined treatment was supported in our study. No radiographic evidence of nephrocalcinosis was found. Serum creatinine remained essentially unchanged up to three years and although there was a small decrease in creatinine clearance at one year, this was not significant in three years. Such small changes in creatinine clearance can be accounted for by problems in collection technique or laboratory variation.

Our data suggest that neutral K-phosphate in the doses prescribed only partially replaces the potassium losses induced by thiazides. Although the decrease in serum potassium is statistically significant, symptomatic hypokalemia was a clinical problem in only two patients. The decrease in serum potassium probably would have been larger without a supplement than with neutral K-phosphate since it supplies approximately 85 mEq of potassium per day. Potassium supplements may be necessary in certain patients on thiazide-neutral-K-phosphate therapy.

We are not recommending combined thiazide and neutral K-phosphate therapy for all calcium stone-forming patients since most respond dramatically to thiazides alone. This study does present evidence that combined treatment is effective in reducing stone episodes generally but will probably be of most benefit to patients continuing to form stones in spite of thiazide therapy. We also feel that a more extensive study of combined therapy is needed before it can be recommended as a primary treatment modality.

Table 3. Thiazide and K-Phosphate Therapy on Stone Episodes

	A	B	C	D
Number of patients	57	16	12	8
Pretreatment interval (pt. year)	486	87	111	68
Pretreatment stone episodes	476	186	140	84
Stone episodes per patient	8.35	11.6	11.7	10.5
Years per patient (pretreatment)	8.52	5.43	9.25	8.5
Stone episode/100 patients/year	98	214	126	124
Treatment interval (pt. yr)	84	15.2	13.6	9.08
Years per patient (during treatment)	1.5	0.95	1.13	1.14
Stone episodes on treatment	12	4	3	2
Stone episodes predicted	83.4	32.5	17.1	11.0
New stone episodes/predicted (%)	14%	12.3%	17.5%	18%
Chi-square (predicted vs. observed)	61.1	25	11.6	7.3

A: Entire study

B: Patients with > 10 stone episodes pretreatment

C: Patients previously on single drug therapy

D: Patients previously on thiazide therapy

REFERENCES

1. W. G. Robertson, M. Peacock, R. W. Marshall, D. H. Marshall, and B. E. C. Nordin, N. Engl. J. Med. 294:249 (1976).
2. E. R. Yendt, and M. Cohanim, Kid. Int. 13:397 (1978).
3. W. C. Thomas, Jr., Trans. Am. Clin. Climatol. Assoc. 83:113 (1971).

4. M. A. Holliday, R. W. Winters, L. G. Welt, M. McDowell, and J. Oliver, J. Exp. Med. 110:161 (1959).

ACKNOWLEDGMENT

Supported in part by grants from the Urolithiasis Laboratory and Don McMillian and Public Health Services Grants USPH 5 R01 AM 20159 and RSA 13-P-59243. Computational assistance was provided by the Clinfo Project, funded by the Division of Research Resources of the NIH under Grant number RR-00350.

PHOSPHATE TREATMENT OF IDIOPATHIC CALCIUM STONE DISEASE

M. Peacock, W. G. Robertson, P. J. Heyburn,
A. E. J. Davies, and A. Rutherford
M.R.C. Mineral Metabolism Unit
The General Infirmary
Leeds LS1 3EX, U.K.

SUMMARY

1. Thirty-nine patients with active idiopathic calcium stone disease were treated with 1g phosphorus/day given as "Phosphate Sandoz." The urinary stone episode rate was calculated and blood and urine biochemistry measured before and on treatment.

2. Three patients increased their stone episode rate and four failed follow-up. In the remainder the stone episode rate was reduced from 0.74 to 0.24/patient year. There was a sustained and significant rise in 24-hour phosphate excretion and fall in calcium excretion. Urine volume, oxalate and pH were unchanged. The urine supersaturation with calcium phosphate increased and with calcium oxalate decreased. Calcium absorption was unchanged and there was no evidence of increased parathyroid hormone secretion.

3. Oral phosphorus treatment, 1g/day, is successful in reducing the stone recurrence rate in the majority of idiopathic calcium stone formers and does not give rise to serious side effects.

INTRODUCTION

Oral phosphate supplements could affect calcium stone formation through at least two independent actions. The first is by reducing urinary calcium and thus reducing urinary saturation levels of the calcium salts. The second is by increasing urinary inhibitors, mainly pyrophosphate, and thus reducing the growth and aggregation of calcium crystals[1].

There are reports that oral phosphate supplements given on a long-term basis reduce the recurrence rate of stone formation in idiopathic calcium stone disease without causing serious side effects[2]. On the other hand not all studies have shown a beneficial effect[3]. The present paper describes our results using 1g of phosphorus/day on the recurrence rate of calcium stone formers.

PATIENTS AND METHODS

Patients

Thirty-nine patients with idiopathic calcium stone disease attending a stone clinic were studied before and on treatment with oral phosphate given as Phosphate Sandoz 0.25 g four times/day. Sixteen of the patients had previously failed to respond to a low calcium/low oxalate diet, the remainder were untreated.

Stone Episode Rate

A stone episode was defined as the surgical removal or passage of a stone and the rate for the group of patients was calculated by dividing the cumulative sum of the stone episodes by the cumulative sum of the patient years.

Methods

Fasting blood and urine and 24-hour urine were collected on a free diet before and at regular intervals on treatment. Radio-calcium absorption was estimated before and on treatment and analysis of the biochemical variables was carried out as previously described[4].

Statistics

The significance of mean differences between data before and on treatment was evaluated by paired Student's t-test.

RESULTS

Four patients failed to attend for follow-up studies within the first year of treatment. Three patients showed an increase in their stone episode rate on phosphate treatment. The stone episode rate in the remaining 32 patients showed a fall from 0.74 episodes/patient year before treatment to 0.24 episodes/patient year on treatment (Figure 1). There was little change in the rate with the period of time on phosphate and 10 of the patients have now been studied for over four years.

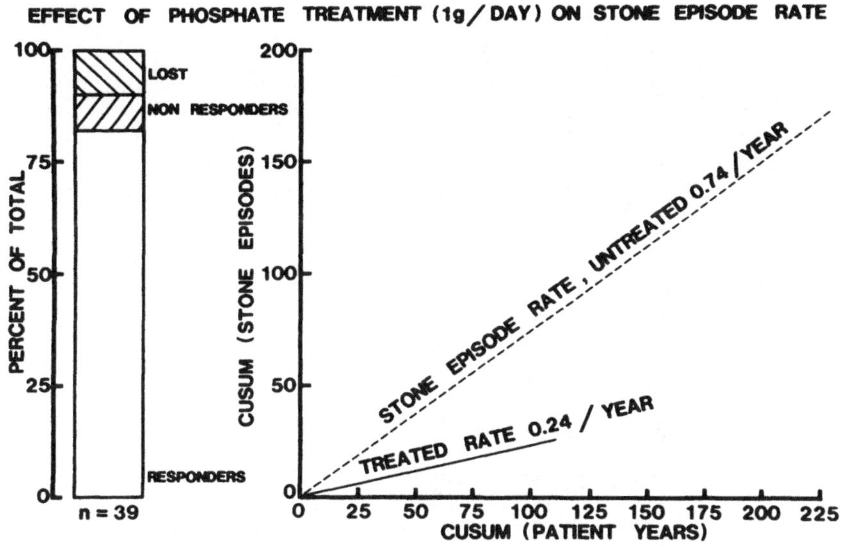

Figure 1. The percentage of patients lost to follow up (lost), failed to respond (non-responders) and who responded (responded) to oral phosphate treatment (left hand panel). The relationship between the cusum of stone episodes and the cusum of patient years before and on treatment with oral phosphate in the group of idiopathic calcium stone formers who responded to treatment.

Table 1 shows the 24-hour biochemistry before and at yearly intervals on treatment with phosphate. There was a sustained and significant rise in urine phosphate excretion and a fall in calcium excretion. Urine volume and oxalate did not change. Urine pH remained above 6 on treatment. The urinary supersaturation levels of calcium oxalate decreased and calcium phosphate increased but not significantly.

Table 2 shows the fasting blood and urine biochemistry and radiocalcium absorption before and in the first and third year on treatment. Plasma calcium, phosphate, parathyroid hormone and radiocalcium were unchanged on treatment. There was a significant rise in alkaline phosphatase and a fall in urine hydroxyproline. The tubular reabsorption of calcium (Tm Ca) was unchanged and tubular reabsorption (Tm P) of phosphate increased.

DISCUSSION

"Phosphate Sandoz" 1g/day in divided doses was well tolerated by all patients and did not give rise to any side effects. In the 35 patients who were followed on treatment only 3 failed to reduce their

Table 1. Effect of Phosphate Treatment on Urine Biochemistry (^{b}untreated, ^{t}treated)

Years on Treatment		Volume (L)			pH			Calcium (mmol)			Phosphate (mmol)			Oxalate (mmol)		
	n	x^b	x^t	p	x^b	x^t	p	x^b	x^t	p	x^b	x^t	p	x^b	x^t	p
1	28	2.2	2.3	ns	6.1	6.3	ns	8.4	6.9	<.02	31	49	<.01	.40	.44	ns
2	33	2.0	2.2	ns	6.1	6.2	ns	8.9	6.9	<.01	29	50	<.01	.39	.43	ns
3	17	2.1	2.4	ns	6.3	6.5	ns	8.8	6.7	<.05	30	49	<.01	.39	.43	ns
4	10	2.0	2.1	ns	6.1	6.4	ns	9.3	5.4	<.01	29	46	<.01	.39	.40	ns

Years on Treatment		Log [CaP]			Log [CaOx]		
	n	x^b	x^t	p	x^b	x^t	p
1	28	.00	.18	ns	.85	.81	ns
2	33	.06	.24	ns	.89	.83	ns
3	17	.09	.38	ns	.85	.77	ns
4	10	.14	.25	ns	.89	.74	ns

Table 2. Effect of Phosphate Treatment on Fasting Plasma and Urine Biochemistry (^{b}untreated, ^{t}treated)

Years on Treatment	Pl. Ca				Pl. PO_4				Pl. Alk. Ph.				Pl. PTH			
	n	x^b	x^t	p	n	x^b	x^t	p	n	x^b	x^t	p	n	x^b	x^t	p
1	39	2.45	2.45	ns	39	0.84	0.83	ns	37	7.3	8.5	<.01	23	154	181	ns
3	24	2.40	2.41	ns	24	0.83	0.85	ns	24	7.0	7.7	ns	-	-	-	-

Years on Treatment	Tm Ca				Tm P				OHP/Cr				Ca^{47} Absorption			
	n	x^b	x^t	p	n	x^b	x^t	p	n	x^b	x^t	p	n	x^b	x^t	p
1	33	1.93	1.94	ns	33	0.94	0.73	<.01	33	.013	0.11	<.05	36	0.98	91	ns
3	24	1.93	1.95	ns	33	0.93	0.75	<.01	24	.014	.013	ns	-	-	-	-

stone recurrence rate on phosphate treatment. These three patients all had a very high stone recurrence rate before treatment and two of them had previously failed to respond to a low calcium and oxalate diet. The reasons for failure in these three patients were not obvious from the urine biochemistry. All fulfilled the criteria for idiopathic calcium stone disease and in particular there was no evidence of hyperparathyroidism, medullary sponge kidney or renal tubular acidosis - conditions which might be expected to have a high stone recurrence rate unresponsive to phosphate treatment. It is interesting, however, that a year after stopping phosphate treatment one of the patients developed hypercalcemia and may have mild primary hyperparathyroidism. Whatever the explanation for the failure of phosphate treatment in these patients they represent a subgroup of idiopathic calcium stone formers in whom stone formation is affected by urinary risk factors other than those examined in the present study.

In 32 patients there was a satisfactory reduction in the stone episode rate. One patient showed rapid growth of a stone in situ which required surgery. Quantitative analysis of the stone, however, showed it to be mainly calcium oxalate. The reduction in the stone recurrence rate was associated with a fall in the supersaturation levels for calcium oxalate and a rise in calcium phosphate mainly due to a fall in urine calcium and rise in urine phosphate. The urinary inhibitory activity was not measured in the present study but from our short term studies where there was a significant increase in urinary inhibitory power[1] it is probably that both saturation and inhibition were altered on long term phosphate treatment.

There was no adverse effect of phosphate treatment on parathyroid function, in agreement with previous studies[2], nor on active intestinal calcium transport.

Our results on stone recurrence rate agree with those showing a reduction in stone episode rate and emphasize the importance of ensuring that the phosphate supplement should be excreted in an alkaline urine to be effective[5].

REFERENCES

1. W. G. Robertson, M. Peacock, R. W. Marshall, C. F. Varnavides, P. J. Heyburn, and B. E. C. Nordin, in:"Urolithiasis Research," H. Fleisch, W. G. Robertson, L. H. Smith, and W. Vahlensieck, eds., Plenum Press, New York/London (1976).
2. L. H. Smith, W. C. Thomas, and C. D. Arnaud, in:"Urinary Calculi: Recent Advances in Aetiology, Stone Structure and Treatment," L. Cifuentes Delatte, A. Rapado, and A. Hodgkinson, eds., Karger, Basel (1973).

3. B. Ettinger, and F. O. Kolb, Am. J. Med. 52:32 (1973).
4. "Calcium, Phosphate and Magnesium Metabolism," B. E. C. Nordin, ed., Churchill Livingstone, Edinburgh/London (1976).
5. K. Lau, C. Wolf, P. Nussbaum, B. Weiner, P. De Oreo, E. Slatopolsky, Z. Agus, and S. Goldfarb, Kid. Int. 16:736 (1979).

PROPHYLACTIC TREATMENT WITH MAGNESIUM HYDROXIDE IN RENAL STONE DISEASE

G. Johansson, U. Backman, B. G. Danielson, B. Fellström,
S. Ljunghall and B. Wikström
Department of Internal Medicine
University Hospital
S-750 14 Uppsala, Sweden

INTRODUCTION

Hammarsten[1] demonstrated 50 years ago that magnesium could increase the solubility of calcium oxalate _in vitro_ and proposed that treatment with magnesium could be used to prevent renal calcium stones. Others[2-3] have shown that magnesium could decrease the incidence of experimental, calcium stone formation. Using a quantitative technique to evaluate the inhibitors of calcium phosphate precipitation in whole urine, Bisaz et al.[4] found that magnesium accounted for approximately 20 per cent of the total inhibitory activity. Experimentally induced, magnesium depletion in the rat has been shown to cause calcification in the proximal tubular cells and the tubular lumen[5].

Magnesium deficiency is apparently not a common feature of renal calcium stone disease[6], but most stone formers seem to have a low urinary excretion of magnesium in relation to calcium[6-9]. It has also been shown in epidemiological studies that a low magnesium/calcium ratio in the urine seems to be an independent risk factor for stone formation[8].

These biochemical and epidemiological findings prompted us to investigate if magnesium could be used for prevention of renal calcium stone formation. In this study we report the biochemical and clinical effects of treatment with magnesium hydroxide during two to three years in renal stone formers in comparison with the natural history of stone disease in a group of patients without prophylactic treatment.

SUBJECTS AND METHODS

Stone Formers

Fifty-six patients with renal calcium stone disease were selected for the treatment. Most of them had experienced frequent recurrences, whereas in some patients an operation due to stone recently had been performed. There were 42 males and 14 females with a mean age of 44 ± 14 years (range 19 - 76 years). Besides routine, clinical work-up, a special program for evaluating the magnesium metabolism was performed[6]. No patient showed evidence of magnesium deficiency.

All patients, except two, had experienced stones during the last two years prior to treatment and altogether 22 patients had been operated at least once due to the stone disease. A new x-ray of the urinary tract was taken before treatment unless the last one had been done during the preceeding three months. Two men had experienced approximately 100 stones each, while the remaining patients had passed 460 stones during 550 patient years, i.e. a stone-episode rate of 0.8 stones/year.

Controls

Forty-three patients with renal stone disease followed at the stone clinic formed a control group. These patients were not on medical treatment, either because it was considered that their stone disease was not active enough for prophylactic treatment or because the patients preferred not to have any medication. There were 35 males and 8 females with a mean age of 45 ± 11 years. The mean stone episode rate was calculated to 0.5 stones/year.

Treatment and Follow-up

After the patients had been informed and their consent had been obtained verbally, treatment was instituted with magnesium hydroxide, 250 mg magnesium, twice daily. Biochemical investigations were performed after 1, 3 and 6 months and thereafter at regular six-month intervals.

RESULTS

Clinical Effects

Forty-seven of the 51 patients have been on treatment for at least three years and 40 of these have during that time been free of stone recurrence (Figure 1). Four of the remaining seven patients have experienced passage of new stones, while in the other three new stones or growing stones were found in the kidneys when the yearly routine x-ray was performed. The mean stone-episode rate was reduced on treatment from 0.8 to 0.05 stones/year/patient.

In the control group, 15 out of 43 patients had formed new stones after two years observation and 15 out of 37 after three years without prophylactic treatment (Figure 1).

Effects of Magnesium and Calcium

The effects of treatment on magnesium and calcium for the 51 patients who completed at least six month's therapy are summarized in Table I. The serum magnesium increased during the first six months, but thereafter returned to the pretreatment level (Figure 2). The urinary magnesium excretion increased by 1.5 - 2.0 mmol/24 hours during the first month, irrespective of the pretreatment level, and remained on this level during the follow-up period. No changes were observed in either the serum or the urinary calcium excretion and consequently, the urinary magnesium/calcium ratio increased and approached the value found in healthy subjects[10].

The magnesium content in muscles was unchanged after two years' therapy, when reinvestigated in 15 patients (Table I).

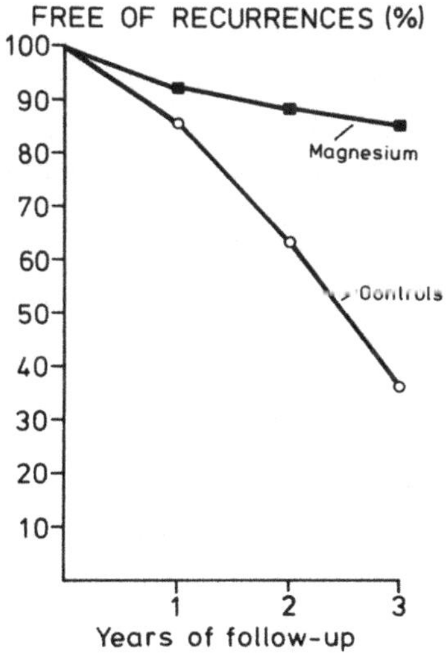

Figure 1. The renal stone recurrence rate in stone formers on prophylactic treatment with magnesium hydroxide in comparison with controls.

Table I. Biochemical Data in 51 Renal Stone Formers on Treatment with Magnesium Hydroxide. Mean ± S.D.

	Before Therapy	On Therapy
Serum magnesium (mmol/l)	0.83 ± 0.06	0.83 ± 0.05
Urinary magnesium (mmol/24 h)	4.6 ± 1.5	6.4 ± 2.5[a)]
Urinary calcium (mmol/24 h)	7.2 ± 2.8	6.3 ± 2.7
Urinary magnesium/calcium	0.7 ± 0.2	1.1 ± 0.5[a)]
Muscle magnesium (mg/100 g FFS)	3.7 ± 0.6	3.4 ± 0.5[b)]
Urinary citrate (mmol/24 h)	2.6 ± 1.4	3.0 ± 1.3[c)]

a) $p < 0.001$ compared with pretreatment values

b) n = 15

c) n = 40, $p < 0.01$ compared with pretreatment values.

Effects on Urinary Citrate

The average urinary citrate excretion increased in 30 out of 40 investigated patients and was on treatment close to that found in healthy subjects, i.e. 3.1 ± 1.2 (S.D.) mmol/24 h[11] (Table I).

Side Effects

Three patients failed to return for follow-up of unknown reason, and another two patients discontinued the therapy during the first

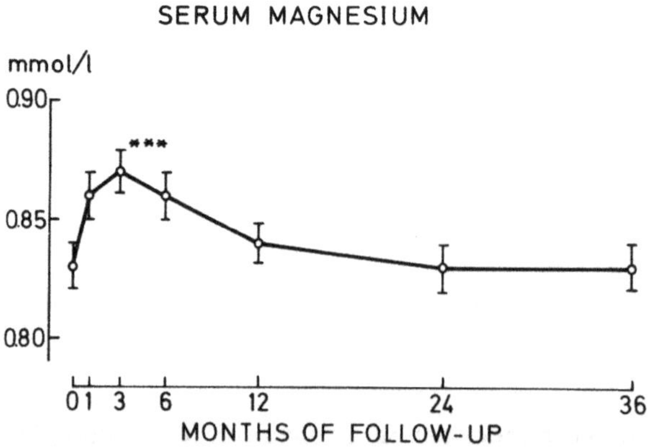

Figure 2. The serum magnesium concentration in renal stone formers before and on treatment with magnesium hydroxide.

six months because of gastrointestinal discomfort. Another few patients experienced mild degrees of gastrointestinal disturbances, but continued the treatment after a temporary reduction of the dose. One of the patients that experienced recurrence on therapy, had frequent lower urinary tract infections prior to therapy. Repeated urine cultures had been negative prior to the start of the therapy. However, after six months of therapy a pyelolithotomy had to be performed due to rapid growth of calculi in one kidney. The possible role of the magnesium treatment as a contributing factor for the stone growth in this case could not be completely ruled out.

DISCUSSION

The present report indicates that magnesium hydroxide has a beneficial effect in prophylactic treatment of patients with renal calcium stones. This is in agreement with results from earlier studies where magnesium oxide was used[12,13]. The results are also comparable with our earlier experience as well as others with thiazides as a prophylactic treatment of renal stones[14,15].

The possible role of magnesium in inhibiting calcium crystallization seems to be dependent rather on the concentration of magnesium in relation to that of calcium, than on the absolute amounts of the electrolytes in the urine. When evaluating the capacity to inhibit stone formation, it therefore seems appropriate to calculate the urinary magnesium/calcium ratio. This was also found to be low in stone formers[6], but normalized on therapy, due to the increased excretion of magnesium and the unchanged excretion of calcium in the urine.

The possibility of a magnesium deficiency in renal stone formers has been suggested[12], due to an observed increased urinary excretion of magnesium during the course of magnesium treatment. This could also be suspected in our patients, because of the increase in serum magnesium during the first six months. However, when the intracellular magnesium concentration was reevaluated in 15 patients after two years therapy, it was found to be unchanged compared to the pretreatment values. This would indicate that magnesium deficiency probably is rare as a common cause of renal stone formation. The observation that the serum values decreased to the pretreatment values after six month's therapy, may be due to some slow-acting magnesium-regulating system.

Adverse effects with the therapy were uncommon. Only two patients discontinued the treatment due to gastrointestinal discomfort, whereas another few temporarily reduced the dose because of mild intestinal disturbance. Possible harmful adverse effects with long-term treatment with magnesium must also be considered, but hypermagnesemia following oral ingestion of magnesium without concomitant disease in the intestine or a renal insufficiency has not been reported[16]. In this study no patient had an impaired renal function as could be judged from the clearance of creatinine or had any sign of intestinal disease. Furthermore, both the serum magnesium and the intracellular magnesium concentration remained unchanged during the follow-up period.

Dietary supplements of magnesium has been shown to increase the urinary excretion of citrate[17]. Urinary citrate excretion in our investigated stone formers was low in comparison with controls, but increased on therapy and approached the value found in our control group. Urinary citrate has, at least *in vitro*, been demonstrated to be a potent inhibitor of the precipitation of calcium salts. An increase in citrate output together with an increased urinary magnesium/calcium ratio may shift the situation in the urine to be less favorable for crystal formation, aggregation and stone growth.

In conclusion, our present experience indicates that prophylactic treatment with magnesium hydroxide reduces the stone recurrence rate in renal calcium stone formers. Side effects are few, but possible adverse effects during long-term treatment has to be evaluated. On therapy, the urinary magnesium/calcium ratio increases due to an increased excretion of magnesium with an unchanged output of calcium.

REFERENCES

1. G. Hammarsten, C. R. Lab. Carlsberg 17:1 (1929).
2. T. A. Borden and E. S. Lyon, Invest. Urol. 6:412 (1969).
3. J. F. Desmars and R. Tawashi, Biochim. Biophys. Acta. 313:256 (1973).
4. S. Bisaz, R. Felix, W. F. Neuman, and H. Fleisch, Mineral Electrolyte Metab. 1:74 (1978).
5. G. E. Bunce and G. A. King, Exp. Mol. Pathol. 28:322 (1978).
6. G. Johansson, U. Backman, B. G. Danielson, S. Ljunghall, and B. Wikström, Invest. Urol. (in press).
7. A. Hodgkinson, Clin. Sci. Mol. Med. 46:357 (1974).
8. S. Ljunghall and A. U. Waern, Scand. J. Urol. Nephrol. Suppl. 41:55 (1977).
9. H.-G. Tiselius, L. E. Almgard, L. Larsson, and B. Sörbo, Eur. Urol. 4:241 (1978).
10. B. G. Danielson, G. Johansson, and S. Ljunghall, Scand. J. Urol. Nephrol. Suppl. 51:49 (1979).
11. B. Wikström, U. Backman, B. G. Danielson, B. Fellström, G. Johansson, and S. Ljunghall, in:"Proceedings Fourth International Urolithiasis Research Symposium," L. H. Smith, B. Finlayson, and W. G. Robertson, ed., Plenum Press, New York (in press).

12. I. Melnick, R. R. Landes, A. A. Hoffman, and J. F. Burch, J. Urol. 105:119 (1971).
13. E. L. Prien and S. F. Gershoff, J. Urol. 112:509 (1974).
14. E. R. Yendt and M. Cohanim, Kid. Int. 13:397 (1978).
15. U. Backman, B. G. Danielson, G. Johansson, S. Ljunghall, and B. Wikström, Br. J. Urol. 51:175 (1979).
16. J. P. Mordes and W. E. C. Wacker, Pharmacol. Reviews 29:273 (1978).
17. S. N. Gershoff and E. L. Prien, Am. J. Clin. Nutr. 20:293 (1967).

EXPERIENCES WITH LONG-TERM USE OF SODIUM CELLULOSE PHOSPHATE FOR PREVENTION OF RENAL CALCIUM STONES

S. Ljunghall, U. Backman, B. G. Danielson, B. Fellström,
G. Johansson, B. Wikström, and O. Wålinder
Department of Internal Medicine,
University Hospital,
S-750 14 Uppsala, Sweden

INTRODUCTION

A high urinary calcium level is common in renal stone patients [1,2]. The majority of hypercalciuric patients appear to have a primary intestinal hyperabsorption of calcium[3,4]. Since the risk of calcium stone-formation is closely related to the urinary calcium output[1,5], a logical approach for prevention of stones should be to reduce the amount of calcium absorbed from the intestine and thereby its excretion through the kidneys. When dietary calcium restriction fails to reduce calcium excretion and stone-formation is of clinical importance drug treatment might be indicated.

Sodium cellulose phosphate (SCP) is an ion-exchange cellulose which binds to intestinal calcium and prevents its absorption. It also in a similar way binds to other divalent cations[6]. During recent years clinical studies have been reported on the use of SCP in patients with recurrent calcium stones[7-10]. In these investigations over shorter periods of time than in our study patients on SCP have usually not formed any new stones. However, comparison with the natural history of stone disease in untreated patients has not been carried out. Since the recurrence rate of stone disease is so variable it is not impossible that the apparent beneficial effects of SCP could have occurred by chance in some instances.

In this study we report on our experiences with treatment of patients with recurrent stones with SCP followed for three years. We compare the outcome of treatment with the course of stone disease among a group of untreated patients.

Particular interest has been directed to the long-term effects of SCP on calcium metabolism since theoretically there is a risk of inducing calcium malabsorption and secondary hyperparathyroidism with a drug that interferes with intestinal calcium uptake.

PATIENTS AND CONTROLS

SCP was administered to 35 patients, 32 males and 3 females with a mean age ± standard deviation of 42 ± 12 years. All of them had a history of recurrent, radio-opaque stones. One of them had passed hundreds of stones during an interval of more than ten years. The remaining individuals had experienced 120 stones during 160 patient years, which yields a mean stone episode rate of 0.7 stones/year.

Recent stone analyses were available in 14 cases. In 11 of them calcium oxalate was the major constituent; 3 patients had pure apatite stones. Intestinal hyperabsorption of calcium was diagnosed using an isotope technique[12]. In addition, all the patients had normal or low values for serum parathyroid hormone (PTH) and/or urinary excretion of cyclic adenosine monophosphate (cAMP). Fasting urinary calcium was within the normal range. Thus the hypercalciuric patients were considered to suffer from primary intestinal hyperabsorption of calcium.

The natural history of stone disease was followed prospectively in a group of 43 patients (35 males and 8 females) with a mean age of 45 ± -11 years and a mean duration of stones of seven years. During this time they had on the average experienced 0.5 stones/year. These patients were not receiving any drug for prevention of stones. Although they had formed recurrent stones many of them were not motivated for medical treatment, in others it was considered that stone disease was not active enough.

All patients and controls were followed at regular intervals (generally each six months) at our outpatient clinic. They received the same type of general advice about the importance of a high fluid intake and moderated reduction of calcium and oxalate intake[12].

SCP was given in a standard dosage of 5 g in sachets within half an hour before meals three times daily.

METHODS

Serum and urinary electrolytes were measured by atomic absorption. Each value for urinary electrolyte excretion was based on two consecutive 24-hour collections. Parathyroid hormone concentrations (PTH) were determined by a commercial method (Medicinsk Laboratorium, Copenhagen). The urinary excretion of cyclic AMP (cAMP) was measured with a radioimmunoassay technique which gives a normal range of 0.2

- 0.6 mol/mmol creatinine[14]. Fasting urinary calcium[3] was determined after an overnight fast. In the same samples of urine hydroxyproline was measured by a colorometric method (Organon, Oss, Netherlands). Urinary citrate was analyzed by an enzyme method (citrate-lyase), with a normal value of 3.1 ± 1.2 mmol/24h.

After three years' therapy, but not before onset of treatment, percutaneous muscle biopsies were taken and analyzed for magnesium and potassium. This procedure is described elsewhere[14,15].

RESULTS

Out of the 35 patients, 13 were followed for three years. Three patients were lost to follow-up during the first year for unknown reasons and another two moved out of our area. Therapy was withdrawn because of side-effects in 11 cases. The reasons for cessation of treatment were usually a combination of mild -to-moderate gastrointestinal discomfort and a reduced tolerance to the taste together with practical problems associated with administrations of the drug, for example, during meals taken outside the home. In addition, therapy was withheld in six patients because of lack of effect.

The effects of SCP on serum and urine parameters are summarized in Table 1. In all the patients except three, SCP caused a reduction in urinary calcium within the first month. This reduction was sustained in all the examined cases during the follow-up period. The reduction of calcium output was most evident in patients with the highest pre-treatment levels but it could also be seen in most normocalciuric individuals. The average reduction of calcium excretion was 30%. Concomitantly with this also magnesium output fell, the average decrease being 40%. Thus the urinary magnesium/calcium ratio fell in almost all the patients during therapy with SCP. Although magnesium absorption apparently was reduced, there were no effects on serum magnesium levels and when the intracellular magnesium concentrations were determined after three years' therapy all the patients studied showed values clearly within the normal range.

There was a non-significant increase in both serum and urinary phosphate (probably due to slight hydrolysis of SCP in the intestine) during the first year of therapy but not thereafter. All patients exhibited normal serum levels of zinc, copper and iron after three years on SCP.

The values for serum PTH and urinary cAMP were unchanged during therapy and there was no evidence of increased bone resorption. A small increase of the serum alkaline phosphatase was seen during the first month but no further rise thereafter.

Table 1. Effects of SCP in Patients with Recurrent Renal Stones (Mean Values ± S.D.)

	Months of Treatment		
	0	1	36
No. of Patients	35	30	15
Recurrent Stones	-	1	9
Serum values			
Calcium (mmol/1)	2.46±0.07	2.46±0.07	2.44±0.06
Magnesium (mmol/1)	0.82±0.05	0.81±0.05	0.82±0.07
Phosphate (mmol/1)	0.92±0.19	0.95±0.15	0.88±0.15
Alkaline Phosphatase (µkat)1)	2.80±0.70	3.10±0.70*	2.93±0.84
PTH (µg/1)	0.38±0.10	-	0.36±0.08
Urine values			
Calcium (mmol/24 h)	8.4 ±3.1	5.2 ±1.6***	5.7 ±1.9**
Magnesium (mmol/24 h)	5.0 ±1.7	3.1 ±1.3***	2.8 ±1.1***
Phosphate (mmol/24 h)	32 ±6	36 ±10	37 ±12
OH-proline (mg/mmol creat)	7.3 ±3.1	-	6.8 ±2.6
cAMP (mmol/mmol creat)	0.34±0.08	0.38±0.10*	0.34±0.11
Citrate (mmol/24 h)	2.2 ±1.2	-	2.0 ±1.1

*) p <0.05; **) p < 0.01; ***) p < 0.001 compared with pre-treatment values (paired t-test)

Altogether 12 patients experienced recurrences during treatment with SCP. The mean stone episode rate during the 64 patient years of therapy was 0.3 stones/year. In the untreated controls during the same period 17 out of 43 patients formed new stones and the mean stone episode rate decreased to 0.3 stones/year. Thus the pattern of stone formation was not different in the SCP-treated group compared to the untreated patients (Figure 1).

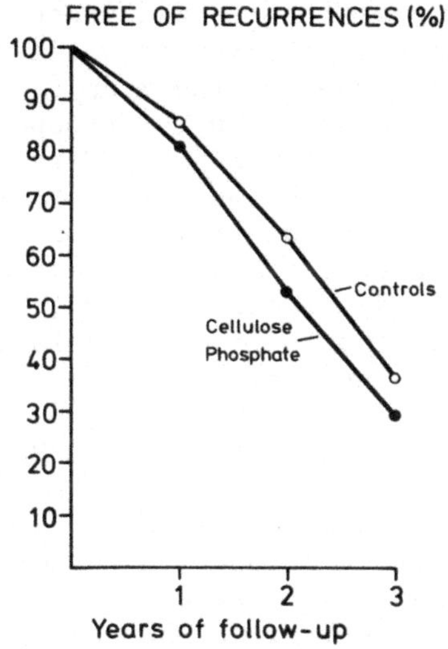

Figure 1. Recurrence of renal stones in stone-patients treated with sodium cellulose phosphate or given only general advice.

DISCUSSION

Patients treated with SCP for a period of up to three years appeared to experience a reduction of the propensity to form stones: The mean stone episode rate decreased from 0.7 to 0.3 stones/year. However, among control patients, followed without treatment, a similar apparent improvement could be seen. The fact that these patients were seen at our clinic and were receiving some general advice could be of some importance. However, among the controls there were no significant changes of the urinary calcium excretion or even of the urinary volume during this period. Therefore it seems unlikely that their stone-forming tendency was actually affected.

It could be questioned if the calculation of a mean stone episode rate yields a representative picture of the course of stone disease. In many patients stone disease is highly variable and longer or shorter symptom-free periods may follow an episode of stones. Since treatment generally is instituted shortly after the passage of a stone there will for this reason only be an apparent reduction of the stone episode rate during the first period of follow-up. This drawback in the assessment of stone activity will be reduced when the duration of follow-up is extended.

Another possible reason for the differences in stone episode rates for both the treated and untreated patients is differences in diagnostic precision. In general, the mean stone episode rate before treatment (or follow-up) is based on a retrospective analysis of stone disease while the corresponding rate during follow-up is made prospectively and there is an obvious risk of bias in judging the symptoms both from the doctor and from the patient. Taken these facts together we believe that there is no evidence to support the view that stone disease was affected during follow-up in the untreated controls. Rather the apparent reduction in the stone episode rate in these patients was artefactual.

If we had not compared the outcome of SCP treatment with the untreated controls, we might have been of the impression that therapy had caused an improvement of stone disease. However, in relation to the controls the effect of treatment was largely disappointing. Despite a clear reduction of calcium excretion stone patients continued to form stones. This lack of therapeutic effect could be due to several different causes. Firstly, the effect of SCP in preventing absorption also of other divalent cations than calcium might be of importance. Urinary magnesium was reduced to a larger extent than was the calcium output. In vitro magnesium is an inhibitor of calcium oxalate crystallization and a high magnesium output seems to prevent against calcium stone formation[1,14]. Secondly, urinary oxalate was not measured in our patients. Calcium and oxalate are normally complexed in the intestinal tract and the excretion of oxalate is therefore to a large extent inversely related to the intestinal calcium content. When the availability of intestinal calcium is reduced (as during treatment with SCP), oxalate should be more easily absorbed. In previous studies significant increases of the oxalate output have been reported[10,15] and the number of calcium oxalate crystals has been found to increase[16].

The effects of SCP on urinary magnesium and oxalate excretion obviously counteract the reduction of calcium output. They could be overcome by dietary restriction of oxalate intake and by the addition of magnesium supplements. In the study by Pak et al.[7], where these measures were instituted, better prophylaxis was reported with 80% of the patients free of recurrences after 2 years of therapy.

However, dietary restrictions are difficult to impose during chronic treatment[12] and when magnesium is added the risk of gastrointestinal symptoms is increased[14].

During the three years of treatment there was no evidence of secondary hyperparathyroidism or increased bone resorption in our patients. In this context it should be pointed out that none of our cases had renal hypercalciuria. If such cases were given SCP further increase in negative calcium balance would be expected. There have been reports about the development of hyperparathyroidism during treatment with SCP which could have come about by this mechanism[17].

From our study it appears that when SCP is used in absorptive hypercalciuria the underlying abnormality is corrected adequately. Calcium homeostasis appears to adapt to the new situation. During the first months there are slight increases in serum PTH and urinary cAMP as well as in serum alkaline phosphatase. After the initial period no further changes appear and a new steady state seems to be achieved.

In order to avoid negative calcium balance in SCP-treated patients an evaluation of calcium absorption and parathyroid activity seems necessary both before and during therapy.

SUMMARY

Sodium cellulose phosphate (SCP) (5 g three times daily) was given to 35 patients with recurrent formation of calcium-containing renal stones, who were followed for up to three years. During treatment urinary calcium was reduced by an average of 30%. There was no evidence of secondary hyperparathyroidism or increased bone resorption. The urinary magnesium decreased but there were no effects on the serum or intramuscular magnesium concentrations.

The effects on stone-formation appeared to be small. Compared to an untreated control group there were no significant changes in the stone episode rate and after three years on SCP, 68% had formed recurrent stones. Gastrointestinal discomfort was common and necessitated withdrawal of treatment in 11 patients.

REFERENCES

1. S. Ljunghall and A. U. Waern, Scand. J. Urol. Nephrol. Suppl. 41:55 (1977).
2. B. E. C. Nordin, M. Peacock, and R. Wilkinson, Clin. Endocr. Metab. 1:169 (1972).
3. C. Y. C. Pak, M. Ohata, E. C. Lawrence, and W. Snyder, J. Clin. Invest. 54:387 (1974).
4. S. Ljunghall, U. Backman, B. G. Danielson, B. Fellström, G. Johansson, and B. Wikström, Scand. J. Urol. Nephrol. Suppl. 54: (1980).
5. C. Y. C. Pak and K. Holt, Metabolism 25:665 (1976).
6. C. Y. C. Pak, J. Clin. Pharmacol. 13:15 (1973).
7. C. Y. C. Pak, C. S. Delea, and F. C. Bartter, New Engl. J. Med. 290:175 (1974).
8. J. Pietrick and F. Kokot, Br. J. Urol. 45:136 (1973).
9. G. A. Rose and A. R. Harrison, Br. J. Urol. 46:261 (1974).
10. R. Hautmann, F. J. Hering, and W. Lutzeyer, J. Urol. 120:712 (1978).

11. S. Ljunghall, U. Backman, B. G. Danielson, G. Johansson, B. Jung, R. Källsen, L. Wibell and O. Wålinder, Scand. J. Urol. Nephrol. Suppl. 41:77 (1977).
12. S. Ljunghall, U. Backman, B. G. Danielson, B. Fellström, G. Johansson, and B. Wikström, Scand. J. Urol. Nephrol. Suppl. 54 (1980).
13. O. Wålinder, S. Ljunghall, and L. Wibell, Scand. J. Urol. Nephrol. 12:67 (1978).
14. G. Johansson, Scand. J. Urol. Nephrol. Suppl. 51 (1979).
15. Y. Hayashi, R. A. Kaplan, and C. Y. C. Pak, Metabolism 24:1273 (1975).
16. P. C. Hallson and G. A. Rose, Br. J. Urol. 48:515 (1976).
17. J. R. Condon, R. A. V. Milsted, and J. R. Nassim, Br. J. Urol. 48:316 (1976).

LONG-TERM EFFECTS OF CAMPANYL IN THE TREATMENT OF PATIENTS WITH RECURRENT CALCIUM URINARY STONES

E. W. Rugendorff[+], H.-J. Schneider[++], and
O. Hallwachs[+++]
+ Department of Urology, Falkeneck Hospital of Braunfels,
++ Department of Urology and O.P.C. University of Jena,
+++ Department of Urology, Municipal Hospital Darmstadt,
University of Frankfurt

The nonabsorbable cation exchange resin Campanyl (Figure 1) complexes with dietary calcium in the gastrointestinal tract and hinders its absorption. Campanyl is 50% amberlite, in the K^+ form, and 46.8% sorbital. It binds 1.935 mEq Ca^{2+}/(g resin). The drug was given orally with meals as a long-term therapy in patients with recurrent calcium urolithiasis[1-4]. After exclusion of primary hyperparathyroidism, an absorptive hypercalciuria could be detected in 40% and a resorptive, mixed (absorptive + resorptive) or renal hypercalciuria in 20% of the patients. The remaining patients were normocalciuric or inconstantly hypercalciuric.

Hyperuricosuria ± hyperuricemia was frequently (approximately 25%) encountered in both hypercalciuric and normocalciuric patients. The differentiation of the various forms of hypercalciuria was achieved by an ambulatory evaluation similar to that described by Pak[5].

Additional information was attained by cation exchange screening. Absorptive hypercalciuria decreases within 48 hours if Campanyl is given orally with meals. This is regarded as an indication for a subsequent treatment of the urolithiasis with cation exchange resins. The dosage of Campanyl is adjusted to the urinary calcium excretion, usually 15g/day. It is well tolerated.

Fifty patients with indications for resin therapy have been given the cation exchange preparation Campanyl for several years, 15 of them subsequently were given Ujolyt. Ujolyt is 88.4% wofalite, in charged with a mixture of H^+, K^+, Na^+, NH^+_4, and Mg^{2+}, and 10.4% amylopectin. Before starting these patients passed at least 2 stones

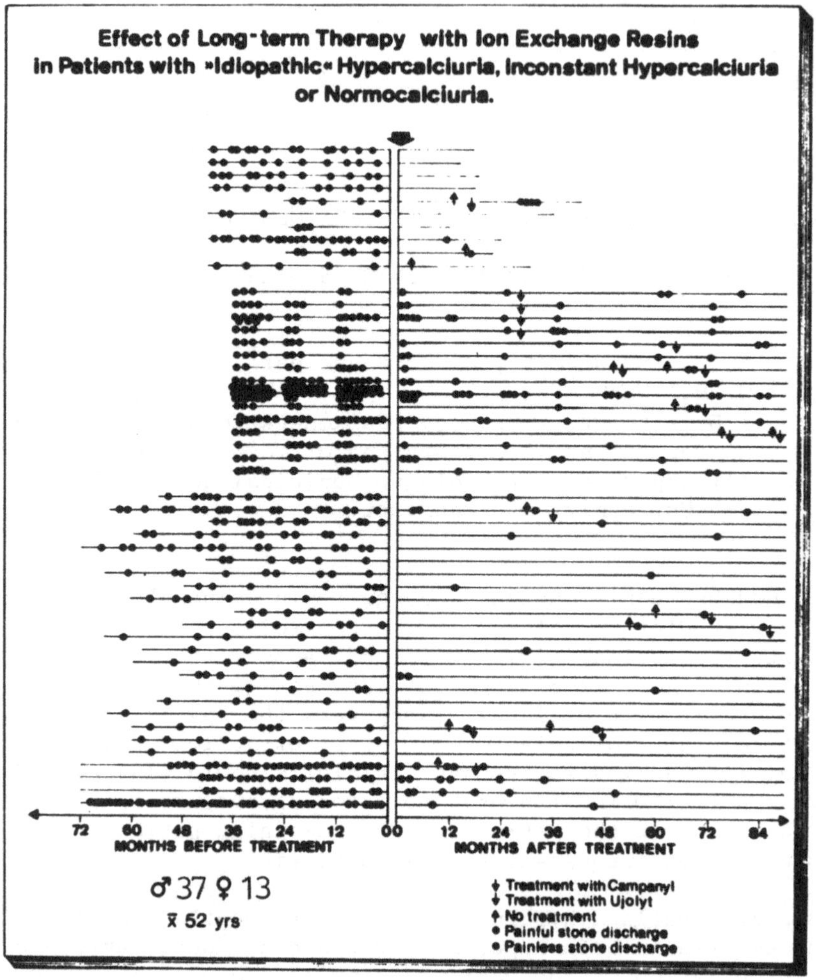

Figure 1.

(sometimes more than 30 calculi) per patient year. The rate of stone occurrence during treatment was reduced to 0.3 stones per patient year (Figure 1). Furthermore, the patients claimed that urinary calculi passed during cation exchange therapy usually were discharged without colic. Some weeks after stopping cation exchange resin therapy many patients discharged urinary stones with renal colic[6,7,8]. The cation exchange resins reduce urinary calcium (Figure 2). Urinary oxalate may consequently rise, probably because of binding of part of the dietary calcium to the cation exchange resin. Since the fall in urinary calcium is usually more prominent, the urinary state of saturation with respect to calcium oxalate does not change significantly. Campanyl therapy causes no significant alterations of serum potassium, calcium, phosphorus and iPTH, even if given over a long period of time[9,10].

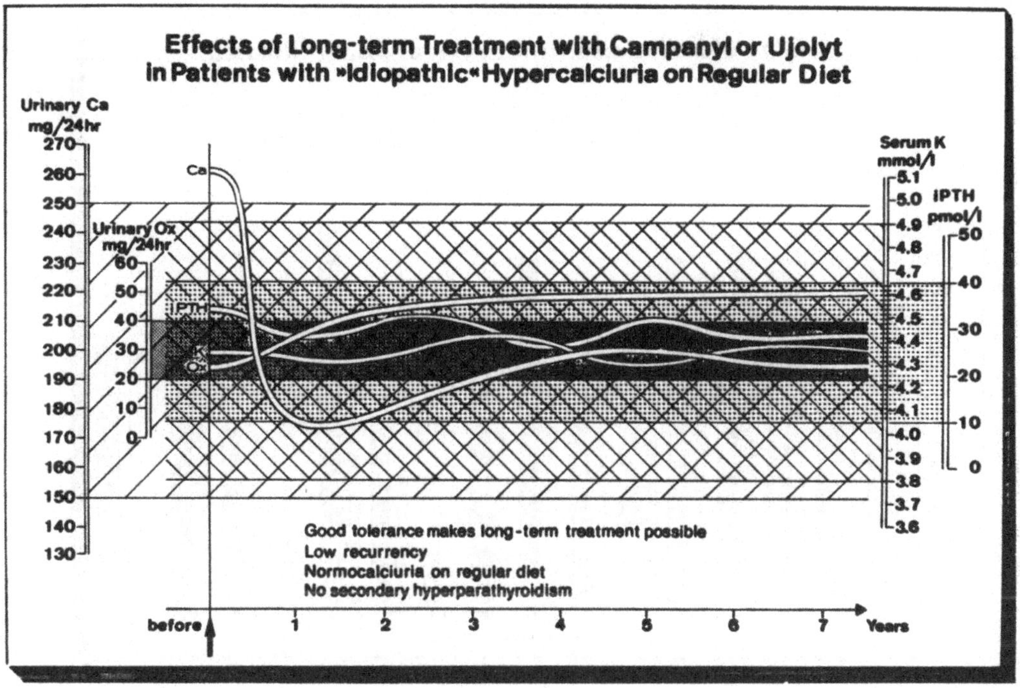

Figure 2.

We have not yet been able to explain the efficacy of the cation exchange therapy in normocalciuric patients with frequently recurring urinary calculi. Stone reduction is as dramatic in patients with normocalciuria as it is in patients with severe calcium overexcretion. Differential renal function studies show that in patients with unilateral stone disease the calcium concentration in urine from the stone forming kidney is less than in urine from the normal kidney. Apparently, even with a low calcium concentration, urine from the calculous kidney can cause crystals to grow and aggregate (Figure 3). Absolute calcium excretion is only an indirect measurement of risk, as urine volume, pH, oxalate excretion and ionic strength all affect the calcium oxalate ion product which may be altered by urine inhibitors, also. This suggests that the main importance of urinary calcium consists in increasing the urine calcium oxalate supersaturation. Since a low urinary calcium greatly decreases the chances of developing calcium stones, a possible explanation for the efficacy of cation exchange resins might thus be the protective effect of relative hypocalciuria which alters the urine from oversaturation to undersaturation in terms of calcium oxalate.

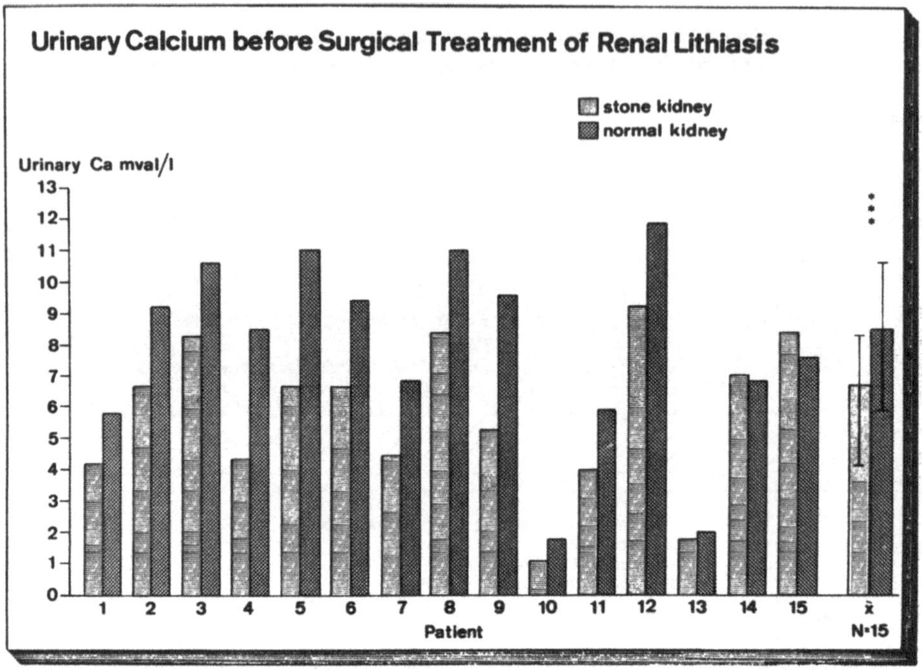

Figure 3.

REFERENCES

1. E. W. Rugendorff, H.-J. Schneider, G. Gundlach, W. A. Behrendt, D. Kuhn, and D. Gundlach, Urologe A 16:197 (1977).
2. E. W. Rugendorff, H.-J. Schneider, D. Kuhn, W. A. Behrendt, and S. Kornmann, in:"Pathogenese und Klinik der Harnsteine V," Dr. Dietrich Steinkopff Verlag, Darmstadt (1977).
3. H.-J. Schneider and G. Stein, Dt. Gesundh.-Wesen 34:2385 (1979).
4. O. Hallwachs, Urologe B 19:293 (1979).
5. C. Y. C. Pak, R. A. Kaplan, H. Bone, J. Townsend, and O. Waters, N. Engl. J. Med. 292:497 (1975).
6. E. W. Rugendorff, Medicamentum 6:234 (1967).
7. Th. Burghele, E. W. Rugendorff, and T. Covaliu, Urologe A 6:234 (1967).
8. O. Hallwachs, in:"Pathogenese und Klinik der Harnsteine VII," Dr. Dietrich Steinkopff Verlag, Darmstadt (1979).
9. E. W. Rugendorff and S. Kornmann, in:"Pathogenese und Klinik der Harnsteine VI," Dr. Dietrich Steinkopff Verlag, Darmstadt (1978).
10. F. Hering, R. Hautmann, and W. Lutzeyer, in:"Pathogenese und Klinik der Harnsteine VII," Dr. Dietrich Steinkopff Verlag, Darmstadt (1979).

HOW TO INCREASE THE LITHOPROTECTIVE AND/OR LITHOLYTIC PROPERTIES OF URINE

P. Leskovar, R. Hartung, M. Hropot, M. Simmel,
R. Allgayer, E. Wellnhofer, and E. Hoffmann
Urologische Klinik und Poliklinik Rechts der Isar der
Technischen Universität München
Munchen, Germany

INTRODUCTION

Recently, several investigators reported that stone patients have a reduced urinary citrate[1,2,3]. This citrate "deficit" in stone formers may be the cause of their recurrent calcium calculi. Bach et al.[1] alluded to the low citrate level and the high calcium concentration in the urine of their stone patients. A high Ca/citrate ratio can be considered as a stone risk factor. The authors emphasized the importance of substances, stimulating the renal citrate secretion, for the prophylaxis of urolithiasis. In accordance with other investigators, the highly significant citrate "deficit" in patients was one of the most pronounced differences between recurrent stone formers and healthy controls that we could find during our six week follow up of the urinary parameters like total and ionized Ca, Mg, Na, Zn, uric acid, creatinine, Pi, urea, citrate, titratable acidity, NH_4[1], Ca- and uric acid- crystalluria, surface tension and microerythruria. We however suggest that stone formers are characterized not only by a reduced citrate secretion but also by a general deficit in urinary organic acids, citrate being one of the main representatives. In our quantitative in vitro experiments by the Coulter Counter Size Distribution measuring technique we could show that citric acid and some other tri- and dicarboxylic acids as acids and as salts not only strongly inhibited the precipitation and the growth of Ca-oxalate and Ca-phosphate crystals out of meta- and unstable solutions but also led to a considerable disaggregation and dissolution of pure stone forming crystals and of native oxalate and phosphate stones. Some of the tested acids showed a surprisingly high efficacy, comparable with that of the citric acid (e.g. tricarballylic acid). Therefore, we were interested in the increase of the Ca^{2+}-binding capacity of urine not only by the stimulation of the tubular citrate secretion but also by the renal secretion of substances that proved in vitro to act litholytically.

The extensive animal experiments, a great many substances in varying doses were tested; here only some few representatives of the substances that proved to be effective are presented. Interestingly, some of the tested substances exerted both effects: they stimulated the tubular citrate secretion and acted additionally by themselves, appearing unchanged in urine. The stimulation of the tubular citrate secretion seems to be a selective process[4-7].

MATERIALS AND METHODS

The following reagents were used: Calcium chloride-2-hydrate, Merck 2382; di-Na-oxalate, Merck 6557; sodium chloride, Merck 6404; sodium hydroxide, Merck 9956; citric acid, Merck 244; Malonic acid, Roth 1-8325; oxalacetic acid, Roth 2-6827; tricarballylic acid, Serva Feinbiochemica; dihydroxyfumaric acid, Roth 2-3599; itaconic acid, Serve Feinbiochemica.

Determination of urinary citrate was made with the Boehringer Test-Kombination Nr. 139076 (Boehringer/Mannheim). In reporting these measurements appropriate corrections were made for urine dilution.

The following instruments were used: Coulter Counter ZF/Channelyzer P 128 (all: Coulter Electronics/Krefeld); Präzisions-pH-Meter E 510/Impulsomat E 473/Dosimat E 535 (all: Metrohm/Herisau); Ca^{2+}-sensitive electrode Orion 93-20/Ionalyzer 801 A (both Colora Meßtechnik/Lorch); Spectralphotometer Beckman 24 (Beckman Instr./München).

The animal experiments are characterized as follows: Wistar rats (Stamm SPF and Hattersheim); normal laboratory diet (Sniff/Intermast); before administration of test substance, 3.0 (2.0) ml water per kg body-weight ("blank"); administration of test substance, 2.0 (1.0) ml test-substance solution + 1.0 (1.0) ml water per kg; urine collection, 4 h - (20 h, 24 h).

Titration of urine samples with 0.01 M KOH after the preacidification to pH < 2.0 should reveal if the test substances, inhibiting the in vitro growth and aggregation of CaC_2O_4 crystals, occur in the urine of treated animals. The comparison of both titration curves before and after the oral administration of Ca^{2+}-binding test-substances allowed the estimation of the resorption rate and renal elimination of tested substances. The global secretion of buffering anions measured in the 4 h urines was additionally related to the weight of rats and expressed as mmol/h/kg. In addition, the Ca^{2+}-

binding capacity of the urine before and after oral administration of test substances was investigated. To 500 µl neutralized urine, 500 µl of the 20 mM $CaCl_2$-standard were added and the volume adjusted (by dist. water) to 2000 µl. The resulting Ca^{2+}-concentration was measured by the Ca^{2+}-selective electrode Orion 93-20, combined with the Orion-Ionalyzer 801A. The results were expressed as direct Ca^{2+}-readings.

RESULTS AND DISCUSSION

In Figure 1, the considerable differences in the consumption of 0.01 M KOH for the titration of preacidified urine from pH 4.0 to pH 6.0 before and after the oral administration of various test substances are pointed out. The increased buffering of the urine after the oral administration of the test substances (hatched columns) heightens the binding capacity of urine for the free Ca^{2+} ions. Figure 2 demonstrates the significantly increased renal citrate secretion in rats after administration of some test-substances. In Figure 3, the absolute Ca^{2+}-values after addition of the "treated" and "untreated" urine to a 20 mM $CaCl_2$-standard solution are depicted graphically. The hatched columns represent the urine after the oral administration of test-substances.

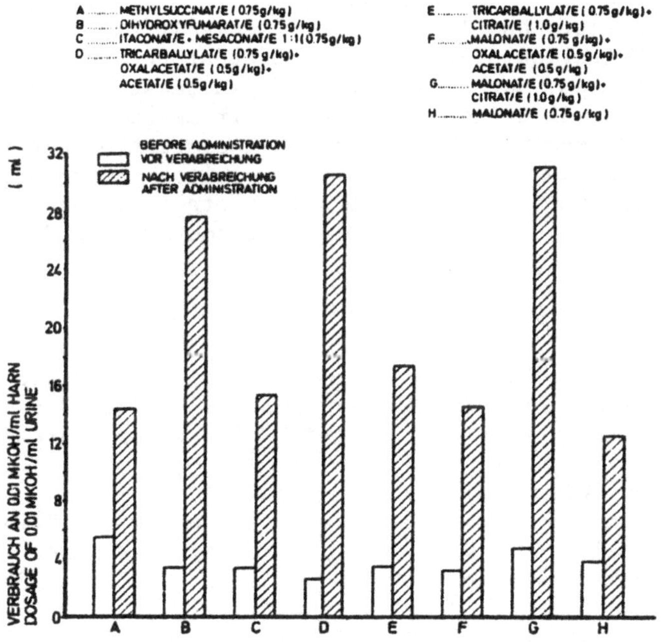

Figure 1. The increased consumption of 0.01 M KOH for the titration of the urine from pH 4.0 to 6.0 after oral application of test-substances, indicating the higher content of org. acids in urine after treatment.

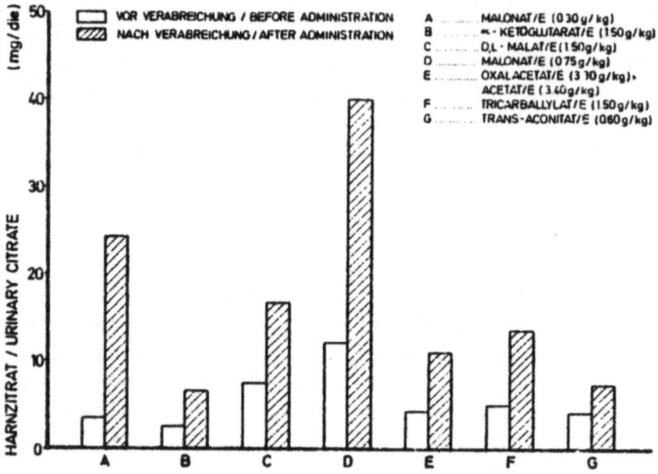

Figure 2. The significantly increased tubular citrate secretion in rats after oral application of various test-substances.

CONCLUSION

From our in vitro and in vivo experiments it can be concluded that oral administration of the described substances as well as some additional substances, not mentioned here, increase the Ca^{2+}-binding capacity of the animal urine, partly by their appearance (in unchanged form) in urine, partly by their stimulating effect of the renal tubular secretion of citrate. The results, though being preliminary, awake the hope that the lithoprotective and litholytic properties of urine could be to some extent modulated and actively influenced.

REFERENCES

1. D. Bach, A. Hesse, W. Schneeberger, W. Vahlensieck, and W. Hamm, in:"Pathogenese und Klinik der Harnsteine VII," G. Gasser and W. Vahlensieck, ed., Dr. D. Steinkopff Verlag, Darmstadt (1979).
2. A. Hodgkinson, Clin. Sci. 23:203 (1958).
3. A. Knappwost and E. Matouschek, in:"Pathogenese und Klinik der Harnsteine III, Dr. D. Steinkopff Verlag, Darmstadt (1975).
4. T. Nielsen and S. Rensen, Acta Med. Scand. 205:303 (1979).
5. H. Otto, Schweiz, Med. Wschn. 29:968 (1957).
6. G. Pylypchuk, U. Ehrig, D. R. Wilson, Can. Med. Assoc. J. 120:658 (1979).
7. B. H. Robinson, J. Oci, S. Cheema-Dhadli, and M. L. Halperin, J. Biol. Chem. 252:5661 (1977).

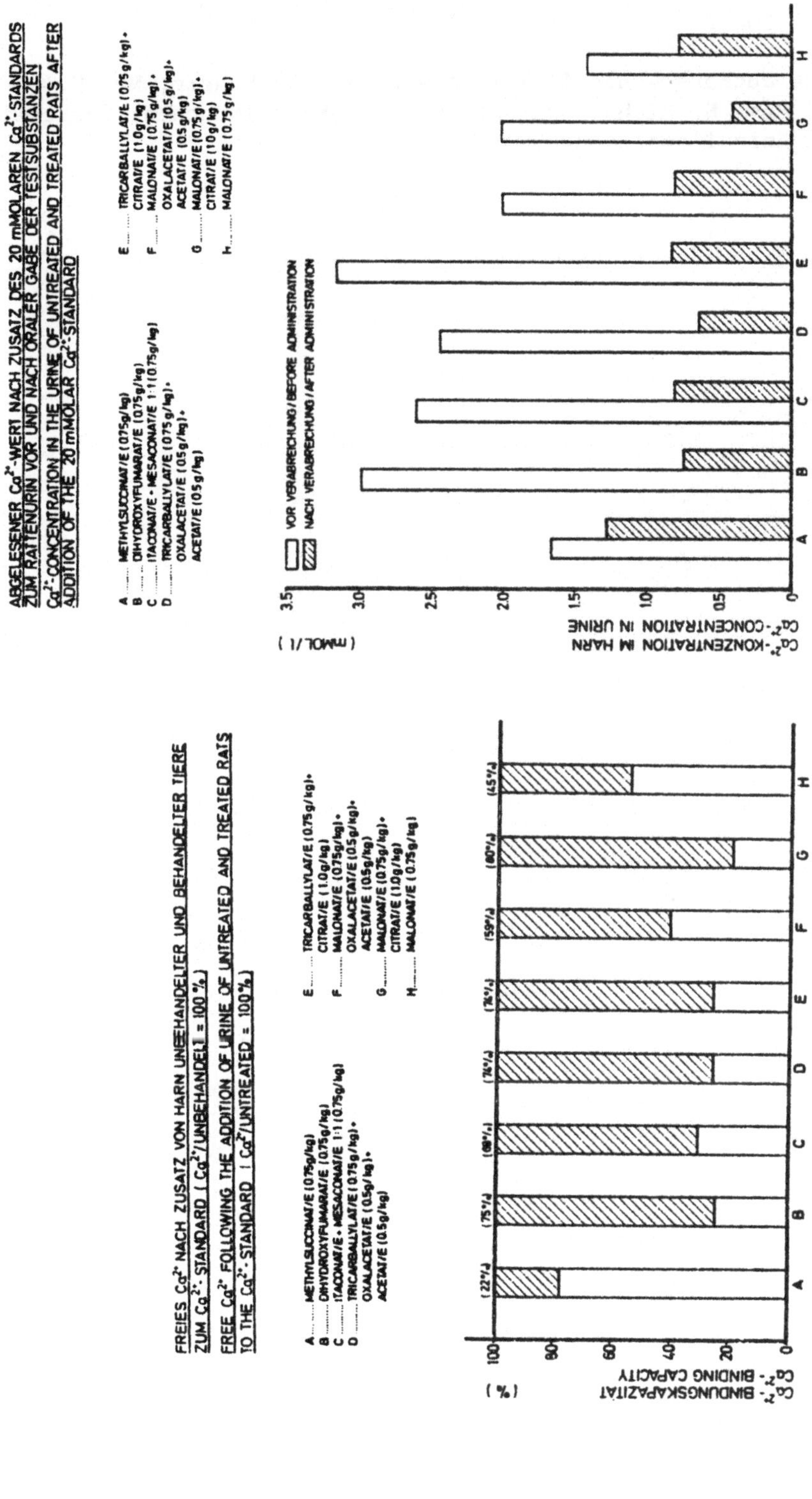

Figure 3. Comparison of the Ca^{2+}-binding capacity of treated and untreated animals.

ACKNOWLEDGMENT

The authors would like to thank Mrs. D. Scherm, Mr. K.-L. Schade, Mrs. H. Richter and Mr. M. Gottinger (München) for their kind technical assistance.

NATURAL VOLATILE OILS IN THE MANAGEMENT OF RENAL CALCIUM STONE DISEASE

E. J. Will, G. D. Bell, M. Taylor, C. Richmond,
A. Middleton, N. Johnson, and B. Dhillon
Nottingham City Hospital and University of Nottingham

Nottingham, U.K.

Volatile (essential) oils derived from plants are used widely in clinical medicine and lay pharmacy. Perhaps the best known examples are the use of menthol as a nasal decongestant, and dill in gripe water as a carminative. There is anecdotal evidence for the effectiveness of natural oils in renal stone disease[1], and European patients not uncommonly turn to "herbal" remedies (e.g. in U.K. - "Dutch drops," "Six-Herb kidney and bladder tablets") to augment more conventional treatment (this is often unadmitted unless interview is particularly thorough). Is there any reason to believe that these are more than fanciful placebos?

The biological properties attributed to various oils include analgesic, antibacterial and antispasmodic activity. Favorable results have been reported from the use of peppermint oil in the irritable bowel syndrome, and a menthol-based mixture ("Rowachol") in biliary stone disease[2,3]. In addition, the metabolites of these compounds may be expected to show inhibitory activity on the crystallization of calcium salts (vide infra)[4]. We have, therefore, studied the properties of Rowatinex (Rowa Ltd., Bantry, Co. Cork, Eire), a mixture of essential oils containing pinene (31%), camphene (15%), borneol (10%), anethol (4%), fenchone (4%) and cineol (3%).

The oils may be oxidized, sulphated, or glucuronidated, or metabolized to unidentified products. Alpha and beta-borneol glucuronide could be detected in the urine after treatment with Rowatinex[5], but no other components were present in their native form. A mean recovery of 80% ingested borneol was obtained in the first 24 h urine - 52% as glucuronides and 28% as sulphate.

The effect of Rowatinex (1.08 g daily for one week) on urinary composition was measured in six healthy subjects (aged 25-35) on a free diet. Table 1 shows data from 24 h urine specimens taken before and on the last day of treatment. There was a doubling of glucuronide excretion but no change in other variables related to the inhibition of crystal growth.

Table 1. The Effect of Rowatinex on the Composition of 24 h Urine

Measurement	Control	After One Week	P
Urine Volume ($ml\ 24\ h^{-1}$)	1548 ±168	1667± 261	>0.50
Creatinine ($mmol\ 24\ h^{-1}$)	16.21±0.47	15.99±0.42	>0.50
Glucuronide - Total[5]	2.49±0.11	4.86±0.61	0.01
($mmol\ 24\ h^{-1}$) Conjugated	2.05±0.11	4.15±0.51	0.02
Inorganic Sulphate ($mmol\ 24\ h^{-1}$)[6]	29.3 ±2	26.0 ±3	>0.20
Glycosaminoglycans ($mg\ 24\ h^{-1}$)[7]	27.3 ±3.5	23.3 ±1.6	>0.20
Inhibition of Calcium Oxalate[8] Crystal Growth (% - urine at 1:20)	48.7 ±2	47.0 ±1	>0.20

In a separate study a single volunteer took Rowatinex 2.16 g daily while on a fixed diet. There was no significant change in urine volume, nor the excretion of creatinine, calcium, phosphate and uric acid. The urines were subsequently examined using a modification of the system of Hallson and Rose[9]. Undiluted samples at pH 5.3 were progressively concentrated in a rotary evaporator at 37°C. ^{14}C-oxalate was used to quantitate crystallization in serial aliquots. Crystallization of calcium oxalate occurred at ca 1000 mOsm Kg^{-1} in all control and test specimens. There was a suggestion of less crystal growth in the test suspensions at each osmolality, but this was not significant.

The model of nephrocalcinosis in the rat devised by Chow et al. was used to assess high dose Rowatinex therapy[10]. Male Wistar rats (180-280 g) were fed glycolic acid (3% w/w) for 6 weeks. Rowatinex (2% w/w) (~0.5 g/kg) and an isocaloric placebo (olive oil) were compared in 2 groups of 6 animals.

All animals were in good condition at sacrifice, the treatment group having gained more weight than controls ($p < 0.01$). There were no abnormal findings at necropsy beyond corticomedullary nephrocalcinosis. There were no significant differences between the groups whether the calcinosis was assessed histologically or by measurement of calcium in the tissue.

The activity of a glucuronide on calcium oxalate crystallization was measured using ammonium menthol glucuronide (AMG) isolated from the urine of rabbits dosed with menthol[11] (99% pure by chromatography, sulphur < 0.5%). Two in vitro systems were employed.

(a) Crystal growth and aggregation[12]. At 10^{-2} mol/l AMG there was significant reduction of growth and aggregation compared with control suspensions, but no effect at lesser concentration.

(b) Crystal growth[8] - AMG at 5 x 10^{-3} mol/l reduced crystal growth at 20 minutes by 50%, and by 25% at 2.5 x 10^{-3} mol/l. These concentrations of glucuronide are barely attainable in vivo (see Table 1).

The effect of Rowatinex (1.08 g/day) on the course of acute ureteric colic is being assessed in a continuing double-blind controlled trial in Nottingham. Preliminary results show slight reductions in the duration of in-patient residence, analgesia and the number of patients coming to surgery. There is a more impressive difference in the number of patients stone-free at three weeks in the treatment (60%, n = 20) compared with the placebo (44%, n = 18) group. None of these differences is statistically significant.

Our studies show that Rowatinex doubles glucuronide excretion and this might achieve levels that would reduce calcium oxalate crystallization. This was not demonstrable in systems using dilute or whole urine samples in vitro. The preliminary results of a controlled trial in ureteric colic suggest some benefit of Rowatinex, particularly in accelerating the passage of calculi.

REFERENCES

1. Culpepers Complete Herbal - 17th Century.
2. W. D. W. Rees, B. K. Evans, and J. Rhodes, Br. Med. J. 4:835 (1979).
3. G. D. Bell and J. Doran, Br. Med. J. 1:24 (1979).
4. C. W. Vermeulen, B. Finlayson, and W. Chapman, J. Urol. 77:685 (1957).
5. G. L. C. methods on file - Rowa Limited, Bantry, Co. Cork, Eire.
6. A. Swaroop, Clin. Chim. Acta. 46:333 (1973).
7. P. Whiteman, Biochem. J. 131:351 (1973).
8. E. J. Will, O. L. M. Bijvoet, and H. te Brake - v.d. Linden, in:"Urolithiasis Research," H. Fleisch, W. G. Robertson, L. H. Smith, and W. Vahlensieck, eds., Plenum Press, New York (1976).
9. P. C. Hallson and G. A. Rose, Br. J. Urol. 50:442 (1978).

10. F. H. C. Chow, M. I. Dysart, D. W. Hamar, and R. H. Udall, Invest. Urol. 13:113 (1975).
11. R. J. Williams, Biochem. J. 32:1849 (1938).
12. H. Fleisch and A. Monod, in:"Urinary Calculi," L. Cifuentes-Delatte, A. Rapado, and A. Hodgkinson, eds., Karger, Basel (1973).

FYBRANTA(R) - A NEW APPROACH TO THE TREATMENT OF IDIOPATHIC HYPERCALCIURIA

P. J. R. Shah, G. Williams, and N. A. Green

Department of Urology, Norfolk & Norwich Hospital,

Norwich, England

INTRODUCTION

Idiopathic hypercalciuria occurs in approximately 50-60% of patients with urolithiasis[1]. It has been shown that the stone recurrence rate can be reduced[2] in the patients by significantly lowering their urinary calcium. Cellulose phosphate and thiazide diuretics have both been used successfully in the treatment of this condition[1,3]. They may be associated with side effects[1], however, and long-term treatment requires supervision.

We have recently shown that unprocessed bran produces an effective reduction in urinary calcium excretion. Unprocessed bran can be taken without any ill-effect, though large doses tend to be unpalatable. FYBRANTA(R) tablets are compressed unprocessed bran which are more palatable than their precursor and may also be taken easily in divided doses. A trial of the treatment of 25 patients with idiopathic hypercalciuria with FYBRANTA tablets is presented.

PATIENTS AND METHODS

Twenty-five patients (23 male and 2 female) with idiopathic hypercalciuria (urinary calcium excretion > 7.5 mmol/24 h) were included in the study. The age range was from 30-75 years with a mean of 50 years.

Six tablets of FYBRANTA were prescribed to be taken in 3 equal doses with meals daily for 2 months. Each patient was asked to remain on a normal diet throughout the study. Serum and 24 h urine collections (for calcium, phosphate, magnesium, urea, creatinine and sodium) were obtained at monthly intervals during treatment and again after treatment had been stopped for one month.

RESULTS

The initial biochemical data of the patients are shown in Table 1. Serum calcium, phosphate and magnesium were within the normal range as were 24 h urinary phosphate and magnesium. The mean 24 h urinary calcium was 10.5 mmol.

Table 1. Results of Treatment of Patients with Idiopathic Hypercalciuria with FYBRANTA(R) (mean values)

		Prior to Treatment	At One Month	At Two Months	After Treatment Stopped
Responders (n=17)	Serum mmol/l				
	Calcium	2.36	2.37	2.40	2.40
	Phosphate	0.90	0.92	0.94	0.88
	Magnesium	0.73	0.73	0.75	0.76
	Urine mmol/24 h				
	Calcium	11.2	8.8	8.38*	8.15
	Phosphate	35	39.2	36.9	31.8
	Magnesium	4.6	4.3	4.2 *	4.3
Non-Responders (n=8)	Serum mmol/l				
	Calcium	2.41	2.43	2.44	2.39
	Phosphate	0.98	0.97	0.92	0.90
	Magnesium	0.73	0.73	0.76	0.74
	Urine mmol/24 h				
	Calcium	9.1	10.8	11.05X	9.08
	Phosphate	31.6	44.4	45.4	35.
	Magnesium	3.6	4.2	4.9 X	4.20

*P < 0.001
X P < 0.01

During treatment with FYBRANTA(R) 17 patients (68%) significantly reduced their urinary calcium excretion (p < 0.001), 8 patients did not respond but increased their urinary calcium levels (p < 0.01) (Figure 1).

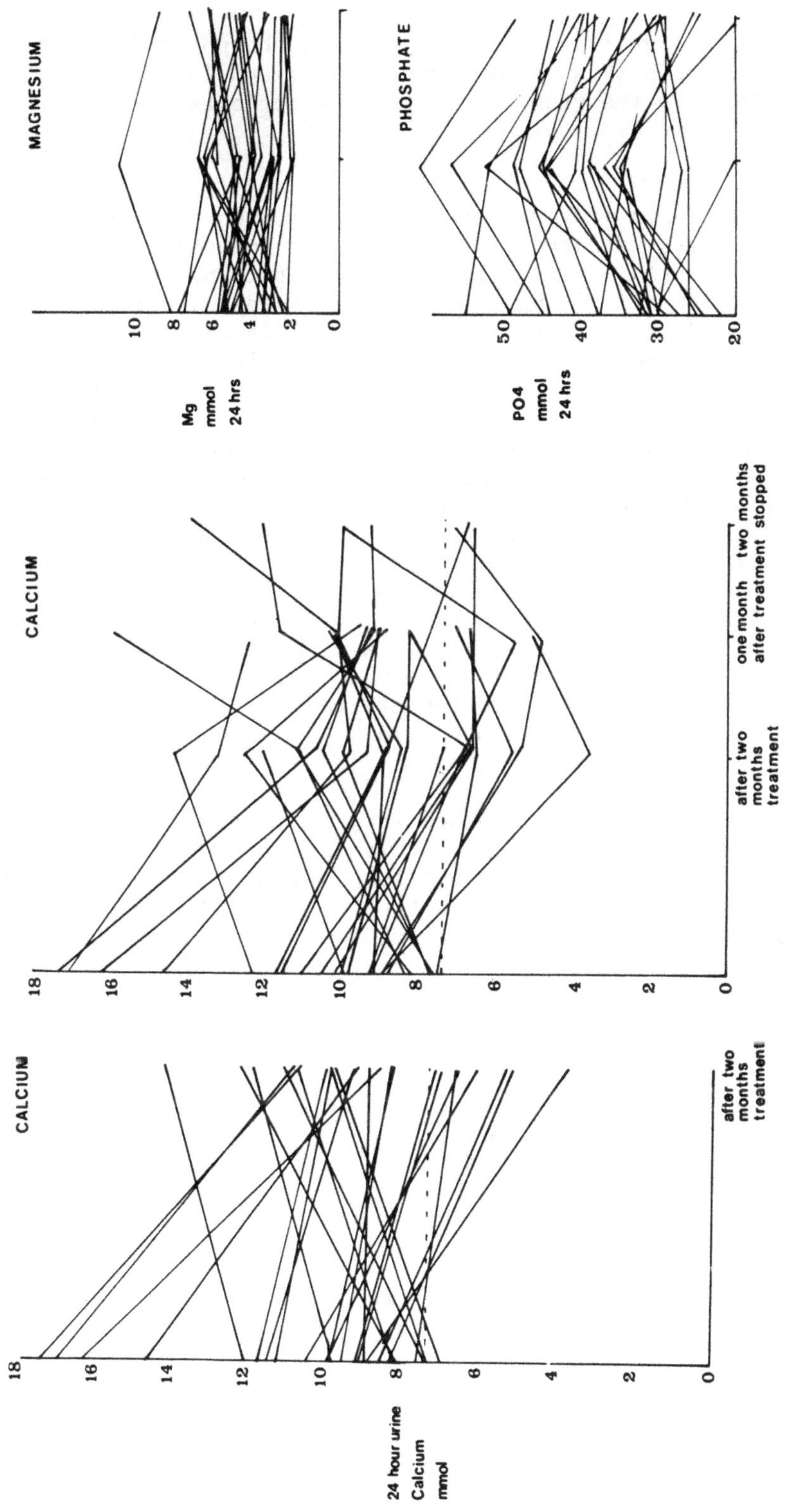

Figure 1. Results of treatment with FYBRANTA in 25 patients with idiopathic hypercalciuria.

There was a significant rise in urinary phosphate during treatment in all patients (Figure 1) and a significant fall in urinary magnesium levels in the group of responding patients.

DISCUSSION

We have shown in previous studies that unprocessed bran effectively reduces urinary calcium excretion in patients with idiopathic hypercalciuria. This effect is thought to be partly due to the binding of intestinal calcium by phytic acid present in bran (1.7g phytic acid in 100g bran). FYBRANTA(R) is unprocessed bran which has been compressed into tablet form to allow ease of consumption at regular intervals. This study shows that FYBRANTA(R) effectively reduces urinary calcium and magnesium excretion in 68% of patients with idiopathic hypercalciuria. The effect on calcium absorption, however, cannot be altogether related to phytate as each tablet contains 100 mg of calcium phosphate. This is included for the purpose of binding phosphate and to avoid calcium depletion in those patients for whom FYBRANTA is primarily designed, i.e. patients with constipation or diverticular disease. It is likely that other factors are involved in the reduction in urinary calcium excretion. A decrease in intestinal transit time will reduce the time available for mineral absorption to occur and may account for the fact that both calcium and magnesium excretion are reduced in the patients responding to treatment. Bran may also have a direct binding action on calcium.

The levels of urinary phosphate were significantly increased during treatment with FYBRANTA(R). This is probably related to the absorption of phosphate from the calcium phosphate included in the tablet. Several patients have been treated with FYBRANTA for periods of up to 6 months and a sustained reduction in calcium excretion has been achieved. It is yet to be seen whether the incidence of stone recurrence is reduced with this treatment.

REFERENCES

1. G. A. Rose and A. R. Harrison, Br. J. Urol. 46:261 (1974).
2. N. J. Blacklock and M. A. Macleod, Br. J. Urol. 46:385 (1974).
3. C. Y. C. Pak, C. S. Delea, and F. C. Bartter, New Engl. J. Med. 290:175 (1974).

ACKNOWLEDGMENT

We would like to thank Mr. M. Scott, Norgine, Ltd. High Holborn, London for his support in providing the FYBRANTA for this study.

II. EPIDEMIOLOGY, NUTRITION AND ENVIRONMENT

A RISK FACTOR MODEL OF STONE-FORMATION: APPLICATION TO THE STUDY OF EPIDEMIOLOGICAL FACTORS IN THE GENESIS OF CALCIUM STONES

W. G. Robertson, M. Peacock, P. J. Heyburn, A. Rutherford,
V. J. Sergeant, and C. P. Bambach*
M.R.C. Mineral Metabolism Unit and *Department of Surgery, The General Infirmary,
Leeds LS1 3EX, U.K.

Within the last few years a new concept has evolved to account for calcium stone-formation in the urinary tract. This attributes the disorder to a combination of "risks" derived from the slightly (or sometimes grossly) abnormal excretion of one or more urinary constituents[1,2]. The six main risk factors identified so far are a high urinary pH, an increased urinary excretion of calcium, oxalate or uric acid, a low urinary volume or a reduced excretion of alcian blue precipitable inhibitors of crystallization (mainly acidic glycosaminoglycans (GAGS)). The relative potency of these risk factors is in the order ↓ volume ≃ ↑ oxalate > ↓ GAGS > ↑ uric acid > ↑ pH > ↑ calcium. Using simple probability theory it can be shown that the overall relative probability of forming a stone (P_{SF}) is given by the expression:

$$P_{SF} = (\alpha_{Vol}\alpha_{Ca}\alpha_{Ox}\alpha_{pH}\alpha_{UA}\alpha_{GAGS})/1 + (\alpha_{Vol}\alpha_{Ca}\alpha_{Ox}\alpha_{pH}\alpha_{UA}\alpha_{GAGS})$$

where α_{Vol} etc. are the contributions from the six risk factors[1,2].

We have previously shown that the values of P_{SF} are higher in idiopathic stone-formers than in normal subjects[1,2]. Recurrent stone-formers have the highest P_{SF} values and these correlate well with the severity of the disease as defined by the stone episode rate of the patient[1]. Single episode stone-formers (SSF) have values intermediate between those of normals and those of RSF. Patients with secondary calcium stones also have abnormally high values of P_{SF}[2].

EPIDEMIOLOGICAL FACTORS IN CALCIUM STONE-FORMATION

Many environmental and metabolic factors influence the rate of calcium stone-formation. The effects of these on the six urinary risk factors and on the overall relative probability of stones has been assessed from personal studies and various reports in the literature. These findings are summarized in Table 1.

(a) Age and Sex: It has been long recognized that idiopathic calcium stones occur mainly in men, the male/female ratio being about 4 or 5 to 1. The peak age of onset is about 28 years but since stones tend to recur, the peak age of occurrence is some years later. In men this is about 35 whereas in women there is a double peak, the first at about age 30 and the second about age 55. The incidence of idiopathic stones in children and in the elderly is very low.

This pattern is paralleled by the relative values of P_{SF} in the two sexes and in the various age groups within each sex. P_{SF} values are lowest in children, slightly higher in women and highest in men[2].

(b) Affluence, Social Class and Occupation: It has often been suggested that calcium stone-formation in the upper urinary tract is a disease of the affluent or industrialized society[3-5]. Indeed, this has recently been confirmed at four separate demographic levels[6]. The more affluent countries, sections of society and individuals spend more of their resources on animal protein. Such a diet, in turn, increases the urinary excretion of calcium, oxalate and uric acid, 3 of the 6 risk factors for calcium stone disease (Table 1). Interestingly, surveys carried out on vegetarians show that they have a low biochemical risk of stones[7] and the prevalence of stones is about one fifth of that in the general population.

(c) Diet: Dietary factors other than animal protein appear to play a lesser role. There are some broad correlations between stone incidence and calcium and fat intake but there are no significant correlations with the intakes of oxalate, magnesium, phosphorus, acid-base balance, total protein or dietary fiber[8]. In particular, there is no consistent relationship with the consumption of refined carbohydrate, contrary to the suggestion of Blacklock[5].

(d) Fluid Intake: Chemically a low urine volume increases the risk of all types of stone-formation. On the risk factor model, the risk of calcium oxalate stones increases rapidly below urine volumes of about 1 liter/day (Table 1)[5,6]. This is supported by data on stone incidence from Israel[9].

(e) Climate: Apart from the influence of temperature on urinary volume it would appear that increased exposure to sunlight may be another risk factor for the disorder. By increasing vitamin D production in the skin, UV light may increase calcium absorption and

Table 1. The Effect of Various Epidemiological Factors on the Relative Probability of Forming Calcium Stones (P_{SF})

Factor	Prevalence of Stones	Urine Biochemistry of Groups at Risk of Stones						
		Volume	pH	Calcium	Oxalate	Uric acid	GAGS	P_{SF}
Age	child<adult>elderly	n	n	↑	↑	↑	n↓	↑↑
Sex	♂ > ♀	n	n	↑	↑	↑	n↑	↑↑
Affluence	rich > poor	n	n↓	↑	↑	↑	?	↑
Social class	I>II>III>IV>V	n	n↓	↑	↑	↑	?	↑
Occupation	sedentary>manual	n	n↓	↑	↑	↑	?	↑
Diet	high animal protein > vegetarian	n	↓	↑	↑	↑	↑	↑↑
Fluid	low > high	↓	n	n	n	n	?	↑↑
Climate	hot > temperature	↓	n↓	↑	n↑	n	?	↑
Season	summer > winter	n↓	n	↑	↑	n	?	↑
Hyperparathyroid	HPT > normal	n	↑	↑	↑	n	n	↑↑
RTA	RTA > normal	n	↑	n↑	n	n	?	↑
Hyperoxaluric	HOX > normal	n	n	n↓	↑↑	n	n↓	↑↑

thereby urinary calcium and P_{SF} (Table 1). This appears to increase the risk of stones in troops moving to hot, sunny environments[10] and in beach life-guards[11].

Apart from climatic factors, seasonal changes in temperature and exposure to sunlight may also be important for increasing P_{SF} (Table 1) and the incidence of stones through effects on increasing urinary calcium and oxalate during the summer months[12].

(f) Metabolic and Genetic Abnormalities: Patients with various metabolic disorders, which predispose to secondary calcium stone-formation, also have abnormal values of P_{SF}. This may be due to increases in urinary calcium (e.g. in primary hyperparathyroidism (HPT) and in some cases of renal tubular acidosis (RTA)), in urinary oxalate (e.g. in HPT and in congenital and enteric hyperoxaluria) or in urinary pH (HPT and RTA).

MODEL OF CALCIUM STONE-FORMATION

Figure 1 summarizes the overall risk factor model of stone-formation. According to this the first prerequisite of stones is a period of abnormal crystalluria during which a particle is formed which is large enough to become trapped in the urinary tract. The formation of abnormal crystals in turn, results from a combination of possible abnormalities in six urinary risk factors giving rise to a high overall relative probability of forming stones. Ultimate-

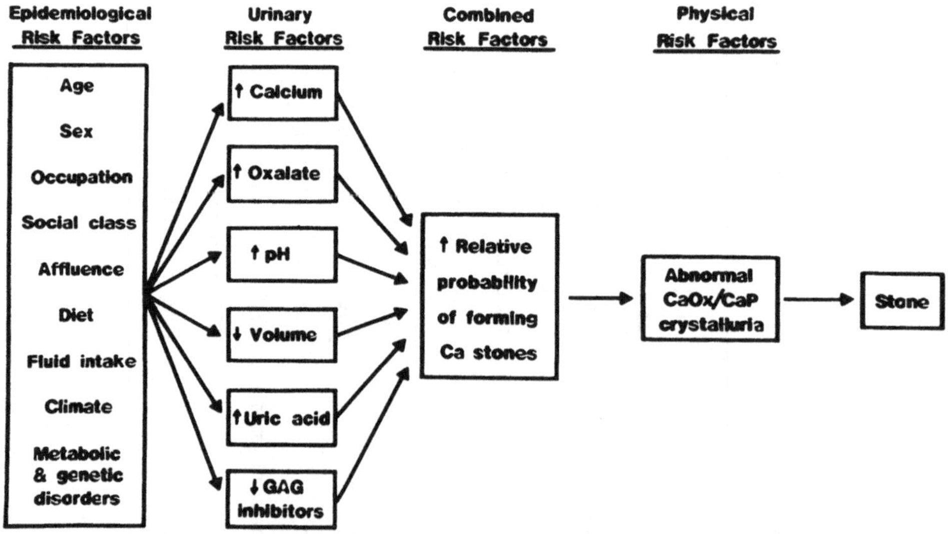

Figure 1. A risk factor model of calcium stone-formation.

ly, there is a set of epidemiological, pathophysiological and environmental risk factors which between them account for the abnormalities in the urinary risk factors.

REFERENCES

1. W. G. Robertson, M. Peacock, P. J. Heyburn, D. H. Marshall, and P. B. Clark, Br. J. Urol. 50:449 (1978).
2. W. G. Robertson, M. Peacock, P. J. Heyburn, and C. P. Bambach, in:"Urinary Calculi, Proceedings of the International Urinary Stone Conference, 1979," J. G. Brockis and B. Finlayson, eds., PSG Publishing Co. Inc., Littleton, MA (1980) (in press).
3. D. A. Andersen, in:"Urinary Calculi," L. Cifuentes-Delatte, A. Rapado, and A. Hodgkinson, eds., Karger, Basel (1973).
4. N. J. Blacklock, in:"Scientific Foundations of Urology," Vol. 1, D. I. Williams and G. D. Chisholm, eds., Heinemann, London (1976).
5. W. G. Robertson, M. Peacock, P. J. Heyburn, D. H. Marshall, and F. Hanes, Fortschr. Urol. Nephrol. 11:5 (1978).
6. W. G. Robertson, M. Peacock, P. J. Heyburn, F. A. Hanes, and R. Swaminathan, in:"Urinary Calculi, Proceedings of the International Urinary Stone Conference, 1979," J. G. Brockis and B. Finlayson, eds., PSG Publishing Co. Inc., Littleton, MA (1980) (in press).
7. W. G. Robertson, M. Peacock, P. J. Heyburn, F. A. Hanes, A. Rutherford, E. Clementson, R. Swaminathan, and P. B. Clark, Br. J. Urol. 51:427 (1979).
8. W. G. Robertson, M. Peacock, and A. Hodgkinson, J. Chron. Dis. 32:469 (1979).
9. M. Frank and A. De Vries, Arch. Environ. Hlth. 13:625 (1966).
10. N. J. Blacklock, in:"Proceedings of the Renal Stone Research Symposium," B. E. C. Nordin and A. Hodgkinson, eds., Churchill, London (1969).
11. O. S. Better, M. Shabtai, S. Kedar, A. Melamud, J. Berenheim, and C. Chaimovitz, Mineral Electrolyte Metabolism 2:208 (1979).
12. W. G. Robertson, M. Peacock, R. W. Marshall, R. Speed, and B. E. C. Nordin, Clin. Sci. Molec. Med. 49:597 (1975).

THE ROLE OF AFFLUENCE IN RECURRENT STONE FORMATION

O. Zechner and V. Scheiber

Department of Urology and Institute for Medical Statistics and Documentation, University of Vienna Medical School, Vienna, Austria

INTRODUCTION

The formation of urinary calculi is a multifactorial disorder and is the end-product of a number of pathogenetic mechanisms. It has been suggested that stone-formation in the upper urinary tract is a disease of the industrialized countries[1]. Recently, Robertson[2], among others, has drawn attention to a possible relationship between urinary stone-formation and environmental factors. The purpose of the present study is to investigate the relationship between aspects of social infra-structure and the incidence of recurrent stone-formation.

PATIENTS AND METHODS

Various epidemiological and biochemical factors were studied in a group of 379 patients registered at the Urology Service, University of Vienna Medical School. The epidemiological data were obtained from questionnaires and blood and urine analyses for calcium, phosphate and uric acid were performed in triplicate with the patients on a free diet. Urinary pH was determined in freshly voided urine. The rêsults were evaluated by computer analysis.

STATISTICAL ANALYSIS

Analysis of variance, single variate analysis, the Pearson Chi-square test and the Chi-square test for regression coefficients were used.

RESULTS

Comparing the monthly net per capita income, no significant difference was found between the urinary stone-formers investigated and the mean value for Austria[3] (Fogure 1).

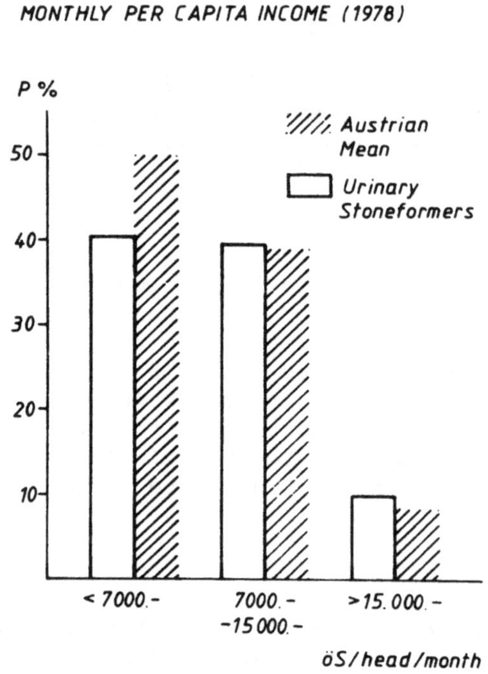

Figure 1. The percentage of stone-formers in three income brackets compared with the average figures for Austria as a whole.

However, more than 40% of the patients spent more per month on food than did the average population in Austria as a whole (Figure 2.).

There was a correlation between the urinary excretion of calcium ($p = 0.01$), uric acid ($p = 0.01$) and inorganic phosphate ($p < 0.001$) and monthly income. In addition, urinary pH was lowest in the group with the highest income ($p < 0.01$) (Figure 3). However these remarkable changes in the urinary excretion of parameters

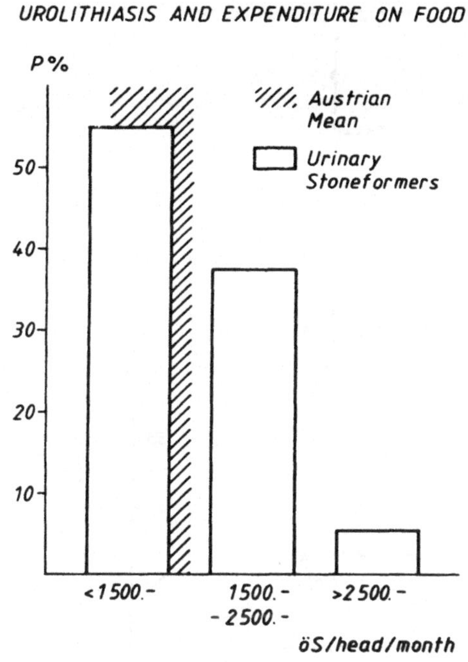

Figure 2. The average monthly expenditure on food in stone-formers compared with the population of Austria as a whole.

usually incriminated as major factors in urinary stone formation did not result in an elevated incidence of recurrent stone-formation.

However, increasing expenditure on food results in a rise of the recurrence rate of stone-formation ($p < 0.05$) and the trend is even more significant ($p = 0.02$) when expressed by the Chi-square of regression coefficient (Table 1).

DISCUSSION

The influence of nutritional factors on the metabolism of calcium, oxalate[4] and uric acid[5] is well known. This study shows that affluence may be one of the underlying factors affecting urine biochemistry and the recurrence of stones. In light of these relationships, the increasing incidence of urinary calculi in the countries of the western hemisphere may be at least partly due to changing life styles in the affluent or industrialized societies.

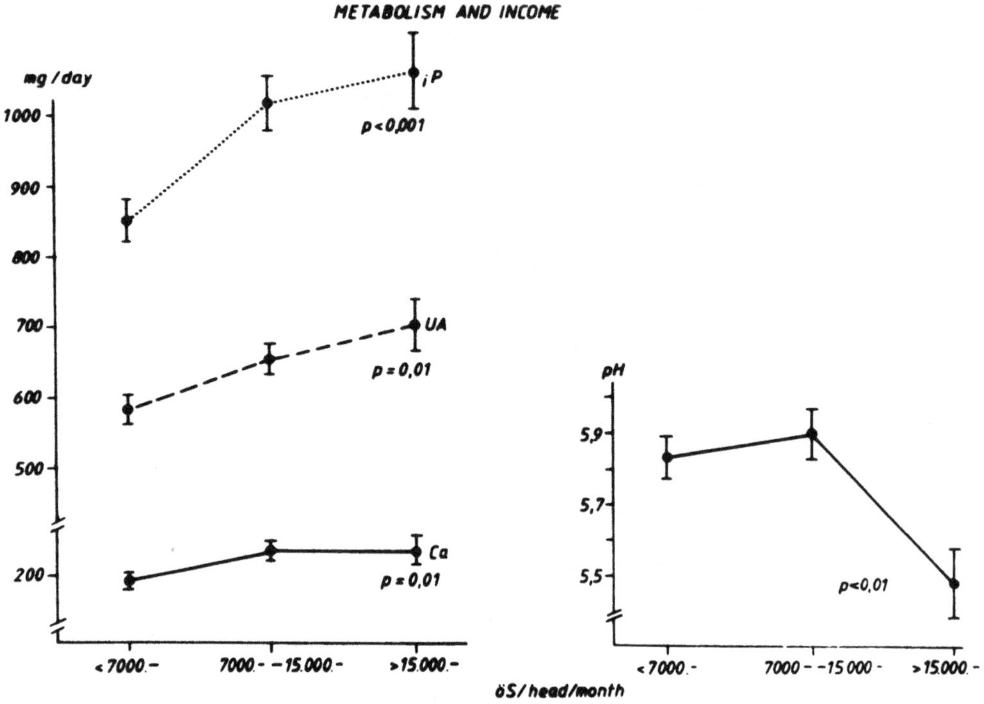

Figure 3. The relationship between urine biochemistry and monthly income.

Table 1.

EXPENDITURE ON FOOD AND RECURRANCE RATE OF STONE FORMATION

Expenditure on Food (öS/head/month)	Recurrance Rate (n/year) Low Rate (< 0,25) n ( )*	High Rate (> 0,25) n ( )*
< 1.500,--	125 (116,11)	32 (40,89)
1.500,-- – 2.500,--	78 (85,79)	38 (30,21)
> 2.500,--	10 (11,09)	5 (3,91)

( )*.... expected cell values

STATISTIC:
PEARSON CHISQUARE $p < 0,05$
Chisquare for Regression Coeff. $p = 0,02$

REFERENCES

1. D. A. Andersen, in:"Proceedings of the Renal Stone Research Symposium," B. E. C. Nordin and A. Hodgkinson, eds., J. & A. Churchill, Ltd., London (1969).
2. W. G. Robertson, M. Peacock, and P. J. Heyburn, in:"Pathogenese und Klinik der Harnsteine VI," W. Vahlensieck and G. Gasser, eds., Dr. D. Steinkopff, Darmstadt (1978).
3. in:"Statistische Nachrichten," 35:12 (1980).
4. W. G. Robertson, P. J. Heyburn, and M. Peacock, Clin. Sci. 57:285 (1979).
5. F. L. Coe, in:"Uric Acid," W. N. Kelley and J. M. Weiner, eds., Springer, Berlin-Heidelberg-New York (1978).

ALCOHOL AS AN EPIDEMIOLOGICAL RISK IN UROLITHIASIS

O. Zechner and V. Scheiber

Department of Urology, Institute for Medical Statistics and Documentation, University of Vienna Medical School, Vienna, Austria

Changing life styles consequent to economic growth and dietary habits have been suggested as factors in the increasing incidence of urolithiasis in industrialized countries. A possible relationship between stone-formation and increased ingestion of animal protein[1] as well as increased sugar consumption[2] have been suggested.

The present study deals with the problem of alcohol as a nutritional risk in urinary stone disease.

PATIENTS AND METHODS

Various epidemiological and biochemical factors were studied in a group of 379 patients registered at the Urology Service, University of Vienna Medical School. The epidemiological data were obtained from questionnaires and blood and urine analyses for calcium, phosphate and uric acid were performed in triplicate with the patients on a free diet. The results were evaluated by computer analysis.

Calculations and Statistical Analyses

Data are expressed as means ± S.E.M. For evaluation both analysis of variance, single variate analysis as reported by Welch and Brown-Forsythe and the Pearson Chi square test were used.

RESULTS

As can be seen in Figure 1 serum uric acid levels increase substantially as a function of the amount of alcohol ingested ($p < 0.01$ and $p < 0.05$, respectively).

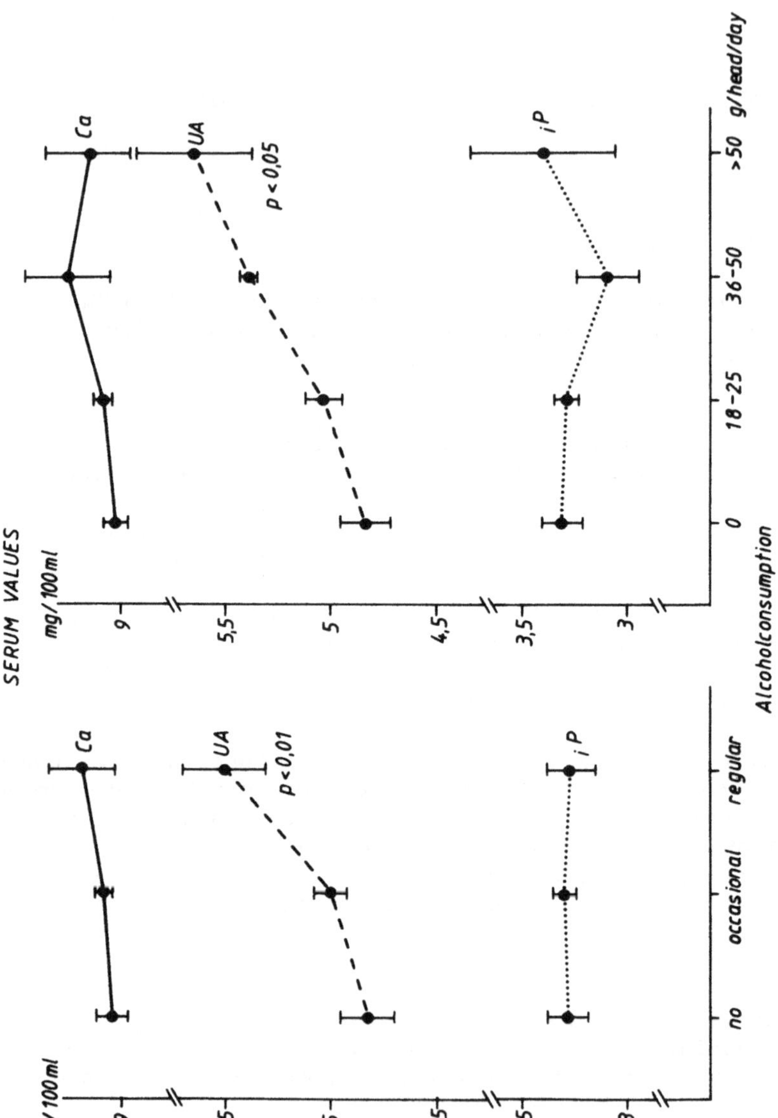

Figure 1. The influence of alcohol consumption on the composition of serum.

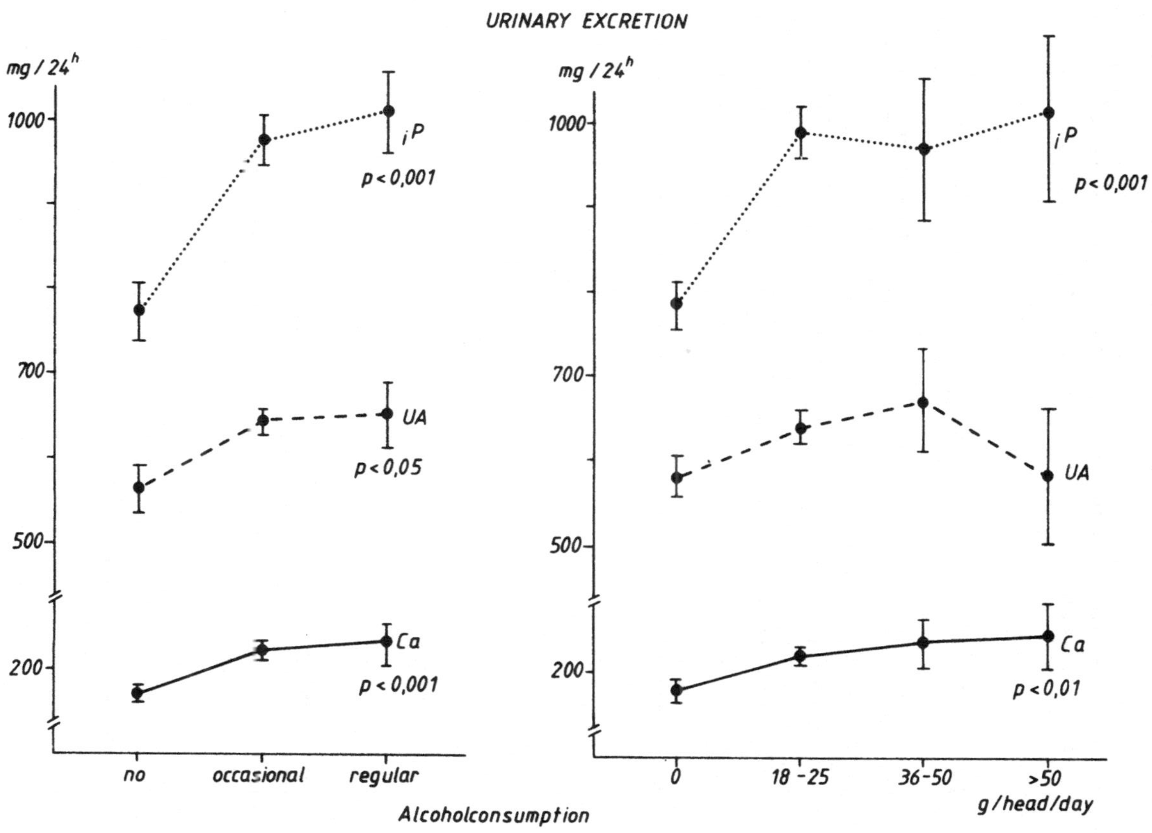

Figure 2. The influence of alcohol consumption on urinary composition.

The urinary excretion of calcium, inorganic phosphate and uric acid are closely correlated with alcohol consumption (Figure 2). Only in patients ingesting more than 50 g of alcohol per day are the urinary uric acid levels lower than in cases consuming less than this amount.

Moreover, increasing amounts of alcohol ingested result in a considerable shift towards urate-containing stones ($p < 0.001$) (Table 1).

Table 1. Alcohol Consumption and Stone Composition

ALCOHOL CONSUMPTION				Mixed Composition	
g/head/day	Ca-Oxalate	Urate	Ca-Phosphate	Ca-Oxalate-Phosphate	Ca-Oxalate-Urate
∅	31 (30)*	6 (8,73)	13 (8,73)	15 (16,36)	7 (5,18)
18 - 25	74 (69,58)	14 (20,24)	28 (27,20)	41 (37,95)	10 (12,02)
36 - 50	4 (8,75)	10 (2,55)	2 (3,42)	4 (4,77)	1 (1,51)
> 50	1 (1,67)	2 (0,48)	0 (0,65)	0 (0,91)	1 (0,29)
	n = 110	n = 32	n = 43	n = 60	n = 19

( )* ..... expected cell values   STATISTIC PEARSON CHISQUARE: $p < 0{,}001$

DISCUSSION

It has been known for some time that increased ingestion of alcohol leads to a rise in serum uric acid concentrations[3]. However, the enhancement of urinary excretion of calcium, inorganic phosphate and uric acid as a function of alcohol consumption represents a new aspect in the etiology of urinary stone formation. In connection with the well-known influence of increased intake of animal protein on urinary excretion of uric acid[4], calcium and oxalate[5], alcohol ingestion may well constitute a potentiating factor for risk of urinary stone-formation. The increasing frequency of urate-containing stones in patients drinking alcohol represents an important aspect to be considered in the prophylactic management of urinary stone disease.

REFERENCES

1. W. G. Robertson, M. Peacock, and P. J. Heyburn, Br. J. Urol. 51:427 (1979).
2. N. J. Blacklock, in:"Scientific Foundations of Urology," D. J. Williams and G. D. Chisholm, eds., W. Heinemann Medical Books Ltd., London (1976).
3. C. S. Lieber and D. P. Jones, J. Clin. Invest. 41:1863 (1962).
4. F. L. Coe, in:"Uric Acid," W. N. Kelley and J. M. Weiner, eds., Springer, Berlin-Heidelberg-New York (1978).
5. W. G. Robertson, P. J. Heyburn, and M. Peacock, Clin. Sci. 57: 285 (1979).

FAMILIAL HYPERCALCIURIC UROLITHIASIS

A. Weinberger, J. Schechter, J. Pinkhas, and O. Sperling

Department of Medicine D and of Clinical Biochemistry, Tel Aviv University Medical School, Beilinson Medical Center, Petah Tikva, Israel

Hypercalciuria is a relatively common etiological factor in calcium urolithiasis[1]. It may be one of the manifestations of various abnormalities, such as hyperparathyroidism, renal tubular acidosis, sarcoidosis and malignancy. However, in the majority of cases it is classified as idiopathic[2]. In a previous study[3] of a large series of patients (50 males and 24 females) with idiopathic hypercalciuric urolithiasis (i.e. idiopathic hypercalciuria associated with urolithiasis) we found that 20% of the examined patients had a family history of renal stones. Only one of these patients had a large enough family to allow a detailed study which is reported in this paper.

PATIENTS AND METHODS

The propositus M.S., a 52-year-old Jew born in Turkey, suffered from recurrent calcium oxalate urolithiasis since the age of 30. He was admitted to our Metabolic Unit for evaluation of recurrent urolithiasis. On admission, the patient was asymptomatic. Physical examination and routine hematological and blood chemistry values were all within the normal range. Serum calcium was 9.5 mg% and serum inorganic phosphate 3.1 mg%. Routine urine examination was normal with a morning pH of 5.4 to 6.2. The urinary pattern of amino acids by paper chromatography showed no abnormalities. The urinary 24 h excretion of calcium was 385 to 425 mg on a diet containing 800 mg of calcium per day, whereas on a low calcium diet (300 - 400 mg per day), it was 230 - 260 mg. Tubular reabsorption of phosphate was 85% to 96 %. Oral ammonium load test lowered the urinary pH from 5.7 to 4.9. A bone survey showed no abnormalities. The chest x-rays and intravenous pyelography were normal. Thirty-nine members of the family of the propositus over three generations, were questioned about the history of renal stone disease and possible cause of hypercalciuria. Two 24 h urine collections were obtained from 13 family members and were analyzed for calcium and creatinine by methods previously described[4].

RESULTS AND DISCUSSION

The family pedigree is presented in Figure 1. As shown, 4 subjects (all males, one of them a 6-year-old boy), were found to have hypercalciuric urolithiasis. Two additional relatives, (one male and one female) were found to have hypercalciuria without urolithiasis, and 4 relatives (2 males and 2 females) were found to have urolithiasis without hypercalciuria. One subject (II-8), with recurrent calcium urolithiasis, died of terminal renal failure. However, we were unable to obtain further information concerning his urinary calcium excretion. There was no evidence of pathologic processes causing hypercalciuria in the family.

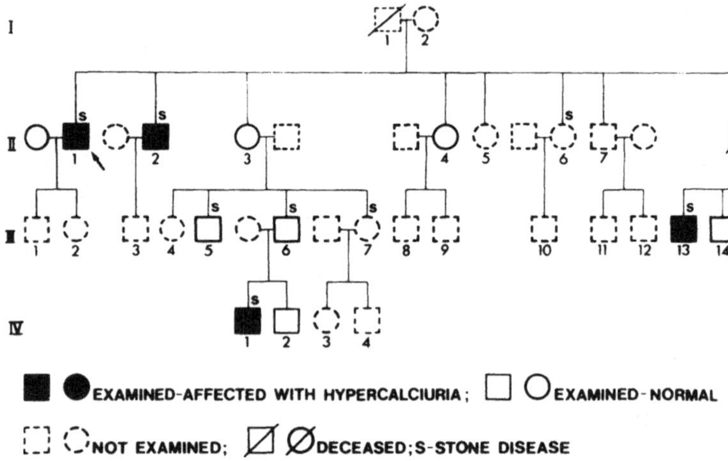

Figure 1. Pedigree of affected family.

In the family reported, several members, spread over three generations, were found to be affected with either idiopathic hypercalciuria or urolithiasis or with both conditions. We believe that all the subjects affected have the same syndrome, i.e. hereditary (idiopathic) hypercalciuric urolithiasis. In this syndrome the idiopathic hypercalciuria is the inborn defect, whereas the urolithiasis is a common accompanying finding which manifests itself clinically. Idiopathic hypercalciuria is classified etiologically into absorptive and non-absorptive types. In the former there are considerable fluctuations in urinary calcium excretion which may be normal or high, depending largely on the dietary calcium intake. The finding that urinary excretion of calcium in the propositus decreased markedly when the patient was on a low calcium diet is compatible with the classification of hyperabsorptive hypercalciuria. Furthermore the finding of four family members with urolithiasis without hypercalciuria is also in accordance with this classification. Two family members were found to have hypercalciuria without urolithiasis. This finding is not unexpected, since the formation of stones depends, in addition to the hypercalciuria, on many other factors such as urine volume and the presence of protecting substances.

In view of the above mentioned considerations, family members affected with hypercalciuria alone, with urolithiasis alone or with a combination of both, should all be considered as similarly affected. Accordingly, the data on this family is compatible with an autosomal dominant transmission of the defect. Both sexes are affected and there is direct transmission from fathers to offspring, both males and females. Consistent with this pattern of transmission, family member II-3 should also have been affected. It is probable that her two urine collections were obtained when she was on a relatively low calcium intake.

The finding of dominant autosomal inheritance of hypercalciuric urolithiasis presently reported is compatible with the results described by Coe et al.[5] in his study of 8 families. The investigation of our series of patients with idiopathic hypercalciuric urolithiasis[3], as well as one of Coe et al.[5] and of others[6], indicate that this inborn defect may be quite common among the patients with renal stones. Since young subjects with this defect suffer from urolithiasis, these findings call for careful investigation of all offspring of patients with this inborn defect, in order to start preventive treatment for renal stones at the earliest possible age.

REFERENCES

1. A. Hodgkinson and L. N. Pyrah, Br. J. Surg. 46:10 (1958).
2. C. Y. C. Pak, M. Ohata, E. L. Lawrence, and W. Snyder, J. Clin. Invest. 54:387 (1974).
3. A. Weinberger, O. Sperling, J. Schechter, U. A. Liberman, J. Pinkhas, and A. de Vries, International Urology and Nephrology 9:213 (1977).
4. O. Sperling, A. Weinberger, I. Oliver, U. A. Liberman, and A. de Vries, Ann. Int. Med. 80:482 (1974).
5. F. L. Coe, J. H. Parks, and E. S. Moore, New Engl. J. Med. 300:337 (1979).
6. R. De Luca and F. Guzetta, La Pediatria 73:613 (1965).

CAUSE OF PRIMARY BLADDER STONE IN ENGLAND - A RETROSPECTIVE EPIDEMIOLOGICAL STUDY

Scott B. Halstead

Department of Tropical Medicine and Medical Microbiology
John A. Burns School of Medicine, University of Hawaii
Honolulu, Hawaii 96816, U.S.A.

Organized studies on primary human bladder stone can be said to have begun on February 20, 1773, when the Board of Governors of the Norfolk and Norwich Hospital in Norwich, England, ordered that the "Apothecary do provide a suitable nest of drawers to deposit the (urinary calculi) extracted in this House to show to strangers, and be referred to occasionally, -- and none suffered to be taken away"[1].

In the 18th and 19th centuries, several important inquiries into the cause of bladder stone in Great Britain were undertaken, principally because of the availability of surgical statistics from the Norfolk and Norwich Hospital[2-7]. These studies documented the marked geographic variation in stone prevalence and the high prevalence of the disease among the urban poor.

In 19th century England, two factors contributed to the practice of giving infants non-milk foods: the high incidence of perinatal maternal mortality and the high rate of absentee mothering due to the excessively large number of young women in the industrial work force. Babies were fed with pap or panada, often composed of bread or other cereal moistened in water, saliva or beer. In 1813, Hamilton[8] wrote "Panada and pap be now almost universally used for the first food of infants, as a substitute for the mothers milk." However, enlightened medical opinion counseled mothers to feed milk to the "hand-reared" infant[9]: "Those who have the means of providing an ass, would do well to give the child three or four meals, in the day, of the milk of that animal; this should be drawn from the udder at the moment it is wanting, and given of the natural heat ... it should not be let to stand, as even a quarter of an hour's contact with air might produce considerable alteration in the quality of the milk ... For those who cannot be provided with ass's milk, that of a cow ... may be substituted."

Since in Thailand, the occurrence of primary bladder stone has been found to correlate with the custom of supplementing newborn infant feedings with glutinous rice[10], we hypothesized that a similar practice in 19th century England was responsible for the endemic bladder stone of that era.

Based upon contemporary sources, it was predicted that the incidence of feeding pap to infants would be highest in those families who were without access to fresh milk from domestic animals. Availability of non-human milk would be expected to vary directly with the abundance of dairy cattle. To test this epidemiologically, per capita density of dairy cattle and the bladder stone admissions per 10,000 hospitalizations were compared in 28 English counties. Data used were those obtained from the first dairy census in England (1866)[11] and Cadge's 1869-1873 hospital survey[7].

Table 1 summarizes these statistics. There is a significant negative correlation ($r = -0.453$, $p = < 0.02$).

Bladder stone of children in England disappeared precipitously in the last two decades of the 19th century[1]. This event was accompanied by the general availability of inexpensive, safe and unadulterated cow's milk as a food for infants. This can be attributed to the discovery of the pasteurization process, the introduction of the milk train and the birth of the science of nutrition and of the practice of pediatrics[12].

Our study supports the hypothesis that carbohydrate feedings given to newborn infants is the single and unitary etiological event in primary bladder stone in children. This conclusion was clearly presaged in 1823[9]: "The custom being generally to give thick victuals to the infant brought up by hand, they do not require to be fed so frequently; but this is a bad practice ... Children, who have not the breast, are apt to have ... a predisposition to gravelly complaints."

Table 1. Bladder Stone Hospitalization Rate (1869-1873) Arranged by Density of Dairy Cattle in 28 Counties of England in 1866

County	Cows or heifers in milk or calf per 100,000 persons (1866 census)[11]	Bladder stone Hospitalizations per 10,000 (1869-1873)[7]	Region of England
Dorset	221.4	15.1	Southwest
Somerset	189.2	0	Southwest
Cumberland	181.9	25.0	Border
Wiltshire	181.6	14.0	Southwest
Shropshire	172.8	38.2	West Central
Derby	159.0	14.5	West North Central
Hereford	155.3	6.4	West Central
North Riding	148.7	22.6	East North Central
Leicester	121.4	42.4	West Central
Devon	98.4	8.5	Southwest
Mean	163.0	18.7	
Lincoln	93.8	28.0	East North Central
Northampton	77.5	35.5	West Central
Berks	72.8	81.7	West Central
Stafford	71.5	65.7	West North Central
Gloucester	69.3	22.6	West Central
Sussex	68.7	41.9	South
Nottingham	64.6	38.0	East North Central
East Riding	62.8	79.0	East North Central
Mean	72.6	49.1	
Norfolk	57.0	167.2	East Central
Suffolk	52.5	62.8	East Central
Cambridge	53.7	82.0	East Central
West Riding	51.1	48.1	West North Central
Northcumberland	48.8	24.9	Border
Hampshire	48.7	26.4	Southwest
Hertford	46.2	40.0	East Central
Warwick	42.4	49.2	West Central
Durham	28.2	49.7	Border
Kent	26.1	52.8	South
Mean	45.5	59.4	

RERERENCES

1. A. Batty Shaw, Med. Hist. 14:221 (1970).
2. M. Dobson, Chester J. Monk, London (1779).
3. A. Marcet, Longman, London (1817).
4. R. Smith, Med. Chir. Trans. 11:1 (1821).
5. J. Yelloly, Phil. Trans. Roy. Soc. 119:55 (1829).
6. W. England, Underwood, London (1830).
7. W. Cadge, Br. Med. J. ii:207 (1874).
8. J. Hamilton, in:"Hints for the Treatment of the Principal Diseases of Infancy and Childhood," Edinburgh (1813).
9. Anonymous (a grandmother), in:"Advice to Young Mothers on the Physical Education of Children," Longman, Hurst, Rees, Orme and Brown, London (1823).
10. S. B. Halstead, A. Valyasevi, and P. Umpaivit, Am. J. Clin. Nutr. 20:1352 (1967).
11. "Ministry of Agriculture," George Edward Eyre and Wellcom Spottiswoode, London (1866).
12. I. A. Abt, in:"History of Pediatrics," Abt-Garrison, eds., W. B. Saunders, Philadelphia (1965).

ACKNOWLEDGMENT

I am grateful to Dr. Anthony Batty Shaw and Mr. Alan Green for providing me access to the records and stone collection of the Norfolk and Norwich Hospital. This study was supported in part by a Fogarty International Fellowship from the National Institutes of Health.

ENDEMIC BLADDER STONES IN INDONESIA

J. G. Brockis, R. C. Bowyer, G. Ryan, T. A. Taylor,
T. Kamardi, and A. Rizal
Royal Perth Hospital and the General Hospital, Padang, Sumatra. The Universities of Western Australia and Andalas, Indonesia.

Bladder stone disease in young children, prevalent in Europe and the United States in the 19th century is now largely confined to a belt of countries stretching from Egypt in the north to Pakistan, India, Burma, Thailand, Vietnam, Southern China, Indonesia and New Guinea. Occasional cases have been found in Australian aboriginals[1]. There are also isolated pockets of the disease in South America, but Central America and most of Africa and the Polynesian islands of the Pacific are not affected. An extensive literature on the subject is well summarized by Andersen[2]. This suggests that there is a broad relationship between cereals in the diet and the incidence of primary bladder stones for many writers remark that the childrens diets are high in plant and vegetable matter and low in animal proteins. Furthermore, Vermooten[3] states that where the main cereal eaten is maize, bladder stones are not found. Other factors common to all areas are poverty, large families (though only often one child is affected), a male-female ratio of 10:1 and a peak age of presentation at about 2 years of age[4].

In our studies in Indonesia we have found that symptoms are confined to the bladder and urethra and about half the cases have infected urine. Urinary reflux is present in many of the young children with stones. This is associated with bladder infections and tends to disappear after the removal of the stone and treatment with antibiotics. It is highly significant that none of these patients suffer from renal colic and it would appear that the stones are formed in the bladder. Working independently, biochemical investigations have taken place in Egypt[5], India[6], Pakistan[7], Thailand[8] and Indonesia[9,10].

Stone analyses in non-infected cases show they consist of ammonium acid urate, uric acid and calcium oxalate with matrix. The stones are characteristically laminated. There is some variation in composition from country to country: oxalate predominates in Thailand, but in Indonesia the centre of non-infected stones is mainly ammonium acid urate. (Table 1). Further, we have found stones in which oxalate could not be demonstrated chemically. The frequency with which ammonium acid urate is found in the centre of stones led us to believe that this was a significant finding, a point previously made by Sutor et al[11]. We believe the explanation is to be found in the excretion patterns of ammonia and urates in young children.

We proceeded to analyze three hourly samples of urine taken from healthy babies in an endemic stone area who were fed by the breast alone and also with rice/water supplements (Table 2). The urinanalysis showed high urinary ammonia levels with a rice diet and a low urinary phosphate at all times.

Table 1.

INDONESIAN BLADDER STONES ANALYSIS (INNER SECTIONS)

FROM CHILDREN WITH STERILE URINE

Patient	Age Yrs	Sex	Uric Acid g/kg	Amm. Ac. Urate g/kg	CaOx g/kg	Total g/kg
AMR	11	M	100	530	250	880
JUL	7	M	380	430	80	890
IRT	4	M	160	430	370	960
SUP	6	M	190	700	0	890
EDR	4	M	250	490	180	920
ROD	4	M	220	690	60	970
TAN	8	M	50	120	650	820
SYA	4	M	240	610	80	930
AMI	4	M	100	240	560	900
BUK	8	M	160	420	320	900
BIS	12	M	80	430	410	920
JAL	3	M	180	570	180	930

COMPOSITION OF STONES

NOTE: PRESENCE OF AMMONIUM ACID URATE IN CENTRAL AREAS

The urinary urates were also quite high compared with those normally obtained in Caucasian children. In normal children uric acid/creatinine ratios are very high at birth but the ratio slowly falls to adult levels by the age of 10 years[10]. High ammonia levels following the feeding of a rice diet is associated with increased total urinary acidity in children not affected by stone disease, but if a child receiving this acid diet develops gastroenteritis or becomes dehydrated, then the formation product of ammonium acid urate is greatly exceeded. Many children have been observed passing muddy urine containing ammonium acid urate crystals. Precipitation of ammonium acid urate does not occur in the kidneys because the process of crystal formation is a time dependent phenomenon and visible crystals do not develop for 2-3 hours. Other investigations by us show that ammonium acid urate precipitation from urine is affected by the ionic strength of urine. An important degree of protection against the precipitation of ammonium urates is provided by the salts of the divalent cations magnesium and calcium. These appear to be particularly potent inhibitors of ammonium urate formation[12]. Rice flour is relatively poor in phosphate content and much is in the form of insoluble phytate. It would appear that the infant kidney does not employ phosphate for buffering purposes to any great extent, hence the high ammonia excretion with an acid diet.

Table 2.

3 HOURLY AMMONIA EXCRETIONS ON DIETS SHOWN. NORMAL INDONESIAN CHILDREN

BREAST ONLY	BREAST AND RICE	BREAST & RICE & EGG
n 48	n 104	n 64
$\bar{x}$ 25.9mmo1/1	31.7	44.7
SD 15.1 += 2.06	SD 18.1 (= 3.74	SD 24.0
	df = 150 p<.05	df = 166 p<.001)

We have attempted to increase the amount of phosphate in urine by feeding hens eggs in addition to the rice as these are rich in phosphate, but the effect of this as is shown in Table 2 is to increase urinary ammonia and the total acid output without appreciably increasing the phosphate excretion. Bean curds on the other hand are known to produce an alkaline urine and also to be rich in phosphate. A program is now underway to evaluate their use as a food supplement in the hope that phosphate excretion will be increased and that as a result, the unfortunate effects on urinary acidity produced by feeding rice when milk is not available at too early an age will be neutralized.

REFERENCES

1. Z. S. Wisniewski and J. G. Brockis, Aust. N. Z. J. Surg. (in press).
2. D. A. Andersen, Br. J. Urol. 34:160 (1962).
3. V. Vermooten, J. Urol. 46:193 (1941).

4. T. Kamardi, A. Rizal, J. G. Brockis, R. C. Bowyer, T. A. Taylor, and Z. S. Wisniewski, Br. J. Urol. 48:617 (1976).
5. A. H. Loutfi, R. Van Reen, and G. A. Hamid, Egyptian J. Med. Assoc. 57:96 (1974).
6. M. Teotia, S. P. S. Teotia, and D. P. Singh, in:"Urinary Calculi, Proceedings of the International Urinary Stone Conference, 1979," J. G. Brockis and B. Finlayson, eds., PSG Publishing Co., Inc., Littleton, MA (1980) (in press).
7. M. A. Rahman and R. Van Reen, in:"Urinary Calculi, Proceedings of the International Urinary Stone Conference, 1979," J. G. Brockis and B. Finlayson, eds., PSG Publishing Co., Inc., Littleton, MA (1980) (in press).
8. S. Dhanamitta, A. Valyasevi, and B. Susilavorn, in:"Idiopathic Urinary Bladder Stone Disease," R. Van Reen, ed., Fogarty International Center Proceedings No. 37, DHEW Publication No. (NIH) (1977).
9. T. Kamardi, Soemanto, A. Rizal, J. G. Brockis, Z. S. Wisniewski, and T. A. Taylor, in:"Urinary Calculi, Proceedings of the International Urinary Stone Conference, 1979," J. G. Brockis and B. Finlayson, ed., PSH Publishing Co., Inc., Littleton, MA (1980) (in press).
10. J. G. Brockis, R. C. Bowyer, R. K. McCulloch, T. A. Taylor, and Z. S. Wisniewski, in:"Urinary Calculi, Proceedings of the International Urinary Stone Conference, 1979," J. G. Brockis and B. Finlayson, eds., PSG Publishing Co. Inc., Littleton, MA (1980) (in press).
11. D. J. Sutor, S. E. Wooley, and J. J. Illingworth, Br. J. Urol. 46:393 (1974).
12. R. C. Bowyer, J. G. Brockis, and R. K. McCulloch, Clin. Chem. Acta. 99:221 (1979).

FUTURE OF TAMARIND AND TARTRATE IN PREVENTING RECURRENCE OF RENAL CALCULI

B. K. Sur, H. N. Pandey, S. Deshpande, R. Pahwa,
R. K. Singh, and Tarachandra
Departments of Biochemistry and Surgery, G.S.V.M.
Medical College
Kanpur, India

It is well known that the incidence of renal calculi is strikingly low in South India as compared to North India[1]. The low incidence of urolithiasis in the South cannot be attributed to the predominance of rice in their diet as urolithiasis is common in several other rice-eating countries[2]. One characteristic regular constituent of the South Indian diet is tamarind which is not used in North. Tamarind is very rich in potassium bitartrate and tartaric acid[3]. Tartrate is a strong chelating agent and may inhibit crystallization of calcium oxalate. The present study was therefore conducted to ascertain if feeding tamarind would lower the calcifying propensity of urine.

MATERIAL AND METHODS

Ten healthy male medical students (age 19 to 23 years) taking food from the same hostel mass were instructed to avoid oxalate-rich foods during the period of study. After 3 days on the mess diet their urine for the period 10 p.m. to 6 a.m. was collected under chloroform for 3 consecutive days. All the subjects were then given 10 g of tamarind pulp each day along with their dinner. After 3 days of tamarind ingestion 8 h urine samples of the subjects were collected for 3 consecutive days. One week after tamarind intake was stopped, 8-h urine samples were collected for one day only.

The urine samples were immediately filtered through Whatman No. 1 filter paper and measured in the inhibitor assay. Volume, pH, Na, Mg, Ca, oxalate, uric acid and creatinine were also measured. For the inhibitor assay the method of Dent and Sutor[4] was made quantitative by measuring the calcium of the calcium oxalate crystallized in 8 h (details to be published elsewhere). Various concentrations of citrate and tartrate were added to synthetic urine (SU) at pH 6.0 and 7.0. Each liter of the synthetic urine consisted of: $(NH_4)_2$ oxalate (0.02 g), NH_4Cl (1.5 g), $(NH_4)_2$ sulphate (0.5 g), $CaCl_2 \cdot 2H_2O$ (0.5 g), $MgCl_2 \cdot 6H_2O$ (1.0 g), NaCl (6.5 g), Na citrate (0.7 g), creatinine (1.0 g), KH_2PO_4 (3.0 g), Na_2HPO_4 (0.6 g), K_2SO_4 (0.8 g), urea (20.0 g), hippuric acid (2.0 g), and uric acid (0.4 g).

RESULTS AND DISCUSSION

Table 1 shows that crystallization of calcium oxalate was strikingly inhibited during the period of tamarind intake. After one week of withdrawal of tamarind from the diet, the crystallization of calcium oxalate returned to the values obtained before tamarind ingestion. Tamarind feeding did not alter significantly any of the other parameters measured in urine.

Table 1. Effect of Ingestion of Tamarind on Urinary Inhibitor Assay (IA) and 8-h Excretion of some Urinary Constituents (Mean ± S.D.)

Vol ml	pH	IA (gCa)	Na mEq	Mg mg	Ca mg	Oxalate mg	Uric Acid mg	Creatinine mg
Cases 10, without tamarind								
570 ±155	5.9 ±0.09	7.11 ±0.42	53.8 ±12.3	45.8 ±12.3	49.4 ±12.6	11.8 ± 4.6	298 ±91.1	446.6 ±146.4
Cases 10, with tamarind								
730 ± 95	5.8 ±0.09	2.57 ±0.53	55.0 ±13.1	59.1 ±13.1	66.9 ±13.2	17.9 ± 6.9	314.4 ± 98.9	669.9 ±140.0
Cases 10, after tamarind withdrawal								
		7.0 ±0.5						

Tamarind pulp contains 11 - 13% tartaric acid[5] and 10 g of tamarind pulp would contain 1 g of tartrate. Within 8 h of feeding, 20%[6] and 6-12%[7] of tartrate have been shown to appear in urine. Thus in the present experiment 0.5 to 2.0 mM tartrate might have appeared in urine. Table 2 shows that, at pH 6.0, 2 mM tartrate is an effective inhibitor. Since tartrate was not quantitatively estimated in the present experiments, it is not possible to state categorically whether tamarind inhibited calcium oxalate crystallization exclusively through tartaric acid. In acetate buffer alteration of pH from 5 to 8 has no effect on rate of crystallization of calcium oxalate[8]. However, Table 3 shows that if the pH of synthetic urine is increased from 6.0 to 7.0, the efficacy of citrate as well as tartrate as inhibitors of calcium oxalate crystallization are considerably increased. The alkalinization of urine (which also increases urinary citrate[9]) caused by tartrate feeding may be useful in preventing the recurrence of calcium oxalate stones. In two human studies, using large pharmacological doses of L-tartrate, there was no evidence of renal toxicity[10].

Table 2. Inhibitory Effect of Citrate and Tartrate

Citrate mM/l	%Crystallization	Tartrate mM/l	%Crystallization	Citrate + Tartrate mM/l	%Crystallization
0.0	100	0.0	100	0.0	100
2.4	89	2.0	92.6	2.4 + 1	98
4.8	96	4.0	63	2.4 + 2	69
10	61			4.8 + 1	95
				4.8 + 2	41
				4.8 + 3	37
				4.8 + 4	50

Table 3. Effect of pH, Citrate, and Tartrate on Calcium Oxalate Crystallization*

Citrate mM/l	+	Tartrate mM/l	% Crystallization pH 6	pH 7
2.4	+	0	100	58
2.4	+	1	90	55
2.4	+	2	64	35

* The synthetic urine used contained 0.2 g/l $CaCl_2$, $2H_2O$ instead of 0.5 g/l.

REFERENCES

1. B. N. Colabawalla, Presented to the I.C.M.R. study group on urolithiasis (1970).
2. V. Benjamin, Presented to the I.C.M.R. study group on urolithiasis (1970).
3. H. C. Wood, The dispensatory of the United States of America 25th edition (1955).
4. C. E. Dent and D. J. Sutor, Lancet ii:775 (1971).
5. The British Pharmaceutical Codex. Council of the Pharmaceutical Society of Great Britain, London (1949).
6. P. Finkle, J. Biol. Chem. 100:349 (1933).

7. C. W. Bauer and R. W. Pearson, J. Am. Pharm. Assoc. 46:575 (1957).
8. S. G. Welshman and M. G. McGeown, Br. J. Urol. 44:677 (1972).
9. M. Butz and H. J. Dulce, in:"Proceedings Fourth International Urolithiasis Research Symposium," L. H. Smith, B. Finlayson, and W. G. Robertson, eds., Plenum Press, New York (in press).
10. V. S. Chadwick, A. Vince, M. Killingley, and O. M. Wrong, Clin. Sci. and Mol. Med. 54:273 (1978).

DIETARY STRUCTURE AND URINARY COMPOSITION IN A STONE-FREE POPULATION

M. Modlin, P. J. Davies and D. Crawford

Department of Urology and Department of Medical Biochemistry, Medical School, University of Cape Town, and Electron Microscope Unit, University of Cape Town

The large number of pure calcium oxalate stones identified by various investigators, coupled with observations that more frequently calcium oxalate forms the major component of stones containing both calcium oxalate and calcium phosphate have been among the reasons for the suggestion that crystals of calcium oxalate nucleate stone formation. Fifty two renal stones were analyzed by infrared spectroscopy. Infrared spectroscopy is particularly sensitive for the detection of phosphate and will detect a calcium phosphate concentration of 1% in a calcium oxalate stone. Forty calcium-stones were identified. All 40 contained meaningful amounts of calcium phosphate. None contained only calcium oxalate. Very small spontaneously passed renal stones represent the nucleus of the stone surrounded by a minimum of crystal deposition. Scanning electron microscopy coupled with chemical microanalysis of the fracture surface of very small spontaneously passed calcium-stones revealed the invariable presence of both calcium phosphate and calcium oxalate. The calcium phosphate occurred either as multiple clusters of conglomerates of crystals (Figure 1), or as a single cluster of conglomerates of crystals, lying among conglomerates of calcium oxalate crystals. The total area occupied by calcium phosphate is smaller than that occupied by calcium oxalate. The probable non-existence of pure calcium oxalate stones, the ubiquity of calcium phosphate, its invariable presence in minuscle calcium-stones, all three of which have been demonstrated by these studies, are consistent with published data which suggest that crystals of calcium phosphate nucleate stone formation and support the proposition.

A report on the rarity of renal stones in South African blacks has previously been presented[1]. The 1970 census figures revealed that 5.1 million black South Africans lived in urban areas along with 4.5 million white South Africans. During the 9 year period 1971-1979, 1 in 510 white patients admitted to Groote Schuur Hospital, Cape Town, had a renal stone as compared with 1 in 44,298 blacks. Clearly, renal stone formation in South African blacks is still very rare. As both groups had been exposed to a similar environment during the nine year period it seemed likely that dietary structure was responsible for the difference in stone incidence. A study of the available data revealed a dietary pattern among urban blacks. The bread eaten is either wholemeal or brown. The intake of animal protein, vegetables, fruit, coffee, tea, milk and sugar is similar to that of the whites. The salt intake is high[1]. Dried beans are a popular item of food. Maize is their staple food. On the average about 680 gm are consumed daily as porridge prepared by boiling either home-produced or coarsely ground maize. Even though a taste is acquired for new foods and irrespective of their economic circumstances, black families continue to eat their traditional maize dishes. As a result they have a high intake of organic phosphorus in the form of phytic (inositol hexaphosphoric) acid. Of 48.8 mmol of P contained in 680 gm of maize[2] 80%, or 39 mmol, exists as phytate p[3]. Brown bread and dried beans contain 2.8 and 7.4 mmol of phytate p per 100 gm respectively[2,3]. The average daily P intake of whites is 50 mmol with a phytate P content of 5%, or 2.5 mmol[4]. Up to 85% of phytic acid derived from cereals is hydrolysed in the gut[5]. Partial hydrolysis of phytic acid can be achieved experimentally, either enzymatically or by acid, with the production of inositol mono-, di-, tri-, tetra-, and pentaphosphate (IP_1, IP_2, IP_3, IP_4, IP_5)[6]. It seems reasonable to assume that the same occurs physiologically. Unspecified phosphorylated inositol, quantitatively related to ingestion, has been identified in urine[7]. As a result of their high intake of phytic acid, chiefly derived from maize, South African blacks could have a high urinary content of various phosphorylated inositols.

The data suggest that black South Africans rarely form stones because of their singular and immutable dietary habits. These result in a urine the composition of which creates a milieu that is inimical to the formation of crystals of calcium phosphate. The specific inimical factors appear to be definable. The urine has a high volume and low concentration. The concentration of both calcium and phosphorus is low (Figure 2). Consequently the formation product of calcium phosphate may seldom be exceeded and the risk of crystal formation is thus considerably reduced. The high urinary content of sodium would increase the solubility of any crystals that formed[1]. IP_2 and IP_3 effectively prevent the formation of hydroxy-apatite crystals from metastable solutions in vitro[8]. It seems likely that black South Africans have a high urinary content of

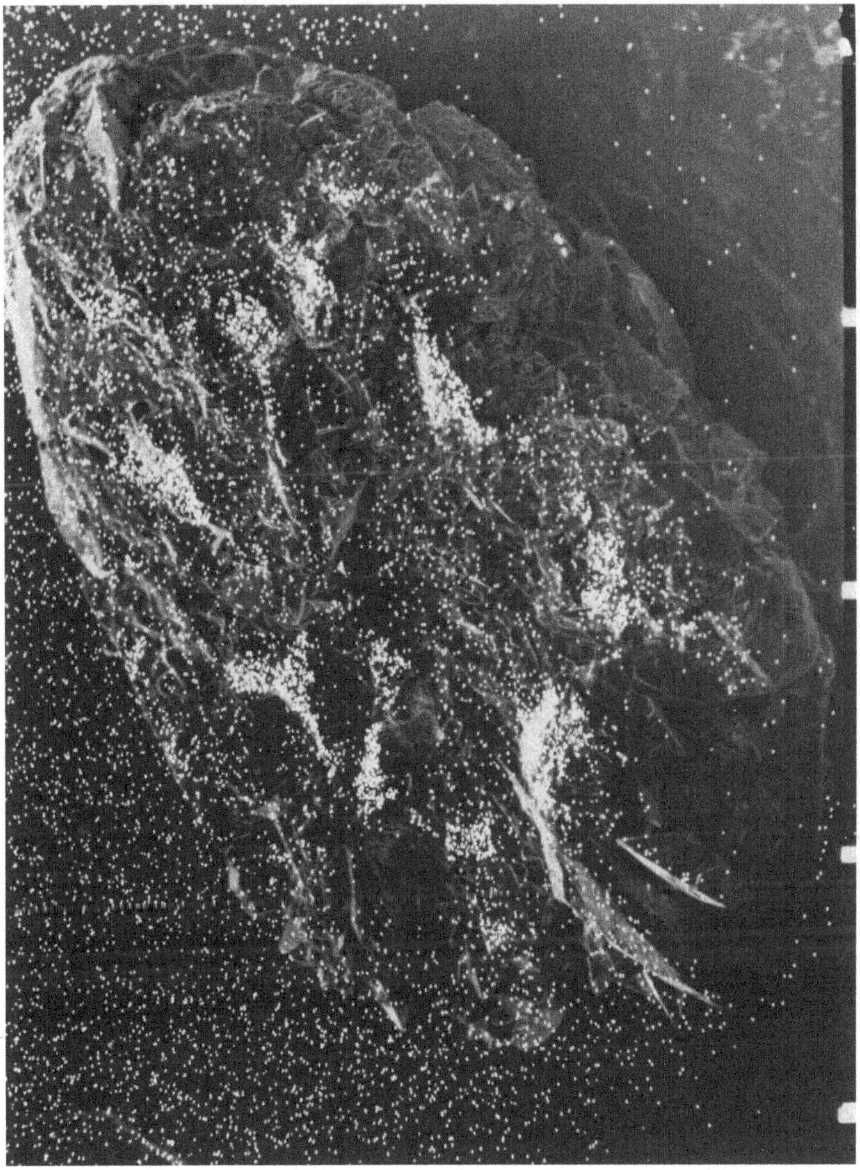

Figure 1. P scan superimposed on scanning electron micrograph of fracture surface of stone showing distribution of clusters of conglomerates of crystals of calcium phosphate (X42. High density areas of white dots represent concentrations of P.)

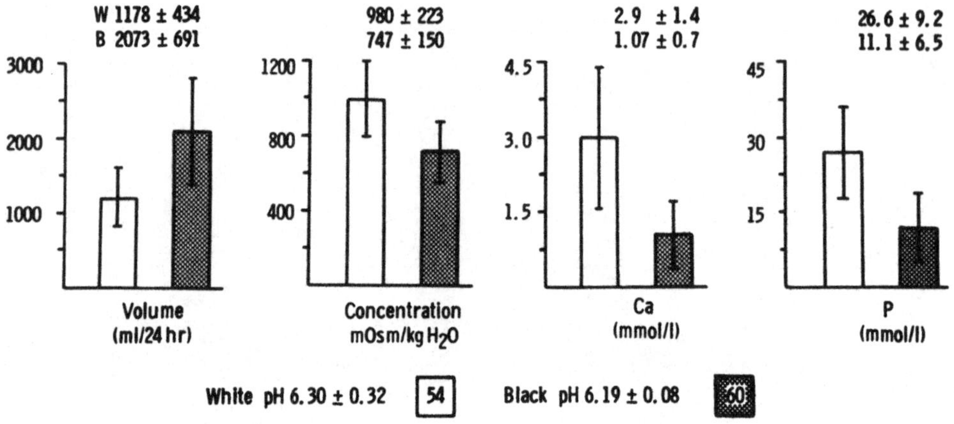

Figure 2. Volume and concentration of urinary constituents. Mean values.

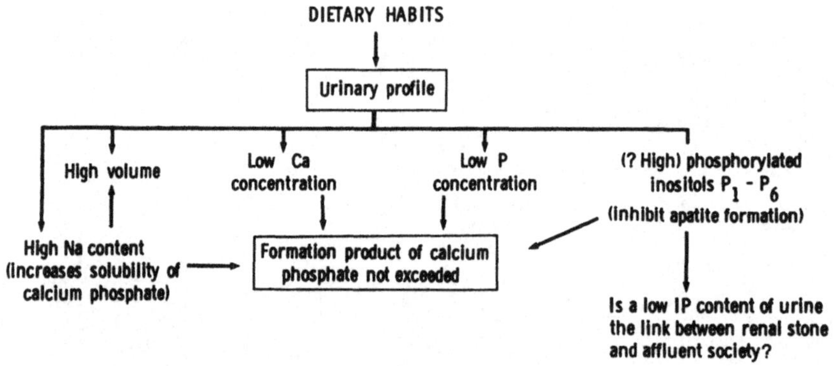

Figure 3. Diet, urinary composition and the genesis of stones.

various phosphorylated inositols which act as potent inhibitors of apatite formation. The biochemical pathway which appears to be discernible between diet, urinary composition and the rarity of stone in the South African black population is outlined in Figure 3.

Unleavened bread, coarse cereals and dried beans, all of which have a high content of phytic acid, form the staple diet of many semi-developed communities in the Middle East and S.E. Asia. Renal stone is less prevalent in these communities than in industrialized and developing communities[9]. The increased incidence of renal stone in the latter more affluent communities of Europe and North America appears to be associated with a reduction in the quantity of phytic acid ingested. This reduction has in the main been due to the elimination of coarse cereals from the diet. Changes in the types of bread eaten have also been responsible. Bread baked with yeast would contain considerably less phytic acid than unleavened bread due to the degradation of phytic acid by enzymes present in the yeast. The process of roller milling of flour was introduced in the industrialized nations in 1870. In this process the grain is crushed and the indigestible fibrous coats are removed as bran. The aleurone layer which is rich in phosphorus is also removed. The degree of extraction, that is the percentage of the whole grain retained in the flour, can be varied widely from 92% in wholemeal to 70% in white flour. Below 80% the loss in minerals is considerable. The use of white flour in baking would further reduce the amount of phytic acid present in bread. The substantial reduction in dietary phytic acid resulting from these changes in dietary pattern would result in a concomitant reduction in urinary phosphorylated inositols. This could be an important factor in the aetiology of renal stones. The interruptions in the increase in the incidence of renal stone that occurred during the two world wars coincided with periods of increased ingestion of phytic acid. An example of this is the introduction in Britain during the last war of the "National Loaf" which contained more of the whole grain. Urinary phosphorylated inositols and their association with renal stones merit further attention.

REFERENCES

1. M. Modlin, Ann. Roy. Coll. Surg. Eng. 40:155 (1967).
2. F. W. Fox, and L. Goldberg, in:"South African Food Tables," South African Institute for Medical Research, Johannesburg (1944).
3. E. L. Wheeler, and R. E. Ferrell, Cereal Chem. 48:312 (1971).
4. R. A. McCance, and E. M. Widdowson, Biochem. J. 29:2694 (1935).
5. V. Subrahmanyou, M. Narayanargo, G. Ramarao, and M. Swaminathan, Br. J. Nutr. 9:350 (1955).
6. A. Desjobert, and F. Petek, Bull. Soc. Chim. Biol. 38:871 (1956).
7. E. Starkenstein, Biochem. Zeitschr. 30:56 (1911).

8. W. C. Thomas, and M. T. Tilden, Johns Hopkins Med. J. 131:133 (1972).
9. D. A. Anderson, in:"Renal Stone Research Symposium," A. Hodgkinson, B. E. C. Nordin, eds., Churchill, London (1969).

ACKNOWLEDGMENT

This study was supported by grants from the South African Medical Research Council and the Harry Crossley Fund.

IDIOPATHIC HYPERCALCIURIA - ITS CONTROL WITH UNPROCESSED BRAN

P. J. R. Shah, G. Williams, and N. A. Green

Department of Urology, Norfolk and Norwich Hospital

Norwich, England

INTRODUCTION

Approximately 50-60% of patients with urolithiasis have a high urinary calcium excretion[1]. In the majority of these patients this is secondary to an increased intestinal absorption of calcium (absorptive hypercalciuria). If a consistent reduction in urinary calcium excretion can be achieved then the incidence of recurrent stone formation is reduced[2]. Current methods of treatment of idiopathic hypercalciuria consist of dietary restriction of calcium, a high fluid intake, sodium cellulose phosphate and thiazide diuretics. Dietary methods are difficult to adhere to as low calcium diets are unpalatable. Cellulose phosphate is a very effective means of reducing urinary calcium excretion but may be associated with side-effects such as diarrhea[1].

An ideal form of treatment is one which is effective, inexpensive, free from side-effects and can be easily tolerated. Henneman et al.[3] showed that sodium phytate reduces urinary calcium excretion in patients with hypercalciuria. It has been suggested that unprocessed bran may effectively reduce urinary calcium excretion by virtue of its phytic acid content[4] (1.7g phytic acid in 100g bran). This study reports on a trial of the treatment of patients with idiopathic hypercalciuria with unprocessed bran.

PATIENTS AND METHODS

Forty-four patients (41 males, 3 females) with idiopathic hypercalciuria diagnosed after 2 consecutive raised 24-h urine calcium levels (normal range up to 7.5 mmol/24-h) whilst on a normal diet were entered into the study. Serum electrolytes, calcium, phosphate, magnesium, alkaline phosphatase, urate and 24-h urinary calcium, phosphate, magnesium, urate, creatinine were estimated prior to treatment and at monthly intervals during treatment. Each patient was prescribed a dose of 24g of fine unprocessed bran daily to be taken in divided amounts with meals. Each patient was advised to remain on a normal diet throughout treatment.

RESULTS

The majority of the patients were in the 40-50 year age group. Serum electrolyte levels remained normal during therapy with bran. In 75% of the patients studied a significant reduction in urinary calcium excretion was obtained (Table 1). There was no change in urinary sodium phosphate or magnesium excretion. Ten patients did not respond.

Table 1. Results of Treatment with Unprocessed Bran (n = 44)

	Before Therapy	During Therapy		Before Treatment Stopped
		One month	Two months	
Serum electrolytes (mmol/l)				
Calcium	2.37±0.08	2.36±0.08	2.35±0.07	2.37± 0.08
Phosphate	0.96±0.16	0.93±0.15	0.88±0.13	0.89± 0.12
Magnesium	0.75±0.16	0.8 ±0.02	0.76±0.02	0.77± 0.04
Urine electrolytes (mmol/24 h)				
Calcium	10.8 ±2.12	8.9 ± 2.4	9.0 ±2.2*	9.7 ± 2.7
Phosphate	37.3 ±8.70	36.0 ±10.7	36.6 ±8.3	36.7 ±10.5
Magnesium	4.6 ±1.00	4.7 ± 1.7	4.9 ±1.5	4.8 ± 1.4

*P < 0.001 compared to pre-treatment values (t-test)

DISCUSSION

In the majority of patients with idiopathic hypercalciuria the high urinary calcium excretion is the result of an increase in the absorption of dietary calcium. Dietary measures and sodium cellulose phosphate have been the mainstays of treatment for many years with considerable success. Dietary restriction of calcium, however, does not produce the consistent reduction in calcium excretion that is expected[5] and a low calcium diet is difficult to adhere to over a long period. Sodium cellulose phosphate has been reported in many studies to be an effective form of treatment of absorptive hypercalciuria[2,6]. However this agent is expensive and side-effects such as diarrhea which may require withdrawal of treatment are not uncommon[1].

An effective dietary regime is the ideal form of treatment without the need for added drug therapy. Previous reports of the effect of sodium phytate on urinary calcium excretion[3] and the knowledge that unprocessed bran may have an effect on reducing intestinal calcium absorption because of its phytate content (1.7g phytic acid in 100g bran) led to a study of the treatment of idiopathic hypercalciuria with bran.

From the results of this study it is shown that unprocessed bran effectively reduces urinary calcium excretion in the majority of patients with idiopathic hypercalciuria. This effect is probably attributable to more than one action. Phytic acid combines with dietary calcium to produce the insoluble compound calcium phytate which is excreted in the faeces. It is suggested that other factors may be responsible for the effect on calcium absorption. A decrease in intestinal transit time may reduce the time available for calcium absorption to occur and bran may have a direct binding effect on dietary calcium. There is also evidence to suggest that bran may inhibit the absorption of glucose which enhances calcium absorption through contact with the intestinal mucosa[7].

The aim of treatment of patients with idiopathic hypercalciuria is to reduce the incidence of recurrent stone formation. Treatment should be prescribed for an indefinite period and should be easily accepted, free from side effects and if possible inexpensive. If it can be shown that unprocessed bran can sustain a reduction in urinary calcium excretion in hypercalciuric patients it could be of significant benefit in their management. Unprocessed bran is inexpensive and entirely non-toxic and may be obtained by patients from any chemist. Apart from the benefits of reducing calcium excretion, an improvement in bowel habit is seen in the majority of patients. In the long-term there may be the added benefits of freedom from diverticular disease and other dietary deficiency diseases.

REFERENCES

1. G. A. Rose and A. R. Harrison, Br. J. Urol. 46:261 (1974).
2. N. J. Blacklock and M. A. Macleod, Br. J. Urol. 46:385 (1974).
3. P. H. Henneman, P. H. Benedict, A. P. Forbes and H. R. Dudley, New Engl. J. Med. 17:802 (1958).
4. K. W. Heaton and E. W. Pomare, Lancet 49 (1974).
5. L. R. I. Baker and W. J. W. Mallinson, Br. J. Urol. 51:181 (1979).
6. C. Y. C. Pak, C. S. Delea, and F. C. Bariter, New Engl. J. Med. 290:175 (1974).

7. M. A. Macleod and N. H. Blacklock, J. R. Nav. Med. Serv. 65:143 (1979).

ACKNOWLEDGMENTS

We would like to thank Mr. M. Scott, Norgine Ltd., High Holborn, London for his support in providing the bran for this study.

UROLITHIASIS - A STUDY OF DRINKING WATER HARDNESS AND GENETIC FACTORS

D. N. Churchill, C. M. Maloney, J. C. Bear, D. G. Bryant,
G. Fodor, and M. H. Gault
Faculty of Medicine
Memorial University of Newfoundland
St. John's, Newfoundland, Canada

A study of the prevalence of kidney stone formers and the relationship of genetic factors and drinking water composition to prevalence was completed in 6 districts in Newfoundland where 82% of stone formers have stones which contain predominantly calcium. One thousand one hundred and twelve adult (age > 25) informants were interviewed in a random sample of households. The mean prevalence of stone formers among males was 15.5% (range 2.3 - 28.6%) and among females, 8.3% (range 3.7 - 11.7%). There was no detectable association between the mean district prevalence (male or female) and the mean district water hardness nor its content of calcium, magnesium, silica, zinc, manganese, iron or copper. However, the range of water hardness values (7 - 89 ppm Ca CO_3) was relatively narrow and did not permit adequate testing of the relationship between drinking water hardness and the prevalence of urolithiasis.

There was a significant excess of affected parents of female stone formers compared to affected parents of female non formers ($p < 0.001$) while the differences were not significant between parents of male stone formers and non-formers ($p > 0.1$).

There was a higher, though not statistically significant, prevalence among the parents of female stone formers as compared to parents of male stone formers ($0.2 > p > 0.1$). The family history data in these first degree relatives of affected and non-affected individuals is consistent with a polygenic mode of inheritance.

	Father %	(N)	Mother %	(N)
Female				
Former	22.2	(54)*	15.4	(52)*
Non-Former	5.8	(608)	4.7	(623)
Male				
Former	11.8	(51)	8.2	(49)
Non-Former	7.7	(287)	4.4	(294)

*$P(X_2) < 0.001$ between formers and non-formers.

URINE CHEMISTRY IN RENAL STONE FORMERS IN AN AREA WITH SOFT DRINKING WATER

D. N. Churchill, D. P. Black, C. M. Maloney,
and M. H. Gault
Faculty of Medicine
Memorial University of Newfoundland
St. John's, Newfoundland, Canada

An association between soft drinking water and a higher incidence of urolithiasis has been reported from several countries [1,2]. A decreased ingestion of calcium could permit an increased gut absorption of oxalate and produce an increased urinary oxalate excretion[3]. A decreased ingestion of magnesium could result in a decreased urinary excretion of this inhibitor[2]. The effect of trace elements in drinking water on the incidence of urolithiasis is unknown although zinc and manganese inhibit while silica facilitates the calcification of an organic matrix in vitro[4].

We have measured the concentration of several elements in drinking water and their urinary excretion in renal stone formers and normal subjects in an area with soft drinking water and a high prevalence of kidney stone disease. Previous studies have shown that 82% of stones analyzed in Newfoundland are primarily composed of calcium in combination with oxalate or phosphate or both[5].

METHODS

The study population comprised all adult residents (> 18 years) of 7 rural communities in Newfoundland. Respondents to a mailed questionnaire had definite urolithiasis if they had either passed a stone, had one removed at operation or identified radiologically. The drinking water from each community was analyzed for calcium, magnesium, manganese, zinc and silica by atomic absorption spectrophotometry.

Twenty-two multiple (> 1 stone) stone formers identified in the survey and 13 control subjects had serum creatinine, phosphorus, uric acid and electrolyte determinations. Two 24 hour urine collections were obtained from each subject, taking no medication, at home on a free diet for measurement of calcium, magnesium, oxalate, silica, manganese and zinc. The average 24 hour values are used in the results.

The urine oxalate was determined by the method of Fraser and Campbell[6]. Urine magnesium, manganese, zinc and silica were measured using the same technique as for drinking water.

RESULTS

The total response rate was 85% (1261 of 1485). The prevalence of renal stone disease ranged from 2.1-13.2% (mean 8.6%) between communities (males 9.6%, females 7.5%). The water hardness values ranged from 5.2-20.6 ppm (mean 12.8 ppm). The mean values and standard deviations for drinking water constituents (mg/l) were: Calcium 3.4 ± 1.4, magnesium 0.96 ± 0.15, silica 0.32 ± 0.20, zinc 0.02 ± 0.01 and manganese 0.02 ± 0.02.

Table 1. Urine Chemistry Results

Value (mg/24 hrs)		Stone Formers 12 male, 8 female Value ± SD	Non-Formers 6 male, 4 female Value ± SD
Calcium:	Male	307 ± 150	184 ± 56*
	Female	187 ± 111	164 ± 53
Oxalate:	Male	21.6 ± 20.5	22.2 ± 21.3
	Female	30.0 ± 30.1	20.2 ± 11.2
Magnesium:	Male	91.4 ± 32.5	90.6 ± 29.8
	Female	56.1 ± 18.1	86.0 ± 29.1*
Manganese:	Male	0.72 ± 0.91	0.26 ± 0.19
	Female	0.24 ± 0.12	0.22 ± 0.07
Zinc:	Male	0.81 ± 0.28	0.86 ± 0.20
	Female	0.64 ± 0.26	0.56 ± 0.20
Silica:	Male	8.67 ± 4.76	8.91 ± 6.93
	Female	8.67 ± 7.65	8.15 ± 1.70

*$p < 0.05$ between stone formers and non-formers.

All residents of 3 communities were descended from English Protestant settlers and the residents of 4 communities were descended from Irish Catholic settlers. The prevalence by religious sect was: Protestant 79/765 (10.3%) and Catholic 27/464 (5.8%), $p < 0.01$.

The mean age of the 22 stone formers was 46.5 years; for the 13 control subjects, 46.9 years. Twenty stone formers and 10 control subjects completed 24 hour urine collections.

There was no significant difference detected ($p < 0.05$) between the groups for serum calcium, phosphorus, uric acid, urea nitrogen, creatinine, or chloride. None had hypercalcemia, hyperuricemia or hyperchloremia. The mean urine chemistry results are given in Table 1. Hypercalciuria, defined as 24 hour calcium excretion > 300 mg (males) and > 250 mg (female) was present in 10 of 20 stone formers (7/12 males and 3/8 females) and 0 of 10 control subjects. The twenty-four hour urine oxalate excretion exceeded 40 mg in 3/20 stone formers and 1/10 control subjects.

DISCUSSION

A stone forming episode had been experienced by 9.6% of male and 7.5% of female respondents. The drinking water in all 7 communities was extremely soft and no correlation with prevalence was found over this narrow range of water hardness. Prevalence studies over a larger range of water hardness values among subjects from a reasonably homogenous ethnic background and in an area without major climatic or socio-economic differences will be necessary to confirm or refute the reported association with soft water[1,2]. The high prevalence among Protestants as compared to Catholics may represent either a genetic factor, considering the geographic isolation of these communities and cultural pressures to marry within ones own religious group[7], or another unrecognized environmental factor.

The very low calcium concentrations in the drinking water did not produce a low urine calcium. The mean urine oxalate excretion was within normal limits for both groups. There was no detectable difference between groups for either urinary manganese or urinary zinc excretion. The zinc excretion reported for normal male subjects[8] was similar to that in this study. Dobbie et al[9], reported 24 hour urine silicon excretion values of 8.9 mg for control subjects compared to 12.0 mg for urolithiasis patients ($p < 0.05$). Values for silicon from our study are similar to the control subjects reported[9].

A decreased urine magnesium excretion has been implicated in the causation of calcium oxalate urolithiasis. We found no detectable difference between male stone formers as compared to control subjects but did find a significantly lower magnesium excretion in female stone formers compared to controls although the number of subjects was small. Daily urinary magnesium excretion has been reported to be 136 mg[10], and 107 mg[11] for normal males and 98 mg for normal females[11]. The mean urine magnesium excretion in this present study was lower than those reported values[10,11]. The excessive loss of magnesium from foods cooked in soft water[12] could produce a decrease in magnesium ingestion despite an apparently adequate diet.

This study does not support the hypothesis that the increased prevalence of urolithiasis in areas with soft drinking water is caused by an increased urinary oxalate excretion. The relatively low urine magnesium values may play a role in the causation of urolithiasis in soft water areas and deserves further study as it could be amenable to dietary supplementation.

REFERENCES

1. D. N. Churchill, D. Bryant, and M. H. Gault, Ann. Intern. Med. 88:513 (1978).
2. G. A. Rose and E. J. Westbury, Urol. Res. 3:61 (1975).
3. P. M. Zarembski and A. Hodgkinson, Clin. Chim. Acta. 25:1 (1969).
4. J. E. Howard and W. C. Thomas, Jr., Am. J. Med. 45:693 (1968).
5. M. H. Gault, W. Cohen, C. Eustace, D. Churchill, and I. Senciall, Clin. Chim. Acta. (in press).
6. J. Fraser and D. J. Campbell, Clin. Biochem. 5:99 (1972).
7. J. J. Mannion, The Peopling of Newfoundland, Institute of Social Economic Research, St. John's (1977).
8. E. R. Yendt and M. Cohanim, Kid. Int. 13:397 (1978).
9. J. W. Dobbie, U. B. Gray, and A. C. Kennedy in:"Abstracts VII Int. Cong. Neph. (Montreal)," (1978).
10. A. Hodgkinson, Clin. Sci. Mol. Med. 46:357 (1974).
11. J. N. Lavan, F. C. Neale, and S. Posen, Med. J. Aust. 2:1049 (1971).
12. R. Masironi, WHO Chronicle 32:382 (1978).

ACKNOWLEDGMENT

Grant Support: Kidney Foundation of Canada

THE IMPORTANCE OF CHRONIC CADMIUM POISONING IN RENAL STONE FORMATION - A FIVE YEAR STUDY

R. Scott, O. P. Fitzgerald-Finch, C. Cunningham,
J. M. Ottoway, and G. S. Fell
Departments of Urology, Radiology and Biochemistry,
Royal Infirmary, Glasgos, and University of Strathclyde,
Glasgow, Scotland

INTRODUCTION

It is now recognized that although cadmium affects a wide variety of tissues the kidney is the organ most susceptible to damage by this nonessential toxic trace element. In early studies of chronic cadmium poisoning it was realized that the subjects had hypercalciuria and along with this an increased tendency to have renal stone disease[1]. Subsequent studies have confirmed that in addition to biochemical effects such as renal tubular acidosis, phosphaturia and amino aciduria indicating renal tubular damage[2,3], hypercalciuria is a prominent feature of chronic cadmium poisoning[4,5]. Very few studies exist however which have followed the progress of stone formation and hypercalciuria in cadmium-exposed workers.

PRESENT STUDY

A group of coppersmiths who had been using brazing rods which contained 20% cadmium were initially studied in 1975. A variety of tests were undertaken to prove that they had chronic cadmium poisoning[6] and these confirmed (a) evidence of renal impairment, (b) significant reductions in serum inorganic phosphate, (c) a prevalence of stone disease of 18.5% (Figure 1) as compared with a normal population (3.5%)[7] and (d) significantly elevated blood and urine cadmium values.

The coppersmiths were reviewed annually between 1975-1979 and at the same time each year. At each visit plain abdominal x-rays were routinely undertaken and IVPs were completed when calcified stone disease was suggested by the plain film. Measurements of blood cadmium and phosphate along with 24 h urine calcium, zinc, protein

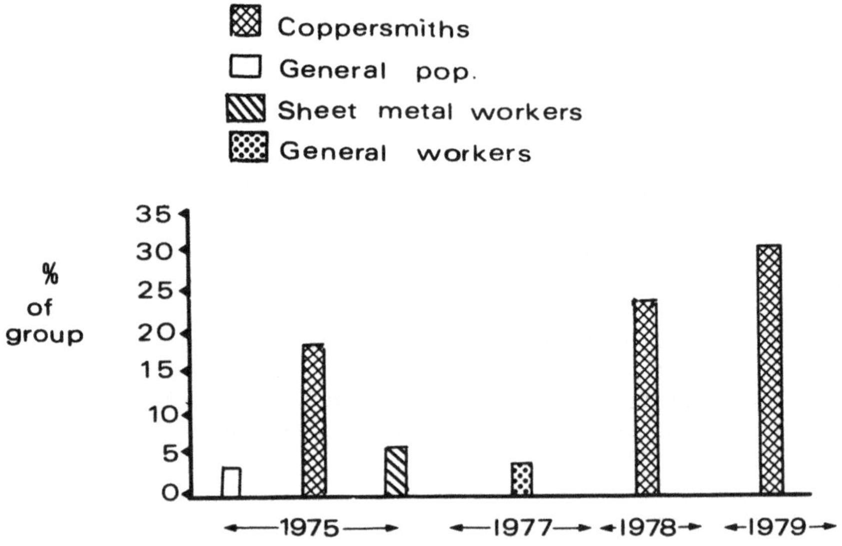

Figure 1. Prevalence of stone disease.

and cadmium were made. These confirmed that mean blood cadmium levels remained elevated (more than 8 μg/l) over the period of study and that the expected increasing incidence of proteinuria occurred within the group (Figure 2). More than 50% of the subjects continued to have hypercalciuria (Figure 2) i.e. urine calcium greater than 6.0 mmol/24 h.

Over the 5 years the excretion of urine calcium has remained above the normal range in the group as a whole but in 6 individuals who were given bendrofluazide in 1976 it has been possible to reduce the total output of urine calcium (Figure 3). In parallel with this reduction of urine calcium, the urine zinc values were also estimated and these have shown a steady fall over the period.

The present study would also suggest that greater attention should be paid to the serum inorganic phosphate levels when assessing suspected cases of chronic cadmium poisoning (Figure 4). When the group was first examined in 1975, 4 of the 5 known stone formers at the outset had serum inorganic phosphate values of less than 0.70 mmol/l. The 3 subjects who developed stones by 1979 were also unique in that their serum inorganic phosphate levels were found to be among the lowest values recorded in 1975 and continued to remain so throughout the study.

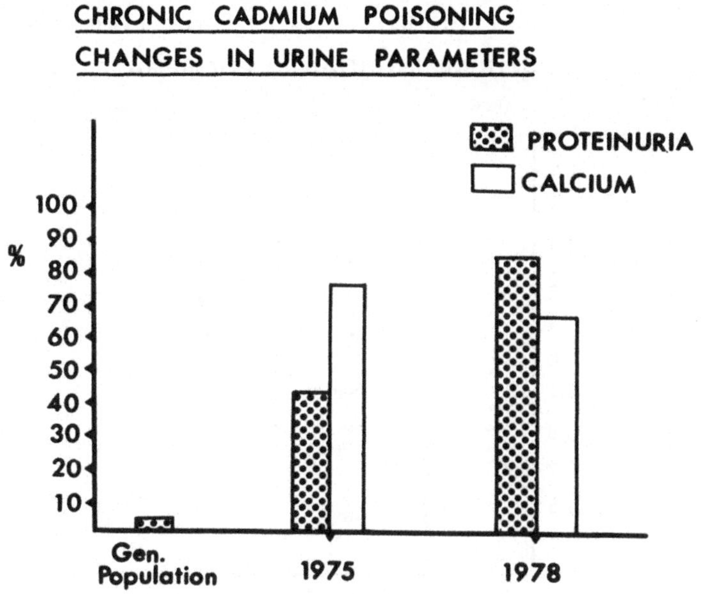

Figure 2. Effect of chronic cadmium poisoning on urinary calcium and protein excretion.

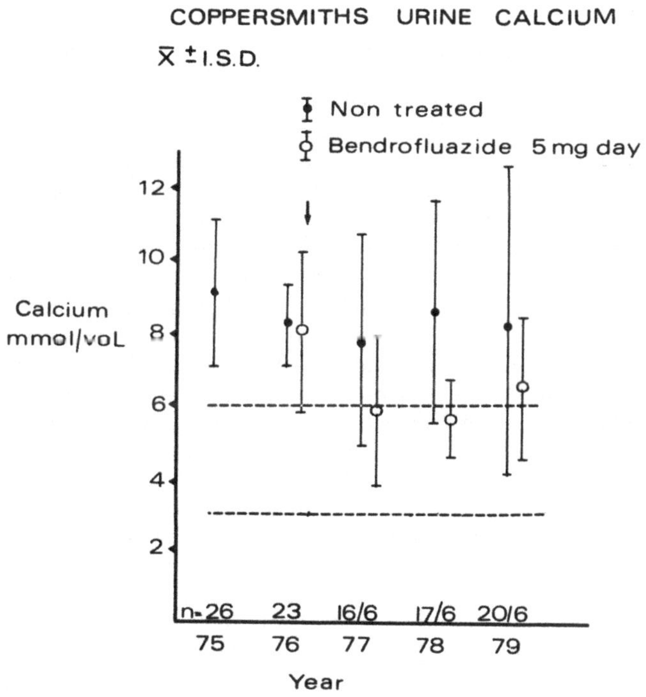

Figure 3. Urinary calcium in coppersmiths in relation to time. (● non-treated; o treated with bendrofluazide)

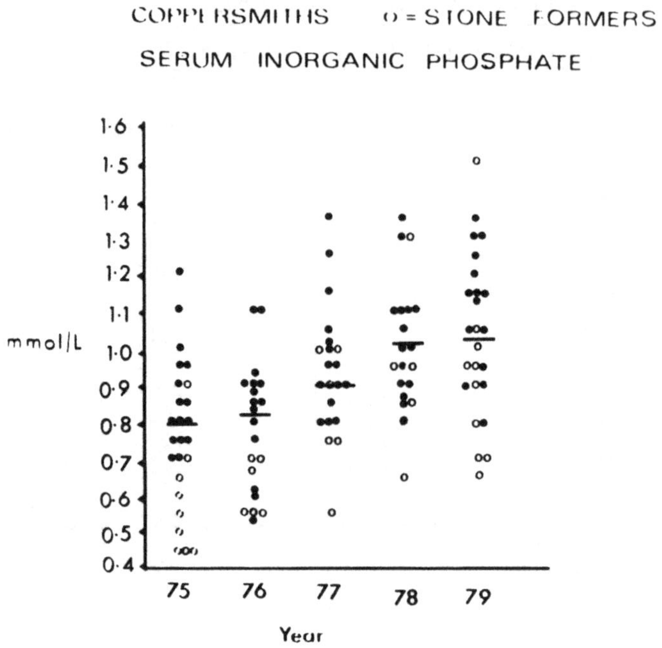

Figure 4. The concentration of serum phosphate in coppersmiths in relation to time.

DISCUSSION

Chronic cadmium poisoning results in a number of recognizable renal and biochemical abnormalities including the excretion of low molecular weight (tubular) protein in urine[8], large molecular weight (glomerular) proteinuria and a variety of other metabolic defects such as altered sodium excretion[9] and amino aciduria[10]. Cadmium metallothionein, the complex in which cadmium is transported to and bound within the kidney, can cause considerable histological damage in kidneys[11]; these changes include tubular atrophy, interstitial fibrosis[12] and calcium deposition[13]. Studies in the experimental animal have shown that cadmium induces a raised calcium excretion and along with this a reduction in 25-hydroxy vitamin D_3 activity in the proximal tubule[14].

In recent years there has been a considerable amount of work undertaken in defining what biochemical parameters are most important in establishing the diagnosis of chronic cadmium poisoning. These debates have centered around the interpretation of the significance of blood and urine cadmium values and whether or not tubular or glomerular proteinuria is the more significant parameter of cadmium poisoning.

In terms of patient care it should be realized that the type of proteinuria merely confirms exposure to the metal and gives an indication of progressive kidney damage. The histological changes[13] induced accompanied by hypercalciuria[4] are considered to be the cause of the increased incidence of stones in such workers. The hypercalciuria has been shown in the present study not to be a transient phenomenon and further evidence of this has been demonstrated by a significant reduction in whole body calcium in these workers[15].

REFERENCES

1. L. Friberg, Acta. Med. Scand. (Suppl) 138:240 (1950).
2. K. S. Williamson, S. A. Roach, D. E. Hickish, M. F. Claydon, J. R. Glover, R. Owen, and D. Turner, Ann. Occup. Hyg. 20:215 (1977).
3. R. R. Lauwerys, J. P. Buchet, H. A. Roels, J. Brouwers, and D. Stanescu, Arch. Environ. Health 28:145 (1974).
4. R. Scott, P. J. Paterson, R. Burns, J. M. Ottoway, F. E. R. Hussain, G. S. Fell, S. Dumbuya, and M. Iqbal, Urology 11:462 (1978).
5. G. Kazantzis, in:"First International Conference on Cadmium," San Francisco (1977).
6. R. Scott, P. J. Paterson, E. A. Mills, A. McKirdy, G. S. Fell, J. M. Ottoway, F. E. R. Hussain, O. P. Fitzgerald Finch, A. J. Yates, A. Lamont, and S. Roxburgh, Lancet 2:396 (1976).
7. R. Scott, R. Freeland, W. Mowat, P. J. Paterson, P. S. Orr, A. J. Yates, and E. A. Mills, in:"Proceedings International Conference on Urolithiasis, Perth," (1979) (in press).
8. H. Welinder, S. Skerfving, and O. Henriksen, Br. J. Industr. Med. 34:221 (1977).
9. J. Lener and J. Musil, Experientia 27:902 (1971).
10. R. A. Goyer, K. Tsuchiya, D. L. Leonard, and H. Kahyo, Am. J. Clin. Pathol. 57:635 (1972).
11. M. G. Cherian, R. A. Goyer, and L. Delaquerrieve-Richardson, Appl. Pharmacol. 38:399 (1976).
12. J. A. Bonnell, J. H. Ross, and E. King, Br. J. Indust. Hyg. 17:69 (1960).
13. E. Aughey and R. Scott, Munich (1977).
14. M. Ando, Y. Sayato, M. Tono-mura, and T. Osawa, Toxicol. Appl. Pharmacol. 39:321 (1977).
15. R. Scott, J. K. Haywood, K. Boddy, E. D. Williams, I. Harvey, and P. J. Paterson, Urology 15:356 (1980).

SHOULD RECURRENT CALCIUM OXALATE STONE FORMERS EAT LESS ANIMAL PROTEIN?

W. G. Robertson, M. Peacock, P. J. Heyburn, F. A. Hanes, D. Ouimet, A. Rutherford, and V. J. Sergeant
M.R.C. Mineral Metabolism Unit, The General Infirmary

Leeds LS1 3EX, U.K.

It has been suggested that calcium stone-formation in the upper urinary tract is essentially a disease of the more affluent countries and sections of society[1,2]. This hypothesis is supported by the observations that the rate of hospitalization for stones has been increasing in industrialized countries over the last 30-40 years[1,3,4] and that calcium stone-formers are found more frequently in the more affluent social classes 1 and 2 than in the less well off sections of society[5,6]. Further studies have indicated that the only dietary factor which is correlated consistently at all demographic levels with affluence is the intake of animal protein, particularly the flesh protein fraction[4,6,7]. Moreover, stone-formers consume more animal protein than normal subjects[7,8]. These observations suggest that the risk of stones in a given population is proportional to the consumption of animal protein.

To test this hypothesis further we have recently studied the effect of feeding diets high and low in animal protein[8,9] and have measured the biochemical risk of forming stones (P_{SF}) using our risk factor analysis procedure[10]. This study showed quite clearly that a high animal protein diet increased the urinary excretion of calcium, oxalate and uric acid and thereby markedly increased the value of P_{SF}. On the other hand, reducing the intake of animal protein from normal lowered the urinary excretion of all three ions and decreased the risk of forming stones. The results of these studies are summarized in the top half of Table 1. They are consistent with the hypothesis that a high animal protein increases the risk of stones and a diet low in animal protein reduces the risk.

What then is the risk of stones amongst practicing vegetarians? The lower half of Table 1 shows the influence of reducing animal

Table 1. The Effect of Different Animal Protein Intakes on the Risk of Calcium Stone-Formation

Group	Animal protein Content of diet (g/day)	Urinary Excretion (mmol/day) Calcium Mean (SEM)	Oxalate Mean (SEM)	Uric Acid Mean (SEM)	Probability of Stones P_{SF} Mean (SEM)
Normals (♂ + ♀)	1	2.19 (0.28)	0.270 (0.016)	2.90 (0.20)	0.190 (0.049)
Normals (")	48	4.39 (0.45)	0.285 (0.015)	3.65 (0.32)	0.290 (0.061)
Normals (")	70	5.52 (0.48)	0.344 (0.016)	4.36 (0.35)	0.427 (0.062)
Normals (♂)	92	7.84 (0.15)	0.387 (0.008)	5.51 (0.11)	0.608 (0.037)
Vegetarians	20	2.57 (0.32)	0.269 (0.016)	2.83 (0.20)	0.120 (0.023)
Normal women	40	3.70 (0.22)	0.259 (0.014)	3.53 (0.10)	0.126 (0.016)
Normal men	49	6.23 (0.39)	0.350 (0.014)	3.94 (0.22)	0.253 (0.033)
Single stone-formers (SSF)	53	7.45 (0.50)	0.380 (0.020)	4.79 (0.24)	0.541 (0.054)
Recurrent stone-formers (RSF)	60	8.92 (0.52)	0.430 (0.022)	5.00 (0.25)	0.689 (0.027)

protein intake from that of recurrent stone-formers through various groups to that of vegetarians. Clearly there is a progressive fall in P_{SF} values through the series with the vegetarians having the lowest predicted risk of stones of all the groups. Comparison with the data in the top half of Table 1, however, shows that the high animal protein diet of the stone-formers only partly accounts for their increased biochemical risk of stones. About 50% of the observed increase in urinary calcium and oxalate and most of the increase in uric acid of the stone-formers can be explained on the basis of their higher intake of animal protein (and accompanying purine). The remainder of the increase in urinary calcium and oxalate is probably due to hyperabsorption of calcium[11] and secondary hyperabsorption of oxalate from the intestine[12,13].

Table 2 shows that the low predicted risk of stones in vegetarians is confirmed by studies on the prevalence rate of stones in various populations. One of the problems of such a study is that vegetarians are members mainly of social classes 1, 2 and 3. To test whether or not the prevalence of stones is lower in this biased population than in the population as a whole comparison should be made with a group of similar social class structure. Since the majority of calcium stone-formers are also in social classes 1, 2 and 3[6] the expected prevalence of stones in a group of this social class structure is about 8.6% in males. The observed rate of vegetarians of 1.9% in males is about one fifth of the expected rate. The rate of stone-formation in vegetarian women is also strikingly lower than that in the population as a whole.

Table 2. Prevalence of Stone Disease in Vegetarians and in the General Population in UK

Group	Prevalence of Urinary Stones Males (%)	Females (%)	Total (%)
General population	3.7	3.9	3.8
Vegetarians (observed)	1.9	0.7	1.2
Vegetarians (expected)*	8.6	-	-
Vegetarians (observed/expected)	0.22	-	-

* Value expected in vegetarians from the bias in social class in this group towards social classes 1 and 2.

In conclusion, it would appear that both practicing vegetarians and normal subjects on a vegetarian diet have a low risk of calcium stone-formation in the urinary tract. It remains to be seen whether or not it will be worthwhile advocating a more vegetarian form of diet as a means of reducing the risk of stone recurrence in patients who have formed multiple stones. Interestingly, inflation - by reducing the purchase and consumption of animal protein appears to be already achieving this goal, since both the number of certified days lost from work owing to renal stones and the annual hospitalization rate for stone disease in the UK fell during the inflationary years 1969-1977[7]. Since then the slight recovery of the economy owing to the flow of North Sea oil has caused a rise both in the consumption of animal protein and in the indices of stone-formation[7].

REFERENCES

1. D. A. Andersen, in:"Urinary Calculi," L. Cifuentes-Delatte, A. Rapado, and A. Hodgkinson, eds., Karger, Basel (1973).
2. N. J. Blacklock, in:"Scientific Foundations of Urology, Vol. 1," D. I. Williams and G. D. Chisholm, eds., Heinemann, London (1976).
3. R. Sierakowski, B. Finlayson, R. R. Landes, C. D. Finlayson, and N. Sierakowski, Invest. Urol. 15:438 (1978).
4. W. G. Robertson, M. Peacock, and A. Hodgkinson, J. Chron. Dis. 32:469 (1979).
5. R. W. White, R. D. Cohen, F. P. Vince, G. Williams, J. Blandy, and G. C. Tressider, in:"Proceedings of the Renal Stone Symposium," B. E. C. Nordin and A. Hodgkinson, eds., Churchill, London (1969).
6. W. G. Robertson, M. Peacock, P. J. Heyburn, D. H. Marshall, and F. Hanes, Fortschr. Urol. Nephrol. 11:5 (1978).
7. W. G. Robertson, M. Peacock, P. J. Heyburn, F. A. Hanes, and R. Swaminathan, in:"Proceedings of the Stone Conference, Perth, 1979", J. G. Brockis and B. Finlayson, eds. (in press).
8. W. G. Robertson, M. Peacock, P. J. Heyburn, F. A. Hanes, A. Rutherford, E. Clementson, R. Swaminathan, and P. B. Clark, Br. J. Urol. 51:427 (1979).
9. W. G. Robertson, P. J. Heyburn, M. Peacock, F. A. Hanes, and R. Swaminathan, Clin. Sci. 57:285 (1979).
10. W. G. Robertson, M. Peacock, P. J. Heyburn, D. H. Marshall, and P. B. Clark, Br. J. Urol. 50:449 (1978).
11. B. E. C. Nordin, M. Peacock, and R. Wilkinson, Clinics Endocrin. and Metab. 1:169 (1972).
12. W. G. Robertson, M. Peacock, P. J. Heyburn, R. W. Marshall, A. Rutherford, R. E. Williams, and P. B. Clark, in:"Oxalate in Human Biochemistry and Clinical Pathology," G. A. Rose, W. G. Robertson, and R. W. E. Watts, eds., Wellcome Foundation, London (1980).
13. W. G. Robertson and M. Peacock, Nephron (in press).

INFLUENCE OF PURINE CONTENT OF DIET AND ALLOPURINOL ON URIC ACID AND OXALATE EXCRETION LEVELS

H. A. Simmonds*, K. J. Van Acker**, C. F. Potter*,
D. R. Webster*, G. P. Kasidas***, and G. A. Rose***
*Purine Laboratory, Guy's Hospital Medical School, London Bridge, London SE1 9RT, U.K.; **Department of Pediatrics, University of Antwerp, Wilvijk, Belgium; ***Department of Pathology, St. Paul's Hospital, London, W.C. 2, U.K.

A defect of the purine salvage enzyme adenine phosphoribosyltransferase (APRT) results in lithiasis in some but not all homozygotes for the defect. The stones are frequently mistaken for uric acid[1], but are really composed of an insoluble analogue, 2,8-dihydroxyadenine (2,8-DHA), excreted in consequence of the defect (see Simmonds et al. this symposium). The present studies were an attempt to establish whether any variation in oxalate or urate excretion with diet could explain the asymptomatic status of one of two male siblings homozygous for the defect. A preliminary study of diet and allopurinol on purine excretion has been reported elsewhere [2]. The rationale for the investigations was based on the association frequently reported between dietary purine intake and increased uric acid levels in oxalate stone formers[3], and the beneficial effect of allopurinol in reducing (a) the absorption of dietary purine in an animal model[4]; (b) the incidence of lithiasis in some oxalate stone formers[5]; (c) any further stone formation on a low purine diet in one of two siblings under investigation[2].

METHODS

The influence of dietary purine and the effect of allopurinol was investigated in control males and compared with the two male APRT-homozygotes and their heterozygous father (previously operated for right-sided lithiasis thought to be oxalate)[2]. An adolescent male homozygote for a deficiency of pyrimidine metabolism (hereditary oroticaciduria, OPRT:ODC deficiency) resulting in the over-excretion of uric acid as well as orotic acid[6], was also studied. The protocol used has already been described[2]. Purine metabolites were measured as previously described[1] and oxalate was determined by an enzymic method[7].

The low purine diet contained less than 100 mg of oxalate and of purine. The high purine regime contained approximately 900 mg purine and 700 mg oxalate. In addition, one healthy adult male was studied on a diet which contained less than 80 mg oxalate throughout the low and high purine regime. In a preliminary study another subject received a single purine additive (600 mg/day) while on a fixed low purine intake throughout for comparison.

RESULTS

Effect of Diet on Urinary Purine Levels

Different results were obtained in each instance. Changes from a low to a high purine diet produced a 2- to 3-fold increment in urinary uric acid in control males, but the increment in APRT-deficient and control children was not as great. By contrast there was no change in uric acid or total oxypurine levels with diet in the OPRT:ODC deficient case (Figure 1).

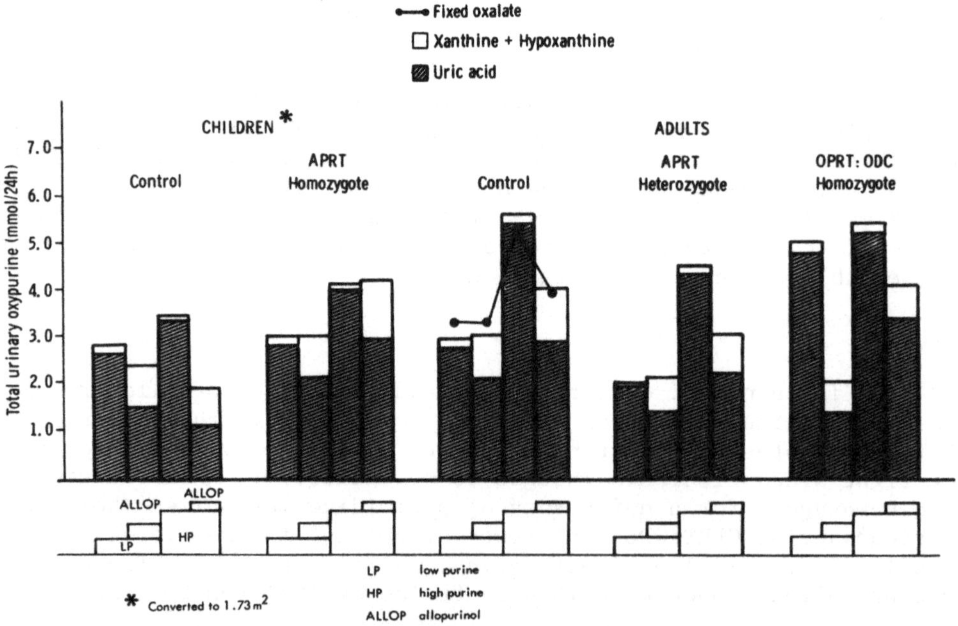

Figure 1. Urinary oxypurine studies.

Allopurinol produced a substantial reduction in the sum of total oxypurine (xanthine + hypoxanthine + uric acid) excreted in all controls on the high, as distinct from the low, purine diet (Figure 1). No such effect was noted in the two young homozygotes for APRT-deficiency, while the effect of allopurinol in OPRT:ODC deficiency was the reverse of that in controls.

Effect of Dietary Purine and Allopurinol on Urinary Oxalate Levels

Urinary oxalate levels were also altered by the different dietary and therapeutic regimes. The changes were identical in both adult and child controls as well as the two separate inborn errors of purine and pyrimidine metabolism (Figure 2), although of smaller magnitude in the children than the adults.

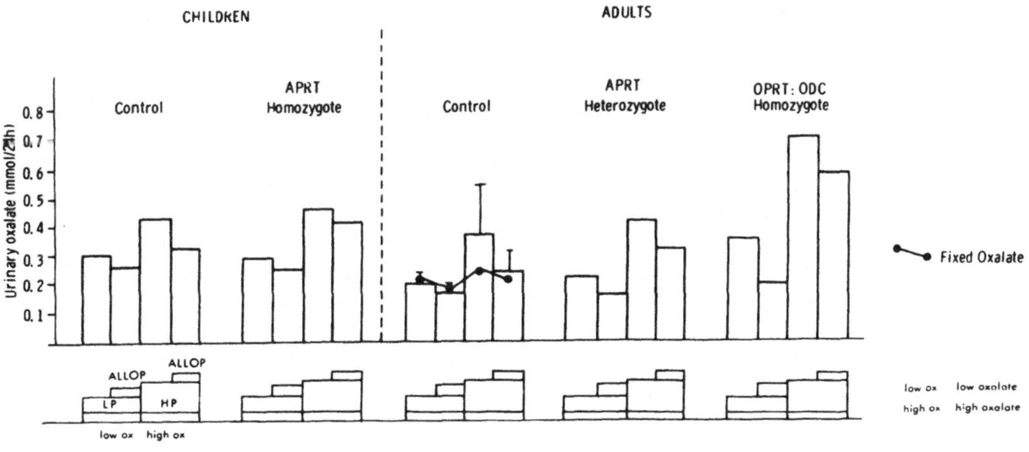

Figure 2. Urinary oxalate studies

The two most striking features were: (a) the approximately 2-fold increment in urinary oxalate with the change from the low to the high purine diet; and (b) the reduction by up to 60% of this dietary purine-induced increment in oxalate when allopurinol was added to the high purine regime. These effects were still seen when dietary purine was varied (with and without allopurinol) whilst the oxalate content of the diet was maintained at a fixed low level (Figure 2).

DISCUSSION

These studies indicate that in APRT deficiency the production and excretion of uric acid and oxalate, and the effect of dietary purine on both of these, is indistinguishable from normal. The latter finding does not substantiate earlier suggestions that urinary uric acid levels may be more sensitive to dietary purine intake in homozygotes for APRT deficiency[2]. The increment in oxalate, but not uric acid, with diet in the case of hereditary oroticaciduria differs from the other subjects, as does the effect of allopurinol, but may be related to the chronic uridine therapy necessary to maintain a clinically normal status in this condition[6].

The concomitant reduction in total urinary oxypurine levels by allopurinol on the high, but not the low, purine regime in healthy controls is identical with that noted by us in an animal model where isotope studies showed enhanced faecal excretion of dietary purine by allopurinol[4]. This is support for an additional beneficial effect of allopurinol in reducing the absorption of dietary purine in the normal adult male[4]. The variation in this pattern in the homozygotes for the two different inborn errors is noteworthy and merits further investigation. It has also been noted in the Lesch-Nyham syndrome[8]. The lack of effect of allopurinol on urinary total oxypurine excretion during the period of excessive dietary purine consumption in the APRT-homozygotes indicates that dietary purine restriction will always be important in this defect.

An association between purines in the diet and increased urinary oxalate excretion has been noted by some[9], but not all workers[10]. It is clearly demonstrated in this study. The reduction in this dietary nucleoprotein-induced increment in oxalate excretion by allopurinol has not been noted previously. A reduction in urinary oxalate excretion by allopurinol has been reported in subjects with blood uric acids in excess of 300 μmol/l[11], but diet was not mentioned. Since this effect was noted only in subjects with the higher blood uric acid levels the possibility that these subjects were also habitual over-consumers of dietary purine would need to be evaluated [3]. Inhibition of dietary oxalate absorption by allopurinol could be invoked for the effect of allopurinol on oxalate excretion noted in this study. However, the single study on a fixed oxalate intake suggests this is not the case, as do preliminary experiments on a fixed low purine diet in the one subject given a single purine supplement, with and without allopurinol. Studies to investigate the reason for these differences are continuing but suggest the involvement of xanthine oxidase and exogenous purines in the process.

SUMMARY

We conclude that although these studies have failed to establish any clearcut differences between asymptomatic and stone forming APRT deficient homozygotes, the concomitant variation in oxalate levels during the different dietary purine and therapeutic regimes is noteworthy. The results suggest an important association between dietary purine and urinary oxalate levels by mechanisms, possibly involving xanthine oxidase, which remain to be defined. If confirmed they suggest a logical explanation for the fact that both gout and oxalate stone formation tend to be associates of affluence[12], as well as the beneficial effect of allopurinol in reducing stone formation in oxalate stone formers[5]. Another important observation is that although dietary purine restriction may not always be so critical in some adults treated with allopurinol, dietary restraint will always be necessary in APRT deficient stone formers.

REFERENCES

1. H. A. Simmonds, K. J. Van Acker, J. S. Cameron, and W. Snedden, Biochem. J. 157:485 (1976).
2. K. J. Van Acker, H. A. Simmonds, C. F. Potter, and J. S. Cameron, New Engl. J. Med. 297:127 (1977).
3. F. L. Coe, E. Moran, and A. G. Kavalich, J. Chron. Dis. 29:793 (1976).
4. H. A. Simmonds, T. J. Rising, A. Cadenhead, P. J. Hatfield, A. S. Jones, and J. S. Cameron, Biochem. Pharmac. 22:2553 (1973).
5. M. J. V. Smith, J. Urol. 117:690 (1977).
6. H. A. Simmonds, D. R. Webster, C. F. Potter, and D. M. O. Becroft, Eur. J. Clin. Invest. (in press).
7. P. C. Hallson and G. A. Rose, Clin. Chim. Acta. 55:29 (1974).
8. C. E. Jones, E. E. Smith, W. Hicks, and J. W. Crowell, J. Lab. Clin. Med. 76:163 (1970).
9. P. M. Zarembski and A. Hodgkinson, Clin. Chim. Acta. 25:1 (1969).
10. C. Y. C. Pak, D. E. Barilla, K. Holt, L. Brinkley, R. Tolentino, and J. E. Zerwekh, Am. J. Med. 65:593 (1978).
11. R. Scott, P. J. Paterson, A. Mathieson, and M. Smith, Br. J. Urol. 50:455 (1978).
12. N. J. Blacklock, in:"Urolithiasis Research," H. Fleisch, W. G. Robertson, L. H. Smith, and W. Vahlensieck, eds., Plenum Press, New York (1976).

INCREASED AVAILABILITY OF DIETARY CARBOHYDRATE: A FACTOR IN THE GENESIS OF IDIOPATHIC CALCIUM OXALATE UROLITHIASIS?

J. A. Thom*, J. E. Morris, A. Bishop, and N. J. Blacklock**
Institute of Naval Medicine, Alverstoke, Hampshire, U.K.; *Now at School of Public Health and Tropical Medicine, University of Sydney, Australia; ** Now at the University Hospital of South Manchester, Nell Lane, Manchester 20, United Kingdom

A characteristic of affluent communities in which idiopathic calcium oxalate renal stone is common is the high nutrient density of the diet compared with that of poorer communities in which it is uncommon. This nutrient density is due to a high intake of animal protein, available carbohydrate and fat. Depletion of dietary fibre contributes to a high calorie density. This study set out to define the influence of increased dietary carbohydrate density on urinary electrolytes and on the calcium oxalate activity product of urine and to determine whether or not such changes could be moderated by increments of dietary fibre.

SUBJECTS AND METHODS

Eighteen healthy male subjects were observed in a metabolic chamber in 2 separate cross-over trials lasting 28 days each. In the first trial (11 subjects) urinary excretion of calcium and oxalate on a "low" carbohydrate diet (LCD) (220 g of available carbohydrate including 110 g sucrose) was compared with that in the same subjects on a "normal" carbohydrate diet (NCD) (450 g of available carbohydrate of which 220 g was sucrose). At the beginning of the period subjects were randomly allocated either to the LCD or the NCD; on day 15 the diets were crossed over.

In the second trial (7 subjects) the 2 experimental diets were the LCD and a "high" available carbohydrate diet (HCD) (600 g available carbohydrate of which 330 g was sucrose. These experimental diets were otherwise standardized for their daily intake of other nutrients - protein (115 g), fat (170 g), calcium (35 mmols), phosphorus (60 mmols) and included approximately 2 liters of water. Subjects were maintained in a steady state of physical fitness.

In the third trial (5 subjects) which lasted for 28 days, urinary calcium and oxalate excretion were compared between an HCD and an HCD with supplements of fiber as wheatbran. The fiber content in the 2 stages of this trial were 20/25 g daily and 60/75 g daily.

Urine was collected as voided, aliquots being taken from each specimen passed and stored at -20°. Analysis of calcium was by atomic absorption spectrophotometry[1,2] and oxalate by colorimetry[3]. Calcium oxalate activity products were determined by nomogram[4].

RESULTS

The calcium and oxalate concentration of individual urine specimens passed in the second week on an LCD were compared with the concentrations in the first week on an NCD (trial 1) and the first week on an HCD (trial 2) (Table 1). Calcium concentration increased significantly in both trials. Oxalate concentration also increased from that on LCD in both trials but this was not statistically significant.

Table 1. Geometric mean and (95 percentile) of calcium and oxalate concentrations of individual urine specimens on LCD compared with NCD (Trial 1) and on LCD compared with HCD (Trial 2).

	Calcium (mmol/l)		Oxalate (mmol/l)	
TRIAL 1				
LCD (2nd week)	5.5 (8.8)	p <0.01	0.18 (0.425)	N.S.
NCD (1st week)	4.6 (11.2)		0.205 (0.525)	
TRIAL 2				
LCD (2nd week)	3.1 (8.2)	p <0.01	0.15 (0.360)	N.S.
HCD (1st week)	4.6 (12.2)		0.715 (0.410)	

These measured values for urine calcium and oxalate concentration in the individual urine specimens in each of these trials were used to determine the logarithmic relative supersaturation[4]. The number of urine specimens in which the calcium oxalate formation product was exceeded is shown in Table 2 as proportions of the total urine specimens voided by all subjects during each of the trials. There were highly significant differences in the frequency with which subjects voided urine oversaturated with calcium oxalate when on either the NCD or HCD compared with the LCD.

Table 2. The number of urine specimens in which the calcium oxalate formation product was exceeded expressed as proportions of the total urine specimens voided by all subjects on LCD compared with NCD and on LCD compared with HCD.

	"Oversaturated" Specimens / Total Specimens	Significance
TRIAL 1 (N = 11)		
LCD	348/929	$Chi^2 = 8.82$
NCD	469/915	$p < 0.01$
TRIAL 2 (N = 7)		
LCD	209/750	$Chi^2 = 20.4$
HCD	312/736	$p < 0.001$

In the third trial individual urine specimens from the 5 subjects were analyzed in the same way and activity products of calcium oxalate were compared between HCD alone and HCD with increments of dietary fiber. The percentage incidence of oversaturation of urine with calcium oxalate in each individual was assessed and plotted against dietary fiber content (Figure 1). There was no significant effect of increments of dietary fiber on the incidence of urinary oversaturation.

DISCUSSION

In these chamber studies we observed considerable spontaneous diurnal variation in urinary concentrations of both calcium and oxalic acid which was more marked in some individuals than others. The number, frequency and amplitude of peaks of concentration were increased the larger the amount of available carbohydrate in the diet. This significantly increased the risk of oversaturation of urine with calcium oxalate in these circumstances. If these changes are accepted as reflecting changes in the risk of calcium oxalate stone nucleation and crystal growth then this study supports the hypothesis that the greater available carbohydrate energy density of the diet in affluent societies is one factor which may account for the increased incidence of idiopathic calcium oxalate nephrolithiasis observed in these communities. The apparent lack of effect of increments of dietary

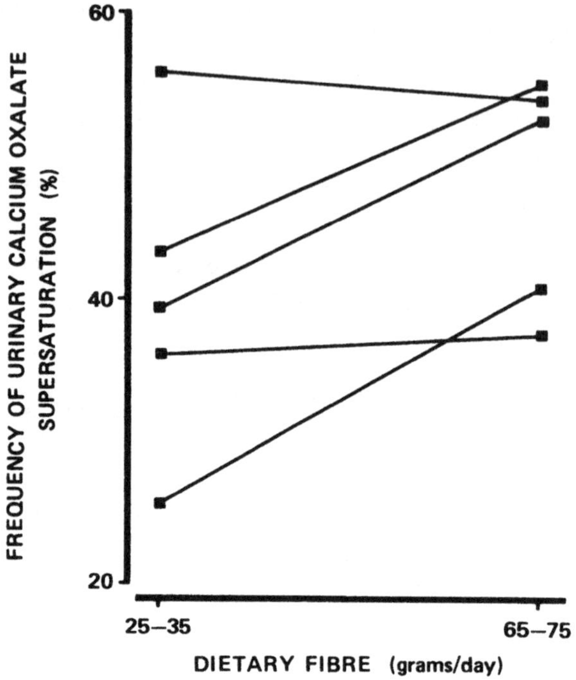

Figure 1. Percentage incidence of urine oversaturation with calcium oxalate in 5 subjects on HCD plotted against dietary fiber content.

fiber in this study suggests that the high available carbohydrate levels were disproportionately large for the cereal fiber to have a "diluent" effect.

SUMMARY

Diets with higher available carbohydrate content significantly increase the frequency of oversaturation of the urine with calcium oxalate. Increments of dietary fiber have no apparent influence on the incidence of urinary oversaturation with calcium oxalate in the presence of a high carbohydrate diet.

REFERENCES

1. J. B. Willis, Anal. Chem. 33:556 (1961).
2. D. L. Trudeau and E. F. Freier, Clin. Chem. 13:101 (1967).
3. A. Hodgkinson and A. Williams, Clin. Chim. Acta. 36:127 (1972).
4. R. W. Marshall and W. G. Robertson, Clin. Chim. Acta. 72:253 (1976).

REDUCTION OF URINARY OXALATE EXCRETION IN PRIMARY HYPEROXALURIA BY DIET

E. R. Yendt, M. Cohanim, and L. Peters

Departments of Medicine and Nutrition Services, Kingston General Hospital and Department of Medicine, Queen's University, Kingston, Ontario, Canada

The medical management of primary hyperoxaluria poses a difficult therapeutic challenge[1]. The administration of pyridoxine, which facilitates the transamination of glyoxylate to glycine occasionally results in a worthwhile reduction of urine oxalate excretion[2-4] but often is without significant effect[2,5,6,7]. Recently Smith has reported encouraging results with the combined use of pyridoxine and orthophosphates which prevented progression of nephrolithiasis and deterioration of renal function in this disease[8].

Attempts to lower urine oxalate excretion by diet in primary hyperoxaluria have hitherto been unsuccessful. Only 2-5% of dietary oxalate is excreted in the urine in this disorder, so that restriction of dietary oxalate has relatively little effect on oxalate excretion[9,10]. Because 40% of urinary oxalate is normally derived from glycine, there have been unsuccessful attempts to reduce the availability of glycine by restricting dietary protein[2,9,10] or by administering sodium benzoate to trap glycine by the formation of hippurate[5,10,11]. The feeding of D-amino acids to compete with glycine for D-amino oxidase has also been unsuccessful[4,12].

We have measured urinary oxalate excretion by 2 methods[13,14] in three female children with primary hyperoxaluria during long-term studies conducted in our Special Investigative Unit while the patients were eating (a) an unrestricted diet, (b) a constant diet containing a normal amoung of oxalate (approximately 100 mg per day) (c) a constant low oxalate diet (10 mg per day) and (d) a constant high oxalate diet (410-530 mg per day). The effects of pyridoxine administration were also assessed.

RESULTS

In Case 1, mean urine oxalate excretion was 155 mg per day on an unrestricted diet but on a constant diet with a normal oxalate content urine oxalate fell gradually over a two week period to approximately 50% of this value; when a high oxalate constant diet was substituted for the normal oxalate diet there was no significant change, but on a low oxalate constant diet, urine oxalate gradually rose again to values similar to those seen during the unrestricted diet (Figure 1). In Case 2, mean urine oxalate excretion on an unrestricted diet was 163 mg per day but on a constant diet with a normal oxalate content, urine oxalate fell by approximately 50%; however in this patient urine oxalate did not change significantly with the high oxalate or low oxalate constant diets (Figure 2). In Case 3, mean urine oxalate on an unrestricted diet was 65 mg per day; no significant changes occurred with the normal or high oxalate constant diets but urine oxalate excretion doubled on the low oxalate constant diet (Figure 3). Pyridoxine administration reduced urine oxalate excretion slightly in Case 2 but had no significant effect in Case 3; in Case 1 its effect was uncertain but probably not great.

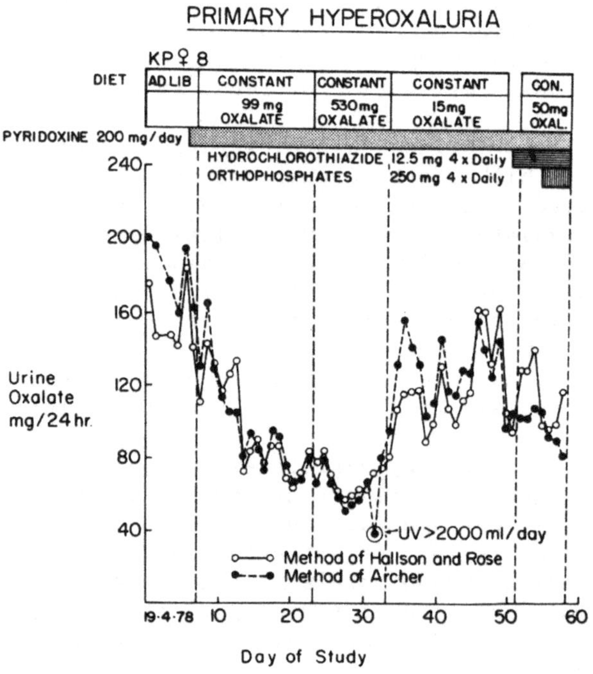

Figure 1. Urinary oxalate excretion during first hospital study in Case 1.

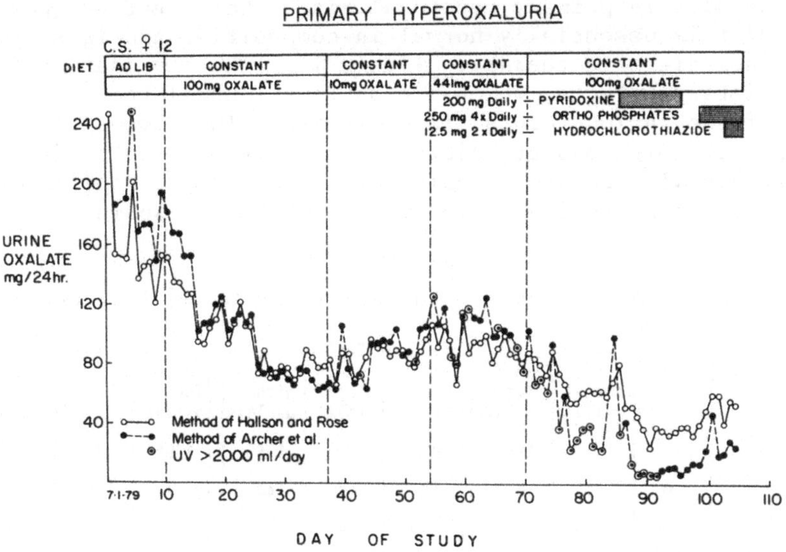

Figure 2. Urinary oxalate excretion in Case 2.

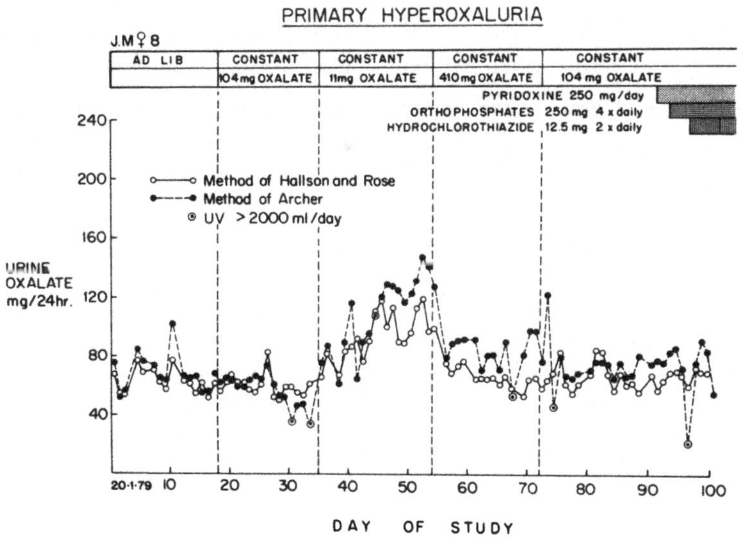

Figure 3. Urinary oxalate excretion in Case 3.

These studies constitute the first demonstration that a therapeutically useful reduction in urine oxalate excretion can be achieved by diet in primary hyperoxaluria. The effective (normal oxalate) diet is essentially normal in composition and is suitable for long term dietetic therapy. (Table 1). The explanation for the observed dietary effects, which are obviously unrelated to the oxalate contents of the various diets, is uncertain. The composition of the normal, low and high oxalate diets did not differ consistently in the three patients with regard to caloric content or the content of protein, fat, carbohydrate, calcium, phosphorus or sodium.

Table 1. Composition of Constant Diets in Cases 1, 2 and 3

	CASE 1			CASE 2			CASE 3		
	low oxalate	normal oxalate	high oxalate	low oxalate	normal oxalate	high oxalate	low oxalate	normal oxalate	high oxalate
Calories	1617	1778	1855	2089	1795	2165	1882	1736	1654
Oxalate mg	15	99	530	10	100	441	11	104	410
Protein gm	78	83	82	86	67	78	65	62	85
Fat gm	79	79	79	107	77	78	83	60	53
Carbohydrate gm	148	195	206	196	214	257	210	221	217
Calcium mg	1288	1314	1405	1421	870	1434	1219	1053	1159
Magnesium mg	182	255	347	211	228	354	200	305	299
Phosphorous mg	1424	1515	1632	1645	1211	1723	1216	1257	1464
Sodium mg	2110	2801	2441	2378	1660	2354	1718	1426	1180
Potassium mg	2232	2985	3288	2027	2664	3398	2145	2735	3433
Ascorbic acid mg	74	149	132						

REFERENCES

1. H. E. Williams and L. H. Smith, Jr., in:"The Metabolic Basis of Inherited Disease," Fourth edition, J. B. Stanbury, J. B. Wyngaarden, and D. S. Fredrickson, eds., McGraw-Hill Book Company, New York (1978).
2. D. A. Gibbs and R. W. E. Watts, Arch. Dis. Child. 42:505 (1967).
3. E. J. Will and O. L. M. Bijvoet, Metabolism 28:542 (1979).
4. L. H. Smith, Jr., and H. E. Williams, Mod. Treat. 4:522 (1967).
5. R. A. Daniels, R. Michels, and P. Aisen, Arch. Dis. Child. 40: 485 (1965).
6. A. W. McLaurin, W. R. Beisel, and G. J. McCormick, Ann. Int. Med. 55:70 (1961).
7. C. E. Dent and T. C. B. Stamp, Arch. Dis. Child. 45:735 (1970).

8. L. H. Smith, in:"Fogarty International Center Proceedings 37," R. Van Reen, ed., DHEW Publication No. (NIH) 77-1063, Washington, D.C. (1977).
9. T. H. Shepard, E. G. Krebs, and L. W. Lee, Pediatrics 25:1008 (1960).
10. H. E. Archer, A. E. Dormer, and E. F. Scowen, Br. Med. J. 1:175 (1958).
11. D. Swartz and S. Israels, J. Urol. 90:94 (1963).
12. C. E. Dent and T. C. B. Stamp, Arch. Dis. Child. 45:735 (1970).
13. H. E. Archer, A. E. Dormer, and E. F. Scowen, Clin. Sci. 16:405 (1957).
14. P. C. Hallson and G. A. Rose, Clin. Chem. Acta. 55:29 (1974).

ACKNOWLEDGMENT

This work was supported by a grant from the Medical Research Council of Canada. (M.T. 681).

III. CRYSTAL FORMATION AND PHYSICAL CHEMISTRY

PREFACE TO PROPOSAL OF STANDARDIZED NOMENCLATURE IN THE STUDY OF CRYSTALLIZATION IN BIOLOGICAL SYSTEMS

Birdwell Finlayson

University of Florida, College of Medicine

Gainesville, Florida

At the 1979 ROCK (Research on Calculous Kinetics) Society meeting, Dallas, Texas, George Drach and Alan Randolph proposed the adoption of a lexicon of terminology concerning crystals and crystal formation. This proposal was committed to manuscript form and then reviewed and amended by an Ad Hoc Committee at the 1980 Williamsburg meeting. The committee members were Bill Gill, Niel and Gretchen Mandel, John Meyer, George Nancollas, Alan Randolph, Bill Robertson, Alan Rose, Gene Schrier, and myself. Several revisions of the manuscript have been subsequently made, circulated, and revised. While nothing is perfect, the following glossary goes a very long way in providing a standard nomenclature that can be used with some precision by urinary stone research workers. Also it will help to correct some conceptual problems that have appeared in the stone literature. It is very much to be desired that this terminology will be adopted and used in reporting urolithiasis research when appropriate. This glossary is not immutable. With usage, the need for emendation may become evident. The next international stone meeting will provide an opportune occasion to review the glossary and its usage and make appropriate changes. Drs. Drach and Randolph merit considerable credit for their persistence in working for a concensus from a cross section of urolithiasis research workers.

A PROPOSAL OF STANDARDIZED NOMENCLATURE IN THE STUDY OF CRYSTALLIZATION IN BIOLOGICAL SYSTEMS, e.g. UROLITHIASIS

Alan D. Randolph and George W. Drach

Section of Urology, Department of Surgery and the Department of Chemical Engineering, University of Arizona, Tucson, Arizona 85724

Scientific reports on chemical equilibria and dynamics of crystallization related to urolithiasis vary greatly in the terminology that they apply to similar processes. As an example, one may see reports of crystal growth rate or crystallization rate in which both rates are derived similarly from the disappearance of some critical ion (e.g. oxalate) from solution over a given period of time[1]. Do these rates refer to the change in dimensions of a single crystal, to the change in mass of the single crystal, or to the total mass transfer rate (from solute to solids) onto crystals in the mother liquor? In many instances the latter is meant and is reported as "crystal growth" or "crystal growth rate". Is there a definition of this concept already in existence? Yes, and it exists in conjunction wich chemical and chemical engineering disciplines. It is the separation intensity factor R, or more widely in industrial parlance, the rate of make, expressed as $mM \cdot min^{-1}$ [2]. The rate of make is in no way a fundamental crystallization parameter but in fact varies with nucleation rate, growth rate, total available supersaturation, crystal size, and the total crystal surface area available for growth. For non-flow batch systems, R is equal to the rate of change of solids concentration, dM_T/dt, and is the variable measured when solids rather than liquor concentrations are observed. Do other fairly standard terms exist that can be applied to studies of crystallization in urine? Yes. Table 1 lists these and we would propose their adoption by other workers in the realm of urolithiasis or any other study of crystallization in biological systems[3].

Certain terms without mathematical definition also arise in discussions of biological crystallization. Some definitions for these are proposed in Table 2. Finally, Table 3 presents an approach to defining inhibition or inversely enhancement of crystallization according to which segment of the crystallization process is being affected.

Table 1. Definition of Terms, Biological Crystallization

Crystal nucleation rate: (birth of new particles), B^o [=] number · ml^{-1} · min^{-1}.

Crystal growth rate (linear): $G[=]$ μm · $min^{-1} = \frac{dL}{dt}$, expressed in terms of crystal size L taken as diameter of equivalent spherical particle.

Formation ion product: (formation product) K_f is the ion product (IP) at the point of spontaneous nucleation with specification of the temperature, pH, time of onset of nucleation, method of detection of nucleation, surface of reaction container, and any other unusual circumstance such as cavitation from stirring and strong magnetic or electric fields and method of supersaturation generation. See definition of ion product.

Growth rate (mass): R [=] mg · min^{-1} · 1^{-1} or mM · min^{-1}, rate of solute depletion in a batch crystallizer. This term is called rate of make in industrial parlance and is a measure of crystallizer productivity.

Ion product: $IP = \alpha_a^{\nu_a} \alpha_b^{\nu_b} \cdots \alpha_n^{\nu_n}$

in which α_i is a concentration expression for the ith ion in the precipitation reaction, e.g. mole fraction, activity, molarity, etc., and ν_i is the number of the ith ions entering into the reaction. If activities are used to express the α_i, IP is an ion activity product (IPa). If molar concentrations are used to express the α_i, IP is an ion molar concentrations product (IP_m). If mole fractions are used to express the α_i, IP is an ion mole fraction product (IP_x), etc. For example, the ion activity product for calcium hydroxy apatite is: IPa (calcium hydroxy apatite) = $(Ca^{2+})^5$ $(PO_4^{3-})^3$ (OH^{1-}) where parentheses indicate molar activity. The ion molar product is IP_m (calcium hydroxy apatite) = $[Ca^{2+}]^5$ $[PO_4^{3-}]^3$ $[OH^{1-}]$ where brackets indicate molar concentrations.

Linear size: L [=] μm, crystal size taken as equivalent spherical diameter.

Mass-weighted mean size: $\bar{L}_{4,3}$[=] μm, crystal size weighted by the fraction of mass occurring at that size[4].

Metastable concentration: Solutions having ion products between Kso and K_f.

Table 1 continued.

Moment (k'th) of population distribution: $m_k = \int_0^\infty nL^k\,dL$ [=] $\mu m^k \cdot ml^{-1}$.

Population density function: n(L) [=] number $\cdot$ ml^{-1} m^{-1}, number of crystals per unit volume per unit size in a crystal suspension[4].

Population - weighted mean size: $\bar{L}_{1,0}$ [=] μm, crystal size weighted by the fractional number of crystals at that size.

Production rate: P [=] g $\cdot$ min^{-1} or mmol $\cdot$ min^{-1}, rate of production of crystalline solute phase, P = V $\cdot$ R where V is suspension volume, ml, and R is mass growth rate (rate of make).

Rate of make or separation intensity factor: R [=] mM $\cdot$ min^{-1} or mg $\cdot$ ml^{-1} $\cdot$ min^{-1}, total inter-facial liquid solid mass transfer rate, equal to mass growth rate as defined above.

Solubility: C_{sol} [=] mg $\cdot$ l^{-1} or mM, total concentration (sum of dissociated, undissociated and complexed) of a species in equilibrium with its solid phase.

Solubility ion product: (solubility product) Kso is the ion product at saturation at a specified temperature. If activities are not used, then the system must be completely specified.

Supersaturation (stoichiometric): s [=] mg $\cdot$ l^{-1} or mM, operationally defined as solute in solution that would precipitate if the solution were held until equilibrium. Equal to total concentration C minus C_{sol}, based on limiting ion. Must be predicted from equilibrium calculations for complex multi-ion systems. Expressed in terms of the phase actually precipitating, e.g., monohydrate or dihydrate form for CaOx. Supersaturation is a dependent variable and cannot be fixed a priori without concentration measurements and feedback control.

Supersaturation (stoichiometric, initial): s_i [=] mg $\cdot$ l^{-1} or mM. As defined above but referring to the initial or feed supersaturation in batch or continuous processes, respectively.

Supersaturation ratio: $S = G + 1 = \frac{IP}{Kso}$ [=] dimensionless. Ratio of actual activity ion product in solution to the thermodynamic equilibrium solubility ion product. Must be predicted from equilibrium calculations for complex multi-ion systems.

Supersaturation relief or yield: $Y = 1 - s/s_i$ where s_i is initial stoichiometric supersaturation. $Y = M_T/s_i$ for MSMPR crystallizer.

Table 1 continued.

Total solids mass concentration: M_T [=] mg · l^{-1}.

Volume shape factor: k_V = volume · size $^{-3}$, equal to $\pi/6$ for spheres. Dimensionless.

Notes to Table 1:

a) The supersaturation driving force s represents the unprecipitated concentration of solute. Mass transfer rates are often proportional to s.

b) The supersaturation ratio, $S = \sigma + 1$, is directly related to free energy changes. This measure of supersaturation is used in expressions describing primary nucleation.

c) The current supersaturation s is a dependent variable and must be determined by analysis of total concentration and solubility concentration or predicted from solution equilibria (from s_i) adjusted by the amount of solute precipitation for both batch and continuous systems.

d) Mass transfer flux to the crystal surface, in mg · $\min^{-1}$. area $^{-1}$, is proportional to the linear growth rate G.

e) The average sizes listed above are forms of the generalized average size $\bar{L}_{i,j} = (m_i/m_j)^{1/(i-j)}$, where m_k is the k'th moment about zero of the population distribution $n^{\circ}(L)$.

f) B^o and G are phenomenological rates and must be expressed as rate laws to obtain growth and nucleation rate constrants. Such kinetic rate laws have been expressed in a variety of forms. We suggest correlations as G(s) and $B^o(S)$.

g) Units notation [=] a·b to read as "the indicated variable has the units of a times b".

Table 2. Additional Definitions in Crystallization Studies

Agglomerate:	Group of two or more particles held together by weak cohesive forces, e.g. electrostatic. Can be broken up by dispersion with shear or solvents.
Aggregate:	Group of two or more particles held together by strong intermolecular forces, e.g. atomic bonds. Cannot be dispersed with shear forces.
Crystal Habit:	Shape of crystals, usually as relative length along axes and/or Relative development of crystal faces with respect to common crystallographic axes.
Crystal Morphology:	External forms of crystals, often used in approximate identification of crystal species[5].
Crystal Magma:	Suspension of crystals in mother liquor.

Table 3. Inhibition of Crystallization: What is Being Inhibited?

Agglomeration or aggregation: at same M_T and S the number of single crystal particles decreases due to increasing crystal-crystal attachment.

Growth inhibition: G declines at constant s.

Nucleation inhibition: B^o declines at constant S, magma properties and external stimuli.

Peptization: at same M_T, number of agglomerated particles in solution decreases by redispersion into smaller particles, thus total particle count ml^{-1} increases.

Notes:

a) Inhibition of growth and nucleation is defined above to exclude the effects of chemical additives which merely change the supersaturation through solution complexing. Inhibitors act to change the precipitation kinetics at the crystal-liquid interface, typically by adsorption on the crystal surface.

b) Agglomeration or aggregation usually appear in MSMPR crystallizer studies as deviate population densities which do not obey the exponential form.

The use of continuous flow, continuously supersaturated systems [3,4] in the study of biological crystallization requires precise definition of what is meant by supersaturation driving forces in the system. (See Figure 1). The constants Kso and K_f of course do not change, but determination of supersaturation driving forces is based on concentrations (activities) in the vessel discharge, rather than feed. The true crystallization driving force in batch systems varies continuously from feed to end-of-run concentrations. Once this difference in operation is appreciated, continuous flow systems gain their advantage in their ability to quantitate nucleation, an aspect of biological crystallization that previously has been difficult to measure. Growth and nucleation rates can also be measured under constant supersaturation driving forces. Finally, the process notations in Figure 2 illustrate the above definitions in reference to the continuous -flow Mixed Suspension Mixed Product Removal (MSMPR) crystallizer.

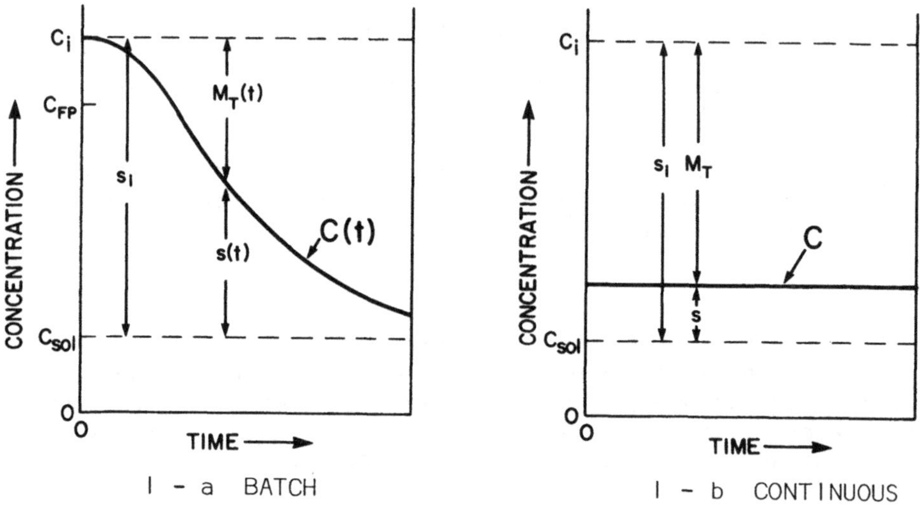

Figure 1. Crystallizer concentration profiles.

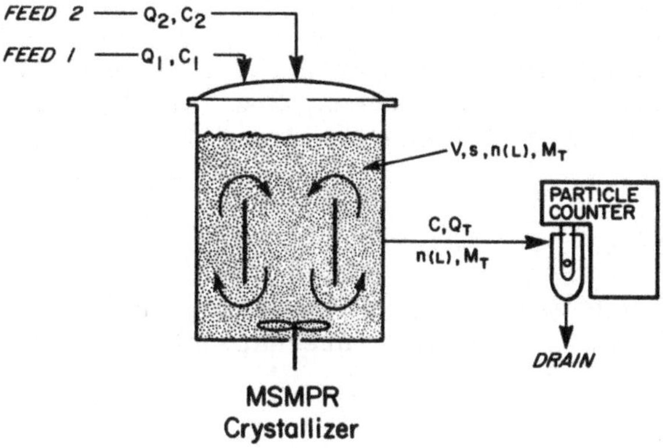

PROPERTIES:

$C_i = [Q_1/Q_T]C_1 + [Q_2/Q_T]C_2$ expressed as mg/ml of precipitating solute

$\tau = V/Q_T$ mean retention time, min.

$n(L) = [B^0/G] \exp\{-L/G\tau\}$ no./ml-μm

$M_T = 6\rho k_v B^0 G^3 \tau^4 = C_i - C = s_i - s$ mg/ml

$P = Q_T \cdot M_T$ mg/min

$$Y = \frac{M_T}{s_i} = \frac{C_i - C}{C_i - C_{sol}}$$

C = concentration in mother liquor. Must be measured. mg/ml or m mol / ml

$\bar{L}_{1,0} = G\tau$ μm

$\bar{L}_{4,3} = 4G\tau$ μm

$R = M_T/\tau$ mg/ml - min or m mol / ml - min

Figure 2. Schematic flow diagram and associated distribution properties for MSMPR crystallizer.

REFERENCES

1. "Urolithiasis Research," H. Fleisch, W. G. Robertson, L. H. Smith, and W. Vahlensieck, eds., Plenum Press, New York (1976).
2. J. W. Mullin, in:"Crystallization," 1st Ed., Butterworth, London (1961).
3. G. W. Drach, A. D. Randolph, and J. D. Miller, J. Urol. 119:99 (1978).
4. A. D. Randolph and M. A. Larson, in:"Theory of Particulate Processes," Academic Press, New York (1971).
5. M. J. Buerger, in:"Elementary Crystallography," Wiley, New York (1963).

ACKNOWLEDGMENT

Doctor Drach was supported by Senior International Fellowship F06-TW00394-01 of the Fogarty International Center, National Institutes of Health.

A CONSTANT COMPOSITION METHOD FOR MODELLING URINARY STONE FORMATION

Mary E. Sheehan and George H. Nancollas

Chemistry Department, State University of New York
at Buffalo
Buffalo, New York

INTRODUCTION

Much attention has been paid recently to the development of an in vitro system for modelling the formation of renal stones. Although one of the major components of the renal stones is calcium oxalate, this may consist of the mono- (COM), di (COD), or tri- (COT) hydrate and the urine may be supersaturated with respect to any or all of these phases. Thus the less stable COD and COT may act as precursors to the formation of COM, precipitating and dissolving transiently. It is generally accepted that urine contains inhibitors to crystallization of calcium oxalates which may be absent in stone formers and studies have focused on the nature and mechanism of the mineralization inhibition of urine.

Finlayson proposed the use of a continuous crystallizer to stimulate the conditions of precipitation and growth of crystallites in the urinary tract[1]. Miller et al.[2] later used this technique together with the measurement of particle size distribution for studying the kinetics of crystallization of calcium oxalate in simulated urine. A supersaturated solution was fed into the reaction cell and the resulting crystal suspension was continuously discharged. The rates of nucleation and growth were determined as a function of size distribution of the particles. In this work, concentrations considerably larger than those found <u>in vivo</u> were required to obtain a measurable quantity of particles and it was therefore difficult to detect small changes in the kinetics of precipitation.

The seeded growth technique developed by Nancollas and Gardner[3] for calcium oxalate and later used by Meyer and Smith[4,5] to study the inhibitory action of urine can be used at a much lower supersaturation. Following the addition of well-characterized COM seed to stable supersaturated solution, the rate of growth was followed by measuring the depletion of calcium ions from solution[4,5], or by monitoring the conductivity[3]. In these studies, the rate of growth was found to follow kinetic equation[1] in which m is the concentration

$$-\frac{dm}{dt} = ks\ (m-m_o)^2 \qquad (1)$$

of calcium oxalate in solution at time t, m_o the corresponding solubility value at equilibrium, k the growth rate constant, and s the surface area of seed crystals available for growth. Since the concentration of calcium oxalate decreased appreciably as the growth reaction proceeded, the driving force for the formation of the different hydrate phases changed markedly during the reaction. Moreover, as the rate of crystallization became smaller near equilibrium, analytical errors made it impossible to obtain reliable estimates of the rate of crystallization.

In the work presented in this paper, a new highly reproducible method is described in which the chemical potentials of calcium and oxalate ions are maintained constant by the simultaneous addition of solutions of calcium chloride and potassium oxalate following the addition of well characterized seed crystals to stable supersaturated solutions of calcium oxalate. The rate of addition is controlled by a specific ion calcium electrode. In conventional seeded growth experiments this electrode does not respond sufficiently rapidly to faithfully reflect changes in calcium concentration. However, in the constant composition approach, the calcium electrode may be used because it has only to maintain the concentration at a constant value. It is interesting to note that a number of different specific ion electrodes can also be employed for such kinetic studies involving other mineralizing systems. This model simulates the relatively constant supersaturation encountered in urine and the kinetics of crystallization at very low degrees of supersaturation can be measured. Moreover, in contrast to the conventional seeded crystal growth model, the molar Ca/Ox ratio can be maintained during the crystallization reaction. Since the calcium activity of the supersaturated solution is monitored, corrections can be made for the calcium ion contained in the urine samples and activity corrections can be made for the formation of coordination complexes with the calcium ion. Moreover, the solution can be selectively supersaturated with respect to any of the hydrate phases. The kinetics of epitaxial growth of one phase or another can also be studied using different renal stone components as seed material.

EXPERIMENTAL

All solutions, prepared using reagent grade chemicals and triply distilled deionized water, were filtered through 0.22 μm Millipore filters. Experiments were performed in a water thermostated double walled cell at 37 ± 0.1°C. The cell was continuously stirred with a magnetic stirrer at about 400 rev/min. Nitrogen gas was passed over the solutions to exclude carbon dioxide. The ionic strength was maintained at 0.15M by the addition of sodium chloride and the calcium ion activity was monitored by means of a specific ion calcium electrode (calcium selectrode Model 72112 Ca, Radiometer Instrument Co.) coupled with a silver-silver chloride single-junction reference electrode (Model 90-01, Orion Research Inc.).

Table 1. Experimental Conditions

	COM	COT
Solution:		
$T_{ca} = T_{ox} (\times 10^4 M)$	4.60	5.90
I	0.15	0.15
$(a_{ca}a_{ox})^{1/2} \times 10^4 M$	1.22	1.56
Titrant $\times 10^3 M$	5.53	11.12
Seed:		
$10^2\ gl^{-1}$	2.48	9.96
specific surface area (m^2g^{-1})	2.94	0.60
avg. particle size (μm)	5	19

A metastable supersaturated calcium oxalate solution was prepared by adding to a premeasured sodium chloride solution known volumes of calcium chloride solution (I = 0.15M). By recording the emf readings for each addition, the calcium electrode was standardized in situ. When the calcium concentration reached the desired value, potassium oxalate solution (I = 0.15M) was added slowly to avoid regions of local high supersaturation. The experimental conditions for both COM and COT growth are listed in Table 1. The solution was allowed to equilibrate for 30 min. before inducing crystallization by the addition of a known quantity of well-characterized seed material. The activity of the solution was kept constant by the potentiostatic controlled addition of solutions containing calcium and oxalate ions using a modified Metrohm Herisau pH-stat (Model Combitrator 3D Brinkmann Instrument Co.) which enabled multiple mechanically-coupled syringes to be driven simultaneously[6]. Samples taken at various times during the reaction and filtered through 0.22 μm Millipore filters were analyzed (Perkin Elmer model 503) in order to verify constancy. The solid phases were characterized using x-ray powder diffraction (Cu Kα radiation, Phillips XRG 3000 Diffractrometer), scanning electron microscopy (ISI Model SMS 2-2, Super II), specific surface area analysis (N_2, BET adsorption, Quantasorb Instrument, Quantachrome Corp.), and particle size determination (Electrozone/Celloscope, Particle Data Inc.). When studying the influence of crystal growth modifiers the additive was introduced prior to the addition of the oxalate solution so that possible complex formation with the calcium ion could be allowed for by making all experiments at the same calcium ion activity. This was especially useful in the experiments with urine.

RESULTS AND DISCUSSION

A typical plot of the moles of titrant added as a function of time for the crystallization of COM is shown in Figure 1. The calcium concentration was constant during the experiments to within ± 1%. The excellent linearity of plots of the rate of crystallization against $(m-m_o)^2$ shown in Figure 2 illustrate the applicability of kinetic equation 1 as was shown for conventional seeded growth experiments with calcium oxalate. Not only was this rate equation followed over a wide range of supersaturation but also for different Ca/Ox molar ratios where m was $(a_{Ca}a_{Ox})^{1/2}$. For the calculation of initial supersaturations in the experiments, it is important to take into account the formation of ion-pairs and complexes and to make corrections for ionic strength effects[6].

Table 2. Calcium Oxalate Monohydrate Crystallization in the Presence of Polyacrylate

Polyacrylate ppm	pH	rate x 10^5 mole min^{-1} lm^{-2}
0	6.0	2.55
.055	6.0	1.98
.055	9.0	1.99
.082	9.0	.93
.164	9.0	.01

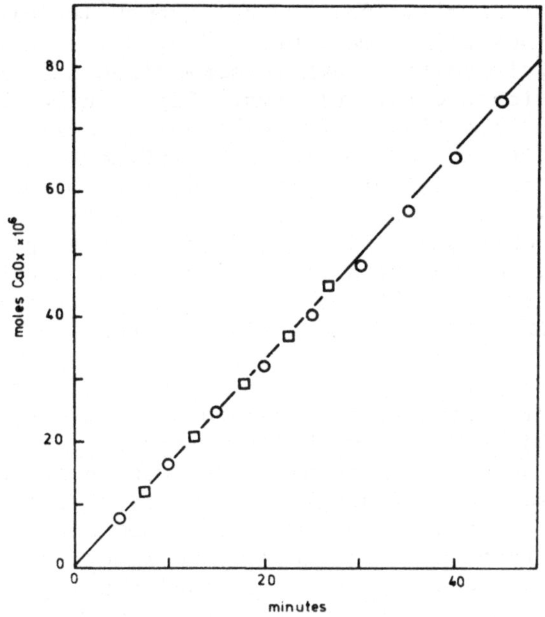

Figure 1. Crystallization of COM. Plot of moles of CaOx crystallized as a function of time. O, Expt. 92; □, Expt. 91.

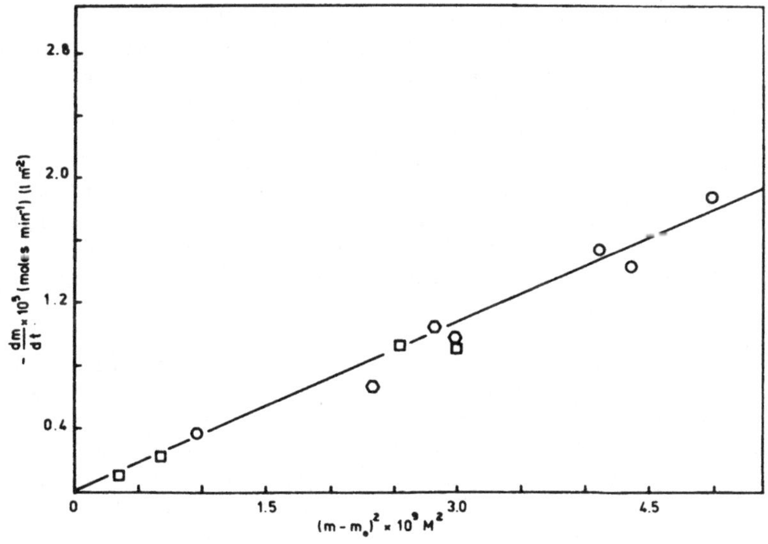

Figure 2. Plot of rate of crystal growth of COM against $(m-m_o)^2$. O, Ca/Ox = 1; □, Ca/Ox ≒ 5, ⬡, Ca/Ox = 3.

The influence of a typical crystal growth inhibitor, polyacrylic acid (Calnox 214DN, mol. wt. ∿ 750, Calgon Corp.) upon the kinetics of crystal growth of COM is summarized in Table 2. The precision with which the rate of crystallization can be obtained by the constant composition technique enables small changes in rate to be observed. It can be seen that the influence of polyacrylate upon the rate of crystallization is independent of pH within the range 6-9. The increase in rate of crystallization during the later stages of the experiments, illustrated in the rate plots of Figure 3 may be attributed to depletion of polyacrylate through adsorption on the growing crystals. It has been shown that the inhibiting effects of polyacrylate can be described in terms of adsorption of additive molecules at the active growth sites on the crystal surface following a Langmuir isotherm[6,7]. In the presence of diluted freshly voided normal whole urine it can be seen in Figure 4 that the rate of crystallization of COM is markedly retarded. An adsorption isotherm following the simple Langmuir model can again be used to represent the results[5]. Although precipitation studies in whole urine indicate the formation of COD[2], only COM was observed to form in these crystallization experiments. The kinetics of crystal growth of COD or COT can, however, be studied using COD or COT as seed material[8]. A typical rate plot for the growth of COT seed crystals shown in Figure 5 indicates the marked increase in rate of reaction in the later stages. Examination of the solid phase formed by x-ray diffraction, indicated the presence of COM and the formation of this phase was also observed in typical scanning electron micrographs (Figure 6). During the crystallization of COT, the greater thermodynamic driving force for the formation of the least soluble COM results in the nucleation of this phase. The results of particle size distribution studies also support this conclusion. A peak at 13-25 μm reflecting the growth of COT seed crystals is joined by another with a much smaller size range, 4-7 μm, at the stage at which COM is detected by x-ray diffraction. The formation of more than one calcium oxalate hydrate phase illustrated by these experiments may have important implications in the formation of calcium oxalates in the urinary tract. The influence of diluted urine on the growth of COT is illustrated in Figure 5 and, as for COM, it can be seen that urine dramatically reduces the rate of COT crystallization.

In vivo it is not uncommon to find stones containing both calcium oxalate and calcium phosphate phases. These mixed solids may form by the epitaxial growth of one phase upon another and the constant composition technique has been used to study these phenomena. It has been shown that hydroxyapatite (HAP) seed prepared as described previously[9], was able to induce the nucleation and subsequent growth of COM[10]. The induction period in these experiments, reflecting the nucleation of COM on the HAP surface, decreased as the supersaturation increased. In terms of the lattice

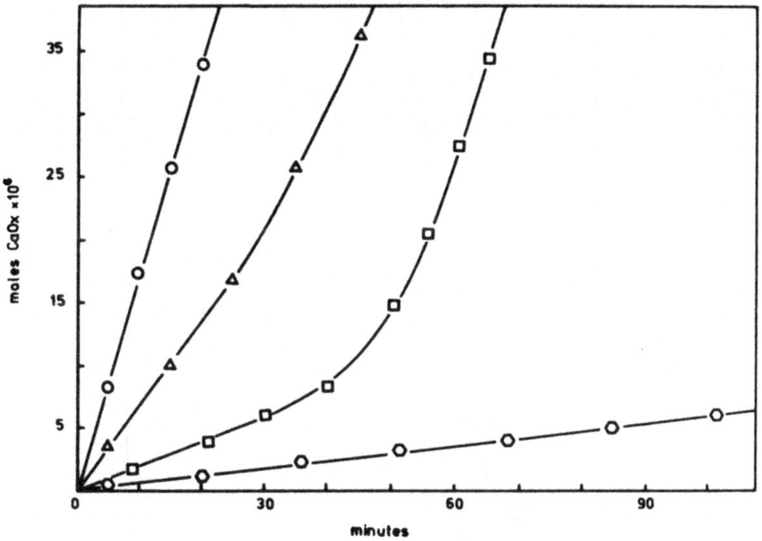

Figure 3. Crystallization of COM in the presence of polyacrylate, A. O, [A] = 0; Δ, [A] = 0.082 ppm, □, [A] = 0.109 ppm; ⬡, [A] = 0.164 ppm.

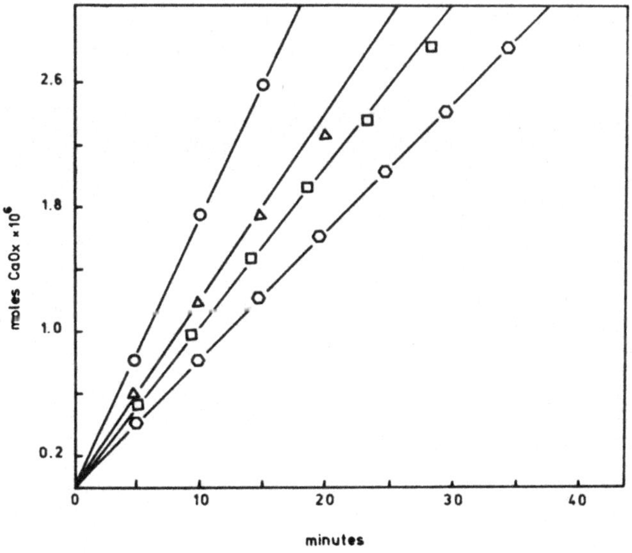

Figure 4. Crystallization of COM in the presence of normal urine. The dilution ratio, DR is the ratio of urine volume to total volume of solution. O, DR = 0; Δ, DR = 5.6×10^{-3}; □, DR = 11.1×10^{-3}; ⬡, DR = 32.4×10^{-3}.

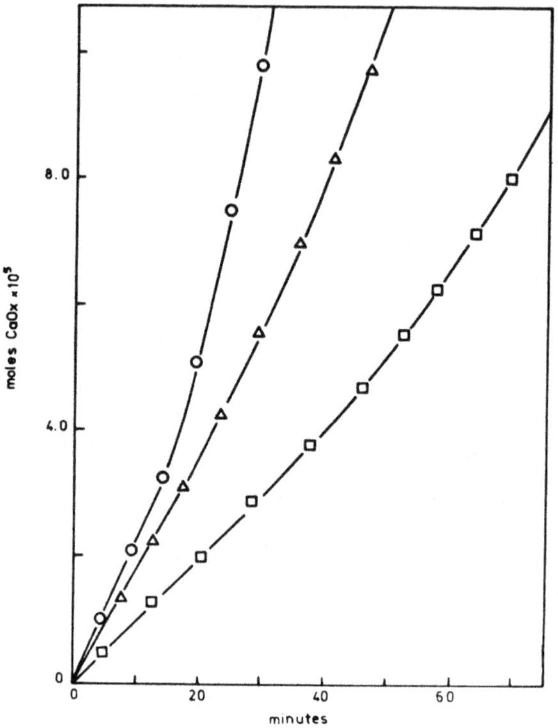

Figure 5. Crystallization of COT in the presence of normal urine. O, DR = 0, Δ, DR = 2.7×10^{-2}; □, DR = 5.4×10^{-2}.

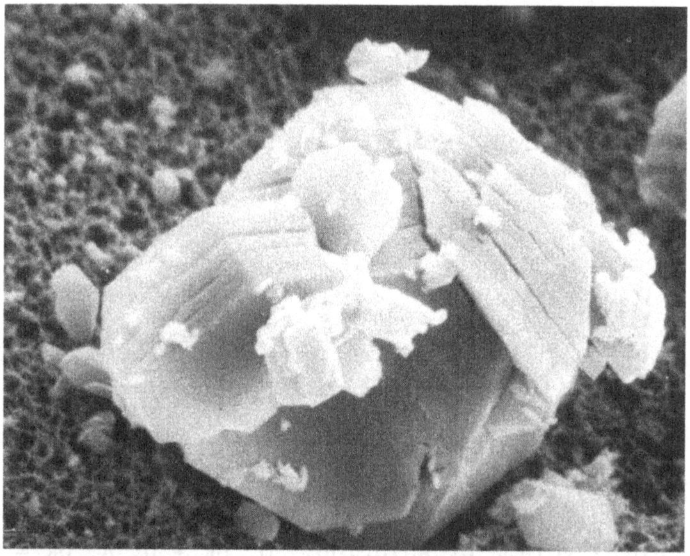

Figure 6. Scanning electron micrographs of the formation of COM in the presence of COT.

matching between HAP and the calcium oxalate hydrates, this variation of induction period may be used to calculate the surface energy of the depositing phases[10]. It is interesting to note that in the reverse process, the growth of HAP takes place only on COT surfaces and not on COD and COM. The lattice matching requirements for epitaxial growth of stone forming minerals may be an important factor in their development in vivo. In addition, urinary macromolecules, which serve as natural inhibitors, may have markedly different effects on the growth of the various mineral phases.

The constant composition method outlined in this paper provides a simple and convenient means for measuring the rate of calcium oxalate crystal growth. The specific ion calcium electrode may be used not only to maintain constant calcium ion activity but also to monitor the extent of calcium ion complexing in the presence of added crystal growth modifiers. Since the activities of solution species are maintained constant during the mineralization experiments, the technique is particularly applicable for the study of solution compositions similar to those in urine.

REFERENCES

1. B. Finlayson, Invest. Urol. 9:258 (1972).
2. J. D. Miller, A. D. Randolph, and G. W. Drach, J. Urol. 117:342 (1977).
3. G. H. Nancollas, and G. L. Gardner, J. Crystal Growth 21:267 (1974).
4. J. L. Meyer, and L. H. Smith, Invest. Urol. 13:31 (1975).
5. J. L. Meyer, and L. H. Smith, Invest. Urol. 13:36 (1975).
6. M. E. Sheehan, and G. H. Nancollas, Invest. Urol. 17:446 (1980).
7. C. W. Davies, and G. H. Nancollas, Trans. Faraday Soc. Land. 51:823 (1955).
8. B. B. Tomazic, and G. H. Nancollas, Invest. Urol. 16:329 (1979).
9. L. C. Bell, A. M. Posner, and J. P. Quirk, J. Coll. Int. Sci. 42:250 (1973).
10. P. G. Koutsoukos, M. E. Sheehan, and G. H. Nancollas, Invest. Urol. (in press).

ACKNOWLEDGMENT

We thank the National Institute of Arthritic, Metabolic and Digestive Diseases for a grant in support of this work (2 ROI AM 19048).

CRYSTAL GROWTH AND AGGREGATION OF CALCIUM OXALATE IN HIGH IONIC STRENGTH SOLUTIONS

H. Füredi-Milhofer, D. Skrtić, M. Marković, and Lj. Komunjer
Laboratory for Precipitation Processes
"Rudjer Bosković" Institute
Zagreb, Yugoslavia

INTRODUCTION

According to the hyperexcretion-supersaturation theory[1], the concentrations of ions in urines of calcium oxalate stone formers persistently exceed the formation product of this salt, and, as a consequence, calcium oxalate crystals are produced by spontaneous nucleation, growth and aggregation. Some of the crystals, or aggregates, are eventually trapped in the kidney and become the nidus for a stone. It has been proposed[2,3] that urines of normal individuals contain inhibitors of crystal growth and aggregation which are decreased or absent in stone formers. Accordingly, much effort has been spent to test potential inhibitors, but most models permit only the measurement of an overall effect, without separating the two precipitation processes. In this study a model system is presented by which the kinetics of crystal growth and aggregation can be followed subsequently and independently in systems in which both processes proceed simultaneously. Quantitative estimates of the rates of crystal growth and aggregation of calcium oxalate from high ionic strength solutions, such as prevail in crystalluria, are given. The proposed model makes it possible to study the effect of inhibitors on both processes simultaneously and independently in the course of spontaneous precipitation.

EXPERIMENTAL METHODS

Reagent grade chemicals and tridistilled water were used. Samples were prepared by mixing equal volumes of equimolar solutions of sodium oxalate (pH 6.5 ± 0.05) and calcium chloride, both 0.3 molar in sodium chloride. All experiments were carried out at constant temperature (25° ± 0.1°C). Solutions used for the preparation and dilution of samples for particle size analysis were additionally purified by filtering twice through 0.22 μm Millipore filters.

The concentration of calcium ions in solution was measured by calcium specific electrode in combination with a calomel electrode. In these experiments mixing of the reactants was achieved by adding a known amount of oxalate solution to an equal amount of the calcium chloride solution within which the selectrode was equilibrated. During the kinetic experiments samples were constantly stirred by a magnetic stirrer. In some experiments crystals were periodically sampled onto glass slides and observed by bright field and polarized light optical microscopy.

Particle number and size analysis was performed in parallel kinetic experiments by a Coulter Counter Mo TA, using 50 μm and 140 μm orifice tubes calibrated with standard monodispersed polyvinyl toluene latexes. For these experiments samples were prepared by direct mixing and stirred mechanically during each run. Counting and sizing was performed at given time intervals by withdrawing the required amount of suspension (0.2 cm^{-3}) directly from the samples. No previous dilution was necessary.

The precipitates formed were characterized by x-ray spectroscopy and thermogravimetric analysis. For this purpose samples were prepared and aged for different time periods (7 min - 60 min) under conditions closely corresponding to those under which growth kinetics were followed by the selectrode. Precipitates were then filtered through 0.22 μm Millipore filters and without previous drying immediately analyzed by either or the above techniques. This way it was possible to avoid structural changes (dehydration) during sample preparation.

TREATMENT OF DATA

For quantitative analysis of the experimental data it was convenient to use the degree of the reaction, α, defined as

$$\alpha = (c_o - c_t) / (c_o - c_s) = V_t / V_{max} \qquad (1)$$

where c_o is the initial total calcium concentration, c_t and c_s are the respective concentrations at time t and at equilibrium, V_t is the total volume of the precipitate at time t and V_{max} is the largest obtainable precipitate volume in each experiment. Since c_t is obtainable by selectrode and V_t by Coulter Counter, a direct comparison between the results obtained by both techniques is possible (eqn. (1)).

The calcium concentration, c_t, was obtained from the Ca^{2+} v.s. time curve (Figure 2, upper diagram) using eqns. (2) and (3), while c_s was calculated according to eqn. (4).

$$c_t = [Ca^{2+}] + [CaOx^o] \qquad (2)$$

$$[CaOx^o] = [Ca^{2+}]\ [Ox^{2-}] \ /\ K_{\mu=0.3} = [Ca^{2+}]^2 \ /\ K_{\mu=0.3} \qquad (3)$$

$$c_s = (Ks_{\mu=0.3})^{1/2} \qquad (4)$$

The association constant, $K_{\mu=0.3}$ and solubility product, $K_{s\mu=0.3}$ were calculated from the respective thermodynamic constants[4,5]. Activity coefficients for the divalent cation and anion were assumed equal and were obtained from the expanded form of the Debey-Hückel equation, proposed by Davies[6].

$$-\log f_z = A_z^2 \left(\frac{\mu^{1/2}}{1 + \mu^{1/2}} - 0.3\ \mu\right) \qquad (5)$$

The quantity V_t could not be directly obtained from Coulter Counter data because of the detection limit of the instrument, which lies at 0.5 µm in volume diameter. However, the function V_t (t) was readily obtained by extrapolation according to a method which was recently developed in our laboratory[7].

The quantity V_{max} was calculated from

$$V_{max} = Mw(c_o - c_s)/p \qquad (6)$$

where Mw is the molecular weight and p is the crystal density.

The kinetic data were interpreted by using Nielsen's approach to surface nucleation controlled growth[8] which shows that for a polynuclear mechanism the rate of crystal growth is defined by

$$d\ /dt = \frac{3k_p\ (c_o - c_s)^p\ \alpha^{2/3}}{r_1} (1-\alpha)^p \qquad (7)$$

In eqn. 7 k_p is a constant, p is the order of the rate controlling surface reaction and r_1 is the largest obtainable particle radius when all matter has been precipitated. At a given initial supersaturation

$$\frac{3\ k_p\ (c_o - c_s)^p}{r_1} = K \qquad (8)$$

and

$$\log (d\alpha/dt \cdot \alpha^{-2/3}) = \log K + p \log (1 - \alpha) \qquad (9)$$

According to eqn. (1)

$$1 - \alpha = (c_t - c_s) / (c_o - c_s) \qquad (10)$$

By introducing eqn. (10) into eqn. (7) and rearranging we obtain

$$d\alpha/dt \cdot \alpha^{-2/3} = K' (c_t - c_s)^p \qquad (11)$$

where $K' = \frac{3kp}{r_1}$, and should be approximately constant in a narrow concentration region.

The interpretation of our results involves eqns (9) and (11) as well as the integral form of eqn. (9)[8]

$$t = k_p \, I_p \, (\alpha) \qquad (12)$$

where I_p is a numerical integral which has been tabulated for values of α between 1×10^{-4} and 0.999.

RESULTS AND DISCUSSION

The solid phases formed in the described experiments had the composition and structure of calcium oxalate trihydrate, $CaC_2O_4 \cdot 3H_2O$. No transformation of this phase during the duration of a typical experiment could be detected. The morphology of the crystals is shown in Figure 1.

All crystals were birefringent and no significant time dependent changes in their morphology were observed.

The results of a typical growth experiment performed by selectrode are shown in Figure 2.

After an initial surge up to a maximum (A), the rate vs. supersaturation curve has a linear part (B) indicating (eqn. 9) that the dominant process is polynuclear crystal growth controlled by a surface process. Eleven experiments performed in the range of supersaturations $(c_o - c_s)/c_s$ between 1.50 and 5.40 and recalculated in terms of eqn. (11) gave the following results: p = 3.80   0.07 and K' = (1.5   1.3) x 10^{-8} dm^{12} $mole^4$ s^{-1}. Scattering of the values of the rate constant K' is due in part to some uncertainty in the detection of the onset of the third part of the rate vs. supersaturation curve (section C in Figure 2).

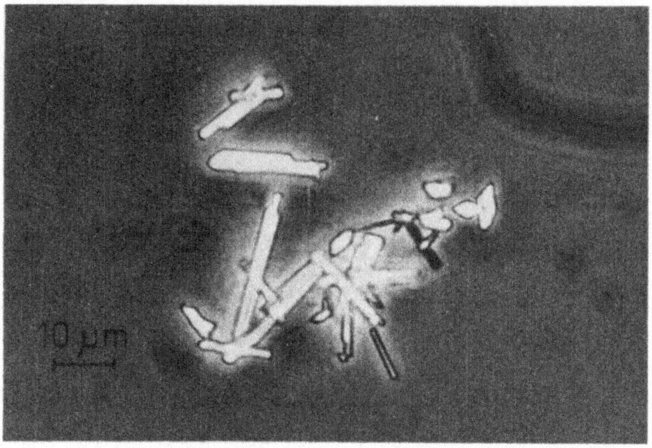

Figure 1. Optical micrograph of precipitate formed during kinetic experiment (calcium electrode). $[Ca] = [C_2O_4] = 1 \times 10^{-3}$ mole dm^{-3}, 0.3 mole dm^{-3} NaCl, 25^oC, sampling time 30 min.

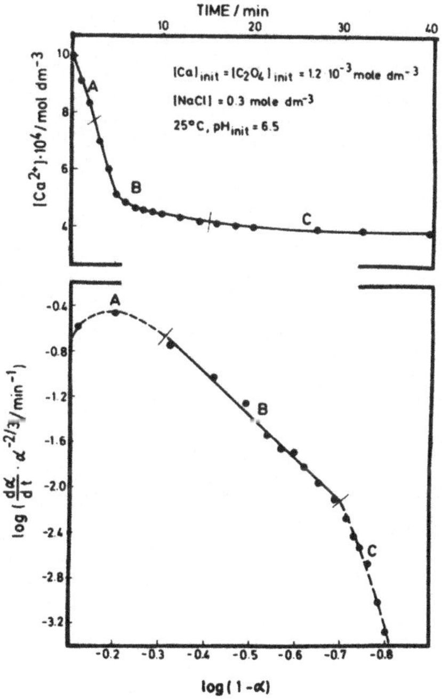

Figure 2. $[Ca^{2+}]$ (t) curve obtained by selectrode (upper diagram) and the corresponding rate vs. supersaturation curve (log scale, lower diagram) calculated after eqn. 11. Sections A,B, and C correspond in time.

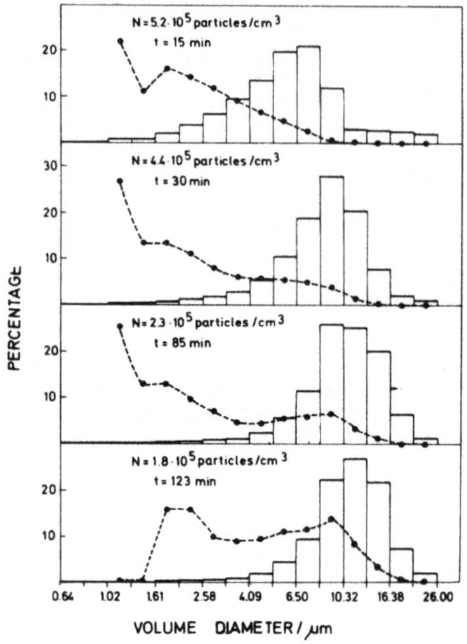

Figure 3. Volume distribution histograms and the corresponding number distribution curves obtained at different sampling times in a kinetic experiment, [Ca] = [C_2O_4] = 9.0 X 10^{-4} mode dm^{-3}, 0.3 mole dm^{-3} NaCl, 25°C.

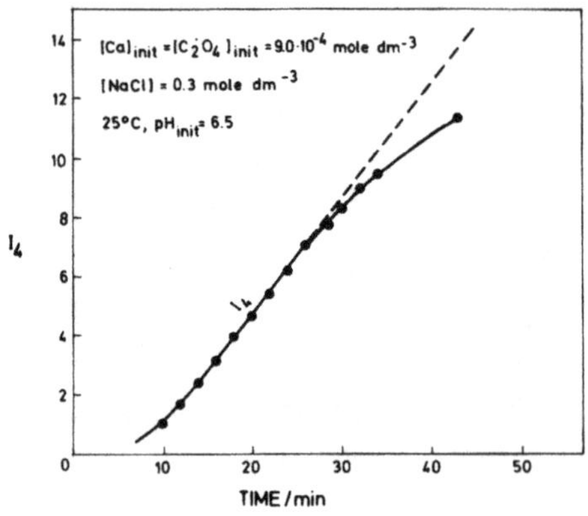

Figure 4. Kinetic experiment followed by selectrode. The chronomal I_4 is plotted as a function of time (eqn. 12).

In this last part of the curve, C, the rate of precipitation decreases faster than expected from eqn. (9). A correlation between the results obtained by selectrode and Coulter Counter shows that this relative decrease in rate corresponds to a decrease in the number of particles. Number distribution curves (Figure 3) are initially unimodal but become bimodal with time, a second maximum appearing at higher volume diameters. This seems to be a positive indication of aggregation of the growing crystallites. It was then assumed that at the time corresponding to section C in Figure 2, crystal growth and aggregation occurred simultaneously, the latter process causing a relative decrease of the rate of crystal growth by decreasing the available surface area.

A quantitative estimate of the magnitude of this influence was obtained by plotting the data in terms of the I_4 chronomal (eqn. 12) as shown in Figure 4. In this plot the relative decrease in the rate of crystal growth becomes apparent by a deviation from linearity at longer time periods (> 30 min). On the assumption that this deviation was caused solely by a decrease in the available surface area, and that the concentration dependence and order of the rate controlling process were unchanged, the I_4 (t) function was extrapolated to longer time periods and I_4 and α values corresponding to undisturbed crystal growth were determined. The experimental α values, corresponding to any given time being known, the effective change in surface area, ΔS, was then calculated from

$$\alpha = \frac{V}{V_{max}} = \left(\frac{S}{S_{max}}\right)^{3/2} \tag{13}$$

$$\Delta S = S_{ext} - S_t = S_{max} \left(\alpha_{ext}^{2/3} - \alpha_t^{2/3}\right) \tag{14}$$

An example, giving time dependent changes in surface area and the number of particles, is shown in Figure 5. The maximum detectable change in the surface area in this experiment amounted to approximately 2% of the total crystal surface, S_{max}.

In order to get a reasonable estimate of the maximum possible loss of surface due to shielding, two models showing possible modes of aggregation are given in Figure 6. The dimensions of the crystals were estimated from micrographs such as shown in Figure 1. If the total surface is $S = 16a^2$, the loss in surface for model a is $\Delta S = a^2$ or 6.25% while for model b it amounts to $\Delta S = 9a^2$ or 56.25%. Thus the above experimental result shows that the mode of aggregation in our systems resembled model a and that crystal growth and aggregation proceeded simultaneously until about 30% of the crystals were aggregated. After this time aggregation prevailed, while crystal growth became insignificant (Figure 5).

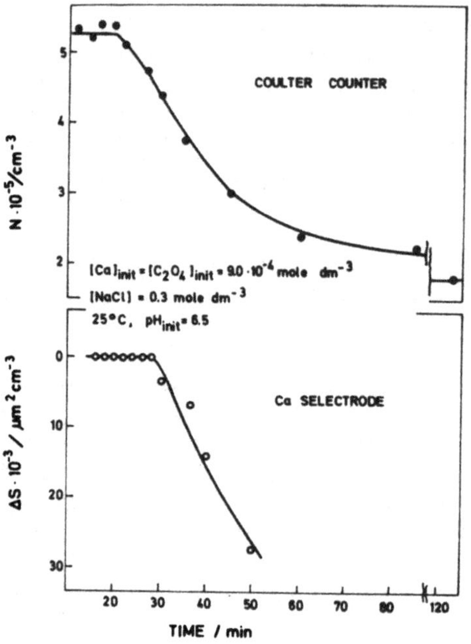

Figure 5. Correlation of two kinetic experiments followed by calcium selectrode (lower diagram) and Coulter Counter (upper diagram) respectively. Calculated changes in crystal surface, ΔS and measured total number of particles, N, as a function of time.

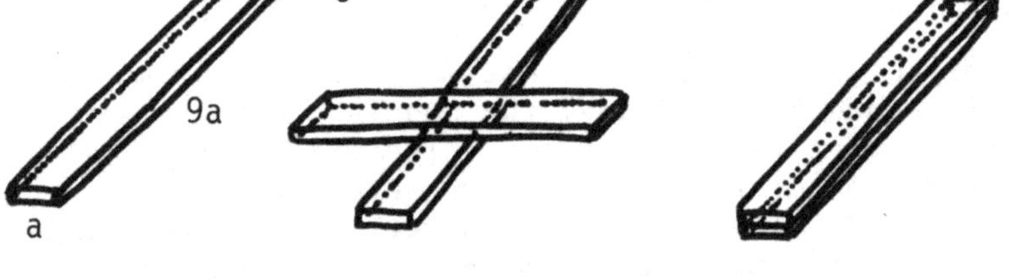

Figure 6. Model, showing two possible modes of aggregation (a and b) of $CaC_2O_4.3H_2O$ crystals. Crystal dimensions are estimated from micrographs (Figure 1).

The results pertaining to crystal growth are in general agreement with earlier authors, who showed that $CaC_2O_4.3H_2O$ is the first solid phase formed from low ionic strength solutions in a comparable range of supersaturations[9] and that crystal growth under these conditions is controlled by a surface process[9,10]. However, no interpretation of a complete precipitation curve, including a quantitative treatment of aggregation, has as yet been attempted.

REFERENCES

1. W. G. Robertson, M. Peacock, and B. E. C. Nordin, Clin. Sci. 40:365 (1971).
2. W. G. Robertson, M. Peacock, and B. E. C. Nordin, Clin. Sci. 43:499 (1972).
3. W. G. Robertson, M. Peacock, and B. E. C. Nordin, Clin. Chem. Acta. 43:31 (1973).
4. B. Tomazić, and G. H. Nancollas, Invest. Urol. 6:329 (1979).
5. G. H. Nancollas, and G. L. Gardner, J. Cryst. Growth 21:267 (1974).
6. W. Stumm, and J. J. Morgan, in:"Aquatic Chemistry," Wiley Interscience, New York (1970).
7. M. Marković, and Lj. Komunjer, J. Cryst. Growth 46:701 (1979).
8. A. E. Nielsen, in:"Kinetics of Precipitation," Pergamon Press, Oxford (1964).
9. G. L. Gardner, J. Cryst. Growth 30:158 (1975).
10. A. E. Nielsen, Acta. Chem. Scand. 14:1654 (1960).

THE ELECTRICAL DOUBLE LAYER AT CALCIUM OXALATE-WATER INTERFACES

P. A. Curreri, G. Y. Onoda, Jr., and B. Finlayson

University of Florida, College of Medicine, Department of Surgery, Division of Urology,
Gainesville, Florida 32610

INTRODUCTION

Crystal growth inhibition and aggregation (coagulation) of calcium oxalate monohydrate crystallites are phenomena of interest in the physical chemistry of stone formation. These phenomena are affected by the presence of adsorbed species at the solid-aqueous phase interface. Inhibitors function by adsorbing at the growing interface. Aggregation tendencies depend on the forces of interaction between particles which are modified by the adsorption of ionic species. Because of the importance of interfacial processes, a study was carried out with calcium oxalate in aqueous suspensions to define better the role of various ionic species in solution. The electrophoretic mobility was used as a measure of the electric potential (zeta potential) near the particle surface. Variations in zeta potential were determined as a function of calcium/oxalate ion activities, pH, and the activities of multivalent ions which are known to function as crystal growth inhibitors.

MATERIALS AND METHODS

Calcium oxalate monohydrate was precipitated by mixing equimolar concentrated solutions of calcium chloride ($CaCl_2$) and sodium oxalate ($Na_2C_2O_4$). Analytical grade chemicals were used. Water was deionized and then distilled in a borosilicate glass still and had a conductivity of less than 1.5×10^{-6} $(\Omega cm)^{-1}$. The precipitate was washed with the purified water until sodium could no longer be detected by atomic adsorption spectroscopy in the wash. X-ray analysis of the dry precipitate confirmed the whewellite form of $CaC_2O_4 \cdot H_2O$. The particles were around 5 μm in diameter, as ascertained by scanning electron microscopy and Coulter Counter measurements.

Suspensions of $CaC_2O_4 \cdot H_2O$ in water were prepared by ultrasonic dispersion at a concentration of 0.35 g/l. The purified water used for the dispersion and solutions showed no evidence of particle contamination by inspection through the electrophoresis microscope. The prepared suspensions were equilibrated for at least 12 h. Final suspensions were made by adding various electrolyte solutions to the dispersion at a ratio of 9 parts suspension to 1 part solution. These solutions were prepared from analytical grade reagents and were passed through 0.22 μm filters to remove undissolved particles. The final suspensions were equilibrated for at least 12 h. The pH values of the various suspensions were measured with glass electrodes.

Electrophoretic measurements were carried out on a commercial instrument*. Except for the electronic components, the electrophoretic apparatus was housed in a constant-temperature chamber, held at 37°C ± 1°C, with glove ports and windows through which the eyepieces of the microscope extended outward. In a preliminary study of the possible effect of suspension concentration on mobility, it was found that mobility did not change over a concentration range of 0.1 - 1.0 g/l; the 0.35-g/l concentration was therefore adopted.

The activities and concentrations of various ions in solution, in the presence of calcium oxalate, were calculated for each experimental condition for which the overall composition was known. An established computer program[1] (EQUILS) uses the Davies modification of the Debye-Hückel theory for activity coefficients, experimentally determined equilibrium constants, and the principles of mass conservation. No corrections were needed for adsorption effects (which are not accounted for in the mass balance), because it was estimated to be negligible, owing to the low surface area of the powder and the low solid:liquid ratio of the suspensions.

RESULTS

Calcium and Oxalate Ions

Ions common to the solid and aqueous phases are Ca^{2+} and $C_2O_4{}^{2-}$. The activities of these two species are related through the solubility constant. The variations in mobility with (Ca^{2+}) were investigated**; $CaCl_2$ and $Na_2C_2O_4$ solutions were used to alter the activity. The (Ca^{2+}) was calculated from the EQUILS program for the known

* Zeta Meter Inc., 1720 First Avenue, New York, New York 10028.

** ( ) = activity (on the molar scale) when applied to ionic species.

additions. The results are given in Figure 1. It should be noted that the ionic strengths varied with the electrolyte added; as shown later, however, this posed no serious problem in analysis, because the EQUILS program characterizes these changes, and they can be taken into account in the analysis of the double layer theory.

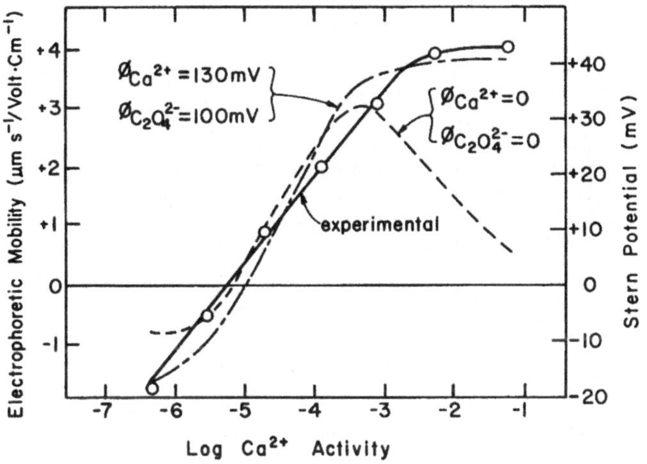

Figure 1. Electrokinetic properties with $CaCl_2$ and $Na_2C_2O_4$ additions as a function of calcium ion activity. Range of pH resulting from addition of electrolyte to system was 6.3 to 7.0. (Mobility is read from left legend; data points and smooth lines drawn through them represent experimental values. Broken lines, curves, and right legend are referred to later in discussion. This is also true for Figures 2 (top), 3, 4, 5 (top), 6 (top), and 7 (top). (Taken from reference 4 with permission.)

The condition of zero mobility at 37°C is found (by interpolation in Figure 1) to be pCa = 5.2, which also corresponds to pC_2O_4 = 3.45 (because pK = 8.65). In the only other known attempt[2] to measure the point-of-zero charge (pzc) of $CaC_2O_4 \cdot H_2O$, the suspension effect was used; the results gave a pzc at 25°C of pC_2O_4 = 2.5 and pCa = 5.11 (where pK = 8.1). Considering the differences in temperature (37°C vs 25°C), the results agree reasonably well.

pH

The variations in mobility with pH, resulting from the addition of HCl and NaOH solutions, are shown in Figure 2 (top). In the intermediate pH range of 5 to 10, the mobility remains approximately constant. This would not be expected if H^+ ions were reacting with the surface (e.g., by hypothesized surface hydroxyl, OH, groups), as in the case of oxides. This supports the interference that ionizable surface OH groups are not present on calcium oxalate surfaces.

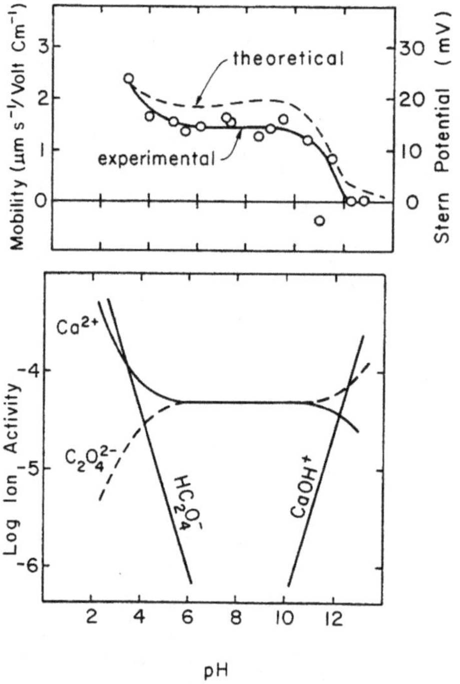

Figure 2. Effect of pH on (top) electrokinetic properties and (bottom) activity of ionic species. (Taken from reference 4 with permission.)

The variations in mobility at low and high pH and the constant values at intermediate pH values appear to relate to variations in (Ca^{2+}) with pH. In Figure 2 (bottom), the activities of the various species present in solution (calculated from EQUILS) are plotted. The shape of the (Ca^{2+})-pH curve is similar to that of the mobility-pH curve. To a first approximation, the variation in mobility with pH could have been predicted by combining the information in Figure 1 with that in Figure 2 (bottom). This correspondence could not be exact, however, because ionic strengths are not comparable. In the analysis of double layer theory, corrections are made for ionic strength to obtain better comparisons.

Electrolytes

The variations in mobility with the addition of 9 electrolytes were investigated; the results are shown in Figures 3 and 4. The data are presented as mobility vs the total concentration of the salt added. Actual activities for the various species at equilibrium resulting from these additions are discussed and presented separately.

The 1:1 electrolytes caused a gradual reduction in mobility with increasing concentration, as expected for indifferent ions. The (Ca^{2+}) remained nearly constant during these additions (from EQUILS).

The addition of sodium sulfate (Na_2SO_4) reduced the mobility to zero at about 4×10^{-3} M and appeared to reverse the sign at higher concentrations, although the data are less reliable at these high ionic strengths. The calcium activity was lowered slightly by the addition of Na_2SO_4, but not enough to account for more than a small fraction of the change in mobility due to the Na_2SO_4 addition. The decrease in mobility with concentration was too fast to be accounted for by the ionic strength when compared with the monovalent electrolyte at comparable ionic strength or as determined by the method described later. Therefore, it suggests that SO_4^{2-}, which is the dominant ionic form of the sulfate (by many orders of magnitude) in the solution, specifically adsorbs to the surface.

The effects of additions of sodium phosphate monobasic (NaH_2PO_4) on mobility (Figure 3) are interesting because of its weak tendency to reduce the mobility. It did not reverse the charge at concentrations as high as 10^{-2} M. This behavior can better be understood by considering the complex ions formed. Under the conditions of this experiment, most of the electrolyte was in the $H_2PO_4^-$ form. The (HPO_4^{2-}) was only a few percent of the $(H_2PO_4^-)$. The (PO_4^{3-}) was lower by nearly 8 orders of magnitude. Consequently, the dominant species was the monovalent species, which was probably functioning as an indifferent counter-ion, whereas only a small amount of HPO_4^{2-} was available to contribute to lowering the mobility by specific adsorption.

Magnesium chloride ($MgCl_2$) additions caused a small increase in the mobility (Figure 4). This suggests that Mg^{2+} (the dominant cation) was specifically adsorbing. To accentuate this effect, the oxalate activity was adjusted to 0.01 M, to create a negative mobility. Further addition of $MgCl_2$ caused an increase in mobility, reversing the sign to positive at 5×10^{-3} M, as shown in Figure 4. For these changes, little variation in (Ca^{2+}) was calculated to occur until 4×10^{-2} M $MgCl_2$ addition. These results indicated the specific adsorption role of Mg^{2+}.

Sodium pyrophosphate ($Na_4P_2O_7$) additions caused a reversal in sign of the mobility at around 1.5×10^{-5} M, as shown in Figure 4.

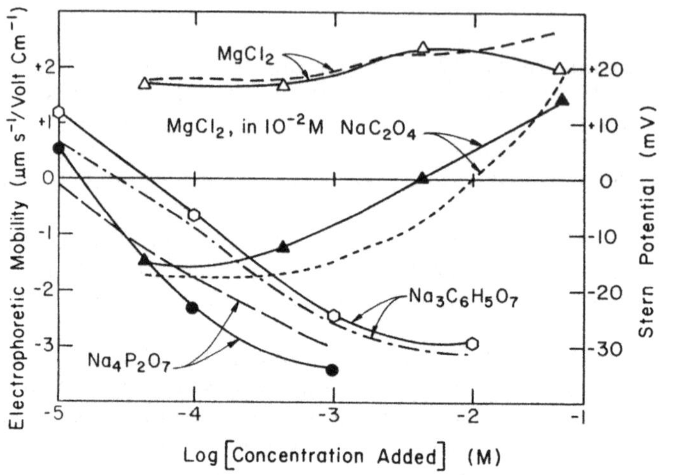

Figure 3. Electrokinetic properties vs logarithm of concentration of electrolyte added. Resulting pH ranges were as follows: NaH_2PO_4, 5.9-5.0; Na_2SO_4, 6.0-6.3; NaCl, 5.9-6.1; KCl, 6.2-6.4; NH_4Cl, 6.6-7.3. Solid lines omitted for monovalent electrolytes for clarity. (Taken from reference 4 with permission).

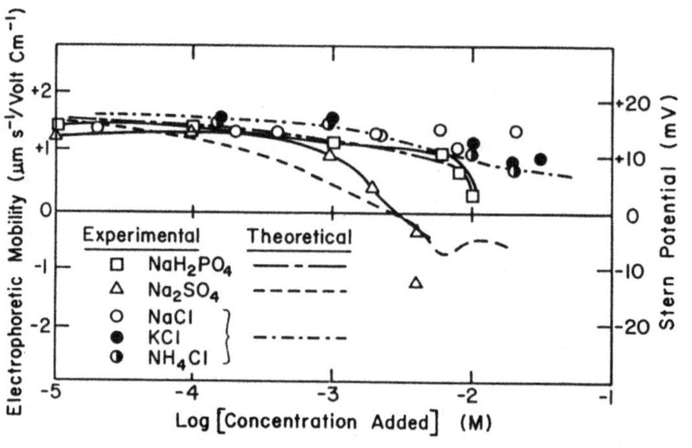

Figure 4. Electrokinetic properties vs logarithm of concentration of electrolyte added. Data points with solid lines are experimental; broken lines are calculated from theory. Resulting pH values were as follows: $MgCl_2$, 6.2-6.0; $MgCl_2$ in 0.01 M $Na_2C_2O_4$, 7.0-6.3; $Na_3C_6H_5O_7$, 6.6 (adjusted with HCl); $Na_4P_2O_7$, 7.1-7.7. (Taken from reference 4 with permission.)

In this case also, the changes in (Ca^{2+}) were not sufficient to expect a charge reversal on this basis alone. Thus specific adsorption of pyrophosphate ion is indicated.

When trisodium citrate ($Na_3C_6H_5O_7$) was added, a reversal in the sign of the mobility occurred at 4×10^{-5} M (Figure 4). In this experiment, the pH was adjusted with HCl titrant to maintain a pH of 6.6. EQUILS revealed that (Ca^{2+}) changed from 4.5×10^{-5} M to 8.6×10^{-6} M when the trisodium citrate concentration varied from 10^{-5} M to 10^{-2} M. This change in (Ca^{2+}) could account, by the use of data in Figure 1, for a reduction of mobility to near zero, but could not account for the larger negative values of mobility obtained. Therefore, it appears likely that specific adsorption is occurring. The principal ionic citrate species in the system were $C_6H_5O_7^{3-}$ and $C_6H_5O_7^{2-}$. Figure 5 (bottom) shows that the calculated activities of these two ionic species underwent large changes in opposite directions in adjusted solutions ranging in pH after equilibration from 4 to 8. In this pH range, for calcium oxalate without $Na_3C_6H_5O_7$, the mobility remains relatively constant as was shown in Figure 2. Therefore, the direction in which the mobility varied with pH, with constant concentration of citrate salt, indicated which of these anions was affecting the mobility. As shown in Figure 5 (top), the mobility became more negative with increasing pH (for the three total concentrations of electrolyte). This can be explained by the increasing $(C_6H_5O_7^{3-})$ shown in Figure 5 (bottom), and not by the decreasing $(HC_6H_5O_7^{2-})$. We conclude, therefore, that the specific adsorption of the $C_6H_5O_7^{3-}$ species was occurring.

"Experimental" and "Theoretical" Stern Potentials

For the calculation of zeta potential, ζ, from electrophoretic mobility we use the Smoluchowski equation:

$$\zeta = \frac{4\Pi\eta}{\varepsilon} U,$$

where η is the viscosity, U is the electrophoretic mobility, and ε is the absolute mermitivity of the aqueous phase.

To relate ζ to double layer theory, we further assume that $\zeta = \psi\delta$. The validity of this assumption has been debated; Lyklama[3] has recently provided some strong arguments for justifying it. The $\psi\delta$ calculated by setting $\zeta = \psi\delta$ and using the Smoluchowski equation will be called the "experimental" Stern potential, in contrast with the "theoretical" Stern potential calculated from theoretical double layer equations. The details of the calculations of theoretical Stern potential will not be discussed here because of space limitations but are available in reference 4. The theoretical $\psi\delta$ can be read from the curves and broken lines - while the experimental $\psi\delta$ calculated for the various mobilities can be read from the

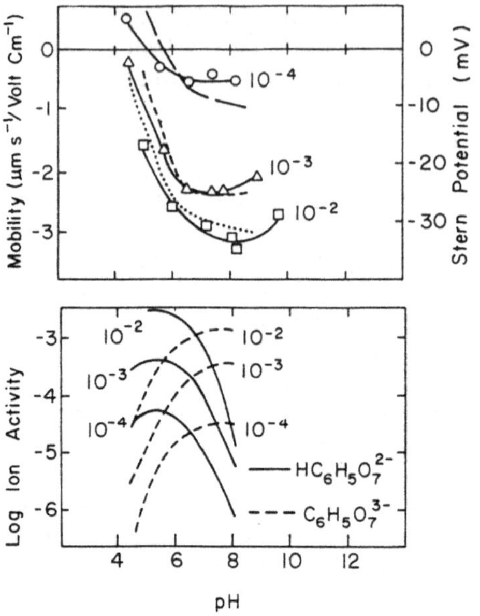

Figure 5. Effect of pH with 10^{-2}, 10^{-3}, 10^{-4} M $Na_3C_6H_5O_7$ additions. Top, electrokinetic properties; data points with solid lines are experimental; broken lines calculated from theory. Bottom, activity of $HC_6H_5O_7{}^{2-}$ and $C_6H_5O_7{}^{3-}$. (Taken from reference 4 with permission.)

data - in Figures 1, 2 (top), 3, 4, 5 (top), 6 (top), and 7 (top) by the right-hand legend. It can be seen that in general the observed data could be fitted quantitatively to the theoretical expressions.

SUMMARY

1. Calcium oxalate in pure water has a positive zeta potential.

2. The zeta potentials were altered by changing pCa. A zero zeta potential was found at a pCa of 5.2. At higher Ca^{2+} activities the zeta potential was positive; at lower Ca^{2+} activities the zeta potential was negative.

3. The influence of pH on zeta potential was found to be due to its effect on altering the calcium ion activity in solution.

4. The effect of the monovalent salts NaCl, KCl, and NH_4Cl upon zeta potential did not indicate specific adsorption.

5. The effect of phosphate, sulfate, pyrophosphate, and citrate ions on zeta potential did indicate chemical adsorption.

6. It was found that the observed data could be fitted nearly quantitatively to classical double layer theory.

REFERENCES

1. B. Finlayson, in:"Calcium Metabolism in Renal Failure and Nephrolithiasis," D. S. David, ed., John Wiley and Sons, Inc., New York (1977).
2. E. P. Honig and J. H. Th. Henyst, J. Colloid Sci. 29:510 (1968).
3. J. Lyklema, J. Colloid Interface Sci. 58:242 (1977).
4. P. Curreri, G. Y. Onoda, Jr., and B. Finlayson, J. Colloid Interface Sci. 69:170 (1979).

CALCIUM ELECTRODE MEASUREMENTS OF CALCIUM OXALATE MINERALIZATION: THE EFFECTS OF URINE AND OTHER INHIBITORS

W. P. Tew and C. D. Malis

Department of Physiological Chemistry, The Johns Hopkins University, School of Medicine
Baltimore, Maryland 21205, U.S.A.

INTRODUCTION

In recent years, investigators in the field of nephrolithiasis have employed numerous *in vitro* assays to measure the kinetics of the formation and crystal growth of hydroxyapatite or calcium oxalate seed crystals in solutions supersaturated with respect to these salts [1,2]. Such assays have proven to be very accurate but their relevance to the formation and growth of urinary calculi is still uncertain. In this connection we have developed a procedure using a Ca^{2+}-specific electrode which measures the rate and extent of calcium oxalate mineralization from initial ion-pair formation to the growth of calcium oxalate crystals.

MATERIALS AND METHODS

The assay system consists of a Radiometer D820 Ca^{2+}-electrode coupled to a Beckman Expandomatic pH meter. The pH of the medium was maintained constant during the assay, with a Metrohm 421 pH/stat automatic titrator.

The standard assay medium was composed of 100 ml of 150 mM KCl, 3.0 mM Hepes-pH 6.0, 200 μM Ca^{2+}, at 37°C. Throughout the assay, the medium was stirred at constant speed. Ca^{2+} activity was standardized by 2.5 μl additions of 1 M $CaCl_2$, followed by sequential additions of $Na_2C_2O_4$ with an automatic pipet. In some experiments pH, temperature, and ionic strength were varied.

RESULTS

Calcium Oxalate Assay

Figure 1 shows the changes in Ca^{2+} activity observed during a typical calcium oxalate mineralization assay. The stock medium was standardized with 2.5 µl additions of 1.0 M $CaCl_2$ to a final concentration of 300 µM. Upon the additions of 500 µl aliquots of 100 mM $Na_2C_2O_4$ there was a decrease in Ca^{2+} activity corresponding to the formation of CaC_2O_4 ion-pairs. Throughout these additions of $Na_2C_2O_4$ sensitive light-scattering measurements did not indicate the presence of any separate CaC_2O_4 mineral phase. After the addition of $Na_2C_2O_4$, there was an induction phase (nucleation and/or aggregation) characterized by no change in Ca^{2+} activity. Following induction, the rapid decrease in Ca^{2+} activity coincided with the appearance of crystals of $CaC_2O_4 \cdot 3H_2O$[3]. The length of the induction period and the rate of crystal formation was a function of the concentration of CaC_2O_4 formed during the addition of $Na_2C_2O_4$ (Figure 2). These conditions provide a convenient induction time with reasonable reproducibility (12 ± 1 min).

Effects of Physical Parameters

Changes in pH (5.5 to 8.0) or temperature (18 to 40°C) of the assay medium had only minimal effect[4] but variations in ionic strength resulted in pronounced changes in ion-pair formation and induction times. Increasing the ionic strength of the medium from 0.075 to 0.300 decreased the formation of CaC_2O_4 ion-pairs and increased the induction time 6-fold (Figure 3).

Effects of Inhibitors

Addition of small volumes of urine (1 to 3 ml) produced significant increases in the induction period without effecting ion-pair formation and with minimal reduction in the rate of crystallization (Figure 4). These effects were proportional to the volume of urine added. The characteristics of small aliquots of urine on calcium oxalate mineralization were duplicated by small amounts of heparin[5]. Pyrophosphate, phosphocitrate and EHDP in µM concentrations had no effect on CaC_2O_4 formation or the induction period but did reduce slightly the rate of Ca^{2+} uptake during the crystallization phase[4].

Epitaxial Nature of Hydroxyapatite

Additions of 1 to 10 mg of hydroxyapatite seed crystals to the assay medium had no effect on ion-pair formation but greatly reduced the induction period and accelerated the rate of crystal formation in a dose-dependent fashion[6]. The presence of µM phosphocitrate, pyro-

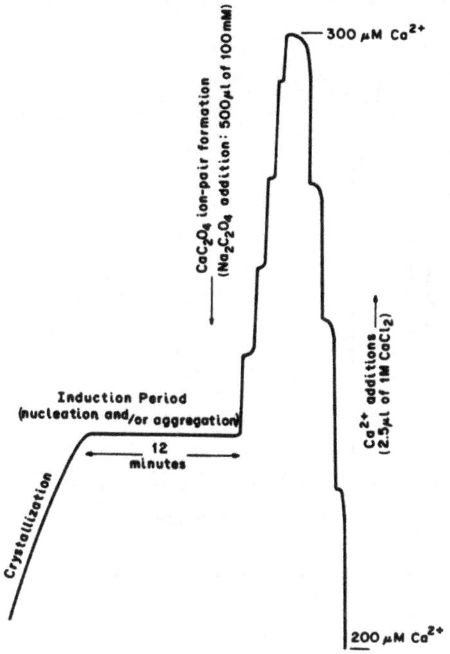

Figure 1. CaC_2O_4 mineralization assay. (See text for details).

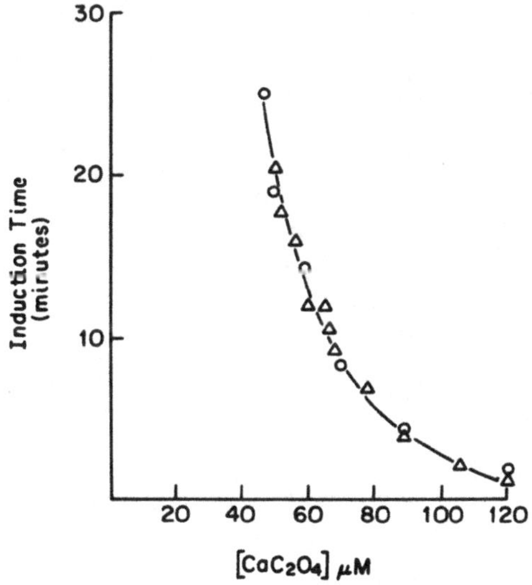

Figure 2. Induction time as a function of CaC_2O_4 ion-pair formation produced by addition of $Na_2C_2O_4$ or $CaCl_2$ to the standard medium containing either 300 μM Ca^{2+} (o) or 2.5 mM oxalate (Δ).

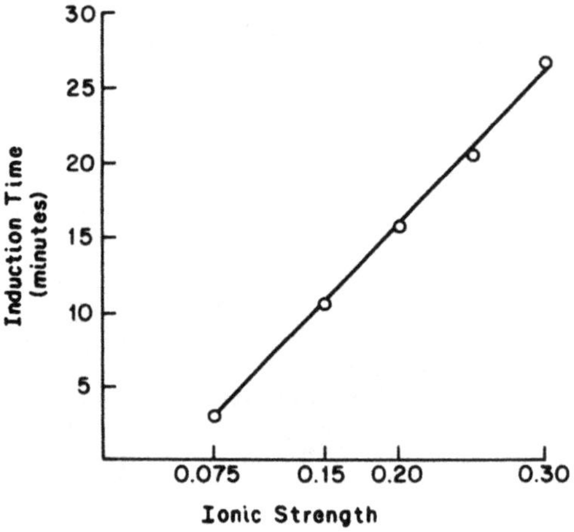

Figure 3. Effect of increasing ionic strength on induction time.

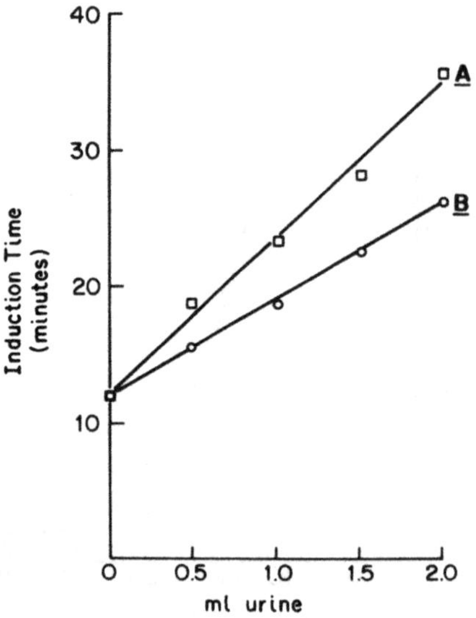

Figure 4. Effect of urine on CaC_2O_4 mineralization. ($Na_2C_2O_4$ was added to a final concentration of 2.5 mM.)

phosphate or EHDP in the assay medium was effective in preventing this (Figure 5).

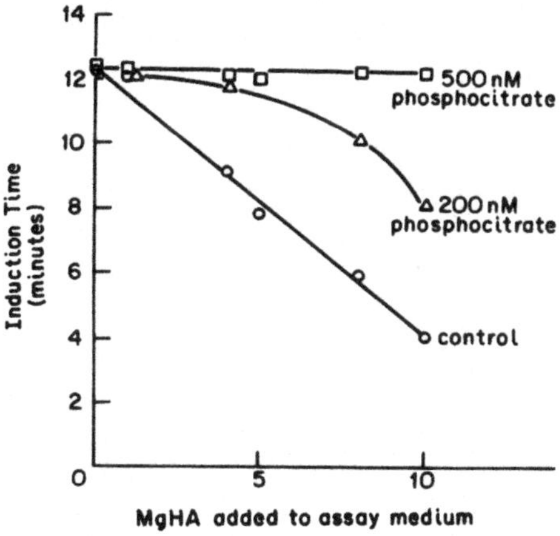

Figure 5. The effect of hydroxyapatite seed crystals on $Ca_2C_2O_4$ mineralization in the presence (□ and Δ) and absence (o) of previously added phosphocitrate.

DISCUSSION

The $Ca_2C_2O_4$ mineralization assay provides in a single rapid determination data on ion-pair formation, nucleation and/or aggregation and crystal growth. The observed effects on calcium oxalate formation of varying physical parameters and crystallization inhibitors are in agreement with measurements made in other CaC_2O_4 mineralization assays and indicate that the Ca^{2+}-electrode can be used with confidence to monitor calcium oxalate mineralization and assay the effects of potential inhibitors, although the limitations of the calcium electrode preclude accurate measurements at Ca^{2+} and oxalate concentrations similar to those of urine.

REFERENCES

1. J. L. Meyer and L. H. Smith, Invest. Urol. 13:31 (1975).
2. J. L. Meyer and E. E. Angino, Invest. Urol. 14:347 (1977).
3. R. H. Doremus, G. L. Gardner, and W. McKay, in:"Colloquium on Renal Lithiasis," B. Finlayson, W. C. Thomas, Jr., ed., The University Presses of Florida, Gainesville (1976).
4. J. L. Meyer, K. E. Lee, and J. H. Bergert, Calcif. Tiss. Res. 28:83 (1977).
5. J. E. Crawford, E. P. Cremety, and A. E. Alexander, Aust. J. Chem. 21:1067 (1968).
6. J. L. Meyer, J. H. Bergert, and L. H. Smith, Clin. Sci. Mol. Med. 49:369 (1975).

EFFECT OF URINARY MACROMOLECULES ON CALCIUM OXALATE DIHYDRATE CRYSTAL GROWTH AND NUCLEATION RATES

Alan D. Randolph, Zlatica I. Kraljevich, and George Drach

The University of Arizona, Section of Urology,

Tucson, Arizona 85724

INTRODUCTION

Two major theories of calcium oxalate urinary stone disease are the hyperexcretion-supersaturation theory and the inhibitor theory. Both are centrally related to the crystallization kinetics of calcium oxalate (CaOx). In the supersaturation theory oxalate stone is a result of persistent overconcentration of Ca^{2+} and/or Ox^{2-} ions in the urine brought about by dietary and metabolic irregularities or inadequate fluid intake. CaOx precipitation (mono or dihydrate form) occurs when the CaOx ion product exceeds the formation product. The supersaturation theory maintains that persistent overconcentration causes excessive crystalluria growth, nucleation, and/or aggregation which raises the probability of a particle eventually lodging in the kidney to become the nidus for a stone. High supersaturations aggravate further growth of the stone by molecular growth, surface nucleation of dendrites and/or aggregation with additional crystalluria. Finlayson[1] demonstrated convincingly using order-of-magnitude calculations that growth of 200μm particles (approximate dimensions of the ducts of Bellini) is virtually impossible solely by molecular accretion on single crystals; agglomeration/aggregation mechanisms are a likely part of the overall stone formation process. Nevertheless, the presence of small CaOx crystalluria sets up these mechanisms and therefore the hyperexcretion-supersaturation theory correctly focuses on the importance of crystallization kinetics.

The inhibitor theory of CaOx stone disease[2-6] assumes the presence in urine of natural inhibitors that slow the growth and/or nucleation of CaOx, thus permitting CaOx excretion as concentrated solution or at least greatly reducing the formation of crystalluria. The presence (or absence) of inhibitor compounds can dramatically affect crystallization kinetics and thus the inhibitor theory of stone disease is also centrally related to CaOx crystallization kinetics and brings into play the vast body of crystallization literature concerned with crystal modifiers.

Organic macromolecular compounds naturally present in human urine are likely compounds which might act as crystal modifiers to allow urinary excretion of CaOx in a benign form (concentrated solution or very small crystalluria). The purpose of the present study was to investigate the influence of such urinary macromolecules (MW > 50,000 D) on the crystal growth and nucleation rates of calcium oxalate dihydrate (COD).

METHOD

A 300 ml continuous-flow mixed suspension mixed product removal (MSMPR) crystallizer system[7-8] was used for this study. Crystallization kinetics of COD was characterized in terms of nucleation rate (B^o), growth rate (G) and total crystal mass concentration (M_T). The MSMPR Crystallizer discharges through an in-line sampling cell. Particle size measurements in the cell were made with a PDI Electrozone/celloscope counter peripherally attached to a microprocessor (PDP8/A32K). Data were automatically regressed by the minocomputer to the well-known exponential population distribution of the MSMPR Crystallizer[7] in order to obtain nucleation and growth rates,

thus: $$n = (B^o/G)\exp(-L/G\tau) \qquad (1)$$

Correlation coefficients of steady state data regressed to Eq (1) were typically in excess of R^2=0.995. Thorson's[8] synthetic urine solution was used as feed, but was modified slightly to allow for the addition of urea. This solution has an osmolarity of 700 mOsm and a pH of 5.8. Calcium and oxalate ions present in the synthetic feed solution correspond to 8.16mM and 0.7mM, respectively, giving a calcium to oxalate ratio of 11.7. COD crystals were mainly obtained at this ratio as verified by birefringence using polarized-light microscopy.

Proteins contained in urine of normal and stone former subjects were separated into MW fractions from 1,000 to 50,000 Daltons by ultrafiltration. (Amincon Corporation, High-Flow Stirred Cell, Teflon coated Model 2000, with Diaflo membranes). Twenty-four hour urine specimens were collected from a group of six healthy subjects (one female) and a group of eight active calcium oxalate stone formers (two females). Of the eight stone forming subjects, two were on a low calcium-low oxalate diet, two were on a low calcium diet, one was on a low oxalate diet, and three were on a free diet. Their age ranged between 31 and 64. The specimens were refrigerated during collection and then centrifuged for 18 minutes at 3500 rpm to eliminate solid material. The volume of each sample was measured and a pooled sample was obtained from each group for pH and osmolarity measurement and ultrafiltration. The filtrate was then refiltered through successively smaller Diaflo membranes. After filtration the residue left on a given membrane was lyophilized (Labconco Freeze Dryer, Model 4451 F, Type J T/c) and stored in sealed vials.

A known amount (10 ppm) of dried residue fractionated from either normals or stone formers was then added to the calcium feed solution and allowed to dissolve before using a MSMPR crystallizer feed. The continuous-flow crystallizer was operated at mean residence times (crystallizer volume divided by total flow rate) of 5, 7, 9, and 12 minutes in order to vary supersaturation driving forces in the system. It is important to note that mother liquor (discharge) supersaturation rather than feed supersaturation is the driving force causing growth and nucleation. Steady conditions in the crystallizer were obtained after about 9-10 residence times. After steady state was reached the crystallizer discharge was filtered through a 3μm millipore filter, the pH was adjusted to pH 1 to 2, and the sample frozen until analysis for oxalate using the double enzymic method for the spectrophotometric determination of oxalic acid in urine due to Costello, Hatch and Bourke[9].

RESULTS

A. Fractionation of Whole Urine

A clear difference in molecular weight distribution of urinary macromolecules was observed between the control group and stone formers. Normal urines contained macromolecules in the range 1 to 30 KD but this size fraction was totally absent in stone formers. Neither group yielded compounds in the range 30-50 KD as shown in Table 1. To verify this result and eliminate the possibility of overlooking too small a residue, we filtered more than one batch of urine (a batch was approximately 1.8 liter) through a given membrane. Still, no recoverable residue was left on the membrane surface in the range 30-50 KD. Resnick and Boyce[10] have reported that some urine specimens showed no evidence of low molecular weight macromolecules. The average yield of macromolecules > 50 KD was 79.6 mg/l for stone formers and 46.4 mg/l for controls. Although no attempt was made to determine physical characteristics of the compounds being obtained, no appreciable differences in terms of color, texture and general appearance was observed between the two groups. The pooled urine specimens from both groups also showed similar pH levels, with an average of 6.2 (min. 5.8, max 7.0). The average osmolarity of stone formers urine was 628 (min. 233, max. 780), and that of normal urine was 535 (min. 523, max. 554).

Table 1. Concentration of Macromolecules in Normal and Stone Former Urines

Urine Type \ MW Range	Concentration of Macromolecules (*) mg/l 1,000 to 30,000 D	30,000 to 50,000 D	>50,000 D
Normal	73	None	46.4
Stone Former	None	None	79.4

(*) Reported as dry substance after lyophilization.

B. COD Growth and Nucleation Rate Measurements

Table 2 summarized values of B^o, G, $\bar{L}_{1,0}$ and oxalate assays for the 12 C, N and SF runs of this study. Figure 1a plots mean (population-weighted) particle size $\bar{L}_{1,0}$ as a function of residence time in the continuous-flow crystallizer (τ = 5 to 12 minutes). Note that over this range of retention times there is virtually no effect on particle size for either controls (C), normal urines (N), or stone former urines (SF). There is only a slight difference in particle size between N and SF runs, but both of these give particles significantly smaller than the control runs (with no urine macromolecules).

Linear crystal growth rate G in the MSMPR crystallizer[7] is related to population-weighted size $\bar{L}_{1,0}$ as $G = \bar{L}_{1,0}/\tau$. Thus for constant $\bar{L}_{1,0}$, growth rate and retention time should be related hyperbolically as illustrated in Figure 1b.

Figure 1c plots oxalate concentrations in the mother liquor as a function of residence time for the C, N and SF runs. Note the inhibition of CaOx growth rate as exhibited directly by the higher residual oxalate concentration in the mother liquor. Note also that except for the value at τ = 7 min there appears to be no change of N or SF assays with crystallizer retention time. All runs were fed the same 0.7 mM oxalate feed concentration. The pooled SF urinary macromolecules (> 50 KD) apparently showed more inhibition (higher oxalate assays in the mother liquot) than the pooled N urinary macromolecules, although this effect is slight compared to the large decrease of concentration with τ shown by the controls.

Figure 2a plots B^o vs τ for C, N and SF runs. Figure 2b plots nucleation rates, B^o, and linear growth rates G, for control runs as a function of residual oxalate concentration in the mother liquor. Growth and nucleation rate for N and SF runs bore no relation to liquor concentration.

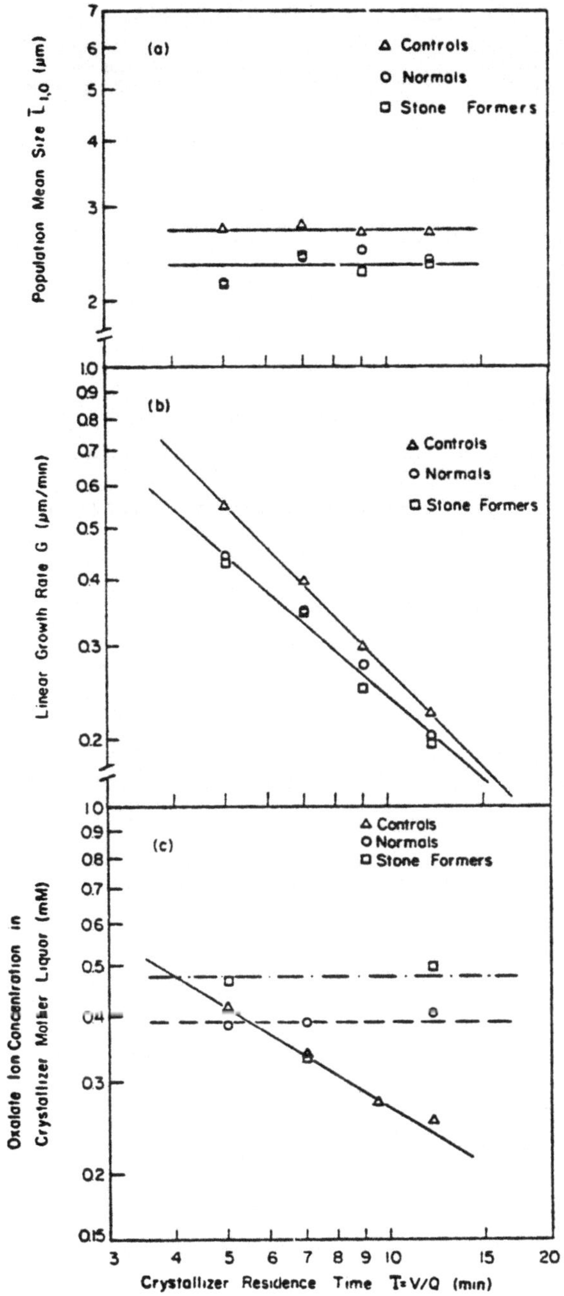

Figure 1. Population Mean Size (a), Linear Growth Rate (b), and Oxalate Ion Concentration in Crystallizer Mother Liquor (c), as a Function of Residence Time.

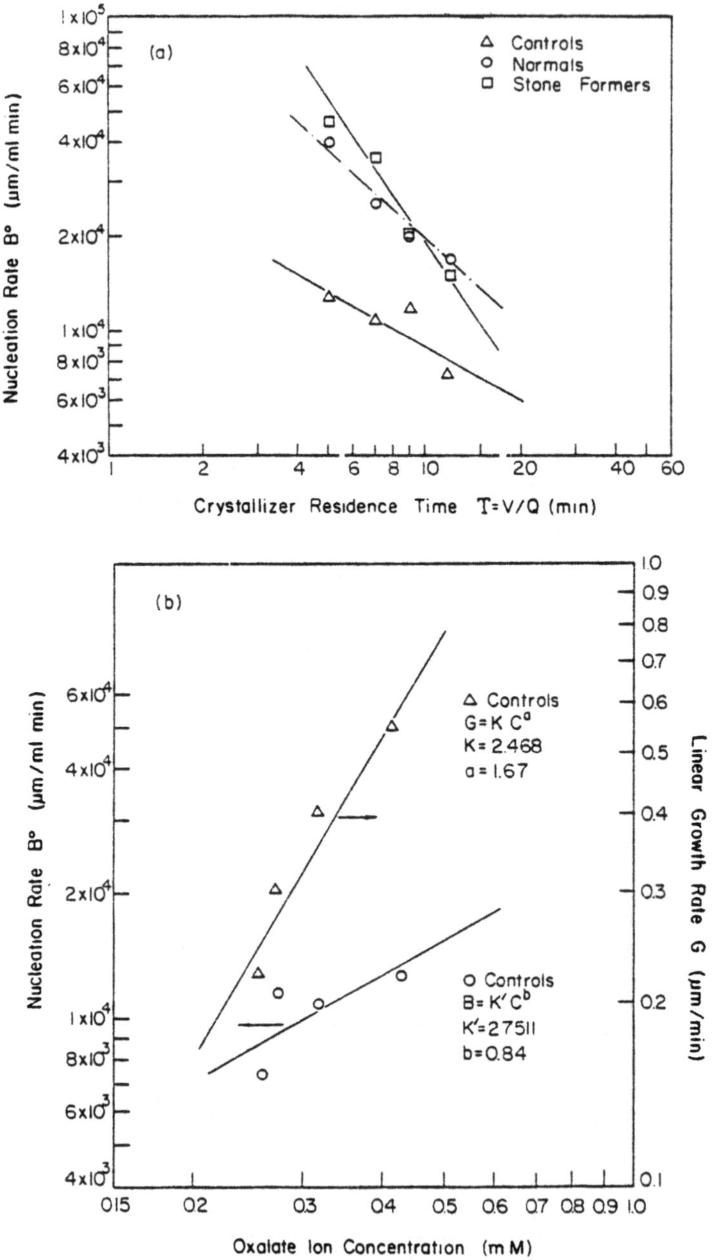

Figure 2. Kinetic Information of COD Crystals
a) Nucleation Rate as a Function of Residence Time;
b) Nucleation and Growth Rate as a Function of Mother Liquor Oxalate Assay

Table 2. Kinetic Data From Control, Normal and Stone Former Runs

Run #	$\bar{L}_{1,0}$ µm	G µm/min	B^o µm/m/-min	Mτ mg/1	Ox Ion mM	Additives 10 ppm	τ min
0409	2.73	0.546	12637	9.02	0.415	C	5
0319	2.76	0.395	10821	11.28	0.318	C	7
0410	2.66	0.296	11583	13.80	0.273	C	9
0414/0520	2.79	0.233	7156	12.93	0.255	C	12
0415	2.14	0.428	39662	13.66	0.381	50 KD/N	5
0326/0327	2.40	0.344	25118	17.27	0.386	50 KD/N	7
0521	2.49	0.276	19680	19.03	---	50 KD/N	9
0417	2.42	0.202	16750	19.87	0.403	50 KD/N	12
0415	2.11	0.422	46509	15.40	0.464	50 KD/SF	5
0320/0322	2.41	0.344	35462	24.30	0.339	50 KD/SF	7
0521	2.25	0.250	20335	14.73	---	50 KD/SF	9
0417	2.34	0.194	14833	16.01	0.494	50 KD/SF	12

DISCUSSION OF RESULTS

Growth and nucleation rates for the control runs were fit to simple power-law correlations of the form:

$$G = k_g \, [C_{ox}]^a \quad \mu m/min \tag{2}$$

and

$$B^o = k_N \, [C_{ox}]^b \quad no./ml\text{-}min \tag{3}$$

A multiple linear regression program was used to fit data from control runs to the above equations, giving the following parameters: $k_g = 2.468$, $k_n = 27511$, $a = 1.67$, and $b = 0.84$.

The relative nucleation/growth rate sensitivity order $i = \frac{b}{a} = 0.50$ is considerably lower than the value of 1.73 reported by Miller[11]. However, our synthetic urine contained urea and had a lower CaOx feed concentration. Miller did not count CaOx particles in situ. His technique was to filter and then resuspent the crystals for measurement with a Coulter Counter.

It was originally planned to regress the N and SF data to similar kinetics correlation models and then compare the rate constants k_g and k_N to enable quantitative documentation of nucleation and/or growth rate inhibition in the system. However, no correlation whatsoever exists between growth or nucleation rates and measured oxalate analyses in the mother liquor for N and SF runs. The dilemma is this: Although changes in system residence time nicely spread the measured values of growth and nucleation rates, no corresponding correlation of oxalate concentration with residence time was observed and thus no correlation of B^o and G with the state of the system (oxalate concentration) can be obtained. The control runs behaved exactly as expected based on the above nucleation and growth rate kinetics; B^o, G and C_{ox} all declined monotonically as τ increased. The N and SF data can only be rationalized by two assumptions, namely

1) The N and SF oxalate assays were grossly inaccurate. Perhaps the urinary macromolecules interferred with the double enzyme oxalate assay.

or

2) Growth and nucleation rates in the presence of urinary macromolecules bear no relation to the state (concentration) of the system.

The latter assertion would demand new crystallization theory.

Assuming the magnitude of the N and SF oxalate assays are at least correct vis-a-vis the control values, then certainly urinary macromolecules do inhibit COD crystal growth rates, as lower crystal growth rates are obtained in the presence of higher oxalate assays. (See Figures 1b and 1c). Furthermore, nucleation rate was always increased in the presence of urinary macromolecules. We cannot say definitely that this represents true enhancement of nucleation or is just the natural consequence of growth inhibition (i.e. higher oxalate concentration in the mother liquor) without having a comparable nucleation kinetics model for the N and SF system. However, if we again assume the magnitude of the oxalate assays are correct then urinary macromolecules do act as nucleation enhancers; the N and SF nucleation data would scatter above the nucleation correlation shown for controls (Figure 2b).

CONCLUDING REMARKS

We have shown that urinary macromolecules (> 50 KD) present in normal and stone former urines significantly inhibit linear growth rate of COD crystals and most probably enhance nucleation rate as well. This dual enhancement and inhibition property probably plays a key role in the body's natural protective mechanism to excrete CaOx in a benign form, i.e. as concentrated solution or very small crystalluria. In this study we found that urinary macromolecules from normals and stone formers differ markedly in their molecular weight distribution; there were virtually no macromolecules < 50 KD in the urines of 8 stone formers investigated. The effect of stone former urinary macromolecules vis-a-vis normals and controls is shown in Table 3.

Table 3. Growth and Nucleation Rate Modification for Stone Formers vs Controls or Normals

	This Study (=5-12 min)		Thorson et al[8] (=7 min)	
	w.r.t.* C	w.r.t. N	w.r.t. C	w.r.t. N
B^o	+185%	+12.6%	+366%	+124%
G	-15.9%	- 3.7%	-48.2%	-20.5%

*w.r.t. = with respect to

Thus the work of Thorson[8] shows a considerably larger degree of crystal modification, although both studies show the same trends, i.e. growth inhibition and nucleation enhancement. The principle difference between the two techniques was that Thorson added a fixed amount (5% aliquot) of human urine while in the present study we added a fixed weight (dry substance) of urinary macromolecules. Our work showed that stone former's urine contains some 72% higher concentration of these active compounds (> 50 KD) than normals. This difference in total amount of active urinary compounds might explain some of the increased modifier activity shown by Thorson's study. On an absolute basis (comparing normals at $\tau = 7$) Thorson's study also showed more urine modifying activity vis-a-vis our work, i.e. B^o = 34,600 vs our 25,000 and G = 0.249 vs our 0.344.

The fact that stone former's urine exceeds that of normals in the dual modifier function suggests the possibility of over-correction in this protective mechanism as a factor in stone disease (Sarig, et al.[12]), perhaps loading to an agglomeration/aggregation mechanism which is aggravated by excessive numbers of crystalluria. Or perhaps the increased amounts of crystal modifiers in SF urines is merely trauma-induced, i.e. a response rather than a cause.

REFERENCES

1. B. Finlayson, in:"Calcium Metabolism in Renal Failure and Nephrolithiasis," David S. David, ed., Wiley, New York (1977).
2. W. G. Robertson and M. Peacock, Clin. Sci. 43:499 (1972).
3. W. G. Robertson, M. Peacock, and B. E. C. Nordin, Clin. Chem. Acta. 43:31 (1973).
4. D. J. Sutor, Br. J. Urol. 41:171 (1969).
5. S. G. Welshman and M. G. McGeown, Br. J. Urol. 44:677 (1972).

6. W. G. Robertson, M. Peacock, R. W. Marshall, D. H. Marshall, and B. E. C. Nordin, N. Eng. J. Med. 294:249 (1976).
7. A. D. Randolph and M. A. Larson, in:"Theory of Particulate Processes," Academic Press, New York (1971).
8. G. W. Drach, S. Thorson, and A. D. Randolph, J. Urol. 123:519 (1980).
9. J. Costello, M. Hatch, and E. Bourke, J. Lab. Clin. Med. 87: 903 (1976).
10. M. I. Resnick and W. H. Boyce, Invest. Urol. 16:270 (1979).
11. J. D. Miller, A. D. Randolph, and G. W. Drach, J. Urol. 117:342 (1977).
12. G. W. Drach, S. Sarig, A. D. Randolph, and S. Thorson, (in preparation).

EQUILIBRIUM-BASED COMPUTER MODEL FOR THE ESTIMATION OF URINE SATURATION

P. G. Daniele and M. Marangella*

Instituto Analisi Chimica Strumentale, Turin University and *Divisione Nefrologia e Dialisi, Ospidale Mauriziano Umberto I, Turin, Italy

Previous computer models for the estimation of urinary saturation of the salts which form renal stones[1,2] are not always reliable because of the use of activity coefficients (at ionic strength higher than 0.1 $mol \cdot dm^{-3}$) and of the difficulty of finding in the literature values of stability constants determined at 37°C. In this paper we present an improved model in which conditional stability constants, determined at 37°C and at the actual ionic strengths of the urine, are used.

METHODS AND MATERIAL

The stability constants of each of the complexes listed in Table 1 were determined experimentally at ionic strengths I = 0.03, 0.05, 0.1, 0.3 and 0.5·mol dm^{-3} by means of potentiometric measurements with glass or Ca^{2+} ion-selective electrodes[3,4]. The stability constants (always referred to Et_4NI ionic medium) are defined as:

$$\beta = \frac{{}^{C}[M_pL_qH_r]}{c_M^p \cdot c_L^q \cdot c_H^r}$$

where c with subscript is the concentration at equilibrium. Their values were correlated as a function of the ionic strength by means of the equation (1), derived from the Debye-Huckel expression for the activity coefficients[5].

$$\lg \beta^{I} = \lg\beta^{I'} - z^*A \frac{\sqrt{I}}{1 + B'\mathring{a}\sqrt{I}} - \frac{\sqrt{I'}}{1 + B'\mathring{a}\sqrt{I'}} + C(I-I') \quad (1)$$

where I is the actual and I' is the reference ionic strength; å and

Ca^{2+}	$[Ca(Cit)H]$	$[Ca(Cit)]^-$	$[Ca(HPO_4)]$	
	$[Ca(H_2PO_4)]^+$	$[Ca(SO_4)]$	$[Ca(Ox)]$	
Mg^{2+}	$[Mg(Cit)H]$	$[Mg(Cit)]^-$	$[Mg(HPO_4)]$	
	$[Mg(H_2PO_4)]^+$	$[Mg(SO_4)]$	$[Mg(Ox)]$	
Na^+	$[Na(Cit)]^{2-}$	$[Na(HPO_4)]^-$	$[Na(SO_4)]^-$	$[Na(Ox)]^-$
K^+	$[K(Cit)]^{2-}$	$[K(HPO_4)]^-$	$[K(SO_4)]^-$	$[K(Ox)]^-$
NH_4^+	$[NH_4(Cit)]^{2-}$	$[NH_4(HPO_4)]^-$	$[NH_4(SO_4)]^-$	$[NH_4(Ox)]^-$
H^+	$[H(Cit)]^{2-}$	$[H_2(Cit)]^-$	$[H_2(PO_4)]^-$	$[H(Ox)]^-$

Table 1. The Various Complexes used in the Calculation of Urinary Saturation

C are arbitrary parameters; A and B' are constant values dependent on ionic medium and temperature; $z^* = pn^2 + qs^2 + r - (pn - qs + r)^2$ for the general reaction: $pM^{n+} + qL^{2-} + rH^+ \rightleftarrows [M_pL_sH_r]^{(pn-qs+r)}$.

Calculation of the equilibrium concentrations of each species was performed simultaneously by a computer program. The method was checked by the direct measurement of one or more species, for instance, by means of ion selective electrodes. Since there is no suitable electrode for measuring oxalate in urine, we made the check with the Orion 93-20 calcium ion-selective electrode. The method was applied to 100 urine samples from 50 fasting healthy controls and 50 stone-formers. The free Ca^{2+} measurements were performed within half an hour after the collection, which had been voided directly into Dewar flasks. The urines were analyzed for pH, Na, K, Ca, Mg, NH_4, sulfate, phosphate, citrate, oxalate, chloride by routine methods.

RESULTS AND CONCLUSION

The results of the analytical determinations are reported in Table 2. The lower concentrations of the stone-formers are due to their higher fluid intakes.

The agreement between measured and calculated free Ca^{2+} concentration was fairly good, the mean error being less than ± 5% (<0.5 mVolts). The data have been calculated using both our own and Robertson's method[6-8]. The results are shown in Table 3. This shows

Table 2. Total Concentrations of Ions in Normal and Stone-Forming Urine. (Mean ± S.D.; $mmol \cdot dm^{-3}$).

	Controls		Stone-formers		P*
pH	5.72	0.42	5.88	0.52	n.s.
Na	143.4	55.4	124.5	47.3	n.s.
K	54.4	26.5	33.6	23.8	<0.005
Ca	6.19	4.1	5.70	3.4	<0.05
Mg	3.63	1.5	3.16	1.3	n.s.
NH_4	51.3	22.0	38.3	20.6	<0.02
Cl	126.3	50.1	117.0	54.6	n.s.
P	31.2	11.9	26.4	11.8	n.s.
SO_4	19.7	4.9	18.3	6.8	n.s.
Cit	4.30	2.20	2.97	1.96	<0.01
Ox	0.30	0.16	0.33	0.14	n.s.

Table 3. Equilibrium concentration products with CaOx and $CaHPO_4$: Comparison between our own and Robertson's method. (C = total concentration; c = free ion concentration; *stone-formers).

I	C_{Ca}	C_{OX}	$-lg(c_{Ca} \cdot c_{Ox})$ Our	Rob.	Δ	$-lg(c_{Ca} \cdot c_{HPO4})$ Our	Rob.	Δ
0.245	17.8	0.36	6.240	6.061	0.18	5.235	5.085	0.15
0.267	3.9	0.70	6.440	6.220	0.22	5.382	5.278	0.105
0.313	9.2	0.38	6.330	6.140	0.19	5.244	5.110	0.13
0.335	5.6	0.26	6.617	6.428	0.19	5.829	5.676	0.15
0.305	7.8	0.37	6.438	6.274	0.16	5.220	5.063	0.16
0.270	3.7	0.46	6.700	6.554	0.15	5.660	5.588	0.07
0.277	3.9	0.43	6.631	6.464	0.17	5.324	5.194	0.13
0.309	3.4	0.22	7.055	6.839	0.22	5.063	4.981	0.08
0.310	7.6	0.13	6.828	6.636	0.19	5.907	5.759	0.15
0.280	8.6	0.24	6.615	6.427	0.19	4.760	4.628	0.13
0.115	2.0	0.08	7.447	7.339	0.11	6.159	6.130	0.03
0.140	1.9	0.21	7.208	7.090	0.12	5.820	5.810	0.01
* 0.286	8.9	0.28	6.470	6.290	0.18	4.955	4.800	0.155
* 0.270	8.8	0.51	6.240	6.057	0.18	4.892	4.754	0.14
* 0.325	6.4	0.55	6.333	6.137	0.20	5.124	4.988	0.14
* 0.290	4.5	0.42	6.555	6.378	0.18	6.002	5.894	0.11
* 0.331	2.4	0.52	6.700	6.483	0.22	5.900	5.790	0.11
* 0.240	7.8	0.31	6.561	6.420	0.14	5.338	5.214	0.12
* 0.320	1.9	0.25	7.050	6.832	0.22	6.400	6.252	0.15
* 0.309	6.9	0.41	6.400	6.216	0.18	5.718	5.555	0.16
* 0.282	6.4	0.50	6.454	6.283	0.17	5.382	5.284	0.10
* 0.288	5.0	0.39	6.200	6.000	0.20	4.938	4.774	0.16
* 0.130	1.9	0.22	7.193	7.098	0.10	6.398	6.397	0.0
* 0.100	4.2	0.11	7.153	7.052	0.11	5.758	5.720	0.04

that the estimates of $-\lg(c_{Ca} \cdot C_{OX})$ and, to a lesser degree, of $-\lg(c_{Ca} \cdot c_{HPO4})$ are lower with our method (mean $\Delta_{CaOX} = 0.19 \pm 0.02$ at $I = 0.3$; $\Delta = 0.110 \pm 0.008$ at $I = 0.1$ mol dm^{-3}; Mean $\Delta_{CaHPO4} = 0.13 \pm 0.027$ at $I = 0.3$; $\Delta = 0.02 \pm 0.018$ at $I = 0.1$) than with Robertson's.

The new approach presented here provides results which significantly differ from those obtainable with Robertson's methods which we chose because it has been previously compared with the methods of Finlayson and Pak[9]. It may be that further improvement of the model will be possible from a better knowledge of the interactions of oxalate with other ions in urine which have not yet been considered.

REFERENCES

1. W. G. Robertson, M. Peacock, and B. E. C. Nordin, Clin. Sci. 34:579 (1968).
2. B. Finlayson, R. Roth, and L. Dubois, in:"Urinary Calculi," Karger, Basel (1973).
3. P. G. Daniele, C. Rigano, and S. Sammartano, (submitted for publication).
4. P. G. Daniele, and M. Marangella, (submitted for publication).
5. P. G. Daniele, C. Rigano, and S. Sammartano, Ann. Chim. 70: 119 (1980).
6. W. G. Robertson, Clin. Chim. Acta. 24:149 (1969).
7. R. W. Marshall and W. G. Robertson, Clin. Chim. Acta. 72:253 (1976).
8. W. G. Robertson, M. Peacock, R. W. Marshall, D. H. Marshall, and B. E. C. Nordin, New Engl. J. Med. 294:249 (1976).
9. C. Y. C. Pak, Y. Yasafumi, B. Finlayson, and S. Chu, J. Lab. Clin. Med. 89:891 (1977).

THE RELATION BETWEEN RELATIVE SUPERSATURATION AND CRYSTAL AGGREGATION IN URINE - AN SEM STUDY AND A COMPUTERIZED CALCULATION OF THE ION EQUILIBRIUM

F. Hering, W. G. Burschardt, N. Pyhel, and W. Lutzeyer

Department of Urology, Department of Electron Microscopy, and Department of Medical Statistics and Documentation
RWTH Aachen, Aachen, West Germany

Using a Coulter Counter technique Robertson et al.[1,2] have shown that the urine of stone-formers contains crystals of calcium oxalate which are larger and more aggregated than those in normal urine. There is, moreover, a relationship between crystalluria and stone recurrence rate.

MATERIAL AND METHODS

Fresh urine specimens from single and recurrent calcium stone formers were passed through Millipore membrane filters (pore size 5 μm). The retained particles were examined as follows: (a) the crystal composition and lattice dimensions were investigated by x-ray diffraction using the technique described by Guinier; (b) crystal formation and aggregation was studied by scanning electron microscopy (SEM). Crystal fragments were analyzed by a microprobe technique (energy dispersive x-ray analysis) and element concentration mapping.

The relative saturation of the filtered urine with respect to calcium oxalate was calculated using an ion equilibrium computer program (in Fortran IV modified from that of Finlayson and Reid[3]) based on the formula:

$$2.2 + (4.1 \times 10^6 \text{ [O X]} - 3 \times 10^4 \text{ [Mg]}) \text{ [Ca]} - 10^3 \text{ [Na] [Citr.]}$$

From this formula the relative saturation of urine can be calculated with an accuracy of 97.3%. The range of the saturation product is 1.7 - 23.2.

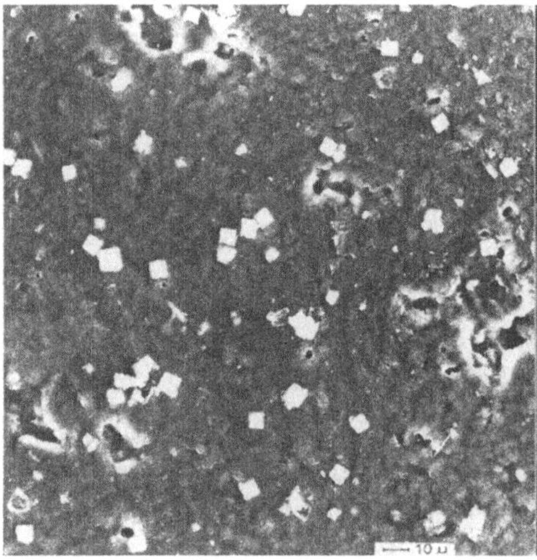

Figure 1. SEM-photomicrograph of urine crystals (relative saturation of urine 5.9).

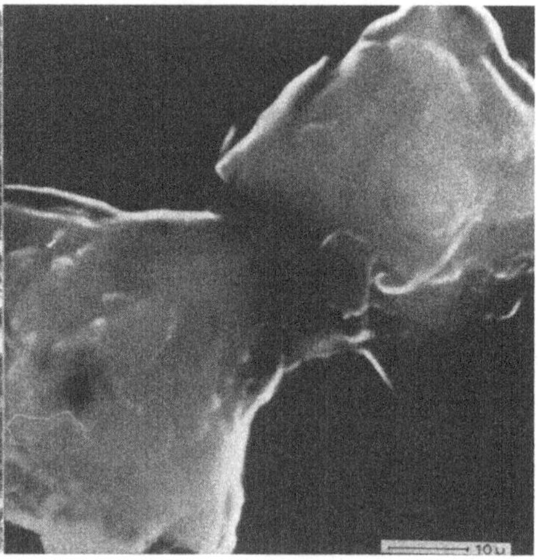

Figure 2. SEM-photomicrograph of urine crystals with connecting bridge (relative saturation of urine 5.9).

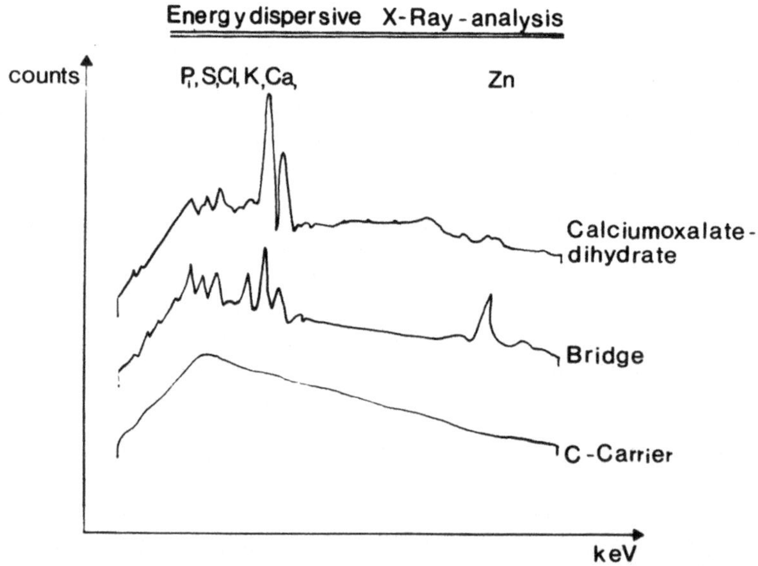

Figure 3. Energy dispersive x-ray analysis of calcium oxalate crystals and connecting bridge.

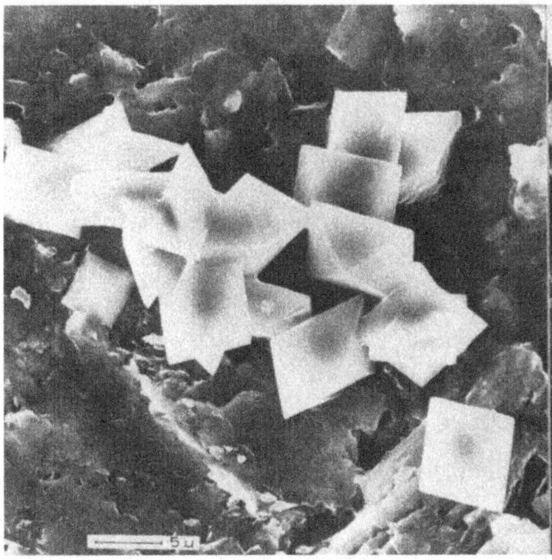

Figure 4. SEM-photomicrograph of urine crystals (relative saturation of urine 11.9).

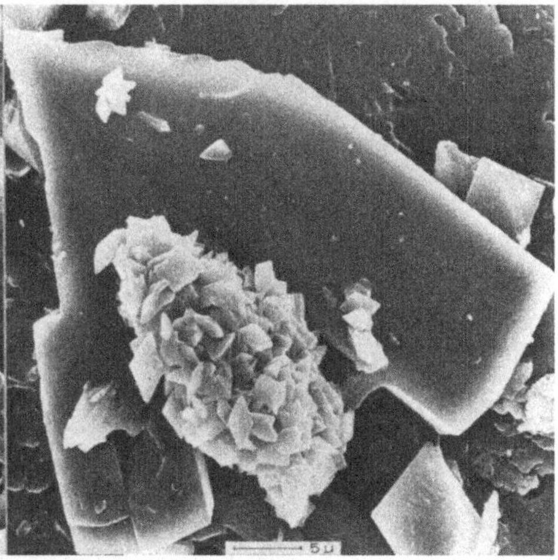

Figure 5. SEM-photomicrograph of urine crystals (relative saturation of urine 15.2).

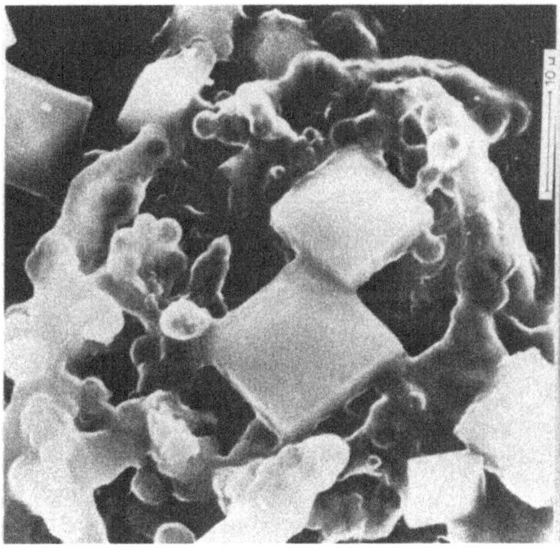

Figure 6. SEM-photomicrograph of urine crystals imbedded in noncrystalline calcium phosphate (relative saturation of urine 11.4).

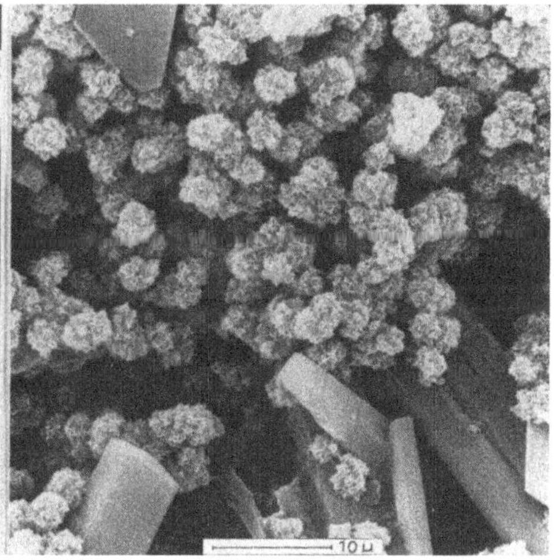

Figure 7. SEM-photomicrograph of urine crystals (relative saturation of urine 34.2).

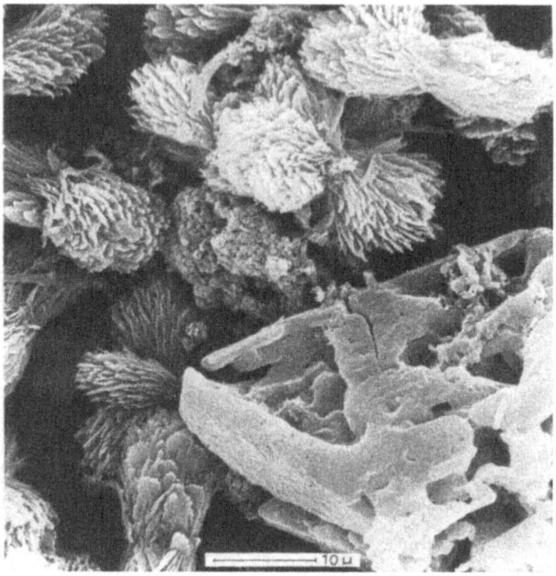

Figure 8. SEM-photomicrograph of urine crystals (relative saturation of urine 28.7).

The aim of our study was to study the relation between the relative saturation of urine with respect to calcium oxalate and the degree of crystal formation, -aggregation and -composition.

RESULTS

A higher degree of crystal formation and aggregation was observed with increasing relative saturation of urine, caused by either an increased concentration of calcium oxalate or both, or a relative lower molar concentration of citrate or magnesium.

In urine of low saturation only single calcium oxalate dihydrate crystals were found (Figure 1). This is a typical feature of non-stone-forming urine. In some cases non-crystalline bridges between calcium oxalate dihydrate particles were observed (Figure 2). Zn was detected in association with these bridges (Figure 3) by energy dispersive x-ray analysis and by element concentration mapping.

In urine of higher saturation calcium oxalate dihydrate crystals grew into one another and formed crystal aggregates between 40 and 80 µm in diameter (Figures 4 and 5). In alkaline urine calcium oxalate dihydrate crystals were imbedded in spheroidal noncrystalline calcium phosphate (size 0.5µm) (Figure 6). The same feature was observed at the contact surface between the various layers of mixed calcium oxalate/phosphate stones. Their importance for crystal aggregation is not yet clear.

In supersaturated urine a characteristic feature was ball-or sheaf-like crystals of calcium oxalate monohydrate (Figures 7, 8).

CONCLUSION

The degree of crystal formation and aggregation was dependent on the relative saturation of urine. Ball-or sheaf-like crystals of calcium oxalate monohydrate were a characteristic feature of highly saturated urine with respect to calcium oxalate. In alkaline urine non-crystalline calcium phosphate formed bridges between calcium oxalate dihydrate crystals. Urine of non-stone-formers showed only single calcium oxalate dihydrate crystals with no tendency to aggregate.

REFERENCES

1. W. G. Robertson, M. Peacock, and B. E. C. Nordin, Clin. Sci. 34:579 (1968).
2. W. G. Robertson and M. Peacock, Clin. Sci. 43:499 (1972).
3. B. Finlayson and F. Reid, Invest. Urol. 15:442 (1978).

DETERMINATION OF THE STABILITY CONSTANT OF THE CALCIUM DIOXALATE COMPLEX

John R. Burns*, Birdwell Finlayson, and Arthur Smith

*Division of Urology, Department of Surgery, University of Alabama in Birmingham, Birmingham, Alabama 35294; Division of Urology, Department of Surgery, University of Florida, Gainesville, Florida 32610

INTRODUCTION

The problem of calcium oxalate (CaOx) urinary calculi is often best understood in terms of the supersaturation of calcium oxalate in urine. Relative supersaturation can be determined by incubation of urine with solid CaOx. An alternative involves measuring various species concentrations and then calculating relative supersaturation with a computer equilibrium program. Minor discrepancies exist between these two methods at low concentrations of calcium and oxalate[1]. At high oxalate concentrations, however, there is a large discrepancy between the two methods: incubation yields a lower relative supersaturation. Such a difference can be accounted for, at least in part, by assuming the existence of a CaOx species not included in the current computational scheme. Studies done with divalent cations, such as magnesium, cadmium, and cobalt, have demonstrated the existence of dioxalate species at high oxalate concentrations[7]. On this basis, a calcium dioxalate species, $Ca(C_2O_4)_2^{2-}$, could be anticipated at high oxalate concentration.

MATERIALS AND METHODS

We prepared [^{45}Ca] calcium oxalate monohydrate ([^{45}Ca] whewellite) by adding 10 mCi of calcium-45 as $CaCl_2$ to 100 ml of 0.1 M $CaCl_2$. We then mixed the labeled $CaCl_2$ solution with 100 ml of 0.1 M $Na_2C_2O_4$ to produce a slurry of labeled CaOx seed crystals. The seed slurry was filtered, washed with double-distilled water, and resuspended. We repeated this process until the concentration of sodium in the filtrate was less than 1×10^{-7} M. A portion of the slurry was filtered and allowed to dry, and the powder was then ground to a uniform consistency. Solubility studies were performed with both the [^{45}Ca] CaOx slurry and the dry [^{45}Ca] CaOx.

For the solubility studies, we added 100 mg of the [^{45}Ca] whewellite powder or 0.2 ml of the [^{45}Ca] whewellite slurry to a series of Erlenmeyer flasks, each containing 15 ml of a sodium oxalate solution ranging in concentration from 10 to 100 mM. The flasks were allowed to stand at 60°C for 5 min before being stoppered and sealed with parafilm. After 1 hr, the temperature was lowered to 38°C, and the flasks were agitated for 72 h. We aspirated the supernatant samples through a 0.22 μm Millipore filter and measured the pH at 38°C. We then determined calcium-45 activity with liquid scintillation by mixing 0.5 ml of supernatant sample in 10 ml of AQUASOL-2, with 5 ml of distilled water added to gel the AQUASOL.

We determined a series of solubilities in distilled water and measured the calcium content with atomic-absorption spectrophotometry. The calcium-45 activity of these samples was determined, and the activity per millimole of calcium was calculated. We used this value to ascertain calcium solubility in oxalate solutions, in which atomic-absorption analysis of calcium is difficult because of interference by the oxalate ion.

RESULTS

The solubility of calcium in the presence of various concentrations of sodium oxalate is shown in Figure 1. The apparent calcium solubility decreases with increasing oxalate concentration until the oxalate concentration reaches 10 mM, after which the apparent calcium solubility slowly rises.

DISCUSSION

In analyzing our results, we assumed the following equilibria:

$$Ca^{2+} + C_2O_4^{2-} \underset{}{\overset{k_1}{\rightleftarrows}} CaC_2O_4 \qquad (1)$$

$$Ca^{2+} + CaC_2O_4 \overset{k_2}{\rightleftarrows} Ca_2C_2O_4^{2+} \qquad (2)$$

$$C_2O_4^{2-} + CaC_2O_4 \overset{k_3}{\rightleftarrows} Ca(C_2O_4)_2^{2-} \qquad (3)$$

$$Na^{+} + C_2O_4^{2-} \overset{k_4}{\rightleftarrows} NaC_2O_4^{-} \qquad (4)$$

$$H^{+} + C_2O_4^{2-} \overset{k_5}{\rightleftarrows} HC_2O_4^{-} \qquad (5)$$

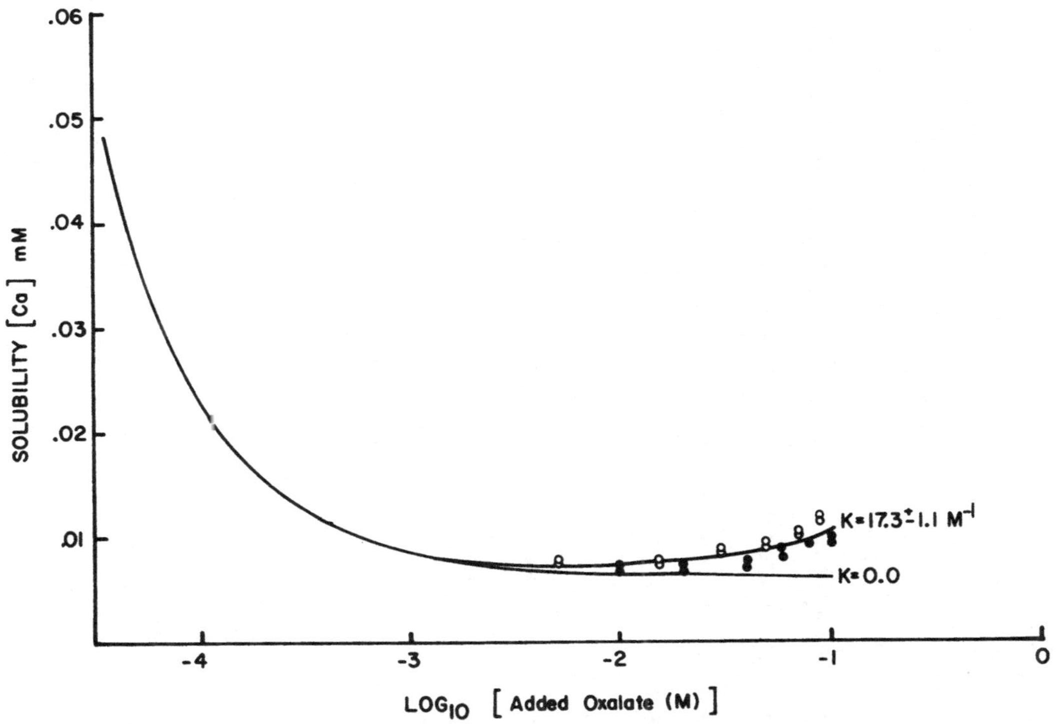

Figure 1. The solubility of $CaC_2O_4 \cdot H_2O$ (at 38°C) as a function of the logarithm of the molar concentration of dissolved oxalate. o indicated solubility measurements using [^{45}Ca] whewellite powder. • indicates measurements using [^{45}Ca] whewellite slurry. The k = 17.3 line was generated with the parameters in Table 1 and Equations 1-12, with the stability constant of $Ca(C_2O_4)_2^{2-}$ set to 17.3. The k = 0 line was generated in a similar manner, but with the stability constant for $Ca(C_2O_4)_2^{2-}$ set to zero.

We determined activity coefficients at 38°C with the Davies equation and coefficients of A = 0.522 and B = 0.286[3]. We also assumed an activity coefficient of 1 for CaC_2O_4. Brönsted stability constants (r_i) were defined as follows: $r_1 = k_1 f_2^2$, $r_2 = k_2$, $r_3 = k_3$, $r_4 = k_4 f_2$, and $r_5 = k_5 f_2$, with f_2 representing the divalent activity coefficient.

We calculated species concentrations by iteratively solving the following equations:

$$[Ca^{2+}] = (\text{Total calcium} - [CaC_2O_4] - r_3[CaC_2O_4]\,[C_2O_4^{2-}])/(1 + 2r_2[CaC_2O_4]) \quad (6)$$

$$[C_2O_4^{2-}] = (\text{Total oxalate} - [CaC_2O_4] - r_3[CaC_2O_4]\,[Ca^{2+}])/(1 + 2r_3[CaC_2O_4] + r_4[Na^+] + r_5(H^+)), \quad (7)$$

with H^+ indicating proton activity ($10^{-pH}/f_1$)

(f_1 represents the monovalent activity coefficient)

$$[Na^+] = (\text{Total sodium})/(1 + r_4[C_2O_4^{2-}]) \quad (8)$$

Other species present were calculated as follows:

$$[Ca_2C_2O_4^{2+}] = r_2[CaC_2O_4][Ca^{2+}] \quad (9)$$

$$[Ca(C_2O_4)_2^{2-}] = r_3[CaC_2O_4][C_2O_4^{2-}] \quad (10)$$

$$[NaC_2O_4^-] = r_4[Na^+][C_2O_4^{2-}] \quad (11)$$

$$[HC_2O_4^-] = r_5[H^+][C_2O_4^{2-}] \quad (12)$$

We solved equations 6-12 repetitively to estimate f_1 and f_2, with a self-consistency of one part per thousand.

This method of determining species concentrations was then used as a function in a nonlinear least-squares program. pH, $[Ca^{2+}]$, and added oxalate were entered as variables, and k_1, k_2, k_4, k_5 and $[CaC_2O_4]$ were considered parameters to be simultaneously fitted to the experimental data. In Figure 1, the k = 17.3 ± 1.1 M^{-1} line is the least-squares fit to our experimental results. If one assumes that a calcium dioxalate complex does not exist, the k = 0 line is generated. On this basis, it appears that a calcium dioxalate complex, $Ca(C_2O_4)_2^{2-}$, exists at oxalate concentrations over 10 mM. The thermodynamic stability constant of this complex is 17.3 ± 1.1 M^{-1}.

Table 1. Parameters Used to Describe Calcium Oxalate Solubility(1)

Parameter	Meaning	Estimated Value±S.E.M.(2)
$[CaC_2O_4]$	Solubility of the complex	6.16 ± 0.38 μM
k_1	Stability constant of CaC_2O_4	2,746 M^{-1}
k_2	Stability constant of $Ca_2C_2O_4^{2+}$	71.6 ± 5.3 M^{-1}
k_4	Stability constant of $NaC_2O_4^-$	13.3 ± 0.4 M^{-1}
k_5	Stability constant of $HC_2O_4^-$	2.153 x 10^4 M^{-1}

(1) Reference (4).
(2) Standard error of mean

REFERENCES

1. C. Y. C. Pak, Y. Hayashi, B. Finlayson, and S. Chu, J. Lab. Clin. Med. 89:891 (1977).
2. J. E. Barney, W. J. Argersinger, and C. A. Reynolds, J. Am. Chem. Soc. 73:3785 (1951).
3. C. W. Davies, in:"Ion Associations," Butterworths, London (1962).
4. B. Finlayson, R. Roth, and L. Dubois, in:"Urinary Calculi: Recent Advances in Aetiology, Stone Structure and Treatment," L. Cifuentes Delatte, A. Rapado, and A. Hodgkinson, eds. S. Karger, Basel (1973).

ACKNOWLEDGMENT

This work was supported by NIH SCOR Grant Urolithiasis AM 20586-03.

CALCIUM OXALATE HYDRATES. DISSOLUTION, TRANSFORMATION AND CRYSTALLIZATION STUDIES

Branko B. Tomazic and George H. Nancollas

Chemistry Department, State University of New York at Buffalo, Buffalo, New York 14214

Many calcium oxalate renal stones consist of an inner core of monohydrate (COM) with an outer surface layer of the thermodynamically less stable dihydrate (COD)[1]. The kinetic relationships between the hydrates may, therefore, be of considerable importance since these phases may form either directly or via a transformation process in the continuously changing urine environment. In vivo, the process of formation and dissolution of kidney stones is complicated by the presence of uncharacterized natural inhibitors and promoters which may markedly influence the nature of the hydrate phase which precipitates. Thus it has been shown that natural urine constituents selectively control the rate of nucleation and crystallization of the calcium oxalates[2].

Highly reproducible kinetic studies have been made of the dissolution and crystallization of COM, COD, and at least thermodynamically stable trihydrate, COT, over a range of temperature (15 to 50°C) and ionic medium (0-0.3M sodium and potassium chlorides)[3,4]. The rate of dissolution is proportional to the relative undersaturation and it can be seen in Table 1 that the first-order rate constants fall in the sequence $k_d(COT)>k_d(COD)>k_d(COM)$. Dissolution appears to be diffusion controlled with an activation energy of 12 to 17 $kJmol^{-1}$.

Both COD and COT readily undergo transformation to the least soluble COM because of the thermodynamic driving forces arising from equilibrium solubilities of the less stable hydrates[4]. The transformation proceeds directly to COM as shown by x-ray and scanning electron microscopic evidence. In contrast to the observed extensive nucleation of COM on COT, the transformation of COD to COM appears to take place through bulk nucleation and growth of COD.

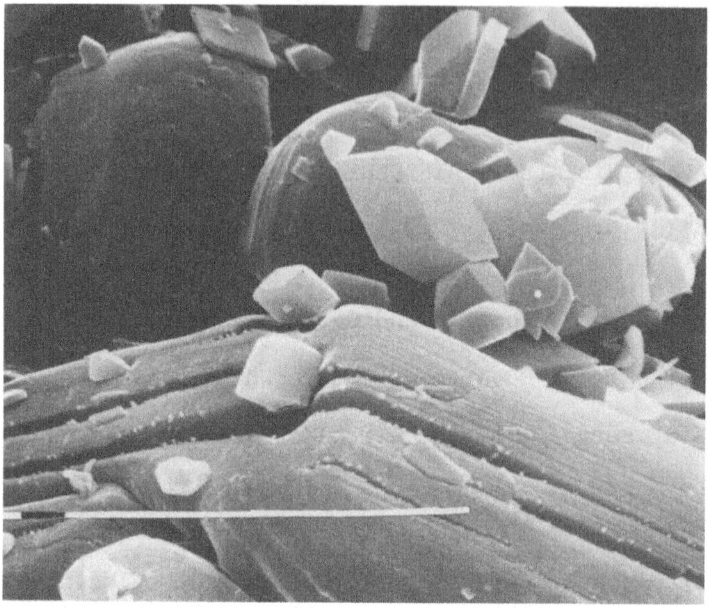

Figure 1a. Scanning electron micrograph: transformation of COT by surface nucleation of COM. White right bar = 5 μm.

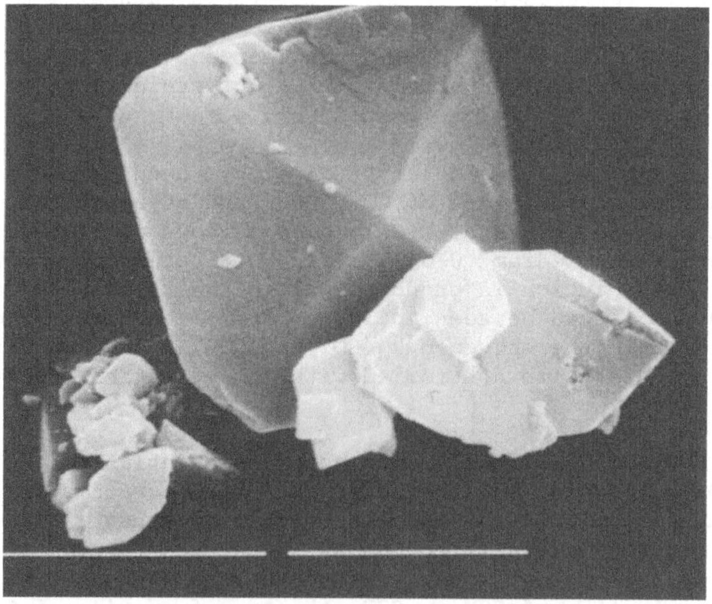

Figure 1b. Scanning electron micrograph: transformation of COD by secondary nucleation of COM 0.15M NaCl, 37°C.

This is illustrated in Figures 1a and 1b. As shown in Figure 2 the transformation process is considerably more rapid for COT and is sensitive to temperature, ionic strength, and ionic medium composition. The transformation appears to proceed through dissolution and subsequent surface or secondary nucleation of the new phase and is also influenced by the presence of traces of crystal growth inhibitors such as polyphosphate, phytate, pyrophosphate and whole urine[5].

Table 1. Dissolution, Growth and Adsorption Reactions

Phase	k_d	k_g	Γ(polyphos)	k_g(in $5x10^{-7}$M polyphos)
	$min^{-1}m^{-2}$	$\ell mol^{-1}min^{-1}m^{-2}$	x $10^7 mol.m^{-2}$	$\ell mol^{-1}min^{-1}m^{-2}$
COM	1.24	$5.87x10^3$	2.71	∿0
COD	1.61	$2.77x10^3$	0.44	5.5
COT	2.28	$2.47x10^4$	1.23	20.0

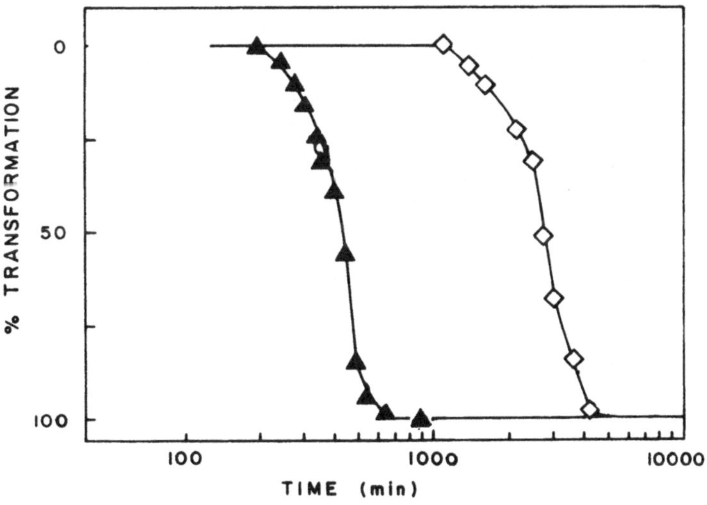

Figure 2. Transformation of hydrates into monohydrates at 37°C. Δ, COT; ◇, COD.

The results of investigation of the extent of adsorption of linear polyphosphate (molecular weight approximately 4500) has shown that the three hydrates differ markedly in their surface adsorbability falling in the sequence Γ(COM)>Γ(COT)>Γ(COD). This may, in part, explain the observed stabilization of metastable hydrates since the formation of stable COM is readily inhibited by the greater surface adsorption of impurity molecules[4]. It is interesting to note that in the presence of polyphosphate, the mechanism of dissolution of all three hydrates appears to become surface controlled with a rate proportional to the square of the relative supersaturation[4].

In the corresponding seeded crystallization reactions from metastable supersaturated solutions of calcium oxalate, (6-7 x 10^{-4}M CaOx in 0.15M NaCl, 37°C), the rate is proportional to the square of the relative supersaturation provided that, in the cases of COD and COT, concomitant transformation to COM is discouraged either by using a high solid/solution ratio or by adding traces of polyphosphate[6]. Plots of calcium concentration, T_{Ca}, against time following

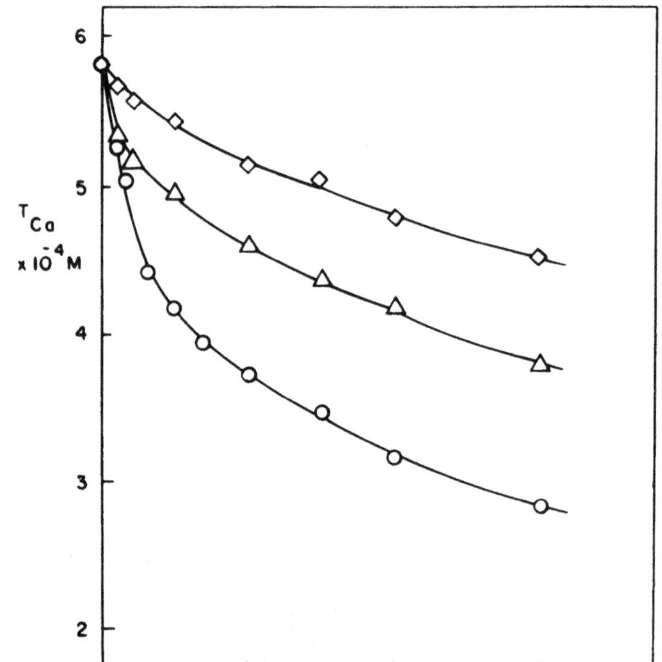

Figure 3. Growth curves of COM, O; COT, Δ; COD, ◊ .

inoculation with each hydrate seed are shown in Figure 3. The second-order growth rate constants are given in Table 1 and it can be seen that they fall in the order $k_g(COT) > k_g(COM) > k_g(COD)$. The evidence points to a surface controlled crystallization and the relatively low rate of COD growth results in the fact that this phase does not precipitate directly from pure calcium oxalate solutions.

In the presence of polyphosphate, the crystal growth of all three hydrates is markedly inhibited. The extent of adsorption of polyphosphate, Γ(polyphosphate), is given in Table 1 together with resulting specific rate constants for crystal growth. The observed differences in inhibitor adsorbability amongst the three hydrates resulting in the complete inhibition of formation of COM and stabilization of the thermodynamically less stable COT and COD, may play an important role in mineralization processes in vivo. However, the overall process of formation of calcium oxalate calculi is the result of competitive kinetic processes such as nucleation, crystal growth, dissolution, and transformation, all of which may be moderated by the presence or absence of natural urine inhibitors. Experiments made in normal whole urine indicate that the transformation of metastable COD and COT into COM is greatly retarded. It is quite possible that the kinetically favored COT may be an active precursor to other stable concretions and especially calcium phosphate phases[5].

REFERENCES

1. J. S. Elliot, J. Urol. 109:82 (1973).
2. G. W. Drach, S. Thorson, and A. D. Randolph, J. Urol. 123:519 (1980).
3. B. Tomazic, and G. H. Nancollas, J. Cryst. Growth 46:355 (1979).
4. B. Tomazic, and G. H. Nancollas, Invest. Urol. (in press).
5. B. Tomazic, and G. H. Nancollas, Invest. Urol. 16:329 (1979).
6. B. Tomazic, and G. H. Nancollas, J. Coll. and Interface Sci. 75:149 (1980).

ACKNOWLEDGMENT

We thank the National Institutes of Health, NIAMDD, for a grant, AM 19048, in support of this work.

ON THE TRANSITION AMORPHOUS CALCIUM PHOSPHATE TO CRYSTALLINE OCTACALCIUM PHOSPHATE

J. M. Garcia Ruiz, V. Lopez-Acevedo, and J. L. Amorós

Departamento de Cristalografia y Mineralogia,
F. C. Geologicas, U. Complutense
Madrid, Spain

INTRODUCTION

Most of calcium phosphates in some hard tissues of living organisms belong to the family of apatites. They crystallize in hexagonal or monoclinic systems, and even non crystalline mineral phases have been detected[1]. Repeated experiments have demonstrated the transformation of amorphous calcium phosphate, ACP, into crystalline calcium phosphate, which is not yet completely understood[2-5]. There are two different hypotheses to explain this transformation[2,3,6]. One hypothesis considers ACP dissolution and subsequent transformation into crystalline phosphate as the main mechanism; while the second hypothesis, ACP constitutes an epitaxic substrate for secondary nucleation of the crystalline phase.

The aim of this work is to show experimental evidence supporting the latter hypothesis. We have applied a method of synthesis which allows the growth of octacalcium phosphate (OCP) crystals and ACP spherulites of a size suitable for characterization.

MATERIALS AND METHODS

Precipitates were obtained by silica gel technique[7] using a U tube arrangement and double diffusion of the reactants. The dimensions of the crystallization apparatus are described in Figure 1. Reacting solutions were introduced in the vertical branches at the ends of the U tube. Figure 2 shows the solutions employed, and the range of experiments carried out varying gel pH and the concentration of the reacting solutions. The precipitates were identified by x-ray diffraction (XRD) (Powder and Lave methods when necessary), and infrared spectroscopy (IR). The morphological study of crystals was carried out under binocular lents, optical microscopy and scanning electron microscopy (SEM). Qualitative chemical analyses were carried out by x-ray energy dispersion in a SEM.

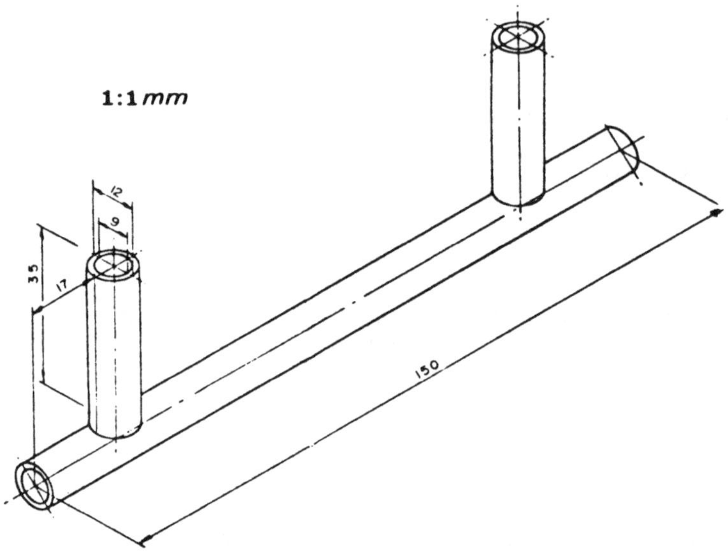

Figure 1

RESULTS

Calcium phosphate precipitates of two different morphologies were obtained: isolated spherulites and Liesegang rings. The results of the different experiments are included in figure 2. Spherulites - In all experiments carried out with gels of pH 6 or 7, a precipitate of spherical morphology took place. By the observation with optical microscopy they appear to be spherical precipitates consisting of thin fibrous crystals in a radial arrangement. The sizes of the spheres are variable, although diameters of 0.5 mm and even larger are most frequent. Due to their relatively large size, we were able to observe certain stages of their evolution in their growing environment with binocular lents and transmitted optical microscopy. At first, some translucent spheres are observed (Figure 3). Then these spheres become opaque and covered with crystallites of acicular morphology which gradually increase their size until they constitute a real spherulite (Figure 4). This evolution can be better understood by sectioning the spherulites, and observing the cut surface with SEM. Figure 5 shows one example in which a nucleus apparently lacking of texture is observed surrounded by acicular crystals in a radial arrangement. Qualitative chemical analysis by x-ray energy dispersion does not detect significant differences between the chemical composition of the nucleus and the

Exp. n°	gel pH				(A)			(B)			(C)	
	4,7	6	7	8	0,1 N	0,5 N	1,0 N	0,1 N	0,5 N	1,0 N	0,25 N	
4.1	●				●			●				
4.2	●				●				●			
4.3	●				●					●		
4.4	●					●		●				
4.5	●					●			●			
4.6	●					●				●		
4.7	●						●	●				
4.8	●						●		●			
4.9	●						●			●		
6.1		●			●			●				Spher.
6.2		●			●				●			
6.3		●			●					●		
6.4		●				●		●				
6.5		●				●			●			
6.6		●				●				●		
6.7		●					●	●				
6.8		●					●		●			
6.9		●					●			●		
6.10		●						●			●	
6.11		●							●		●	
6.12		●								●	●	
7.1			●		●			●				L.r. and Spher.
7.2			●		●				●			
7.3			●		●					●		
7.4			●			●		●				
7.5			●			●			●			
7.6			●			●				●		
7.7			●				●	●				
7.8			●				●		●			
7.9			●				●			●		
8.1				●	●			●				L.r.
8.2				●	●				●			
8.3				●	●					●		
8.4				●		●		●				
8.5				●		●			●			
8.6				●		●				●		
8.7				●			●	●				
8.8				●			●		●			
8.9				●			●			●		

A : PO_4H_3 ; B : Cl_2Ca ; C : $PO_4HNa_2 . 12 H_2O$

Figure 2

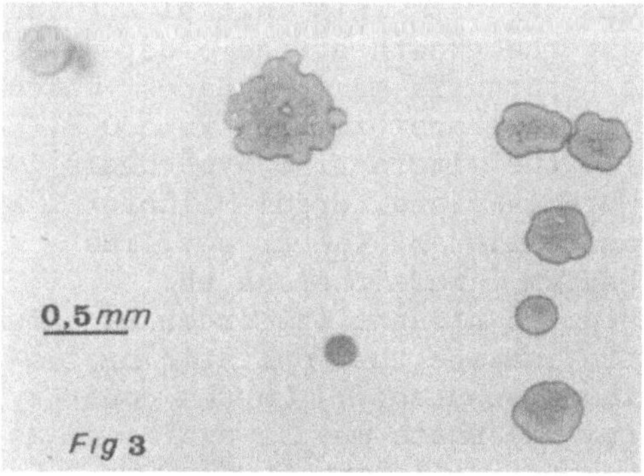

Figure 3

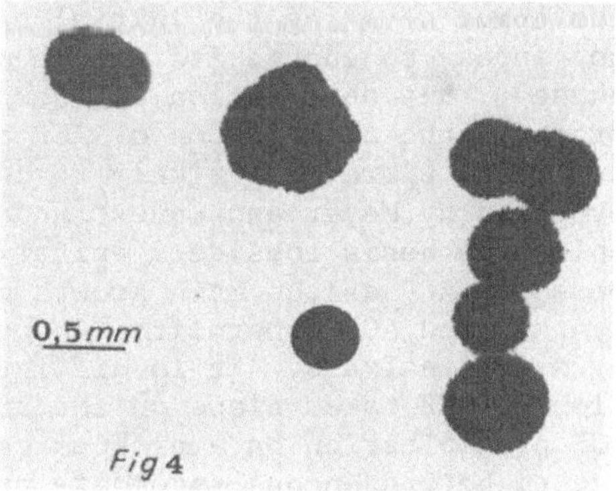

Figure 4

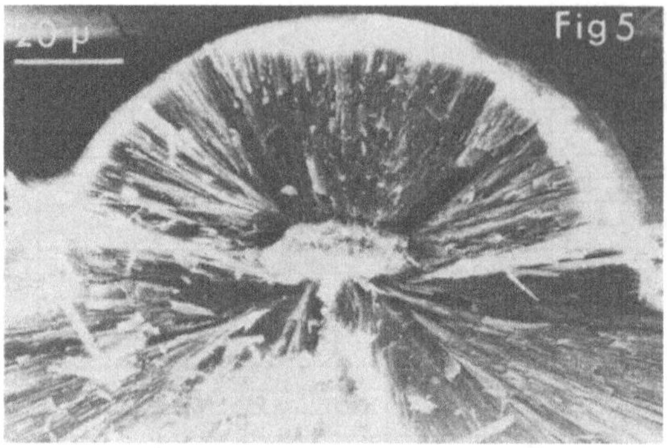

Figure 5

same of crystalline external part of the spherulite. XRD patterns of the completed spherulites shows the main reflections of the OCP (Figure 6), and the IR analysis shows (Figure 7) the typical absorption bands of the OCP[8]. The XRD patterns of the translucent spheres (Lave method) does not show any reflection, and the IR spectra (Figure 7) corresponds to one of the apatitic family, characterized by non stochiometric composition and low crystallinity, i.e. tricalcium phosphate, which has been considered as amorphous calcium phosphate[9,10].

DISCUSSION

From the results of this study an evolution hypothesis of calcium phosphate precipitation can be inferred: the translucent spheres do not show texture under SEM nor XRD; after a certain period (about 2 days) an ordered phase nucleates over them. This phase, structurally identified as OCP, takes the form of enlarged prismatic crystals (Figures 8a, b) oriented in all directions of the space covering the initial nucleus of ACP. This initial ACP does not appear to change its volume during the growth of the ordered phase. This observation opposes the hypothesis made by Eanes[2] which predicts the dissolution of ACP and later transformation into OCP. Our results are more likely to confirm the alternative hypothesis proposed by Meyer and Eanes[6] and by Brecevic and Furedi-Milhofer[3]. This hypothesis considers epitatic nucleation of the crystalline phase on ACP as the main growth mechanism. Nevertheless the synthetized ACP spherulites do not seem to present any order as shown by x-ray analysis. It is difficult to imagine that epitatic nucleation of OCP takes place on the amorphous substance. On the contrary, OCP precipitation on amorphous calcium phosphate may be explained as due to heterogeneous secondary nucleation. OCP formation is explained as a consequence of a drop of the calcium phosphate concentration due to the prior precipitation of ACP.

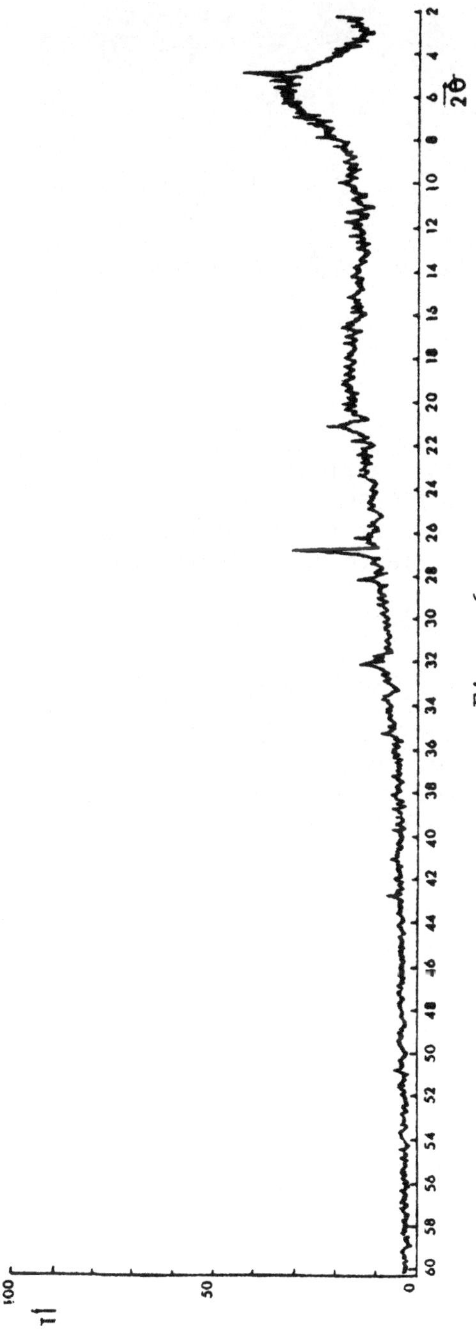

Figure 6

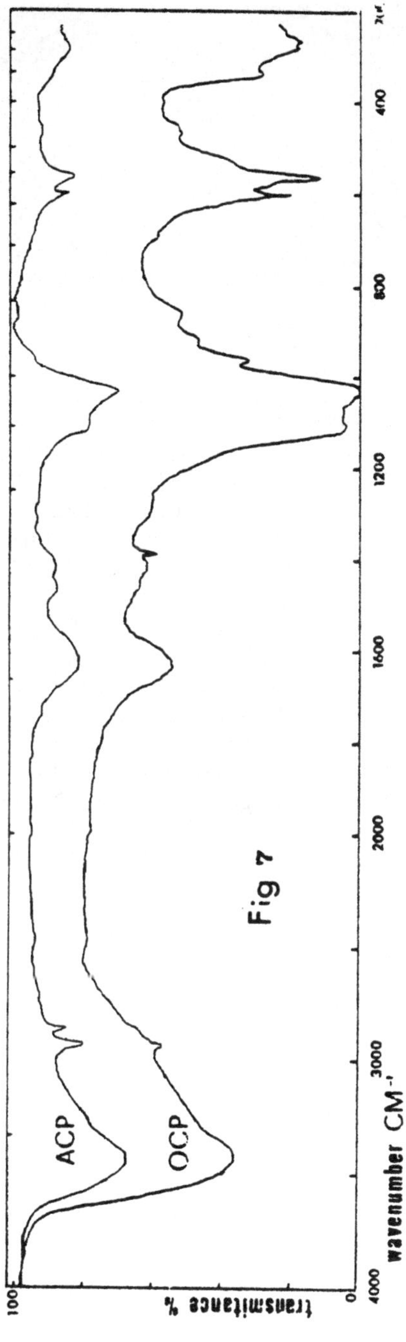

Figure 7

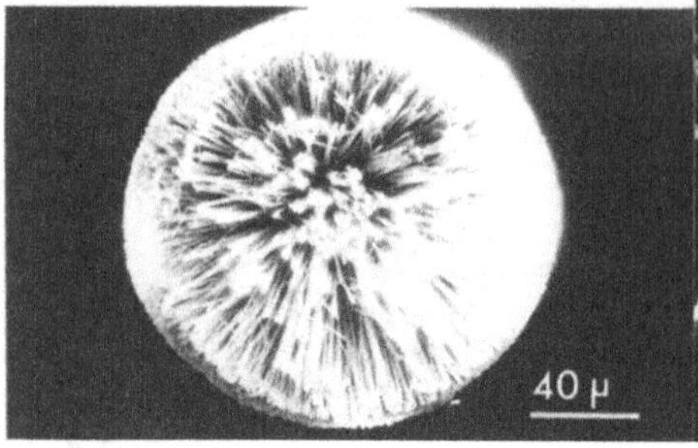

Figure 8a

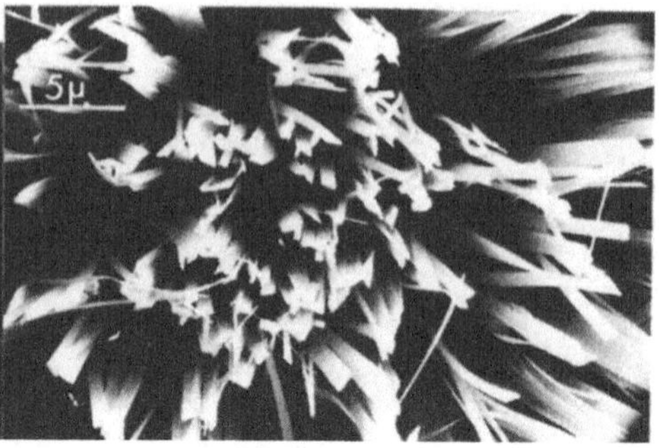

Figure 8b

REFERENCES

1. G. Montel, Coll. Int. C.N.R.S. 230:13 (1975).
2. E. D. Eanes, Coll. Int. C.N.R.S. 230:295 (1975).
3. L. J. Brecevic and H. Füredi-Milhofer, in:"Industrial Crystallization," J. W. Mullin, ed., Plenum Press, New York and London (1976).
4. A. S. Posner and F. Betts, Metab. Bone Dis. Rel. Res. 1:179 (1978).
5. B. Pokrić and Z. Pucar, Calcif. Tiss. Intl. 27:171 (1979).
6. J. L. Meyer and E. D. Eanes, Calcif. Tiss. Res. 25:59 (1978).
7. J. M. Garcia Ruiz, Fac. Geol. U. Complutense. (1976).
8. R. Z. Legeros and P. Morales, Inv. Urol. 2:12 (1973).
9. R. Z. Legeros, W. P. Shirra, M. A. Miravite, and J. P. Legeros, Coll. Int. C.N.R.S. 230:105 (1975).
10. M. Santos, C.S.I.C. 1:247 (1979).

STABILIZING FACTORS FOR URIC ACID DIHYDRATE - A CONTRIBUTION TO URIC ACID STONE FORMATION

R. H. Börner, H.-J. Schneider and W. Berg

Clinic of Urology, Friedrich-Schiller-University

Jena/GDR, Lessingstraße 1

Recently several authors, by investigations of the topographical phase distribution in uroliths, were able to demonstrate uric acid dihydrate (UAD) in the outer parts of uric acid concrements[1] analogous to weddellite in calcium oxalate stones. Scanning electron microscopic studies by our team[2,6] also suggest that initially dihydrate is formed, similar to a mechanism suggested for calcium oxalate stone genesis. In the opinion of other authors, one or several urine components can stabilize the metastable UAD phase within a certain pH range[3,4]. This was an essential starting point for the investigations under discussion.

We first studied the influence of synthetic and native urines on uric acid and UAD precipitation in the pH range between 3.0 and 5.5 by changing the qualitative and quantitative composition. The results showed that different ion contents have no significant influence on the uric acid percentage in the precipitate. Nor was it possible to demonstrate different trace element concentrations in the uric acid and UAD stone substances by means of mass spectroscopy and Laser micro analysis.

If high molecular organic substances are added to the "synthetic urines", the formation of UAD is markedly decreased (Table 1).

Starting from these results we dialysed pooled urines and studied trends of formation of UAD in the dialysis solution as well as in the dialysate.

In Figure 1 the uric acid proportion of UAD resulting from the presence of dialysate and dialysis solution are compared with those of non-dialysed pooled urines.

Table 1. Influence of High Molecular Organic Compounds on UAD-Precipitation from Synthetic Urine

Model Solution	Macro Molecular Compounds Added	UAD (%)
1	-	94
1	Heparin/hyaluronic acid	80
1	Chondroitin sulfate	80
1	Urine proteins M > 10,000	40
5	-	98
5	Chondroitin sulfate	85

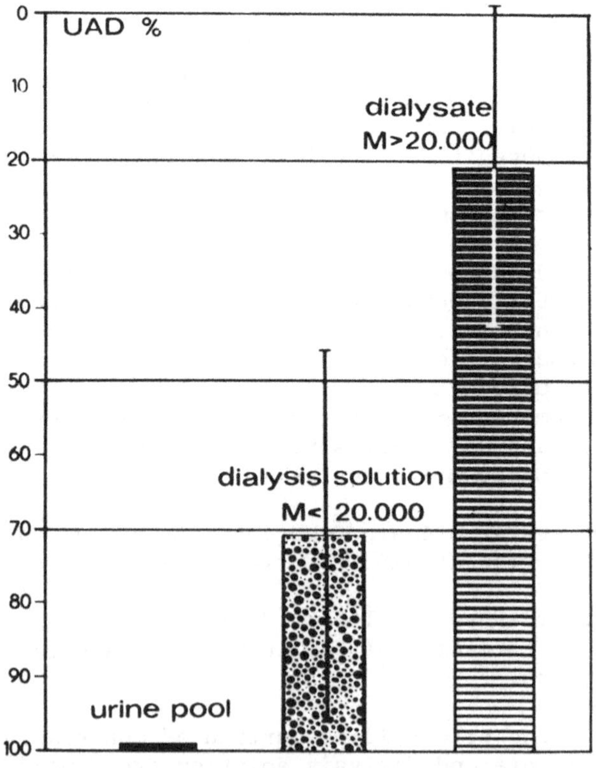

Figure 1. Influence of organic substances on UAD precipitation.

As Figure 1 shows, the brown precipitate from the dialysates have a markedly higher uric acid content (58 - 100%) than corresponding precipitates from nondialysed pooled urines, i.e. an increasing concentration of macromolecules with mol masses > 20,000 results in a decreasing stabilization of the unstable UAD phase. Hence, increased concentrations of high molecular compounds, especially of proteins, might support the transformation of original UAD microliths into uric acid.

Amino acid analyses show that the mean total amino content in uric acid stones (2.77 weight %) is higher than in UAD stones (1.95 weight %). In this connection, the good amino acid correspondence with mucoprotein in UAD precipitates from native urines (1.84 weight %) is remarkable, as shown in Figure 2.

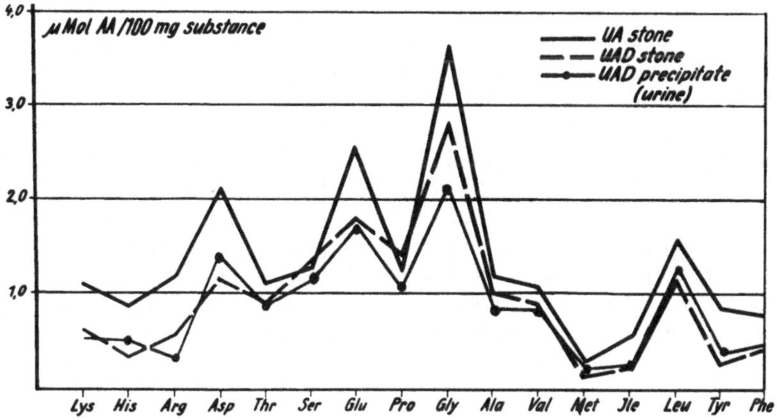

Figure 2. Mean amino acid composition in UAD uroliths.

The importance of organic urine components for the stabilization of UAD is emphasized by the following result. UAD stone substances dehydrate during thermal analysis between 40 and 140°C. This results in a weight loss of about 17%, corresponding to a loss of 2 molecules of crystal water.

UAD precipitates from native urines having a similar percentage of amino acids and identical composition (Figure 2) behave in the same way during thermal analysis. This is in contrast to the behavior of UAD precipitates from model solutions, which do not contain organic substances. Here, loss of crystal water starts at room temperature and ends at 35-40°C.

Table 2. Influence of Low Molecular Organic Substances on UAD-Precipitation

Denotation		UAD %
ML 1	all ions contained in the urine plus urea and creatinine	90
ML 8	ML 1 + bilirubin	94
ML 11	ML 1 without urea	88
ML 12	ML 1 without creatinine	99
ML 10	ML 1 without urea and creatinine	91

Studies of the influence of certain low molecular organic substances on UAD precipitation showed a slight increase of UAD in the precipitate (Table 2).

Interestingly enough, these results are consistent with the stone formation hypothesis at Charlton[5], which makes a decrease in the proteolytic activity of the urine responsible for a trend of increased stone formation. Our results suggest a connection between a decrease of "normal" proteolytic activity and an increased occurrence of high molecular substances in the urine, i.e. the rapid transformation of metastable UAD microliths into the stable uric acid phase.

REFERENCES

1. G. Brien, C. Bick, and G. Schubert, Jenaer Harnsteinsymposium, Wissenschaftliche Beitrage der Friedrich-Schiller-Universitat, Jena S.76 (1977).
2. W. Berg, A. Hesse, and H.-J. Schneider, Jenaer Harnsteinsymposium, Wissenschaftliche Beitrage der Friedrich-Schiller-Universitat, Jena S.101 (1977).
3. C. J. Laue, G. H. Nancollas, and S. J. Ko, Invest. Urol. 15:473 (1978).
4. A. Hesse, H.-J. Schneider, W. Berg, and E. Hienzsch, Invest. Urol. 12:405 (1975).
5. J. G. Jediny, Allunionskongreß fur Urologie, Kiew S.391 (1978).
6. A. Hesse, W. Berg, and C. Bothor, Int. Urol. Nephrology 11:13 (1979).

EPITAXIS BETWEEN STONE-FORMING CRYSTALS AT THE ATOMIC LEVEL

Neil S. Mandel and Gretchen S. Mandel

Department of Medicine, The Medical College of Wisconsin, and The Research Service, Wood Veterans Administration Medical Center, Milwaukee, Wisconsin 53193

Numerous treatises have been published on the common components of renal calculi and on the most frequent combinations of those crystalline materials in multicomponent stones. These studies have utilized the techniques of optical microscopy, electron microscopy, chemical analysis, and x-ray crystallography. The most common stone components are summarized in Table I. Renal calculi are frequently composed of more than one crystâlline component, and, as shown in Table II, there is a higher degree of incidence for some admixtures than others[1]. When these multicomponent stones are sectioned, the different crystalline entities are seen to lie in distinct layers, and each distinct layer is, in general, homogenous in crystalline composition.

One of the major questions still unanswered in renal calculi research concerns the mechanisms of growth in multicomponent stones. Since the multicomponent stones do not contain substantial levels of protein, researchers have suggested that epitaxy might play a major role. This manuscript explores the possible epitaxial relationships between renal stone crystals, especially at the atomic level.

The bonding forces involved in the growth of a single crystallite are very similar to those bonding interactions occurring at the interface between two or more crystallites of the same crystalline material. Within a paracrystalline sample, which is composed of clusters of paracrystalline arrays, the crystal structure and crystallographic symmetry is identical within every finitely defined single crystalline domain. As a crystal grows, molecules from the solution phase become oriented in the proper crystallographic orientation, form the necessary chemical contacts and become an integral

Table 1. The Crystalline Substances Most Frequently Occurring in Renal Calucli

MINERAL NAMES	CHEMICAL NOMENCLATURE	CHEMICAL FORMULA
WHEWELLITE	CALCIUM OXALATE MONOHYDRATE	$CaC_2O_4 \cdot H_2O$
WEDDELITE	CALCIUM OXALATE DIHYDRATE	$CaC_2O_4 \cdot (2{+}x)H_2O$
HYDROXYAPATITE	BASIC CALCIUM HYDROGEN PHOSPHATE	$Ca_5(PO_4)_3(OH)$
BRUSHITE	CALCIUM HYDROGEN PHOSPHATE	$CaHPO_4 \cdot 2H_2O$
WHITLOCKITE	β-TRICALCIUM PHOSPHATE	β-$Ca_3(PO_4)_2$
STRUVITE	MAGNESIUM AMMONIUM PHOSPHATE HEXAHYDRATE	$Mg(NH_4)(PO_4) \cdot 6H_2O$
	URIC ACID	$C_5H_4N_4O_3$
	URIC ACID DIHYDRATE	$C_5H_4N_4O_3 \cdot 2H_2O$
	MONOSODIUM URATE MONOHYDRATE	$Na\ C_5H_4N_4O_3 \cdot H_2O$
	ℓ-CYSTINE	$S_2C_6H_{12}N_2O_4$
	OCTACALCIUM PHOSPHATE	$Ca_8H_2(PO_4)_6 \cdot 5H_2O$

Table 2. An Analysis of 1,000 Urinary Calculi by Optical Inspection, Chemical Analysis, and X-ray Powder Diffraction in England in the Early 1960s[1].

COMPONENTS	PERCENTAGE OCCURRENCE
PURE WHEWELLITE	13.7
PURE WEDDELITE	0.4
WHEWELLITE + WEDDELITE	18.6
WHEWELLITE + APATITE	7.2
WEDDELITE + APATITE	4.7
WHEWELLITE + WEDDELITE + APATITE	22.4
PURE APATITE	3.4
PURE URIC ACID	4.7
URIC ACID + OTHER SUBSTANCES	1.1
PURE CYSTINE	2.2
CYSTINE + OTHER SUBSTANCES	-0-

part of the crystalline lattice. Those chemical contacts include van der Waals interactions, hydrogen bonding such that most, if not all, available hydrogen bond donor and acceptor atoms are hydrogen bonded, and electrostatic interactions such as cation--anion coordination polyhedra. When the cation is calcium, the number of calcium--anion coordination interactions ranges from 5-9. If a molecular dislocation occurs in the process of single crystal growth, a new crystallite begins to grow with a new preferred crystal growth direction. There are, of course, many environmental parameters which could influence preferred crystal growth and therefore induce new crystallite formation on the original single crystal lattice.

It is possible to extrapolate from ideal homogenous cocrystallization to the heterogeneous systems frequently observed in multicomponent renal calculi. Within the two-component stone such as hydroxyapatite/whewellite, the crystalline lattices of the two respective crystalline structures are in contact, and "sense" each other at the molecular level. Within the three-component stone such as hydroxyapatite/whewellite/weddelite, the crystalline lattice of calcium oxalate monohydrate is in molecular contact with two different crystalline structures. If the different crystalline lattices interact with each other at the atomic level, the molecular distributions at the contact faces in both lattices must be chemically complementary. For a stable crystalline complex to be formed, the molecular bonding of the two different structures must be supportive of each other at the contact zone. The process of orientated overgrowth of one crystalline lattice onto another crystalline lattice is termed "epitaxy" and is the subject of the second half of this manuscript.

Since the contact zone in an epitaxial system involves the interactions of the atoms of the two different crystal structures and since these interactions must satisfy the bonding requirements of both structures simultaneously, we must first understand the various bonding interactions evidenced in each of the stone's single crystal structures. The crystal structures covered in this manuscript[2] are calcium oxalate monohydrate (whewellite), calcium oxalate dihydrate (weddelite), uric acid and hydroxyapatite.

WHEWELLITE

A crystallographic molecular packing drawing of the structure of calcium oxalate monohydrate[3] (whewellite) is shown in Figure 1a. The calcium atoms in the drawing are denoted by the smaller circles, and the calcium coordination is indicated with dashed lines. The calcium atoms in the structure bind to oxalate oxygen atoms and to the water molecule of crystallization. The major bonding forces involved in forming the structure is the calcium coordination, with some added strength from water hydrogen bonds to oxalate oxygens.

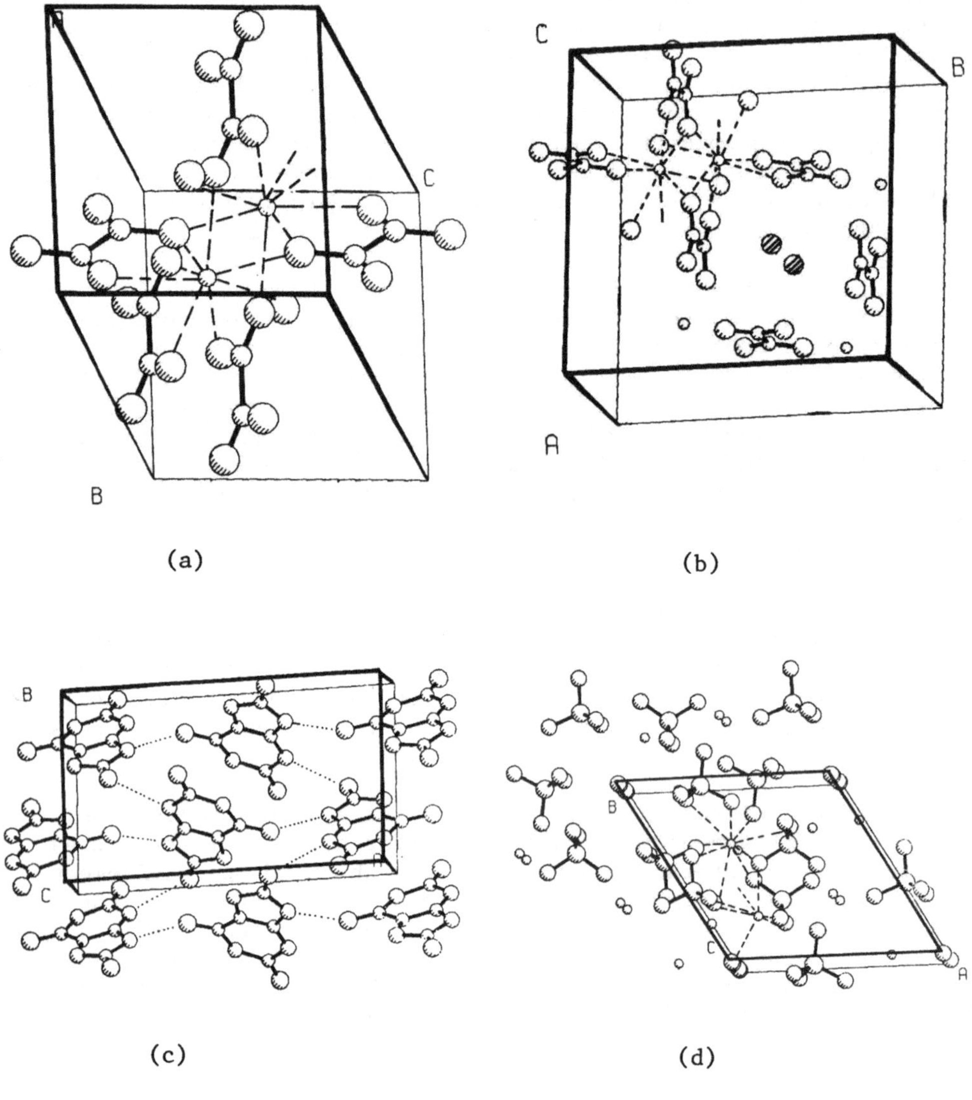

Figure 1. The molecular packing drawing of the structure of (a) whewellite--calcium oxalate monohydrate, (b) weddelite--calcium oxalate dihydrate, (c) uric acid, and (d) hydroxyapatite.

The two unconnected Ca--contacts indicate two Ca--O contacts between the calcium atom and an oxalate anion above the plane of the drawing.

WEDDELITE

The molecular packing drawing for calcium oxalate dihydrate[4] (weddelite) is shown in Figure 1b. The calcium atoms are denoted by the smaller circles, and the calcium coordination is indicated with dashed lines. For clarity, the coordination polyhedra about the calcium atoms are not shown in their entirety; however, as in the whewellite case, the direction of the remaining Ca--O contacts are noted with dashed lines. The calcium coordination forms the major force holding the structure together. The two water molecules, which are in contact with the calcium atoms, form hydrogen bonds to oxalate oxygens.

Even though the weddelite structure is referred to as calcium oxalate dihydrate, the chemical formula, as determined by single crystal x-ray crystallography, is $CaC_2O_4 \cdot (2+X)H_2O$. The additional water of crystallization denoted by the X can be seen as the two striped atoms in the center of Figure 1b. The oxalate anions form a channel which runs throughout the crystal and contains these X water molecules. The water molecules in the channel are structurally disordered; that is, instead of occupying one stable position in the lattice, the water molecule occupies different positions within the channel. At one point in the structure the water molecule will occupy a different position than in another part of the structure, and it is therefore impossible to quantitate how much water of crystallization resides within the channel.

URIC ACID

The three-dimensional structure of the purine uric acid[5] is shown in Figure 1c. This structure, in contrast to the previous structures, is held together exclusively through an elaborate hydrogen bonding network. The purine molecules form sheets with each neighboring molecule being inclined by 60 degrees to each other. The molecules therefore form rows of co-planar molecules where the rows are held together and in place by hydrogen bonds. The hydrogen bonds are denoted with dotted lines; they are formed by nitrogen-hydrogen--oxygen contacts (N-H--O).

HYDROXYAPATITE

The structure of hydroxyapatite[6], as shown in Figure 1d, was left for last due to its complicated molecular packing and bonding interactions. The structure contains two independent calcium atoms, denoted by the small circles in the drawing. One calcium atom coordinates to nine phosphate oxygen atoms, and the second calcium atom coordinates to six phosphate oxygen atoms, and the anion residing in the anion channel. The channel may contain hydroxyl, chloro, fluoro, or other anions, and can be seen in the corners of the repeating structural unit defined by the prism in the figure. The primary force holding the structure together is the calcium coordination.

The anion substitution channel is in contact distance to only one calcium atom. If the ion is a hydroxyl group, the structure becomes disordered; that is, for the hydroxyl group to form hydrogen bonds to the phosphate oxygens, it will be forced to occupy an atomic position different from a fluorine atom, destroying the crystallographic symmetrical repeat. This atomic coordinate shift is termed "disorder" and hinders the determination of accurate atomic positions for the atoms sitting in the anion substitution channel.

EPITAXY

Epitaxial growth, as described earlier, is the oriented overgrowth of one crystalline lattice onto another. In the multicomponent stone, the atoms on the surface of the substrate crystalline lattice must bind the molecules of a new chemical substance in a very specific way for the growth of a new crystalline lattice on that substrate. The two crystalline lattices are in molecular contact with each other, and the atomic arrays at the epitaxial contact zone must be both chemically and structurally compatible. The degree of complementarity in the two crystalline lattices probably need not extend beyond the layer of molecules at the contact zone.

There is no direct evidence for the definitive proof that epitaxis is the major mechanism for the growth of multicomponent renal calculi. Scanning electron microscopic studies[7-9] have shown that, at least in some of the multicomponent systems, seed crystals of the substrate enhance the crystallization of the second crystalline phase.

X-ray crystallographic research on epitaxy in renal calculi has to date been limited to comparison of the dimensions of the prominent crystal growth faces in the common stone components. The most recent study[10], published in 1968, was limited to two prominent crystal growth faces in uric acid as the substrate and did not calculate the percent misfit in contact faces for any other common match. The number of excellent fits in the dimensions of uric acid, uric acid dihydrate, whewellite, and weddelite were too numerous to be coincidental, and it was concluded that epitaxis was definitely possible in stones containing these substances.

We have extended the calculation of the percent misfit for the common stone components, relaxing all restrictions of preferential growth directions. The criteria[11] used in our calculation of lattice misfit included: 1) the lengths of the two lattice vectors in the selected two-dimensional slice through the three-dimensional structure; 2) the angles between these two lattice vectors defining the possible contact face; and 3) a parameter indicating the general complexity of the associated atomic pattern on the possible contact plane. The complexity of the atomic array is assessed by assigning a unit area to a cation, an anion, or a molecule and estimating the density of these molecular fragments on the contact surface. Thus, lattice nets with large network areas yield higher values of the atomic density index. Possible epitaxial matches are sorted on the sum of the generalized misfit and the effective atomic density (the sum of 1, 2 and 3), with the matches having the lowest values of the sum ranking the highest in potential for epitaxis (see Table 3).

Table 3

CRYSTAL LATTICE A	CRYSTAL LATTICE B	NO. OF MATCHES WITH ERRORS		
		<15%	<10%	<5%
WHEWELLITE	URIC ACID	110	26	2
	URIC ACID DIHYDRATE	68	12	3
	MONOSODIUM URATE MONOHYDRATE	245	18	0
	WEDDELITE	32	4	0
	CALCIUM OXALATE TRIHYDRATE	47	47	2
	HYDROXYAPATITE	9	3	0
	BRUSHITE	85	13	0
	STRUVITE	118	9	0
	WHITLOCKITE	0	0	0
	OCTACALCIUM PHOSPHATE	29	6	0
	CYSTINE	18	2	1
HYDROXYAPATITE	BRUSHITE	14	1	0
	WEDDELITE	2	1	0
	URIC ACID	8	2	0
URIC ACID	WEDDELITE	13	1	1
	URIC ACID DIHYDRATE	42	8	2
	MONOSODIUM URATE MONOHYDRATE	134	13	0

The large number of matches, as shown above, seem to indicate that there are large numbers of possible epitaxial matches in multi-component stones. It is also noteworthy that the number of possible matches markedly drops as the allowable percent misfit is reduced from 15 to 10%, and approaches zero when the cutoff is 5%. The results of these dimensional calculations are by no means consistent with clinical findings. For example, the stone of high frequency -- apatite/whewellite/weddelite -- would not have been predicted to exist (insofar as epitaxis is concerned) due to the lack of any matches at or below the 5% misfit cutoff. In contrast, the admixture of whewellite/cystine is predicted to have one fit below 5%, even though the clinical incidence is extremely low. The number of false negative and positive dimensional matches strongly suggest that additional parameters must be analyzed for the determination of epitaxis in multicomponent calculi. The additional parameter which must be included is an analysis of the atomic structures of the two contacting crystal lattices.

To represent the atomic interactions at the epitaxial interface, we have prepared a series of gray-line overlays of the molecular structures. In these figures, the substract crystal lattice is denoted in gray, and the epitaxially deposited lattice is black. We have examined most of the potential dimensional matches reported at 10% misfit using these atomic overlays, and have successfully determined the most probable atomic match. In general, the number of possible epitaxial matches has been reduced to one or two molecular orientations of the two crystal lattices.

We have imposed stringent molecular bonding and molecular contact constraints in the molecular overlay studies. In systems which contained calcium cations, we required that the calcium coordination environment be maintained with substitutions of oxygen atoms from the epitaxially deposited crystal lattice. In systems containing water of crystallization, we required that the hydrogen bonding potential of the water be continued at the molecular interface. Similarly, when the epitaxially deposited layer contained molecules which had additional hydrogen bonding capabilities, we required that all possible hydrogen bonding be complete. Finally, in systems which contained identical cations and/or anions, we required that these ions not be in atomic positions which would create charge repulsion. In most cases, this restriction necessitated that the cations and anions be in similar positions in both lattices so that atomic substitution was possible.

A molecular overlay of weddelite on whewellite is shown on the following page (Fig.2). The gray-line drawing is whewellite and the black lattice conforms to weddelite. In this drawing, the calcium atoms are the smaller circles, with those on the surface of the structure being darkened. The oxygen atoms of the oxalate anion on the surface are striped, and the water oxygen atoms are crossed. The oxalate anions are seen to lie in very similar positions in both structures, and the calcium atoms are also in positions for atomic substitution; that is, the calcium atoms in the weddelite lattice could be substituted (at the interface zone) for the calcium atoms on the surface of the whewellite structure. The oxalate anions are also easily substituted. The water molecules in both lattices are in

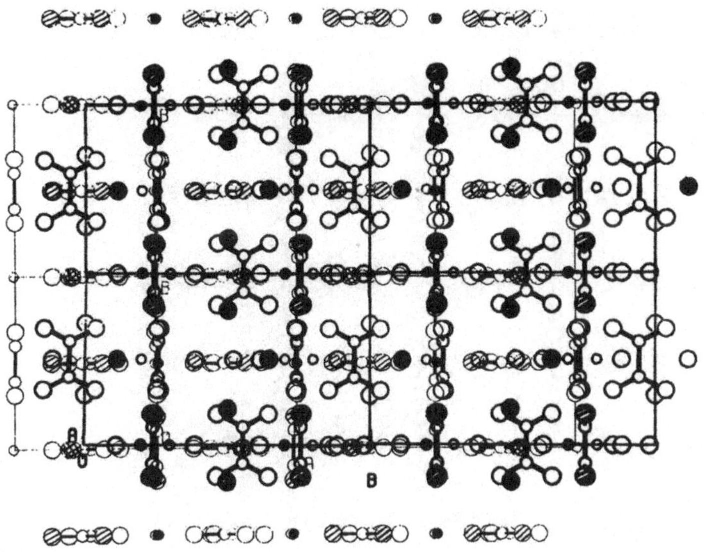

Figure 2. Molecular overlay of weddelite on whewellite.

perfect atomic positions for hydrogen bond contacts to the oxalate oxygen atoms of the other lattice. The atomic match using these two crystallographic lattice nets, which were calculated to have less than 10% dimensional misfit, is excellent. The remaining three lattice matches with less than 10% dimensional misfit were not epitaxially complementary at the atomic level.

The best atomic match between the whewellite and uric acid lattices is shown on the following page (Fig. 3). Uric acid has been used as the substrate lattice and is shown in gray-line. The calcium atoms are the smaller circles, with those on the surface of the whewellite lattice being darkened. The surface oxygen atoms of the oxalate anion and of the purine ring are striped, and the surface purine ring nitrogen atoms are crossed. In the specific molecular orientations depicted in the drawing, the purine rings and oxalate ions are inclined at approximately 40 degrees, an ideal orientation for hydrogen bond formation between the oxalate oxygen atoms and the purine ring nitrogen atoms (N-H--O hydrogen bonds). The calcium coordination is maintained by substituting some of the oxygen atoms in the oxalate system with the oxygen atoms of the purine ring system. The structure at the interface is therefore supported by continued calcium coordination and hydrogen bonding between the purine rings and the oxalate anions. The atomic overlay is excellent in the whewellite/uric acid system.

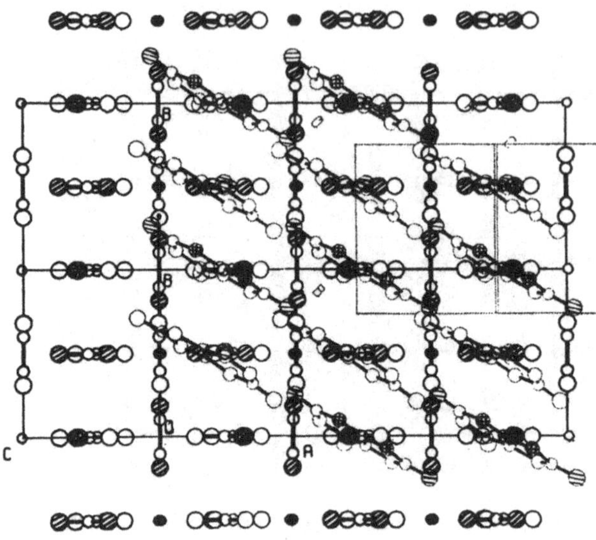

Figure 3. Atomic match between the whewellite and uric acid lattices.

One of the atomic matches predicted from the dimensional misfit calculations for hydroxyapatite and whewellite, with the apatite lattice being the substrate and denoted in gray-line, is shown below (Fig. 4). All three-dimensional misfits with an error less than 10% did not yield atomic matches that were complementary. In no orientation could the calcium coordination be maintained with atomic substitution as in the case of whewellite/weddelite, and in no case could charge repulsion be avoided. It therefore appears that hydroxyapatite does not form an epitaxial match with whewellite, but rather serves as a nucleating site for secondary crystal growth.

SUMMARY

An analysis of the crystal structures of the common components of renal calculi has shown that the cation containing structures such as whewellite, weddelite, and apatite all have well-defined cation--anion interactions. These cation coordination polyhedra play a major role in the bonding forces which hold the crystalline lattices together. In the non-cation containing structure of uric acid, the major force holding the crystalline lattice intace is an elaborate hydrogen bonding network.

A comparison of the dimensions of possible contact faces in these structures has indicated a large number of dimensional matches. It is possible to predict if any of these matches are epitaxially mediated using computer generated atomic overlays. In the whewellite/weddelite and whewellite/uric acid systems, the two

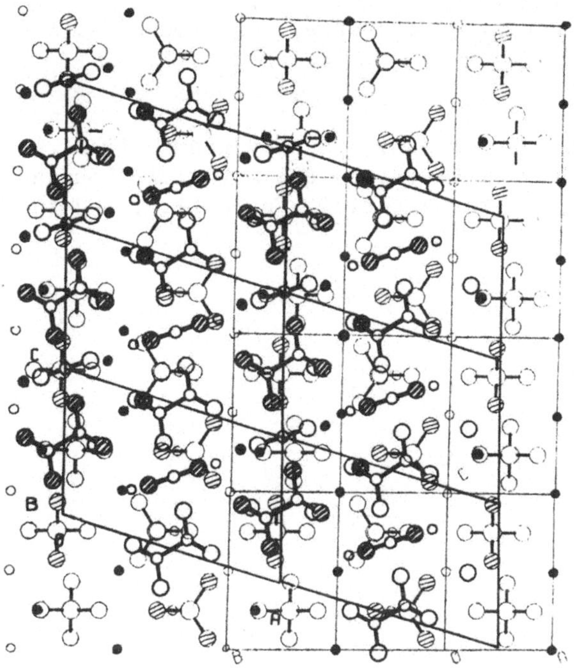

Figure 4. Atomic match between hydroxyapatite and whewellite lattices.

interacting crystal structures are totally supportive of each other at the atomic level. These interactions allow for anion and/or cation substitutions, and strong hydrogen bond interactions. The apatite/whewellite system, however, does not appear to be epitaxially mediated, since the two atomic structures are not supportive. These studies are being extended to include the remaining possible epitaxial matches in multicomponent renal calculi.

REFERENCES

1. B. T. Murphy and L. N. Pyrah, Br. J. Urol. 34:129 (1962).
2. G. Mandel and N. Mandel, Am. Crystal. Assoc. Mtg. (abstract) (1979).
3. S. Deganelo, private communication (1979).
4. C. Sterling, Acta. Crystallographica 18:917 (1965).
5. H. Ringertz, Acta. Crystallographica 20:397 (1966).
6. M. I. Kay, R. A. Young, and A. S. Posner, Nature 204:1050 (1964).
7. J. L. Meyer, J. H. Bergert, and L. H. Smith, Clin. Sci. Mol. Med. 49:369 (1975).
8. J. L. Meyer, J. H. Bergert, and L. H. Smith, Invest. Urol. 14:115 (1976).
9. J. L. Meyer, J. H. Bergert, and L. H. Smith, Clin. Sci. Mol. Med. 52:143 (1977).

10. K. Lonsdale, Nature 217:56 (1968).
11. B. Dickens and L. W. Schroeder, NBS Technical Note 893 (1976).

ACKNOWLEDGMENTS

This work is supported in part by grants from the Kroc Foundation for Medical Research, the Arthritis Foundation, the Wisconsin Chapter of the Arthritis Foundation, and the Veterans Administration.

THE EFFECT OF SEED CRYSTALS ON CALCIUM OXALATE NUCLEATION

John R. Burns* and Birdwell Finlayson

*Division of Urology, Department of Surgery, University of Alabama in Birmingham, Birmingham, Alabama, 35294 and Division of Urology, Department of Surgery, University of Florida, Gainesville, Florida 32610

INTRODUCTION

It has been well documented that renal stones are often non-homogeneous in composition[1,2]. The small areas of additional mineral phases often found have led to theories invoking epitaxy as an important factor in stone formation. Both Coe et al. and Pak et al. have demonstrated an increase in calcium oxalate heterogeneous nucleation by sodium acid urate seed crystals[3,4,5]. Meyer et al. have shown an increase in calcium oxalate nucleation by seed crystals of hydroxyapatite[6]. All these studies have been performed with solution-depletion techniques. We have chosen to study the heterogeneous nucleation of calcium oxalate by examining actual calcium oxalate particle production. This approach allowed us to study not only changes in particle production, but also shifts in particle size distribution.

METHODS AND MATERIALS

Reagent-grade chemicals were used throughout. All solution were prepared with distilled water passed through a 0.45 μm Millipore filter. A calcium chloride solution was rapidly mixed with a solution of potassium oxalate in the presence and absence of various seed crystals. The resulting solutions were kept mixed by continuous overhead stirring. After 15 min, we analyzed the precipitated calcium oxalate crystals for both total count and size distribution with a Coulter Model TA II counter. All experiments were carried out in double-walled Pyrex beakers maintained at 38°C with a circulating water bath. The pH was recorded, but not adjusted. The final solution volume was 100 ml.

Calcium Oxalate Nucleation Without Added Seeds

The test solution contained 1mM calcium and 1mM oxalate and had a pH of 6.2-6.8. Precipitation with this solution was repeated until a reproducible total particle count and a reproducible particle distribution curve were obtained (N=32). We then determined the effect of seed crystals by comparison with this unseeded system.

Calcium Oxalate Nucleation With Calcium Oxalate Seed Crystals

The test solution contained 1mM calcium, 1mM oxalate, and 10 cc of calcium oxalate seed. Calcium oxalate seed crystals were prepared by the rapid addition of 50 cc of 100 mM calcium chloride to 50 cc of 100 mM potassium oxalate. The calcium oxalate precipitate was stirred for 15 min and then allowed to settle. Particles remaining in suspension at the end of this time were siphoned off and used as seeds. Because the seed crystals were unstable after more than about 2-3 h, we prepared them freshly for each experiment. A sample of the seed crystal solution was passed through a set of Nuclepore™ filters ranging in pore diameter from 0.03 to 0.8 µm. The number and size of the seed crystals were determined from scanning electron micrographs of the particles trapped on the 0.03 µm filters.

Calcium Oxalate Nucleation With Sodium Acid Urate

Sodium acid urate suspension was filtered through a 0.45 µm Millipore filter, and the filtrate used as a seed crystal solution. As outlined previously, scanning electron micrographs were used to determine particle size and number. To prevent possible particle dissolution, we prepared the potassium oxalate solutions with a saturated sodium acid urate solution previously passed through a 0.05 µM Millipore filter. We tested calcium oxalate nucleation at two calcium-to-oxalate ratios. The first test solution contained 1 mM calcium, 1 mM oxalate, and 10 cc of sodium acid urate seeds (N=11). The second contained 0.2 mM oxalate, 5 mM calcium, and amounts of 10-40 cc of sodium acid urate seeds (N=9). The pH was 7.1-7.5.

Calcium Oxalate Precipitation With Hydroxyapatite Seed Crystals

The hydroxyapatite crystals formed agglomerates 1-3 µm in diameter. The final test solution consisted of 1 mM calcium, 1 mM oxalate, and hydroxyapatite seeds numbering 6.3 x 10^6 per cubic centimeter. The pH of the solutions averaged 7.8.

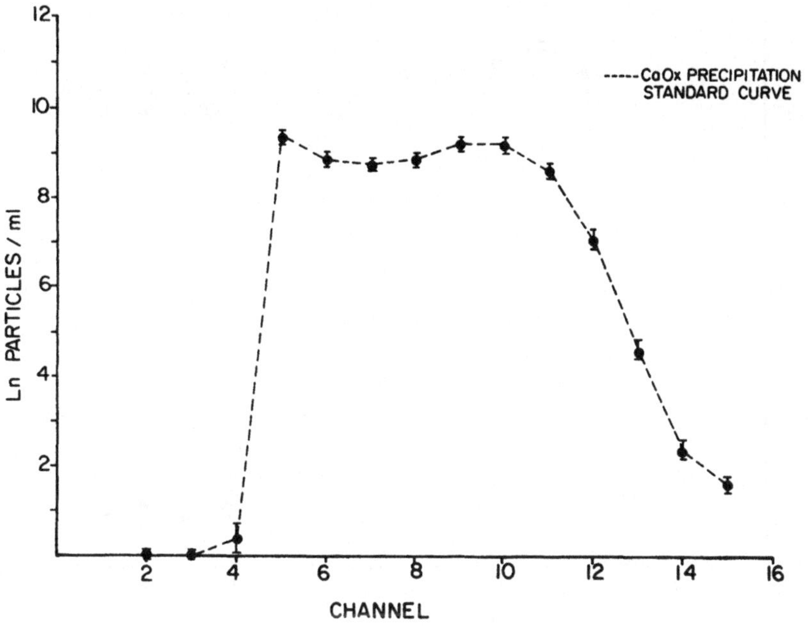

Figure 1. Calcium oxalate precipitation without added seed crystals. Ln total particles, 11.02 ± 0.34. Error bars represent standard error of mean (S.E.M.).

RESULTS

Calcium Oxalate Nucleation Without Added Seeds

Figure 1 shows the standard curve for calcium oxalate nucleation in the absence of seed crystals. Each particle counted is thought to represent at least one nucleation event. Each successive channel indicates a doubling of the particle volume, with channel 2 representing a diameter of 1.78 μm. As stated previously, all particles were counted 15 min after mixing. Although equilibrium had not been achieved by 15 min, previous (unpublished) data had shown that a plateau in total particle number is usually reached within 15 min. For the calcium oxalate nucleation in this experiment, calculations indicate 51% completion at 15 min. The average volume of calcium oxalate particles precipitated was 3.09×10^7 μm^3.

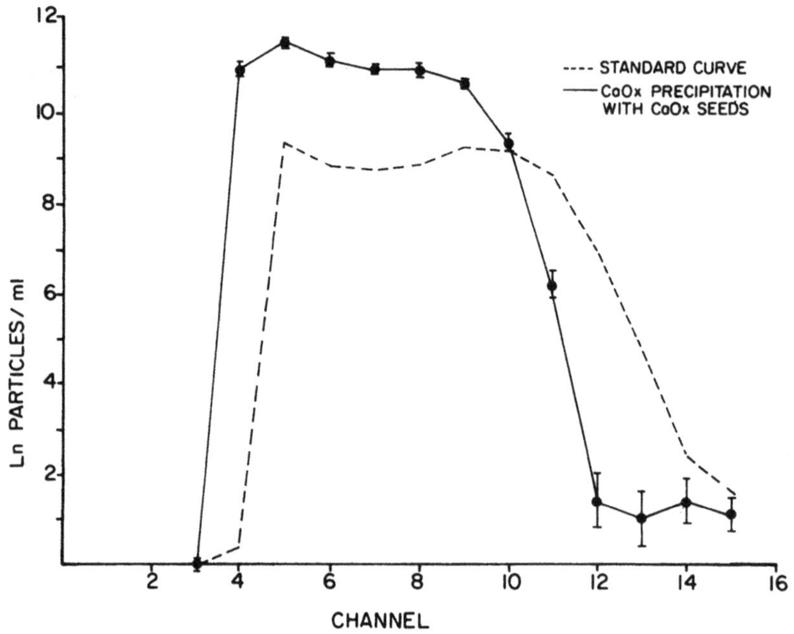

Figure 2. Calcium oxalate precipitation with added calcium oxalate seed crystals. Ln total particles, 12.96 ± 0.23. Error bars represent S.E.M.

Calcium Oxalate Nucleation With Calcium Oxalate Seed Crystals

The number of seed crystals added was estimated to be approximately 2.31×10^6 per milliliter in the test solution with an average diameter of 0.7 µm. Figure 2 shows the effect of the addition of calcium oxalate seeds. There is a marked increase in the total particle count ($p < 0.001$). The curve shows a shift to the left, indicating the production of an increased number of smaller calcium oxalate crystals. After subtraction of the volume of the seed crystals themselves, the average volume of newly precipitated calcium oxalate is 4.9×10^7 µm. This volume is significantly increased over that of the unseeded system ($p < 0.001$), indicating that the calcium oxalate seeds in some way increase the rate of the reaction toward equilibrium. Although the total particle count (Figure 2) increased by 3.64×10^5 particles/cc, this increase represents only 16% of the 2.31×10^6 seed crystals/cc added. As to efficiency, apparently less than one in six of the calcium oxalate seed crystals are functioning as effective nucleators.

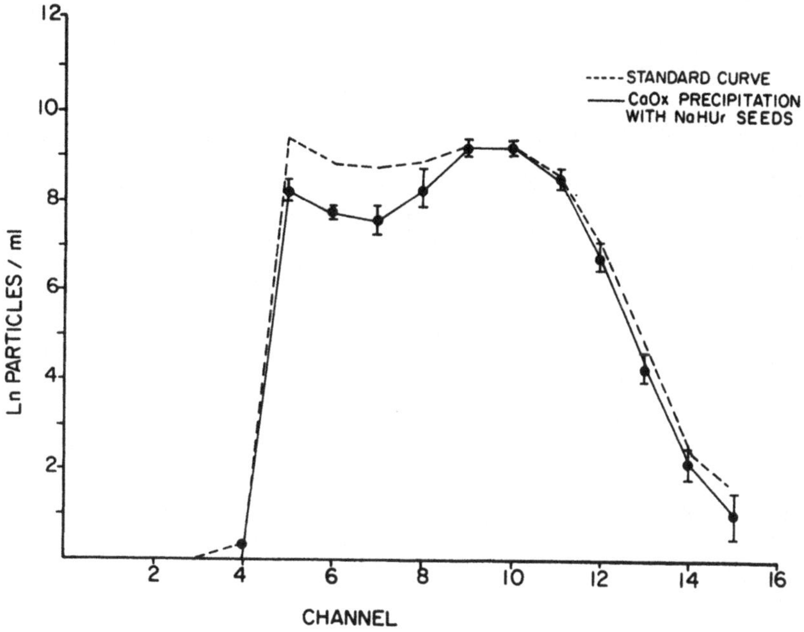

Figure 3. Calcium oxalate precipitation with added NaHUr seed crystals. Ln total particles, 10.69 ± 0.44. Error bars represent S.E.M.

Calcium Oxalate Nucleation With Sodium Acid Urate Seed Crystals

The sodium acid urate seed crystals were rod-like, with dimensions of 3 x 0.3 µm. With a solution of 1 mM calcium, 1 mM oxalate, and 1.0×10^6 sodium acid urate seeds/ml, there is no evidence of enhancement of calcium oxalate nucleation (Figure 3). This is, rather, a small but significant ($p < 0.05$) decrease in the number of calcium oxalate particles precipitated. Calculations indicate that less than one in 1,000 of the seed crystals could be functioning as effective nucleators. With a computer equilibrium program described elsewhere[7], we estimated the initial relative supersaturation of the solution at 65. In solutions consisting of 0.2 mM oxalate, 5 mM calcium, and various amounts of sodium acid urate seeds (Figure 4), there is an increase in nucleation by the sodium acid urate seeds. The increase appears to be directly related to the number of seeds added. We estimated the initial relative supersaturation of this test solution at 21. Although the sodium acid urate seeds in this second test solution significantly increased calcium oxalate nucleation ($p < 0.001$), apparently only 0.5% of the seeds were acting as effective nucleators.

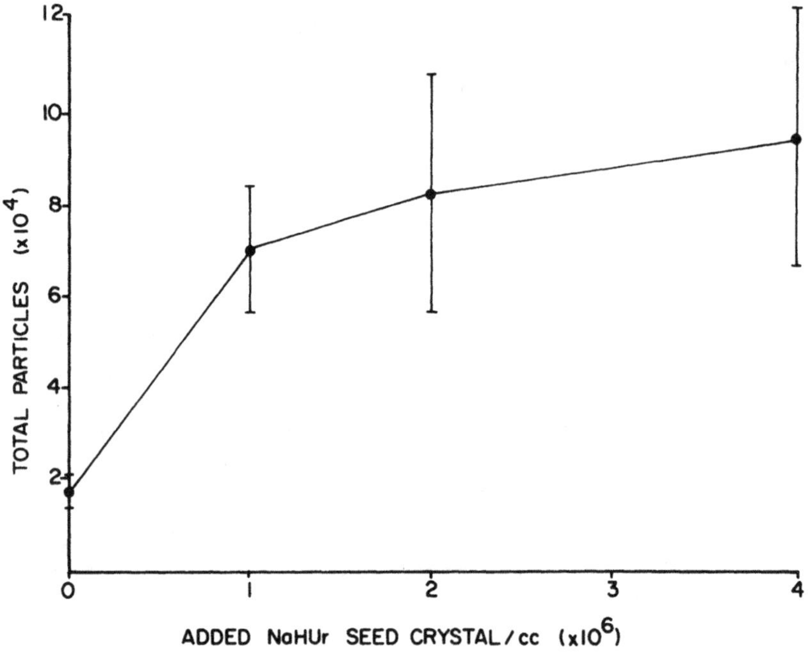

Figure 4. Calcium oxalate precipitation with various numbers of added NaHUr seed crystals. Error bars represent S.E.M.

Calcium Oxalate Nucleation With Hydroxyapatite Seed Crystals

The addition of hydroxyapatite seeds resulted in an apparent increase in the number of calcium oxalate particles precipitated. However, if the contribution of the seeds alone to the total count is excluded (Figure 5), the number of calcium oxalate crystals precipitated is 52% less than the control value.

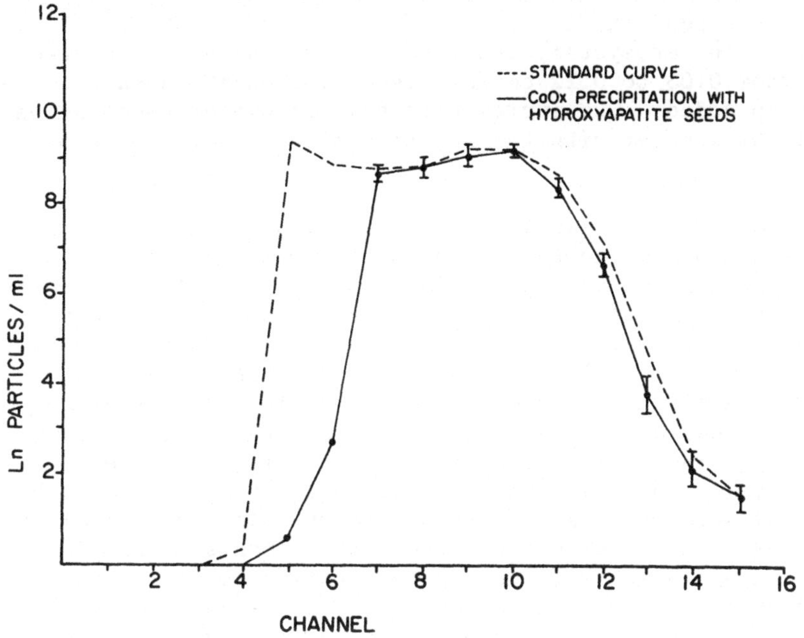

Figure 5. Calcium oxalate precipitation with added hydroxyapatite seed crystals (background seed count subtracted). Error bars represent S.E.M.

DISCUSSION

The process of heterogeneous nucleation is probably important in the formation of all calcium oxalate calculi. It is still unknown, however, what substances in urine are able to function effectively as heterogeneous nuclei. Because the epitaxial growth of one substance on another is in part a function of the degree of registry match between lattice faces, calcium oxalate crystals should serve as ideal nucleators for calcium oxalate precipitation. However, only one of every six calcium oxalate seed crystals in our solutions was able to serve as a nucleator.

The ability of sodium acid urate seed crystals to function as nucleators appears to be related to several factors. The surface area of the added seed crystals in the system is probably of major importance. Other investigators in this field have used sodium acid urate seeds with a total surface area of 10-40 cm^2/ml of solution. In our system, the total surface area of the seeds varies from 0.03 to 0.12 cm^2/ml, depending on the amount of seed suspension added. The increase in calcium oxalate nucleation would probably be greater with the addition of a larger amount of surface area.

The degree of relative supersaturation may also be important in heterogeneous nucleation. In our experiments, there was no increase in calcium oxalate nucleation at high relative supersaturation (1 mM calcium, 1 mM oxalate). There was, however, an increase in the system with lower relative supersaturation (0.2 mM oxalate, 5 mM calcium). At least two possible mechanisms can be invoked to explain this phenomenon. The high concentrations of calcium and oxalate may in some way poison the sodium acid urate seeds, rendering them incapable of functioning as nuclei. Alternatively, there may be an unequal competition of mass between the sodium acid urate seeds and other heterogeneous nuclei at high relative supersaturation. Whatever the mechanism, it appears that, even at physiologic relative supersaturation, sodium acid urate is not a particularly effective nucleator, inasmuch as only about one in 200 seed particles were capable of nucleating calcium oxalate.

With hydroxyapatite, we were unable to show any increase in calcium oxalate nucleation. That may be related to the size of our crystals, the relative supersaturation of our test solution, or other factors.

REFERENCES

1. E. L. Prien and C. Frondel, J. Urol. 57:949 (1947).
2. L. C. Herring, J. Urol. 88:545 (1962).
3. F. L. Coe, R. L. Lawton, R. B. Goldstein, and V. Tembe, Proc. Soc. Exp. Biol. Med. 149:926 (1975).
4. C. Y. C. Pak and L. H. Arnold, Proc. Soc. Exp. Biol. Med. 149:930 (1975).
5. C. Y. C. Pak, Y. Hayashi, and L. H. Arnold, Proc. Soc. Exp. Biol. Med. 153:83 (1976).
6. J. L. Meyer, J. H. Bergert, and L. H. Smith, in:"Colloquium in Renal Lithiasis," B. Finlayson and W. C. Thomas, Jr., ed., University Presses of Florida, Gainesville (1976).
7. B. Finlayson, in:"Calcium Metabolism in Renal Failure and Nephrolithiasis," D. S. David, ed., John Wiley and Sons, New York (1977).

ACKNOWLEDGMENT

This work was supported by NIH SCOR Grant in Urolithiasis, AM 20586-03.

THE EFFECT OF URINARY pH ON THE SATURATION OF CALCIUM AND OXALATE AND ON URINARY CRYSTAL FORMATION

John G. Gregory, Michaela M. Hoy, Ki Y. Park, and Alex Feigl
Section of Urology, St. Louis University, School of Medicine
St. Louis, Missouri

Alteration of urinary pH within the physiologic range has little effect upon previously formed calcium oxalate crystals or stones. Nevertheless, calcium oxalate crystallization appears to be quite sensitive to small pH changes with a preferential point of crystallization being 5.0.

The relationship between urinary pH and urinary saturation of calcium oxalate has been explored in an intact dog model and the findings applied to a group of hyperoxaluric small bowel bypass patients.

METHODS

Animals - Catheterized dogs were infused simultaneously in separate extremities with solutions of calcium carbonate and sodium oxalate. Solutions of either ammonium chloride or sodium bicarbonate were intermittently infused into a third extremity. Urine was collected at 15 minute intervals. Determinations were made of urinary volume, pH, total calcium and oxalate[1], the amount of calcium oxalate in crystal form, and the calcium oxalate concentration product ratio[2].

Small bowel bypass patients - A group of hyperoxaluric stone formers were instructed to collect the total urine volume excreted for 24 hours while on a regular diet and on no medication. These patients were then instructed to ingest alkalinizing agents; sodium bicarbonate, Polycitra, Citrolith, until a urinary pH of 8.0 was achieved, after which time a 24 hour urine was again collected. Measurements identical to those performed on the dog were carried out on these human urine specimens.

RESULTS

The continuous infusion of calcium carbonate and sodium oxalate with intermittent infusion of ammonium chloride resulted (Figure 1) in: 1) the maintenance of a urinary pH less than 5.9, 2) prompt appearance of urinary crystals, 3) a progressive increase in the calcium oxalate crystal fraction, 4) concentration product ratios for specimens with calcium oxalate ion products more than 5.83, recorded as negative log of the ion product, were 10 or greater.

Urine Sample	Urine pH	Calcium µg/ml	Oxalic acid µg/ml	Wt. of CaOx crystals µg/ml	Types of crystals	-log IP	CPR
1	5.8	76	26	0	x	6.26	2.9
2	5.9	81	65	11	Oct	5.83	9.8
3	5.8	98	149	89	Oct	5.39	31.4
4	5.8	96	161	120	Db & Oct	5.37	42.5
5	5.9	128	278	200	Db & Oct	5.01	47.4
6	5.8	88	406	250	Db & Oct	5.00	28.0

Db = Dumbbell and biconcave oval.

Oct = Octahedral, dodecahedral and bipyramidal.

IP = Ion product obtained from total calcium and oxalate.

CPR = Concentration product ratio.[2]

Fig. 1. Dog infused with calcium carbonate, sodium oxalate, ammonium chloride.

The continuous infusion of sodium oxalate and calcium carbonate with intermittent infusion of sodium bicarbonate resulted (Figure 2) in: 1) the maintenance of a urinary pH between 7.8 and 8.1, 2) ion products comparable to those seen in the acid urine preparation were achieved by crystallization did not occur until relatively higher ion products were reached, 3) calcium oxalate crystal fractions remained relatively low, 4) concentration product ratios of specimens with calcium oxalate ion products less than 5.08, again recorded as negative log of the ion product, were less than 2.5.

The urine of 4 small bowel bypass stone formers were alkalinized with Polycitra and Citrolith and the amount of urinary calcium, oxalate and crystals compared to that obtained in the pretreatment period (Figure 3). In these patients alkalinization dramatically reduced the crystal fraction and at the same time seemed to reduce urinary calcium.

Urine Sample	Urine pH	Calcium µg/ml	Oxalic acid µg/ml	Wt. of CaOx crystals µg/ml	Types of crystals	-log IP	CPR
1	8.0	116	39	0	x	5.90	1.2
2	7.9	88	72	0	x	5.75	1.1
3	7.8	94	124	0	x	5.49	1.3
4	7.8	96	161	14	Db & Oct	5.37	1.4
5	8.0	100	256	33	Db & Oct	5.15	1.8
6	8.1	70	431	49	Db & Oct	5.08	2.5

Db = Dumbbell and biconcave oval.

Oct = Octahedral, dodecahedral and bipyramidal.

IP = Ion product obtained from total calcium and oxalate.

CPR = Concentration product ratio.[2]

Fig. 2. Dog infused with sodium oxalate, calcium carbonate, sodium bicarbonate.

Patient	Date	Urine pH	Alkalinizing Agent	Microscopic Observation	Oxalate µg/ml	Calcium µg/ml	Percent Crystals
D.G.	8-9-79	5	Polycitra-K	+	165	132	60
	9-11-79	8		0	89	44	2
R.R.	9-29-79	5	Polycitra-K	0	64	168	8
	10-20-79	8		0	44	84	2
N.W.	4-3-79	5	Citrolith	+	85	84	34
	9-11-79	8		+	97	58	6
D.W.	10-1-79	5	Citrolith	0	149	12	1
	10-15-79	8		0	220	14	0

Fig. 3. Small bowel bypass stone formers following alkalinization.

A group of 20 small bowel bypass patients have been maintained on an alkalinization regimen. (Figure 4) The length of followup varies, but there is an apparent decrease in the stone formation coincident with the initiation of alkalinization.

The apparent pH effect upon calcium and oxalate crystallization we postulate to be due to the fact that at a urinary pH of less than 6.0 calcium oxalate crystal formation can occur because at this pH the predominant stable salt of calcium is calcium oxalate.

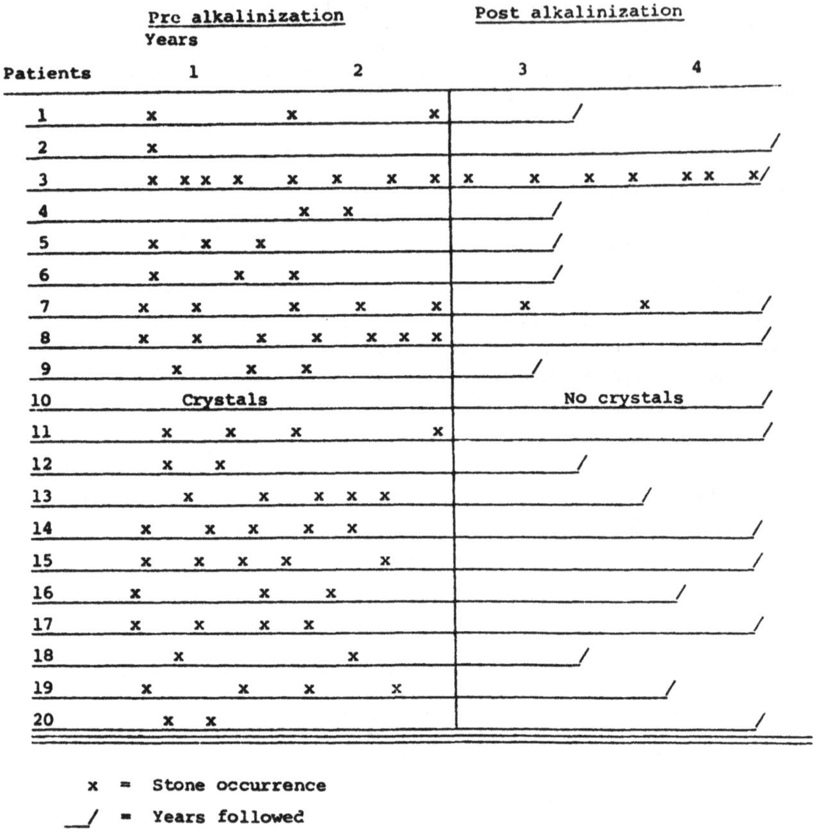

Fig. 4. Stone occurrence in 20 small bowel bypass patients.

At an alkaline pH calcium oxalate crystal formation is inhibited because in this environment conversion of urinary acids to anionic forms takes place. A certain percentage of these ions which are cleared, by the kidneys, compete with oxalate for calcion and form stable soluble salts.

This work suggests that alkalinization may be of therapeutic benefit in the treatment of calcium oxalate stone disease.

REFERENCES

1. K. Y. Park and J. G. Gregory, Clin. Chem. 26:1170 (1980).
2. C. Y. C. Pak, and M. Ohata, Kid. Int. 7:154 (1975).

HYPERURICOSURIA IN CALCIUM OXALATE UROLITHIASIS AND ITS POSSIBLE RELATIONSHIPS WITH STONE MATRIX FORMATION

J. G. Brockis and R. C. Bowyer

Royal Perth Hospital and University of Western Australia

Perth, Western Australia

The association of calcium oxalate stone formation with hyperuricosuria and hypercalciuria has been the subject of a number of papers[1,2,3]. It has been known for a considerable time that patients prone to forming recurrent calcium oxalate stones may on occasion form calculi composed of uric acid and the association is clearly more than fortuitous. The explanation for this association has proved quite formidible to resolve, but the importance of this is clear since it has been suggested that lowering urate excretion by the administration of allopurinol may prevent recurrent urinary stone formation[2]. The studies on this subject are fraught with difficulty because of the time lag needed before any form of therapy for recurrent stone formation can be regarded as successful and in the absence, as yet, of properly performed controlled trials of this drug in stone disease.

That the association of hyperuricosuria with calcium oxalate stone formation may be dietary has been suggested by Fellstrom et al.[4] and indirectly by Robertson[5] who includes hyperuricosuria as a risk factor in the production of recurrent urinary calculi. He has further shown (Robertson[6]) that the high protein meat diet of Western civilization accounts for the high incidence of calcium oxalate stones by causing increased excretion of calcium, oxalate and urate ions in the urine. If the increased urate excretion rate is not an incidental finding in patients forming calcium oxalate calculi, then it is logical to examine the hypothesis that excess urate in the urine affects calcium oxalate crystal growth and aggregation. Theoretically, it could do this in a microcrystalline or colloidal form as sodium, calcium or magnesium urate or in solution as urate ion and these possibilities are now examined. If a microcrystalline state of sodium acid urate, calcium urate or magnesium urate were to form in urine, then these substances will absorb the known inhibitors of crystal growth and aggregation present in urine on to their surface[7,8]. Alternatively it has been alleged that sodium urate will enhance the epitaxial growth of calcium oxalate[9]. There are, however, serious objections to both these hypotheses because they depend upon the demonstration of urates in microcrystalline or colloidal state. Unfortunately, conductivity studies, dialysis, ultrafiltration and Tyndall effects show that solutions of sodium urate up to 16 mmol/l are non-colloidal[10]. Ultrafiltration evidence for a macroscopic form of urate[2] may be explained by the properties of the filters used to study the urine specimens. A further objection to this hypothesis is that sodium urate has only very rarely been found as a constituent of stones and is also relatively soluble in water.

Calcium and magnesium urates have been proposed as alternatives being somewhat less soluble and particularly the suggestion has been made that they might form complexes. We have shown, however, calcium urate does not form a complex in aqueous solution and that if the ionic strength of other ions present using the Davis equation is allowed for, then there is no evidence for complexing. That calcium urate and magnesium urate will absorb glycosaminoglycans in solid phase has been clearly demonstrated by Finlayson[8]. However, it appears to be a quantitative problem because glycosaminoglycans seem to be normally present in excess in urine and a modest reduction in concentration would have little effect on the ability to inhibit urinary crystal growth. Furthermore, Sallis and Bichler[11] have only been able to demonstrate reductions in urinary glycosaminoglycans in patients with infected staghorn calculi and not in the ordinary oxalate recurrent stone former, though this work contradicts that of Robertson[7].

There remains an alternative proposition that urates are active in solution and there are three possible ways in which this could happen.

(1) That they combine in solution with crystal growth inhibitors, particularly the chondroitin sulphates. There is however, no evidence that chondroitin sulphates combine with urate when placed in dialysis sacs even in the presence of magnesium and calcium ions [10]. Any movement that occurs across the membrane can be readily accounted for by the ionic strength of the ions present.

(2) In the polymerisation of urinary proteins into protein matrix the presence of urate may be important particularly as Boyce[12] suggested years ago, the mucoprotein is an essential part of stone formation. In support of this too is the evidence of the presence of urates in stone matrix[13]. More indirectly there is evidence of deposits of protein in renal tubules during the formation of calcium

oxalate crystals[13]. Rose[14] has also shown that when urine is evaporated oxalate crystals appear to aggregate in the presence of uromucoids. Pinto[15] also commented on the effects of urinary mucoproteins on the nidation of stones but neither he nor Rose specify any role of urate in this respect.

(3) There remains the possibility that urate in someway, not understood, affects the change which comes about when soluble urinary protein is transformed into insoluble matrix, possibly by enzyme action in the renal tubules, a process in which sialic acid appears to be lost.

This review shows clearly the missing links in the present chain of investigation and these are:

(1) Confirmation is needed that the presence of urate is not merely an associated phenomenon induced by the same factors which cause calcium oxalate stone formation i.e. particularly a high protein diet.

(2) That microcrystals of urate do exist in urine as these have yet to be effectively demonstrated and if present that the surface area is adequate to absorb the amount of glycosaminoglycans that would be necessary to alter crystal growth of oxalate.

(3) Whether urates affect uroproteins during the process of the laying down of stone matrix.

The first question would appear to be only partly answered, but if as is alleged by Pak et al.[2] that allopurinol reduces urate excretion without at the same time affecting oxalate excretion and does really reduce the incidence of stones, the concentration would then certainly seem to be established. Certainly all early reports are in this direction, but controlled trials are needed and if confirmed, questions (2) and (3) require answers before this problem is finally resolved.

REFERENCES

1. F. L. Coe and A. G. Kavalach, N. Eng. J. Med. 291:1344 (1974).
2. C. Y. C. Pak, D. E. Barilla, K. Holt, L. Brinkley, R. Tolentino, and J. E. Zerwekh, Am. J. Med. 65:593 (1978).
3. W. G. Robertson, M. Peacock, P. J. Heyburn, D. H. Marshall, and P. B. Clark, Br. J. Urol. 50:449 (1978).
4. B. Fellstrom, U. Backman, B. G. Danielson, S. Ljunghall, and B. Wikstrom, in:"Proceedings of Fourth International Symposium on Urolithiasis Research," L. H. Smith, B. Finlayson, and W. G. Robertson, eds., Plenum Press, New York (in press).

5. W. G. Robertson, M. Peacock, P. J. Heyburn, and C. P. Bambach, in:"Urinary Calculi, Proceedings of the International Urinary Stone Conference, 1979," J. G. Brockis and B. Finlayson, eds., PSG Publishing Co. Inc., Littleton, MA (1980) (in press).
6. W. G. Robertson, M. Peacock, P. J. Heyburn, F. A. Hanes, A. Rutherford, E. Clementson, R. Swaminathan, and P. B. Clark, Br. J. Urol. 51:427 (1979).
7. W. G. Robertson, F. Knowles, and M. Peacock, in:"Urolithiasis Research," H. Fleisch, W. G. Robertson, L. H. Smith, and W. Vahlensieck, eds., Plenum Press, New York (1976).
8. B. Finlayson and J. Du Bois, Clin. Chim. Acta. 84:203 (1978).
9. C. Y. C. Pak, O. Waters, L. Arnold, K. Holt, C. Cox, and D. Barilla, J. Clin. Invest. 59:426 (1977).
10. R. K. McCulloch, R. C. Bowyer, and J. G. Brockis, in:"Urinary Calculi, Proceedings of the International Urinary Stone Conference, 1979," J. G. Brockis and B. Finlayson, eds., PSG Publishing Co. Inc., Littleton, MA (1980) (in press).
11. K.-H. Bichler, J. Sallis and S. Broring, in:"Urinary Calculi, Proceedings of the International Urinary Stone Conference, 1979," J. G. Brockis and B. Finlayson, eds., PSG Publishing Co. Inc., Littleton, MA (1980) (in press).
12. W. H. Boyce, Am. J. Med. 45:673 (1968).
13. B. Finlayson and J. J. Leal, Invest. Urol. 14:278 (1977).
14. G. A. Rose and P. C. Hallson, Lancet 1:1000 (1979).
15. B. Pinto, in:"VI Jena Urinary Stone Symposium," (1980).

CALCIUM OXALATE CRYSTALLIZATION IN UROTHELIAL-LINED SYSTEMS

W. B. Gill, K. W. Jones, K. J. Ruggiero, M. C. Fromes

University of Chicago
Department of Surgery (Urology)
Chicago, Illinois

INTRODUCTION

The liquid/solid interface is of fundamental importance in the crystallization of solutes from aqueous systems. Nucleation preferentially occurs at interfaces that inherently present energetically favored sites for the initiation of crystallization[1,2]. Most crystallization studies have dealt with the nature of the solute and/or the solvent[2,4] and have usually ignored consideration of the containers and the nature of the solid surfaces enclosing the systems.

Urolithiasis research has traditionally involved studies of crystallization in glass or plastic containers[5,6]. We have previously reported a pronounced inhibitory effect of urinary macromolecules on calcium oxalate crystal nucleation and adhesion to glass test tubes[7,8]. We herein describe systems to study crystallization in the living urothelial-lined container of the catheterized female rat bladder. This setting more closely approaches that of the in vivo disease situation of urolithiasis wherein crystalline masses frequently adhere to transitional urothelium.

In these studies, the status of the container surface (normal or injured urothelium or glass) markedly affected crystal adhesion to the surfaces of the container and the metastable limit for nucleation. Chemically injured urothelium and glass tubes were accompanied by significant adhesion of calcium oxalate crystals to the container surface, but normal urothelium permitted only intraluminal free crystals without any adherence to the urothelial surface. Normal urothelium resulted in an elevation of the metastable limit and absence of container surface nucleation/adhesion for calcium oxalate crystallization as compared to glass containers.

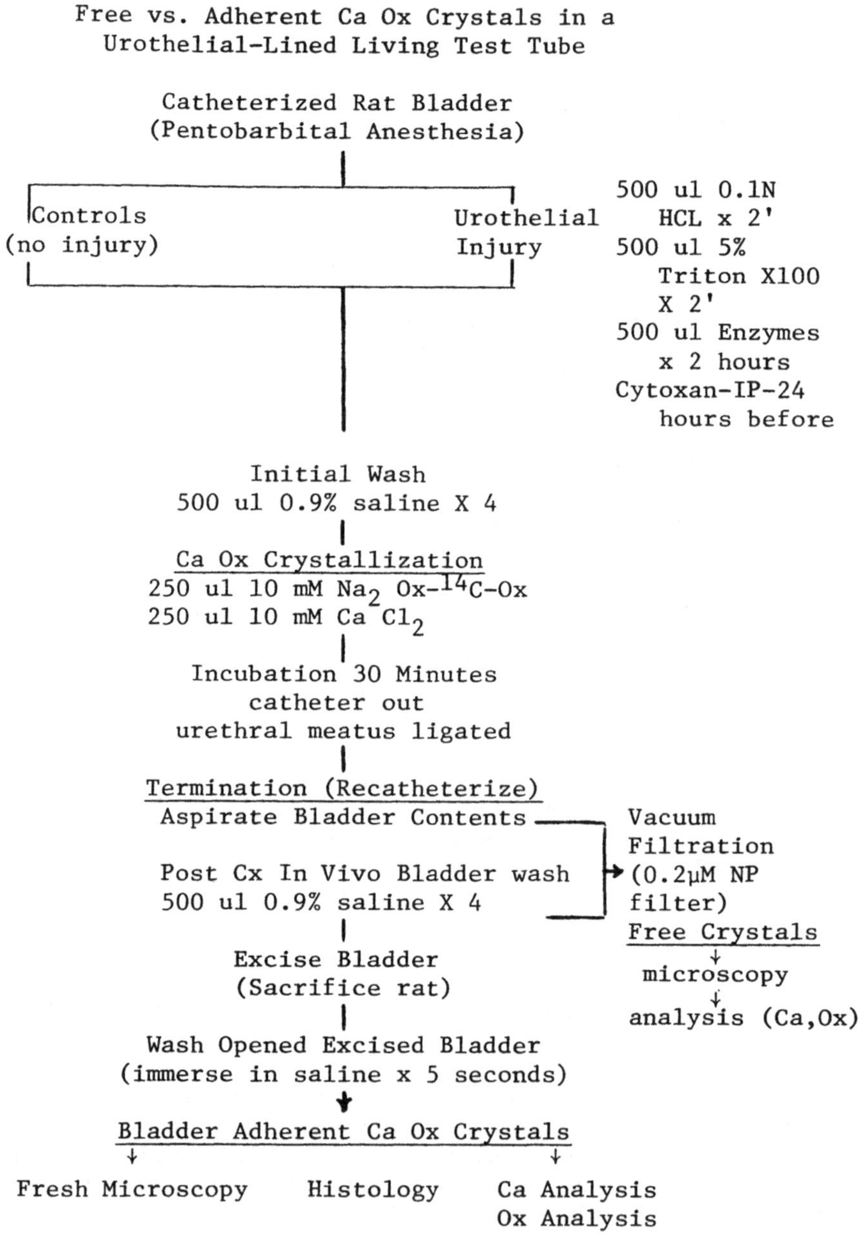

Figure 1

Schematic flow chart of methods to differentiate free from container-adherent calcium oxalate crystals in urothelial-lined systems (bladder).

I Crystal Adhesion Studies

Figure 1 is a schematic flow chart of the methods to differentiate free (intraluminal) from container-adherent calcium oxalate crystals formed by active crystallization from supersaturated saline solutions within urothelial containers. Identical steps were also employed with glass screw top tubes (nonpyrex, Rochester Scientific). Young adult female rats were anesthetized with intraperitoneal sodium pentobarbital and both ureters were ligated and divided at their midpoints through midline abdominal incisions. PE 50 polyethylene catheters were easily passed up the urethra to a 2 cm mark on the catheter which insures against mechanical injury from passing the catheter too far[9]. After instilling the desired solutions, the catheters were withdrawn and ligatures were placed around the external urethral meatus to insure that the bladder contents remained in place during the test periods.

Injuries of the urothelium were produced by one of the following methods: 1) 500 ul of 0.1 N HCL acid intravesically for 2 minutes, 2) 500 ul of 5% Triton X-100 (a nonionic detergent) in a 0.9% saline intravesically for 2 minutes, 3) cyclophosphamide, 300 mg/kg, given intraperitoneally 24 hours before the intravesical induction of crystallization, 4) papain 400 ul of 10% papain (African papaya, Calbiochem) in 0.1M acetate buffer pH 6.5, plus 100 ul of 0.1% EDTA for activation intravesically for 2 hours before induction of crystallization, 5) Neuraminidase (vibrio cholerae) 30 units in 500 ul of pH 5.5 acetate buffer 0.1M with [2mM] $CaCl_2$ for activation.

At the conclusion of the test periods, the meatal ligatures were removed or the screw top caps removed from glass tubes and a new catheter was passed for aspirating the contents and washing the containers (bladders or glass tubes) with 500 ul aliquots of saline. After microscopic examinations of the opened bladders and filters, each was placed in a fresh glass tube with 1.0 ml. of 1 N HCL for dissolution of any crystalline material. Duplicate 50 ul aliquots were taken for determination of calcium by atomic absorption spectrophotometry and ^{14}C-oxalate by liquid scintillation spectrometry. From the original total mass and radionuclide concentrations of oxalate plus the final quantity of ^{14}C-oxalate, calculations were made of the total oxalate mass on the containers or the filters by standard isotope dilution techniques.

For the second type of crystal adhesion study, preformed crystals were prepared by rapidly mixing 250 ul of 10mM $CaCl_2$ in 0.9% saline (NaCl) with 250 ul of 10mM Na_2 oxalate plus ^{14}C-oxalate tracer in 0.9% saline in glass screw top tubes and incubating for 48 hours at 37°C in a shaking (40 cycles, 2 cm stroke) water bath. These 500 ul volumes of crystal slurries were then instilled through PE 50 catheters into either rat bladders or glass tubes.

After the incubation period of 30 minutes, the containers were aspirated, filtered, and "physiologically washed" as in the previous sections with active crystallizations.

Table 1. Crystal Adhesion Study 1 (Active Crystallization)

Distribution of calcium oxalate crystals following 30 minutes of active crystallization from supersaturated saline solutions within urothelial or glass containers.

	n	Container Adherent Crystals Ca Ox .1H_2O $\bar{x}$, nM/container	Free Filterable Crystals Ca Ox .1 H_2O $\bar{x}$, nM/filter
Bladders			
Normal	10	0	1031
0.1 N HCL Injured	9	327	190
5% Triton X-100 Injured	11	898	68
Cyclophosphamide Injured	5	420	293
Papain alone	5	8	968
EDTA alone	6	0	1166
Papain + EDTA Injured	8	879	109
Neuraminidase	8	13	1234
Glass Tubes	12	268	1272

Table 1 shows the distribution of calcium oxalate crystals following 30 minutes of active crystallization from supersaturated saline solutions of 5mM initial concentrations of calcium and oxalate within urothelial or glass containers. Spectacular differences were noted between normal urothelium and injured urothelium or glass. With normal, uninjured bladders, there were no detectable calcium oxalate crystals adherent to the surface (Fig. 2), but a great number of free, intraluminal crystals were filterable on 0.2μM Nucleopore filters (Fig. 3).

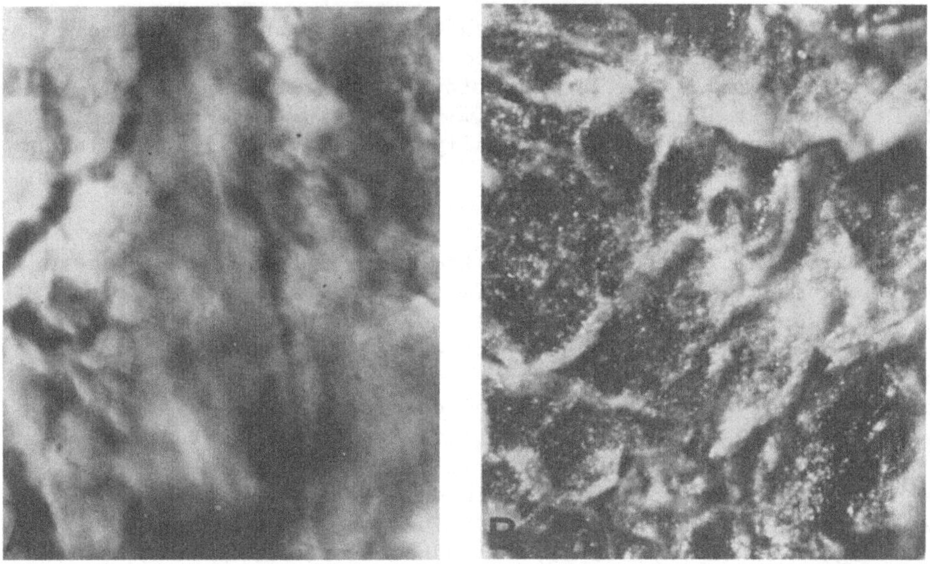

Figure 2. Photomicrographs of bladder surfaces (reflected light 25 x). A. Normal, uninjured, urothelium showing absence of crystals. B. Triton X-100 injured bladder demonstrating diffuse crystalline masses ranging from single crystals to large polycrystalline masses in ridges and mounds over the injured urothelial surface.

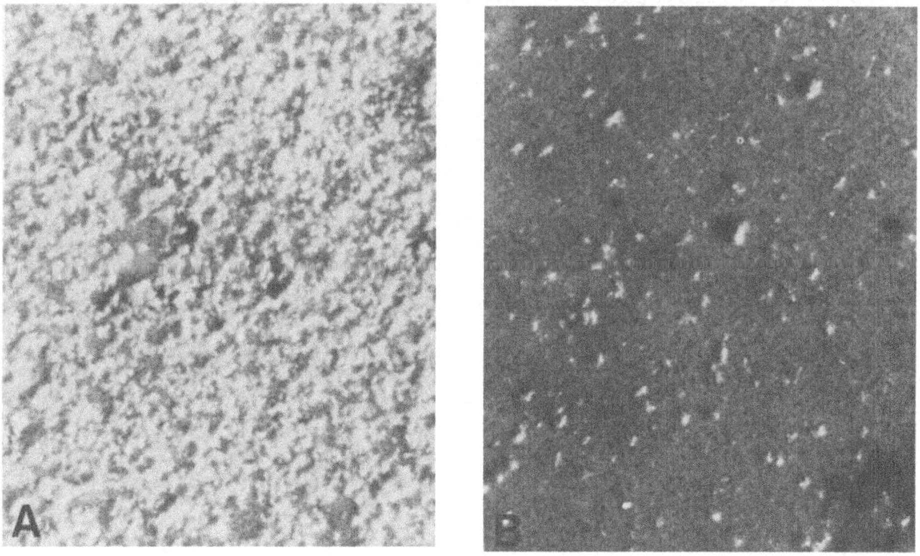

Figure 3. Photomicrographs of free crystals on Nuclepore filters (oblique reflected light 40 x). A. Numerous, uniform-size crystals from uninjured rat bladders. B. Fewer, variable size crystals from Triton X-100 injured rat bladder.

Chemically injured urothelium showed a pattern of moderate to marked adhesion of calcium oxalate to the bladder surface (Fig. 2) with a correspondingly smaller quantity of free, filterable crystals (Fig. 3). Qualitatively similar results were obtained whether the injury was produced locally by intravesical instillation or systemically (cyclophosphamide with subsequent urinary excretion of an injurious metabolite).

Enzymatic injuries produced by the proteolytic enzyme, papain, in the presence of its activator EDTA produced significant urothelial damage with subsequent crystal adherence. Neither papain alone or EDTA alone produced significant injuries as detectable by microscopic appearance or calcium oxalate chemical analyses. The papain/EDTA injury resulted in marked calcium oxalate crystal adherence from either active crystallization in supersaturated solutions (Table 1) or from the instillation of preformed calcium oxalate crystals (Table 2). Neuraminidase, which attacks the sialic acid constituents of glycoproteins, or glycosaminoglycans, did not significantly affect crystal adherence to urothelium (Table 1).

Table 2. Crystal Adhesion Study 2 (Preformed Crystals)

Distribution of calcium oxalate crystals following 30 minutes of intravesical or intraglass incubations of preformed crystals in a saline slurry.

	n	Container Adherent Crystals Ca Ox $.1H_2O$ $\bar{x}$, nM/container	Free Filterable Crystals Ca Ox $.1H_2O$ $\bar{x}$, nM/filter
Bladders			
Normal	10	0	806
0.1 N HCL Injured	8	169	603
5% Triton X-100 Injured	9	581	139
Papain alone	6	0	692
EDTA alone	5	0	596
Papain + EDTA Injured	6	432	282
Glass Tubes	12	8	1105

Table 2 shows that preformed calcium oxalate crystals also adhere to injured urothelium. Whether this is a direct adhesion of the 3 to 30 micron-sized crystals or dissolution/reprecipitation of the preformed crystals is debatable. The preformed crystals were the ones left free in glass tubes after 48 hours crystallization from 500 ul of 5mM $CaCl_2$ and 5mM Na_2 Ox in saline. Surprisingly, the preformed crystals adhered considerably more to the papain/EDTA and Triton X-100 injured bladders than to the acid injured bladders or glass tubes; whereas with active crystallization (Table 1) the container adherent crystals were considerably greater in quantity and showed less variation between groups or urothelial injuries and glass tubes.

II Crystal Nucleation Studies

Studies were made of the metastable limits of calcium oxalate supersaturation in both glass tubes and urothelial-lined rat bladders from a solvent system consisting of 0.9% saline [0.154mM NaCl]. Both bladders and glass tubes were treated identically with all solutions being introduced and removed through PE 50 catheters. Each of a series of glass tubes and rat bladders received various quantities of [10mM] sodium oxalate with a tracer dose of ^{14}C-oxalate in [0.154M] NaCl, [10mM] calcium chloride in [0.154M] NaCl, plus intervening quantities of [0.154M] NaCl to make a total volume of 500 ul. Table 3 shows the initial concentrations of calcium and oxalate ranging from [0.4mM] through [1.0mM] at [0.1mM] increments.

The levels of calcium and oxalate necessary for detectable crystallization at 30 minutes in glass and urothelial containers are compared under crystallization frequency in Table 3. Note that crystallization occurred first and continued most prominently as adherent calcium oxalate crystals to glass tubes. In urothelial-lined bladders, however, adherent crystals did not occur at even the highest concentrations of calcium and oxalate. Only free, filterable crystals occurred at [0.9mM] levels and higher in the urothelial-lined system. Detectable crystallization by 30 minutes occurred at [0.6mM] initial concentrations of calcium and oxalate in glass tubes, but it usually took a [0.9mM] level to produce crystallization in the urothelial-lined bladders. Therefore, the 30 minute metastable limit for calcium and oxalate in [0.154M] NaCl was between [0.5mM] and [0.6mM] in glass tubes and between [0.8mM] and [0.9mM] in urothelial-lined bladders.

Crystal quantitation data is also presented in Table 3. The mean total calcium oxalate precipitates which were recovered per container or per filter are given in nanomoles (nM).

Table 3. Effects of Container/Saline Interfaces on Metastable Limits and Sites of Calcium Oxalate Nucleation

Initial Concentrations calcium & oxalate in [0.154M] NaCl		Glass/Saline Interfaces: filterable free crystals	Glass/Saline Interfaces: container adherent crystals	Urothelial/Saline Interface: filterable free crystals	Urothelial/Saline Interface: container adherent crystals
[0.4mM]	Cx frequency*	0/6	0/6	0/5	0/5
	Ca Ox .1H_2O, $\bar{x}$, nM	0	0	0	0
[0.5mM]	Cx frequency*	0/7	0/7	0/6	0/6
	Ca Ox .1H_2O, $\bar{x}$, nM	0	0	0	0
[0.6mM]	Cx frequency*	8/11	9/11	0/10	0/10
	Ca Ox .1H_2O, $\bar{x}$, nM	9.8	29.8	0	0
[0.7mM]	Cx frequency*	12/12	12/12	0/11	0/11
	Ca Ox .1H_2O, $\bar{x}$, nM	23.6	75.4	0	0
[0.8mM]	Cx frequency*	11/11	11/11	2/11	0/11
	Ca Ox .1H_2O, $\bar{x}$, nM	30.8	130.1	2.5	0
[0.9mM]	Cx frequency*	12/12	12/12	10/11	0/11
	Ca Ox .1H_2O, $\bar{x}$, nM	25.6	172.9	31.0	0
[1.0mM]	Cx frequency*	13/13	13/13	11/11	0/11
	Ca Ox .1H_2O, $\bar{x}$, nM	44.5	224.7	49.6	0

*crystallization frequency = number of times crystals detected/number of trials

Table 4. Mechanisms of Urothelial Container on Elevation of Metastable Limits of Calcium Oxalate Nucleation (Saline/Urothelial Interface vs. Secretions into Solution)

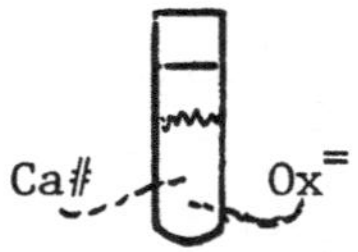

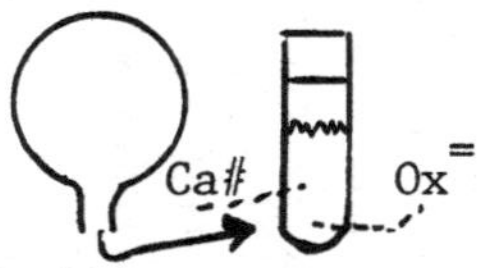

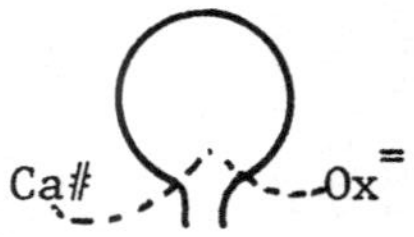

Initial Concentrations calcium and oxalate in [0.154M] NaCl		Glass: filter free crystals	Glass: container adherent crystals	Bladder Glass: filter free crystals	Bladder Glass: container adherent crystals	Bladder: filter free crystals	Bladder: container adherent crystals
[0.7mM]	Cx frequency*	3/5	5/5	4/5	5/5	0/5	0/5
	Ca Ox $.1H_2O$, $\bar{x}$, nM	18.1	78.9	14.5	48.3	0	0
[0.8mM]	Cx frequency*	6/6	6/6	5/5	5/5	0/5	0/5
	Ca Ox $.1H_2O$, $\bar{x}$, nM	18.5	101.4	36.0	69.8	0	0
[0.9mM]	Cx frequency*	6/6	6/6	6/6	6/6	5/5	0/5
	Ca Ox $.1H_2O$, $\bar{x}$, nM	49.1	138.3	18.4	138.5	38.4	0
[1.0mM]	Cx frequency*	5/5	5/5	5/5	5/5	5/5	0/5
	Ca Ox $.1H_2O$, $\bar{x}$, nM	23.6	184.4	67.9	148.2	56.2	0

*crystallization frequency = number of times crystals detected/number of trials

The calcium oxalate crystals were consistently monohydrate (whewellite) as determined by optical crystallography. Attention should again be focused on the fact that with glass tubes, the bulk of calcium oxalate crystals were adherent to the container, but only free, filterable crystals occurred in the urothelial-lined systems.

What could account for the differences in the metastable limits for nucleation between glass and living urothelial-lined systems? Great care was taken, insofar as possible without damaging the living urothelial-lined bladder, to obviate extraneous factors from entering into the comparison of liquid/solid interfaces. Such factors as residual urine in the bladder or urine production entering the bladder were obviated by ligating the ureters and washing the bladder prior to nucleation/crystallization experiments. pH measurements of the terminal aspirates also did not show differences between the glass and urothelial systems (pH meter values ranged from 6.1 to 6.3). Controls of either calcium chloride alone or sodium oxalate alone at the various concentrations used in 0.5 ml of saline were placed in rat bladders for 30 minutes. Aspirations revealed a 5% to 8% decrease in recoverable volumes, but the concentrations of calcium or oxalate were increased by amounts which paralleled the decreased volumes. Therefore, not only was there not a selective decrease in calcium or oxalate by urothelial removal, but the actual concentrations of calcium or oxalate in the urothelial-lined system after 30 minutes were actually slightly higher than the initial instillations.

The mechanisms by which the urothelial container elevated the metastable limit of nucleation as compared to glass containers could be due to: 1) secretion(s) from the urothelial surface which would change the solvent characteristics, or 2) the nature of the urothelial/saline interface.

This question as to the urothelial mechanism of action was answered by experiments in which 500ul aliquots of 0.9% saline were placed in rats bladders without additions of calcium or oxalate. After 30 minutes in the rat bladders, the saline aliquots were removed and placed in glass tubes and only then were calcium and oxalate added. If this bladder to glass group behaved like glass alone, then the nature of the urothelial/saline interface would seem to be the differentiating factor. Whereas, if secretion from the urothelium to alter the solvent characteristics obtained, then this bladder to glass group would be similar to the straight bladder group.

The bladder to glass group behaved similar to glass alone (Table 4); as if the saline had never been in the rat bladders. Therefore, the nature of the urothelial/saline interface, especially the characteristics of the urothelial solid surface, was crucial in altering the site of nucleation from the solid surface of glass to intraluminal when the urothelial surface bounded the system. In keeping with a shift from heterogeneous surface nucleation to homogeneous intraluminal nucleation[2] in the urothelial system, an elevation in the solute concentration was required to induce crystallization.

From the results presented, it would appear that the differences in the metastable limits and sites of crystallization (glass surface vs. intraluminal in urothelial container) are a function of the liquid/solid interfaces with heterogeneous surface nucleation on the glass tubes and homogeneous intraluminal nucleation or heterogeneous nucleation on intraluminal "foreign particles" within the urothelial-lined bladder.

DISCUSSION

This in vivo system of crystallization in a urothelial-lined, "living container" approaches the system in which crystallization may be of clinical importance, namely, human urolithiasis. The urothelium lining the urinary bladder of the rat is quite similar to the human urothelium lining the renal papillae, calyces, and pelvis as well as the bladder[10].

Two general possibilities could explain crystal adhesion to injured urothelium: 1) the removal of a normal protective non-sticking surface coating, the glycocalyx, or 2) the presence of a gluing substance produced by the injured cells or leaking from the blood or lymph vessels. Two dimensional surface histochemistry with cationic and anionic dyes demonstrating differences between the various types of injured and normal urothelium.

These results suggest that the structure of the urothelial surface may play a vital role in determining nucleation and whether calcium oxalate crystals will adhere to the urothelium and thus remain in the urinary tract where further "fixed particle"[12] growth into a macroscopic stone could occur. Further studies are needed to substantiate or refute this hypothesis of an abnormal urothelial surface to explain the development of otherwise "idiopathic" urolithiasis.

REFERENCES

1. A. Van Hook, in:"Crystallization Theory and Practice," Reinhold Publishing Corporation, New York, p. 8, (1961).
2. V. K. LaMer, Ind. Eng. Chem. 44:1270 (1952).
3. A. G. Walton, in:"The Formation and Properties of Precipitates," Interscience Publ. (J. Wiley), New York, p. 7 and p. 24, (1967).

4. H. Buckley, in:"Crystal Growth," J. Wiley & Sons, New York, p. 43, (1951).
5. C. W. Vermeulen, E. S. Lyon, and W. B. Gill, Invest. Urol. 1:370 (1964).
6. B. Finlayson, Invest. Urol. 9:258, 1972.
7. W. B. Gill and J. W. Karesh, in:"Urolithiasis Research," H. Fleisch, W. G. Robertson, L. H. Smith and W. Vahlensieck, ed., Plenum Press, New York, p. 277, (1976).
8. W. B. Gill, J. W. Karesh, L. Garsin, and J. J. Roma, Invest. Urol. 15:95 (1977).
9. W. B. Gill, K. J. Ruggiero, and F. H. Straus, II, Invest. Urol. 17:257 (1979).
10. B. Monis and H. D. Dorman, J. Histochem. Cytochem. 15:475 (1967).
11. S. Levin and W. Richter, Cell Tiss. Res. 158:281 (1975).
12. B. Finlayson, Urol. Clin. N. Am. 1:187 (1974).

ACKNOWLEDGMENT

Supported by National Institutes of Health Grant No. IP50 AM 20585 and the Edward and Sarainne Andrews Foundation.

INTRARENAL CALCIUM AND OXALATE CONCENTRATION GRADIENTS IN HEALTHY AND STONE FORMING KIDNEYS - THE RENAL PAPILLA AS THE PRIMARY NUCLEATION SITE

R. E. Hautmann, A. Lehmann, and H. Osswald

Department of Urology, Institute for Organic Chemistry and Department of Pharmacology, Rheinisch-Westfälische Technische Hochschule Aachen, West-Germany

Many investigators have attempted to identify causative factors influencing the pathogenesis and growth of calcium oxalate stones. Calcium and oxalate excretion patterns, urinary proteins, saturation/inhibition indexes, natural inhibitors of crystallization and a host of other metabolites have been studied but none of these parameters unequivocally separates the stone former from the non-stone former. Like numerous predisposing factors better defined risk factors are neither a sufficient nor a necessary cause of calcium oxalate stone formation.

In the past the attention has been focused on the calcium and oxalate concentrations in urine and plasma (Figure 1). The oxalate and calcium content of the area between plasma and urine has been largely ignored.

Therefore the objects of this paper are to report the concentrations of oxalate, calcium, sodium, and potassium in the papilla, medulla, and cortex of healthy and stone forming human kidneys and to compare these figures with the corresponding concentrations in the urine. Furthermore, an attempt was made to calculate the absolute calcium and oxalate concentrations within the different compartments of the papilla.

MATERIAL AND METHODS

Fresh human renal tissue was obtained at surgery from 10 subjects, in whom a nephrectomy had been carried out for a small papillary carcinoma of the renal pelvis or for a small hypernephroma.

Within two minutes after nephrectomy, the kidney parenchyma was cut into two parts by an off center longitudinal incision to expose the papillae.

One or two full thickness sections, each containing a papilla with adjacent medulla and cortex, were excised with as little disturbance as possible to retain any solute gradients which might exist. To avoid any fluid loss, the renal pedicle clamp was not released before the pyramid was excised.

The methods used have been published in detail[1,2]. After weighing, the samples were lyophylized and defatted. The residue was then extracted with hydrochloric acid and the acid extract was retained for analysis. The whole procedure was carried out in silica crucibles.

Sodium and potassium were measured by flame emission spectrophotometry. Calcium was measured by flame emission spectrophotometry from the acid extract as well as by atomic absorption spectrophotometry. For this purpose, the calcium concentration was measured in further tissue specimens, obtained from representative regions in each kidney after the method of Gains[3]. For the oxalate determination we prefer ^{14}C-oxalate methods and, therefore used the radioenzymatic procedure, described in 1978 by Bennett and co-workers[4]. Using this method, the urinary oxalate determination is not so simple, accurate and economical as the authors state. However, results obtained from artificial urines, oxalate solutions and acid tissue extracts reveal, in our hands, satisfactory reproducible results.

RESULTS

Table 1 exhibits the concentrations in mmol per kg wet weight of tissue of oxalic acid, calcium and sodium in papilla, medulla and cortex in 9 pyramids out of 7 healthy human kidneys. Significance was calculated using Student's t-test for unpaired data. Each p value indicates the degree of significance between the values on either side of it.

A significantly higher concentration of oxalate was observed in the papilla compared with the medulla of these normal kidneys. The medulla in turn contained a higher oxalate concentration than the cortex. However, this difference was not significant. Calcium showed a similar gradient between papilla and medulla of the kidney. There was, however, no significant change in the calcium concentration in the cortex. Potassium did not show a concentration gradient.

Measuring the solute concentrations of the stone forming papilla is not without problems. Usually the papillary tip then is calcified and has to be separated from the remainder of the papilla. The removal of that calcified cap is admittedly arbitrary and not a clearly defined procedure.

Table 1 also compares the concentrations of oxalate and calcium in the pyramids of the healthy kidneys with those of 4 pyramids out of 3 stone forming kidneys. The stone formers demonstrate a comparable concentration gradient for calcium as well as oxalate. The solute concentrations in the stone forming papilla seem to be somewhat lower than in the normal kidneys. However, the stone forming papillae were investigated after removal of their calcified papillary tip.

Table 1 permits a comparison of the gradients of solute concentration in healthy and stone forming kidneys. For the renal medulla and cortex no major difference has been observed and these gradients have been demonstrated in other mammals[3,5,6]. The significant difference between a normal and a stone forming papilla is the tremendous oxalate and calcium content of the papillary tip in the stone forming kidneys.

Table 1. Concentrations of Oxalic Acid, Calcium and Sodium in the Renal Tip, Papilla, Medulla, and Cortex of Man

Constituent[a]	Tip	Papilla	P	Medulla	P	Cortex
		Site of Probability				
Normal[b]						
Calcium	-	16.9± 2.4	<.05	1.6± 0.3	NS[c]	2.0±0.4
Oxalic acid	-	5.5± 0.8	<.05	0.4± 0.08	NS	0.3±0.06
Sodium	-	178.6±19.9	<.05	113.2±10.2	NS	93.5±5.2
Stone former[d]						
Calcium	27.4±6.0	11.3± 3.2	<.05	1.3±0.4	NS	1.7±0.6
Oxalic acid	14.9±4.2	4.5± 0.9	<.05	0.9±0.1	NS	0.8±0.1

a Constituent quantities expressed as mmol/kg (wet weight), mean ± standard error of mean.

b 9 pyramids from 7 kidneys were analyzed.

c NS = not significant.

d 4 pyramids from 3 kidneys were analyzed.

Figure 1 shows the over all concentrations of calcium, oxalate, sodium and potassium in papilla, medulla and cortex of the seven healthy kidneys as well as in the urine and plasma of these patients. The data are shown in mol per liter for urine and plasma or in mol per kg wet weight of tissue. All of these data - except for the plasma values - are measured concentrations and not

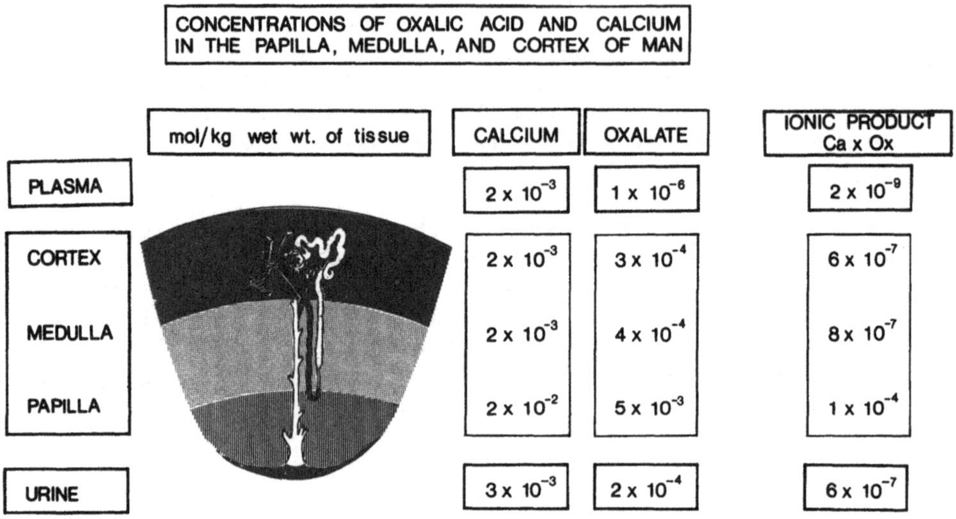

Figure 1.

Geometry of the Papilla (Volume Fractions in per cent)

VASC.	INTER STIT.	CELLS	C.DUCT LOOPS	
20	20	35	25	Literature

Solute Content (mol/ kg wet wt. of tissue)

		calculated	Literature	measured		total content (measured)
OX	max	$1.2 \cdot 10^{-2}$	10^{-3}	$2 \cdot 10^{-4}$	◀	$5 \cdot 10^{-3}$
	min	$1.1 \cdot 10^{-2}$	10^{-6}			
Ca	max	$4.8 \cdot 10^{-2}$	10^{-3}	$3 \cdot 10^{-3}$	◀	$2 \cdot 10^{-2}$
	min	$4.7 \cdot 10^{-2}$	10^{-6}			
Na		$1.0 \cdot 10^{-1}$	$3 \cdot 10^{-2}$	$1.5 \cdot 10^{-1}$	◀	$2 \cdot 10^{-1}$

Figure 2.

calculated activities. The oxalate and calcium concentrations are appreciably higher even in the normal papilla than in the urine. A comparison of the tissue and urine data shows that the oxalate concentration is about twenty-five times higher in the normal papilla than in the urine, while calcium is approximately six times higher.

DISCUSSION

An open, but interesting question is: What are the absolute solute concentrations within the different compartments of the papilla? Quantitative anatomical data describing the mammalian kidney is presently available from a number of sources[7,8]. The volume fractions of the papilla that we use are a rough estimate from the literature, using results obtained from different authors in various mammals. Data from man are not available. Our calculations are based on a ratio of 20 percent vascular structures, 20 percent interstitium, 35 percent cells, and 25 percent collecting ducts, ducts of Bellini and loops of Henle. Our measured overall concentration in the normal papilla for oxalate is 5×10^{-3}, for calcium 2×10^{-2} and for sodium 2×10^{-1} mol/kg wet weight of tissue. These solutes are distributed in three spaces (Figure 2). In the renal tubes the concentration was assumed to be equal to that of the final urine. These figures were measured from our patients. In the cells the values for sodium and calcium were obtained from the literature[9]. The upper calcium value represents the total cellular calcium, the lower one the physiologically acting calcium concentration. For the intracellular oxalate concentrations no figures are available in the literature. In comparison with the calcium values, we calculated with an assumed maximum of 10^{-3} and a minimum of 10^{-6} mol/kg wet weight of tissue. For purposes of calculation, the vascular space and the interstitium were considered as one single compartment. The oxalate, calcium and sodium concentrations within that space were calculated from measured and estimated concentrations in the other compartments. The maximum concentration of oxalate and calcium in the papilla then must be located in the interstitial space.

These results support evidence that in view of these high concentrations, particles can be formed in the interstitial space and can migrate into an intraluminal position (Figure 3). The possible relevance of our findings to human calcium oxalate stone formation is of interest. It is well recognized that calcific deposits occur in every kidney and have been identified either as calcium phosphate or calcium oxalate[10,11]. Ordinarily, microscopic calcium deposits are found in both the renal tubule and the renal interstitium. In an autopsy series, microscopic crystal deposits that stained with alizarin have been found in every kidney. In most series, the spatial frequency of calcium deposits increases as the papillary tip is approached. These findings are in accordance with our observation, that the concentration maximum of the oxalate and calcium gradients is localized in the inner medulla or papilla.

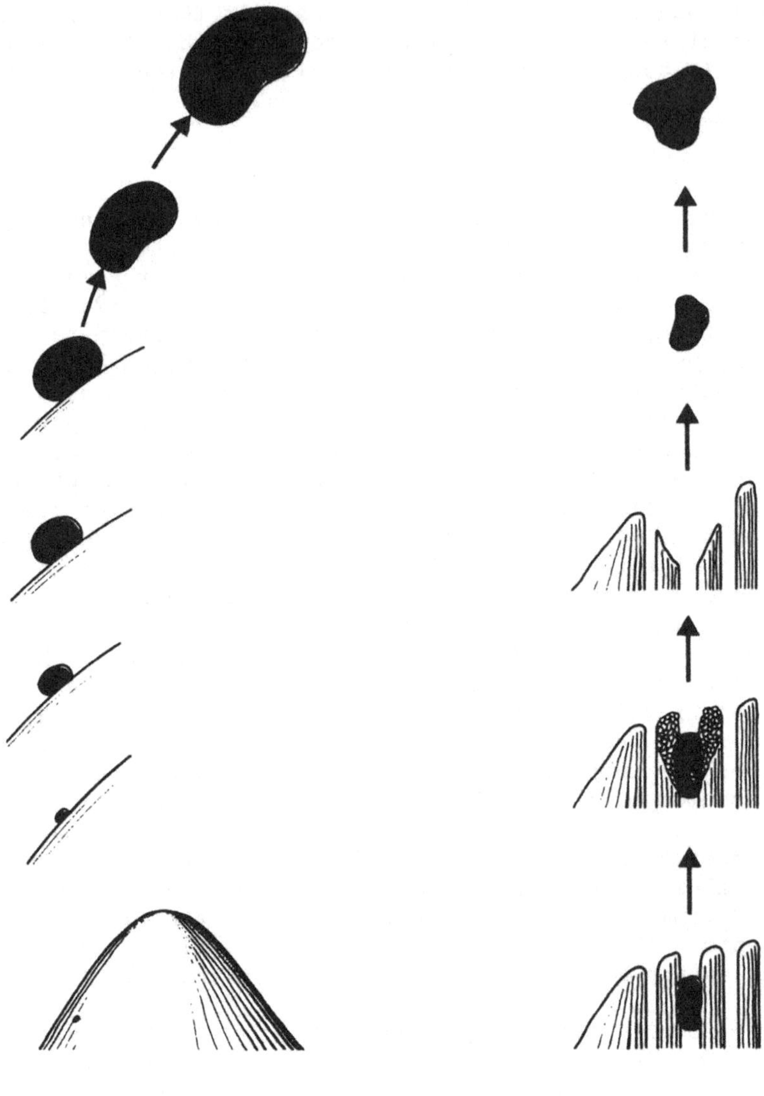

Figure 3. See text.

On the basis of what is known about the renal tube dimensions, tubular flow velocities[12], urinary supersaturation of calcium and oxalate, and about the renal handling of oxalate by three micropuncture studies[13-15] it seems, that free particle stone disease cannot occur in the renal tubule[12]. In the theory of fixed particle nucleation it is suggested, that, because of excessive concentration of calcium and oxalate in certain areas of the kidney, precipitation of crystals may occur in the renal papilla either within the tubular lumen or beneath the surface of the papilla[16-18].

We suggest that the high concentrations of oxalate and calcium which have been found in the human papilla, in particular in the papillary cap of the stone forming papilla contribute to the formation of calcium deposits which are the basis for stone formation, starting from fixed crystalluric particles. Our experiments have further emphasized the importance of the renal papilla as the site of early stone formation.

REFERENCES

1. R. Hautmann, A. Lehmann, and S. Komor, J. Urol. 123:317 (1980).
2. R. Hautmann, A. Lehmann, and S. Komor, Eur. J. Clin. Invest. 10:173 (1980).
3. N. A. Gains, C. W. Michaels, M. Z. Thwaites, and J. R. Trounce, Nephron 5:352 (1968).
4. D. J. Bennett, F. E. Cole, E. D. Frohlich, and D. T. Erwin, J. Lab. Clin. Med. 91, 5:822 (1978).
5. R. J. Wright and A. Hodgkinson, Invest. Urol. 5:369 (1972).
6. K. J. Ullrich and K. H. Jarausch, Pflügers Arch. Ges. Physiol. 262:537 (1956).
7. W. Pfaller and M. Rittinger, Mikroskopie Georg Fromme Verlag, Wien (Oesterreich) 33:74 (1977).
8. M. A. Knepper, R. A. Danielson, G. M. Saidel, and R. S. Post, Kid. Int. 12:313 (1977).
9. F. H. Epstein, Am. J. Med. 45:700 (1968).
10. R. C. Haggit and J. A. Pitcock, J. Urol. 106:342 (1971).
11. J. L. Bennington, L. S. Haber, J. V. Smith and N. E. Warner, Am. J. Clin. Path. 41:8 (1964).
12. B. Finlayson and F. Reid, Invest. Urol. 6:442 (1978).
13. R. Hautmann and H. Osswald, Naunyn-Schmiedeberg's Arch. Pharmacol. 304:277 (1978).
14. R. Greger, F. Lang, H. Oberleithner, and P. Deetjen, Pflügers Arch. 374:243 (1978).
15. E. J. Weinman, S. J. Franfurt, A. Ince, and S. Sansom, J. Clin. Invest. 61:801 (1978).
16. A. Randall, in:"VII Congress of the International Society of Urology," 186 (1939).
17. C. W. Vermeulen, E. S. Lyon, J. E. Ellis, and T. A. Borden, J. Urol. 97:573 (1967).
18. E. L. Prien, Sr., J. Urol. 114:500 (1975).

ACKNOWLEDGMENT

This work was generously supported by the Martin-Brinkmann-Foundation, Bremen, West-Germany.

RAT RENAL PAPILLARY STRUCTURE IN OXALATE-INDUCED MICROLITHIASIS, A SCANNING ELECTRON MICROSCOPE STUDY

S. R. Khan, B. Finlayson, and R. L. Hackett

University of Florida, College of Medicine

Gainesville, Florida, U.S.A.

Most commonly, renal stones are found in the renal calyces or pelvis and several of the hypotheses concerning calculogenesis implicate the papilla as having a central role. Attention was first focused on this region of the kidney by Randall[1,2,3], who described minute calculi and calcium plaques on and within renal papilla. Vermeulen et al.[4,5] extended these observations in a series of experiments which suggested that the papillary tip was critical in the formation of various types of stones. However, few current studies are available which explore changes in the renal papilla during experimental calculogenesis. To extend further the knowledge of papillary involvement in lithogenesis we examined structural alterations of the papillary surface during calcium oxalate crystalluria.

METHODS

Male Sprague-Dawley rats, 250-350 g, were injected intraperitoneally with 0.22M sodium oxalate in 0.9% saline using a dose of 7 mg/100 g rat body weight. At 15 min, 1 h, 6 h, 24 h, 48 h, and 7 days following the injection, kidneys were fixed with a formaldehyde-glutaraldehyde mixture by retrograde aortic perfusion. The papillae were isolated, post-fixed in osmium tetroxide and dehydrated. Specimens were critical point dried using carbon dioxide and mounted on aluminum stubs. After being coated with gold-palladium in a sputter coater, the papillae were examined by scanning electron microscopy.

RESULTS AND DISCUSSION

As previously described[6-8], the oxalate challenge is toxic but not lethal. In this model crystallization of calcium oxalate starts within 15 min of the sodium oxalate injection and by 1 h the crystals can be identified in all segments of the nephron[7,8]. Calcium oxalate is present in the papilla in pure or mixed aggregates of monohydrate and dihydrate crystals. Viewed under the scanning electron microscope, the normal rat papilla is a smooth, conical structure. The covering urothelium is composed of uniform cells with distinct cell borders and surfaces marked by short, blunt microvilli. The expanse of epithelium is interrupted only at the papillary tip where the ducts of Bellini open into parallel furrows (Figure 1). The furrows are usually slightly curved and vary from 7-12 in our material.

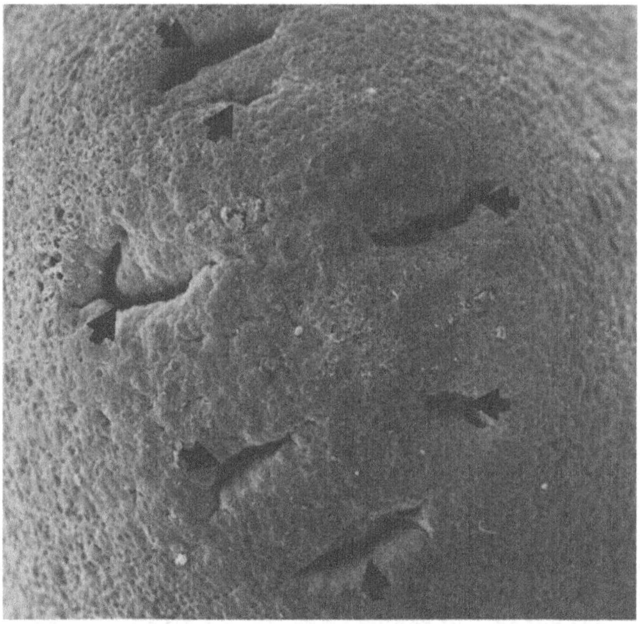

Figure 1. Papillary tip of a normal rat. Seven furrows can be identified (arrows) on the surface (Bar = 150 μm).

In the experimental animals, progressive distortion of papillary architecture occurs eventually resulting in severe structural alterations. For the first hour papillary surface appears normal even though crystals are present in the papillary ducts. However, sometimes crystal aggregates can be seen occluding the furrows. By 6 h the papillary furrows are grossly deformed (Figure 2) and the surface urothelium is torn revealing the protruding crystals (Figure 3).

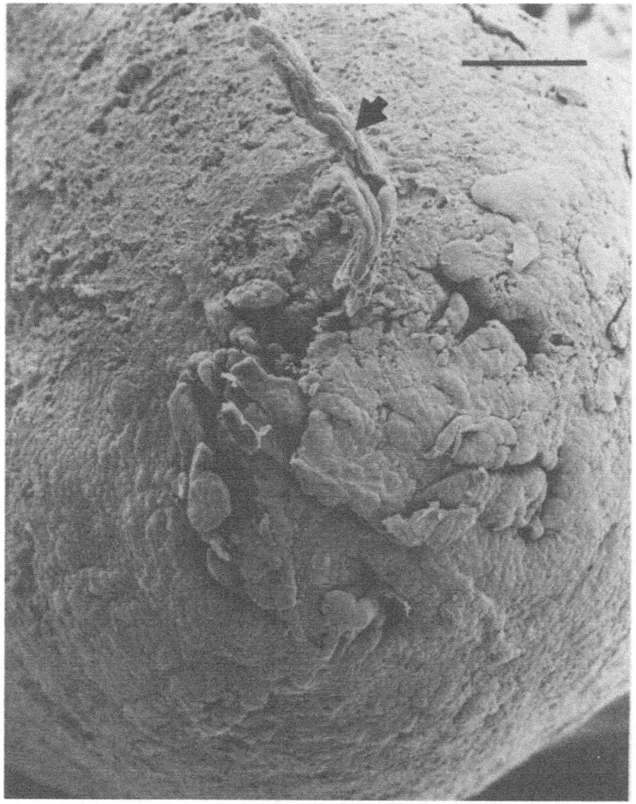

Figure 2. Papillary tip 6 h after sodium oxalate injection. Papillary furrows are grossly deformed. Torn urothelium appears to be hanging (arrow) from the surface of the papillary tip. (Bar = 100 μm).

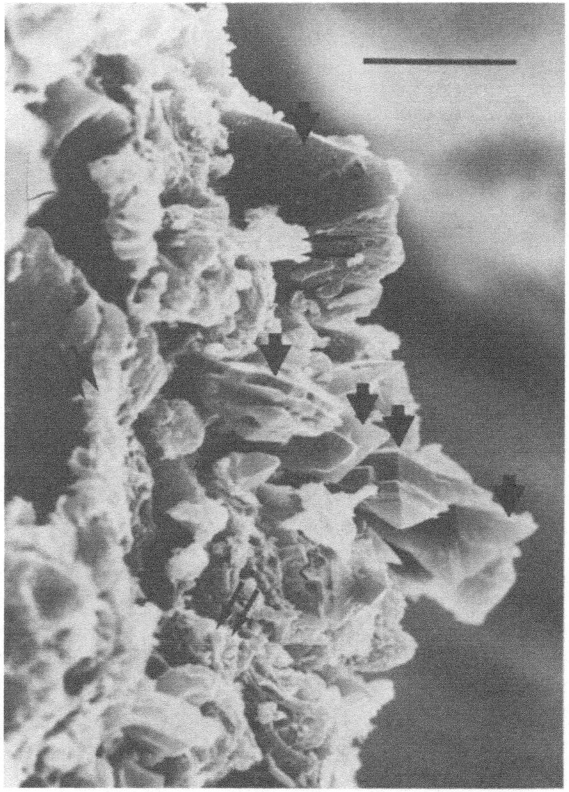

Figure 3. Dihydrate crystals (arrows) protruding on the papillary surface. Crystals are covered with necrotic epithelium (double arrows). (Bar = 17 μm).

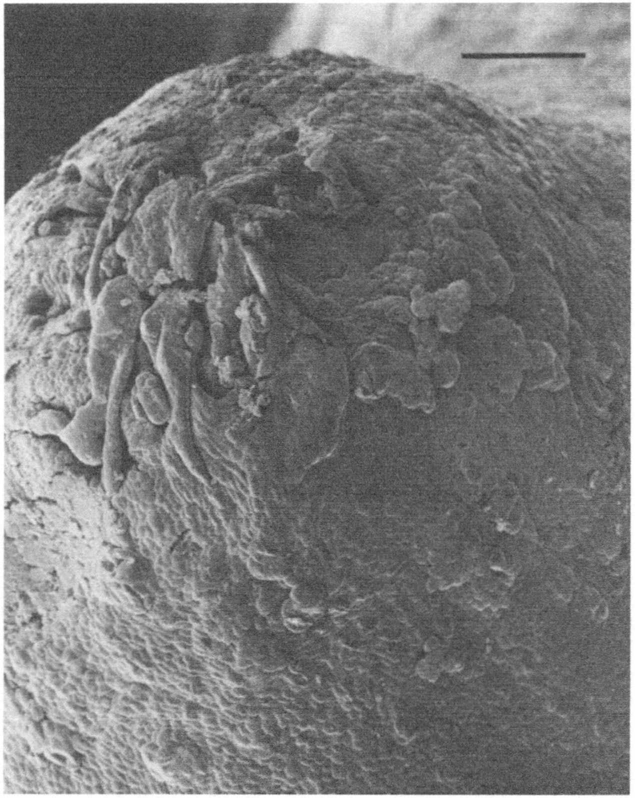

Figure 4. Papillary tip 48 h after sodium oxalate injection. (Bar = 17 μm).

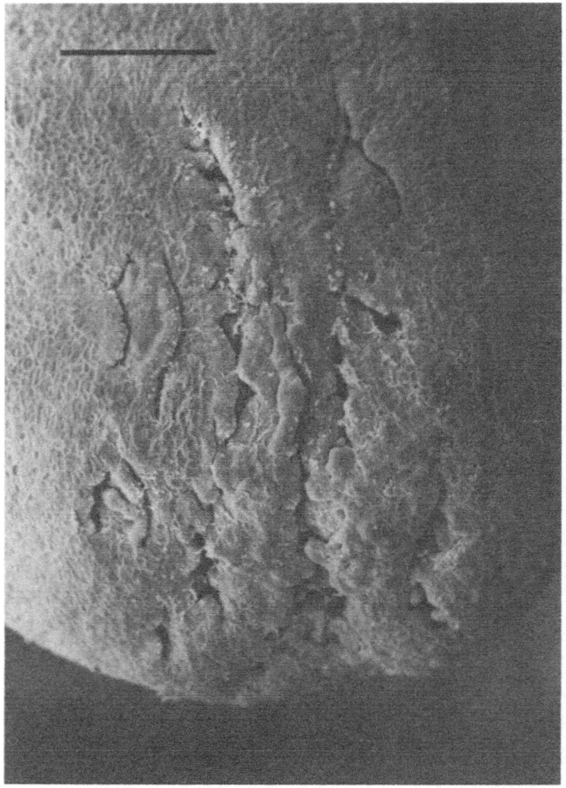

Figure 5. Papillary tip 1 week after sodium oxalate injection. Papillary epithelium appears to be regenerating. The furrows can be identified. (Bar = 200 μm).

By 48 h the process is amplified and extended (Figure 4). The papillary furrows are difficult to identify, the urothelial cells are destroyed and fragments of torn epithelium line the jagged perimeters of the furrows (Figures 2, 4). One week after the oxalate injection the papillary structure appears to be recovering (Figure 5). Parallel furrows can again be identified even though their outlines remain distorted. The epithelium lining the furrows appears to be regenerating.

The results of these experiments show that papillary structure is severely altered in this model of calcium oxalate microlithiasis. Papillary tip alterations appear to be a combination of urothelial necrosis and the distortion of the furrows. The ulcerated areas on the papillary surface where the urothelium is torn and the crystals are exposed can be compared to Randall's plaque.

REFERENCES

1. A. Randall, New Engl. J. Med. 214:234 (1936).
2. A. Randall, Ann. Surg. 105:1009 (1937).
3. A. Randall, J. Urol. 44:580 (1940).
4. C. W. Vermeulen, E. S. Lyon, and T. A. Borden, Trans. Am. Assoc. Genito-Urinary Surgeons 58:30 (1966).
5. C. W. Vermeulen, E. S. Lyon, J. E. Ellis, and T. A. Borden, J. Urol. 97:573 (1967).
6. M. J. Dykstra and R. L. Hackett, Kid. Int. 15:640 (1979).
7. S. R. Khan, B. Finlayson, and R. L. Hackett, Invest. Urol. 17:199 (1979).
8. S. R. Khan, B. Finlayson, and R. L. Hackett, Lab. Invest. 41:504 (1979).

THE ULTRASTRUCTURE OF RAT RENAL TUBULES IN EXPERIMENTAL CALCIUM OXALATE NEPHROLITHIASIS

Saeed R. Khan, Birdwell Finlayson, and Raymond L. Hackett

University of Florida
College of Medicine
Gainesville, Florida

Formation of calcium oxalate crystals in the rat kidney was induced by a lithogenic challenge made by intraperitoneal injection of various amounts of sodium oxalate utilizing 0.22M sodium oxalate solution in 0.9% saline. The rat kidneys were fixed by retrograde aortic perfusion with a glutaraldehyde-paraformaldehyde mixture at different time intervals following the lithogenic challenge. The kidneys were sliced into small pieces and processed for transmission and scanning electron microscopy. Normal rat kidneys were fixed and used as controls. Two major problems were encountered in the ultrastructural study of renal tubules containing calcium oxalate crystals. First, the small number of crystals in the renal tissue of animals injected with the lesser doses of sodium oxalate made systemic study difficult. Second, crystals could not be infiltrated with plastic and caused sectioning problems for transmission electron microscopy. This problem was solved by treating the crystals with hydrochloric acid or EDTA, which resulted in their partial digestion facilitating plastic infiltration.

Calcium oxalate crystals appeared first in the lumens of proximal tubules within fifteen minutes of the sodium oxalate challenge. At early times crystals were never seen in the tubular cells or the interstitium. Based on morphology two types of crystals were identified by SEM. Calcium oxalate monohydrate crystals were present as aggregates of monoclinic prismatic plates while calcium oxalate dihydrate crystals appeared as tetragonal bipyramids present individually or in aggregates. Transmission electron microscopy confirmed our earlier observations[1,2] about the adherence of crystals to the luminal surface of the tubular epithelium. Polarity of calcium oxalate monohydrate crystal aggregates shown earlier by SEM[1,2] was also seen by transmission electron microscopy. TEM also revealed a membrane-like covering around the crystals.

A number of morphological changes were observed in the renal tubular cells. It is remarkable that most cells exhibiting changes were in epithelium lining tubules that contained crystals. Few cellular changes were seen in the first 30 minutes of the oxalate challenge. The alterations became obvious 1 hour after the oxalate challenge and were pronounced within 6 hours of the challenge.

The first noticeable cellular change occurred in the shape of the luminal surface of the epithelium lining the proximal tubules. Although all three segments of the proximal tubule were involved, the changes in the S-2 segments were more pronounced. The micro-villous brush border was distorted by the formation of blebs which were revealed by the transmission electron microscopy to be the protoplasmic projections of the epithelial cells. The blebs usually contained the same contents as the main cell body, sometimes even a nucleus. Some of the microvilli appeared club-shaped with swollen tips while others appeared vesiculating. Endocytic apparatus of the pars convoluta of the oxalate challenged animals was very extensive and contained a large number of tubular profiles. The basement membrane of the S-2 segment of the proximal tubules appeared to be slightly thickened.

Cellular necrosis was seen in all parts of the nephron. Luminal cell membranes of the necrotic cells appeared to have burst releasing their contents into the tubular lumen. In some cases the cells appeared to be sheared away from the tubular basement membrane. Cellular debris was seen in the lumens of all parts of the nephron. The debris consisted of necrotic cellular organnelles and amorphous substance. There was an intimate association between the crystals and the debris and amorphous material appeared to be deposited on the surface of the crystals.

After an oxalate challenge, there was an increase in the number of lysosomes in all parts of the nephron, some of which appeared to be autophagic vacuoles. There also was an increase in the elements of Golgi apparatus in all parts of the nephron particularly in the epithelial cells of the distal tubules. The intercellular spaces between the epithelial cells also appeared to be enlarged.

All the changes in the renal tubular ultrastructure following sodium oxalate challenge appear to be non-specific and are similar to changes in renal tubular ultrastructure following other types of toxic injuries[3]. Whether these changes are the result of the presence of crystals of calcium oxalate or the homeostatic imbalance brought about by sodium oxalate injections is unresolved. We think that the crystals are toxic to the epithelial cells because most of the changes resulting from sodium oxalate challenge appeared to be limited to the tubular parts that contained the crystals. Whether the crystals nucleate on the epithelial surface or they attach themselves to the epithelium after their formation in the tubular lumen is also unresolved. Gill et al.[4] (personal communication) in their studies of calcium oxalate crystallization in female rat bladders have shown enhanced adherence of crystals to the urothelium following acid and Triton X 100 injuries. In their view adherent crystals were nucleating on the injured epithelium while the free crystals had intraluminal nucleation. A similar phenomenon may explain the presence of free and adherent crystals in our model.

REFERENCES

1. S. R. Khan, B. Finlayson, and R. L. Hackett, Invest. Urol. 17:199 (1979).
2. S. R. Khan, B. Finlayson, and R. L. Hackett, Lab. Invest. 41:504 (1979).
3. B. F. Trump, M. L. Jesudason, and R. T. Jones, in:"Diagnostic Electron Microscopy," B. F. Trump and R. T. Jones, ed. John Wiley & Sons, New York (1978).
4. W. B. Gill, K. Ruggiero, and F. H. Straus, II, Invest. Urol. 17:257 (1979).

CRYSTAL FORMATION IN THE RENAL TUBULES OF RATS INDUCED BY ETHYLENE GLYCOL ADMINISTRATION AND MAGNESIUM DEFICIENCY

H. Gil Rushton, Myron Spector, Allen L. Rodgers,
and Christian E. Magura
Medical University of South Carolina

Charleston, South Carolina

INTRODUCTION

Many previous studies have employed diet-inducing hypomagnesemic or hyperoxaluric protocols in experiments with rats and other animals to investigate aspects of renal calculus disease. Several early investigators focused on the renal tubules and papillae in an attempt to delineate the earliest histological and ultrastructural stages of hydroxyapatite deposition induced by hypomagnesemic protocols[1]. Later investigators employed vitamin B6 deficient diets and ethylene glycol administration to induce hyperoxaluria and subsequent renal tubular calcium oxalate crystal formation[2,3,4]. More recently intraperitoneal injection of sodium oxalate has been used to induce calcium oxalate intranephronic calculosis[5,6,7]. The objectives of the present study were to investigate the combined effects of hyperoxaluric and hypomagnesemic protocols in the rat kidney and to describe ultrastructural features of the formation of the experimentally induced crystals.

MATERIALS AND METHODS

Fifty-four male Sprague-Dawley rats weighing 225-325 gm were used for the study. Group 1 was administered 1% ethylene glycol drinking water; group 2 was fed a magnesium deficient diet containing less than .0005% magnesium; group 3 was placed on a combined regimen of the above. A fourth group was maintained as a control. Rats were sacrificed at intervals ranging from 1-9 weeks. Kidney specimens were allocated for conventional paraffin processing, plastic embedment and section preparation by grinding, and scanning electron microscopy (SEM). When present, calculi were removed from kidney specimens after dissection and processed for x-ray diffraction analysis and SEM. Intratubular crystals for x-ray diffraction studies were removed under the dissecting microscope from 10 μm thick deparaffinized sections of kidneys.

RESULTS

X-ray diffraction studies of tubular crystal deposits and calculi from groups 1 and 3 revealed the monohydrate form of calcium oxalate. Crystalline deposits in group 2 were identified as hydroxyapatite. Tubular deposits and calculi composed of calcium oxalate monohydrate (COM) were also identified in group 2 kidneys after 9 weeks.

Light microscopy revealed that COM crystals appeared at earlier time periods and were markedly more extensive in the combined group than in the ethylene glycol group alone (Figures 1a and b). Both individual crystals and fan-shaped aggregates were intraluminal and were found predominantly within proximal tubules.

Histochemical analysis of COM deposits revealed positive staining with alcian blue. These deposits were PAS negative. Hydroxyapatite crystal deposits were both alcian blue and PAS positive.

SEM demonstrated individual, coffin-shaped, hexagonal COM crystals lying within the lumen of renal tubules in groups 1 and 3. At times smaller COM crystals were seen growing from the surface of others. In other areas, fan-shaped aggregates of COM were observed completely obstructing tubular lumens. In kidney specimens from group 2, clusters of small ill-defined crystallites, often in spherical aggregates, were seen within and often obstructing tubular lumens. Sheet-like and strand-like organic material was frequently found emanating from the tubular wall epithelium and adsorbed to the surface of both COM and hydroxyapatite crystals, appearing to attach these to the tubular walls (Figure 2).

Renal calculi 0.5-2 mm in diameter were present in the kidneys of 12 test animals, either lying free in the renal pelvis or attached to the papilla; several kidneys had multiple stones. The cleaved surface of small stones consistently revealed a central core with a porous appearance surrounded by a thick outer shell consisting of tightly packed, radially oriented crystals (Figure 3). These calculi were composed of coffin-shaped COM crystals ranging from 2-25 microns in length. Smaller rosette patterns of crystals reminiscent of those seen occluding the renal tubules were frequently found in the core of the stones.

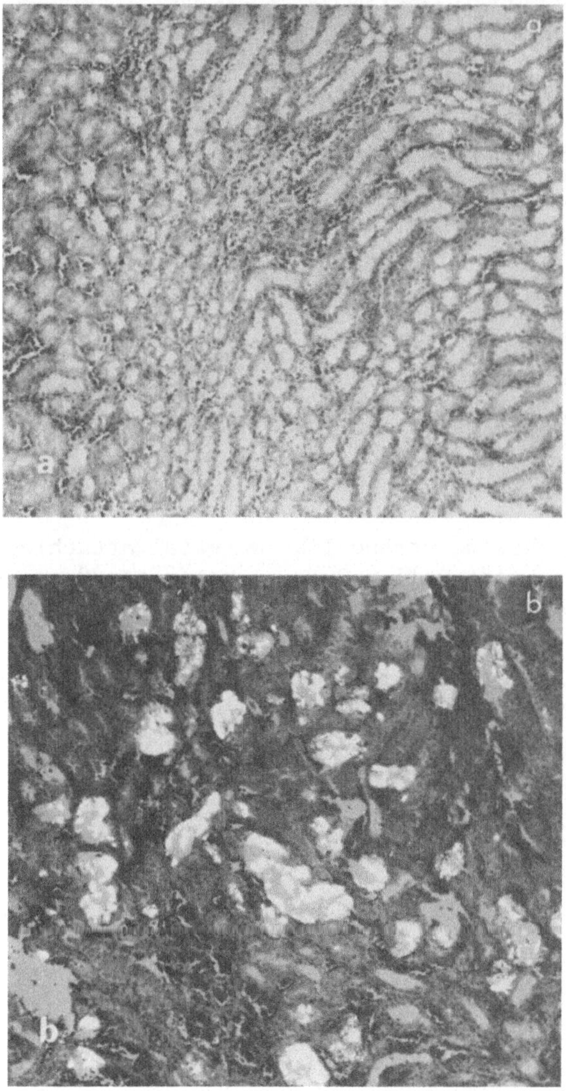

Figure 1. Partially polarized light micrographs of kidneys from rats in a) group 1 and b) group 3 after 9 days. Note extensive calcium oxalate crystal formation in the kidney in (b). 10X.

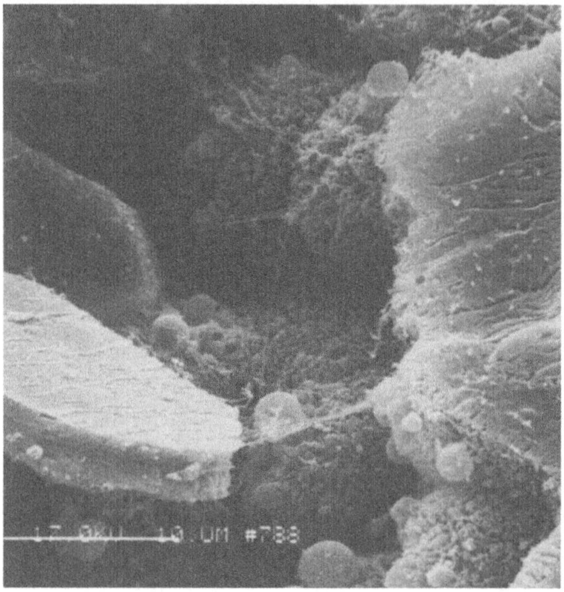

Figure 2. SEM showing strand-like material attaching COM crystals to tubular wall. Group 1 rat after 8 weeks. Perfusion fixed. 2,500X.

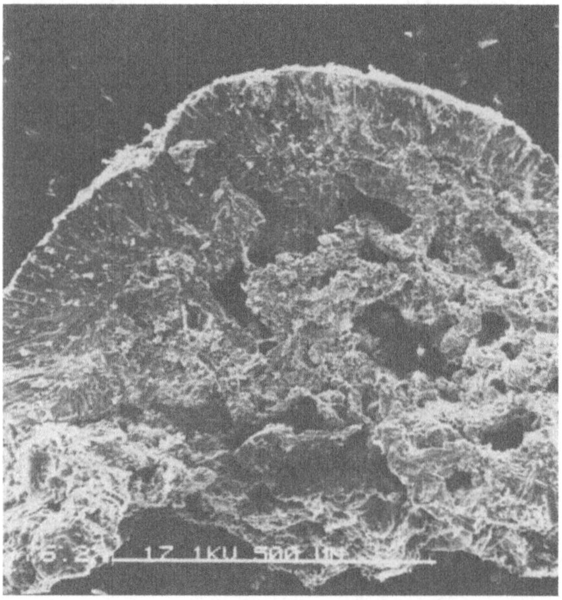

Figure 3. Cleaved surface of renal stone from kidney of a rat from group 3 after 9 weeks. 80X.

DISCUSSION

Previous studies in both man and animals have suggested a significant role for magnesium amongst the parameters involved in the multi-etiological problem of renal stone disease. In the present study, magnesium deficiency was found to enhance markedly calcium oxalate renal tubular deposition in hyperoxaluric, stone-forming rats. The effect of magnesium deficiency was to accelerate the renal tubular crystal deposition and secondary histopathological changes induced by ethylene glycol alone.

One hypothesis of calculus disease, emphasizing the importance of the site and mechanism of formation and retention of renal tubular crystals, proposes that a crystal fixed to the tubule wall would be predisposed to further growth and aggregation with other crystals to form microliths[8]. In the present study, SEM revealed the presence of strand and sheet-like organic material which appeared to attach renal tubular crystals to the renal tubular walls. Histochemical analysis demonstrated this material to be alcian blue positive indicating the presence of acid glycosaminoglycans and PAS negative, indicating the absence of glycoprotein. This substance may be significant in the retention of crystals to the tubular walls, providing fixed particles for further aggregation and growth.

Rosette-shaped aggregates of COM reminiscent of those occluding renal tubules were frequently found within the central core of renal calculi. These ultrastructural similarities suggest a possible sequence of events whereby dislodged intratubular deposits may pass through the collecting system of the kidney to enter the pelvis where they serve as the nidus for subsequent stone formation.

CONCLUSIONS

The results of the present study suggest 1) magnesium deficiency increases the propensity toward calcium oxalate formation in hyperoxaluria, and 2) a mucoid-appearing substance serves to attach calcium oxalate and hydroxyapatite crystals to the tubule walls.

REFERENCES

1. J. Oliver, M. McDowell, R. Whang, and L. G. Welt, J. Exp. Med. 124:263 (1966).
2. S. N. Gershoff and S. B. Andrus, J. Nutr. 73:308 (1961).
3. E. J. Lyon, T. A. Borden, and C. N. Vermeulen, Invest. Urol. 4:145 (1966).
4. J. A. Roberts and B. Finlayson, in:"Colloquium on Renal Lithiasis," B. Finlayson and W. C. Thomas, Jr., ed., University Presses of Florida, Gainesville, Florida (1976).

5. B. van't Reit and R. L. Bowe, in:"Colloquium on Renal Lithiasis," B. Finlayson and W. C. Thomas, Jr., ed., University Presses of Florida, Gainesville, Florida (1976).
6. S. R. Khan, B. Finlayson, and R. L. Hackett, Invest. Urol. 17:199 (1979).
7. M. J. Dykstra and R. L. Hackett, Kid. Int. 15:640 (1979).
8. B. Finlayson and F. Reid, Invest. Urol. 15:442 (1978).

ACKNOWLEDGMENTS

The technical assistance of J. T. Eldridge and J. C. Lilga is gratefully acknowledged. Dr. Spector was supported by NIH-NIDR Research Career Development Award DE00067.

A NEW VIEW OF STONE FORMATION UNDER THE ASPECT OF FLOW DYNAMICS

E. Schulz and H.-J. Schneider

Urologische Klinik und Poliklinik der Friedrich-Schiller-Universität
69-Jena, Lessingstr. 1/GDR

With decreased activity of certain inhibitors, or if the urine is supersaturated in stone forming salts, homogeneous or heterogeneous nuclei in the urinary system may grow into uroliths[1,2].

Yet the question is open, why these nuclei in stone formers are not excreted by the urine flow.

The first nuclei are found in the tubular regions (minimal diameter about 10 μm) or in the papillary ducts (maximal diameter about 300 μm), respectively.

The sizes of uroliths in the pyelo-calyceal system however, are as much as 1 cm.

It can be suggested that the urine stream may become pathologic in the complicated forniceal-pelvic system. Areas rich in vortices or with a slow urine flow may result in retention periods long enough for stone formation from nuclei[3,4]. Hydrodynamic studies (electromanometric and x-ray cinematographic)[5] and technical calculations[4] resulted in Reynolds number less than 500 in the pyelocalyceal system. This proves the existence of laminar flows (Figure 1).

Flow velocity v is very small near the walls of the tube and is zero immediately on the wall. An analysis of the velocity (v) - pressure (p) course in a closed pipe system with different diameters results in the picture shown in Figure 2.

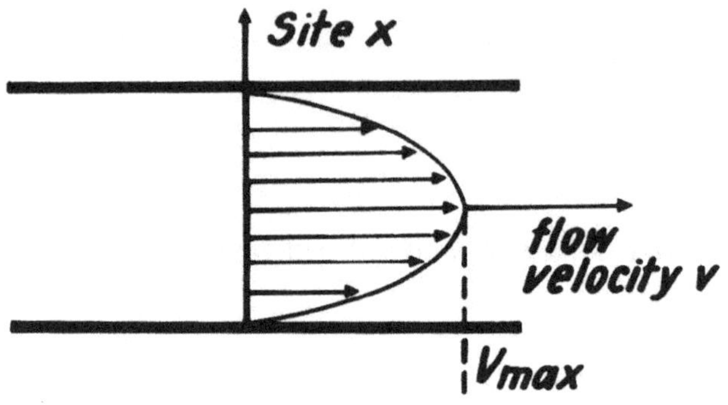

Figure 1. Course of flow in laminar flow.

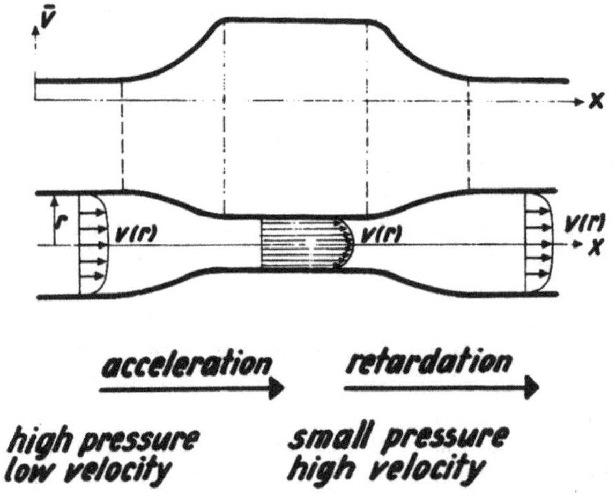

Figure 2. v-p course in different pipe diameters.

This leads to the following conclusions: a) areas with very low flow velocity such as dead zones or vortex regions have good fixation of nuclei, poor transport of substances, and slow stone growth; b) areas with rapid flow have poor fixation of nuclei, good transport of substances, and rapid stone growth.

There exist exact patterns of flow in laminar regions for liquids flowing in technical pipe systems of different geometrical forms. From these patterns, interesting conclusions can be drawn about urodynamic systems[6].

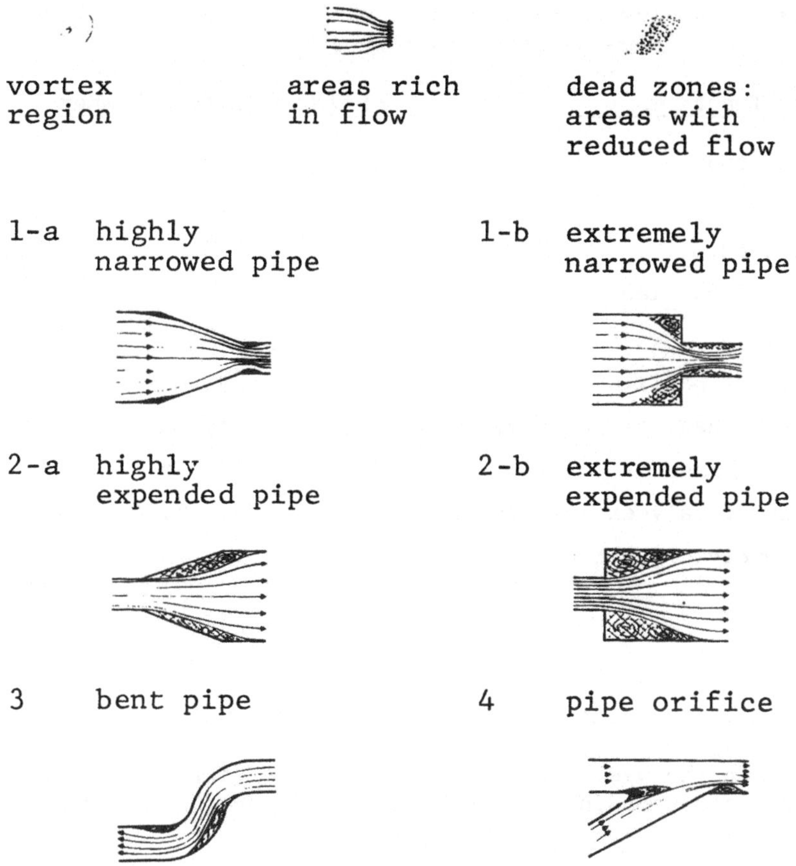

Figure 3. Flow courses in technical pipe systems.

Figure 3 shows some patterns of flow profiles for various geometries. Table 1 draws some analogies between the patterns in Figure 3 and what might be expected in the urinary tract.

During the change between filling and emptying-stages the forms of flow in the calyces and pelvis may change according to the respective geometrical conditions.

The expectation of these risk zones and their differences in flow compared to the surroundings is highest in the pyelocalyceal system with certain conditions of pressure and geometry. Congenital or acquired pathological changes of certain parameters of the urinary system (shape of the pelvis, pressure, peristalsis rhythm, etc.) may produce an increase in risk regions and may support stone formation.

Table 1. Analogous Relations in the Flow Courses of Technical Pipe Systems and in the Urinary Tract

Urinary Tract		Flow Course Type Number
Proximal tubule		3
Loop of Henle		1a, 2a, 3
Distal tubule		3
Collecting tubules		4
Papillae		2b
Entrance of papillae into calyces		2a, 4
Calyces:	Phase of contraction	1a, 2a
	Phase of dilation	2a, 2b
Entrance of calyces into the pelvis		2a, 2b, 4
Uretero-pelvic-junction		1a, 1b

SUMMARY

From the present study, the following conclusions may be drawn:

1. In the pyelo-calyceal system great differences in the flow patterns corresponding to type 1-4 (see Figure 3) must be taken into consideration.

2. Dead zones and zones with poor flow occur near the walls and between different flows near orifices or in pipes with changes in direction. Here fixation is easily possible.

3. Vortex regions form between different flows, especially entrances of several pipes (calyces into pelvis etc.).

4. A closed type renal pelvis shows a greater risk of particle retention than an open one.

5. Factors affecting the flow pattern in the renal pelvis are diuresis, stages of contractions, position of kidney, forms of pelvis and calyx (size), number of calyces and papillae, entrance angle, and entrance cross-sections.

REFERENCES

1. W. G. Robertson, in:"Urolithiasis Research," H. Fleisch, W. G. Robertson, L. H. Smith, and W. Vahlensieck, ed., Plenum Press, New York/London (1976).

2. A. Preisinger, in:"Pathogenese und Klinik der Harnsteine 5," W. Vahlensieck, ed., Steinkopff-Verlag, Darmstadt (1975).
3. H.-J. Schneider and H. Seyfarth, Eur. Urol. 5:32 (1979).
4. E. Schulz and H.-J. Schneider, Z. Urol. Nephrol. 59:915 (1979).
5. H. Schmidt, in:"Motilität der Oberen Harnwege," Springer-Verlag, Berlin(W)-Heidelberg-New York (1978).
6. M. Hackeschmidt, in:"Grundlagen der Strömungstechnik Bd. I Deutscher Verlag für Grundstoffindustrie, Leipzig (1970).

RATES AND MECHANISMS OF DISSOLUTION OF RENAL CALCULI. I. RATES AND MECHANISM OF DISSOLUTION OF PURE CALCIUM OXALATE MONOHYDRATE IN ACID AND EDTA SOLUTION

John Pawelchak, Douglas R. Flanagan, and
Anthony P. Simonelli
University of Connecticut, School of Pharmacy
and Institute of Materials Science,
Storrs, Connecticut 06268

In the past there has been varying degrees of clinical interest in dissolving renal calculi by some type of in situ irrigation technique. The physical-chemical rationale for the selection of the best irrigation solutions has been based on the equilibrium solubility of calcium oxalate or other stone minerals in the particular medium without regard to other possible factors which may govern the dissolution process.

In this paper we will compare the dissolution properties of pure calcium oxalate monohydrate (COM) discs with those of sectional renal calculi. It is our purpose to determine how important the intrinsic solubility and diffusional properties of COM are to the release patterns from renal calculi.

EXPERIMENTAL

Dissolution studies[1] were conducted in an apparatus depicted in Figure 1 which provides a constant surface area for release and constant hydrodynamics because the stirrer is maintained at a constant distance from the disc surface and its speed is controlled by a constant speed synchronous motor. Sink conditions (i.e., bulk concentration of COM < 5% of its solubility) were maintained by using sufficiently large medium volumes (150-400 ml) and by exchanging the entire medium at regular intervals for fresh medium.

Real renal calculi were sectioned, the surface ground flat and then mounted in the dissolution apparatus such that release was obtained from one surface. Pure COM discs were prepared by a precipitation technique which involved producing a fine COM precipitate which, when filtered and sucked dry in the filter funnel, generated a solid cake which could be shaped into 19 mm diameter discs. Dissolution studies were conducted at 25°C with samples being removed from the media at regular intervals which were assayed for calcium by atomic absorption spectrophotometry. As mentioned earlier, the medium was often exchanged entirely at periodic intervals to maintain sink conditions.

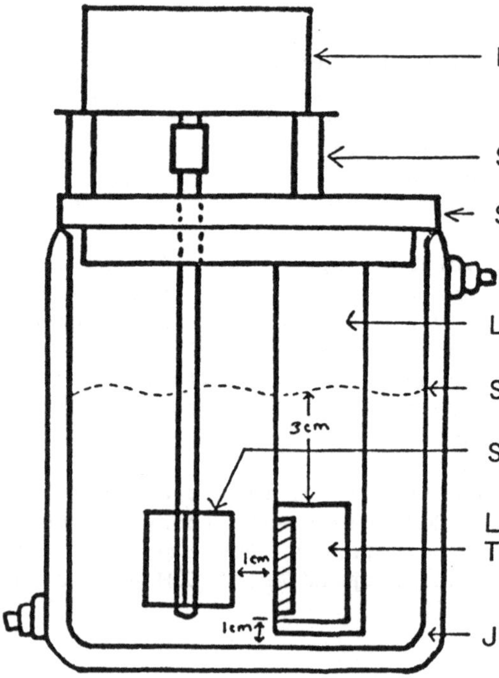

Figure 1. Apparatus

RESULTS AND DISCUSSION

Figures 2 and 3 show the dissolution profiles of pure COM discs in various pH media and in various concentrations of EDTA. As can be seen these profiles exhibited a linear time dependency which follows the simple diffusion-controlled model described by the following equation:

$$Q = \frac{D_a C_s t}{h}$$

where D_a is the aqueous diffusion coefficient of COM, C_s is the solubility of COM, h is the diffusion layer thickness, t is time, and Q is the amount of COM released/cm^2. The increase in slope of these plots will either decrease in pH (Figure 2) or increase in EDTA concentration (Figure 3). Analysis of the data showed that the dissolution rate was proportional to solubility as predicted by the diffusion-controlled model.

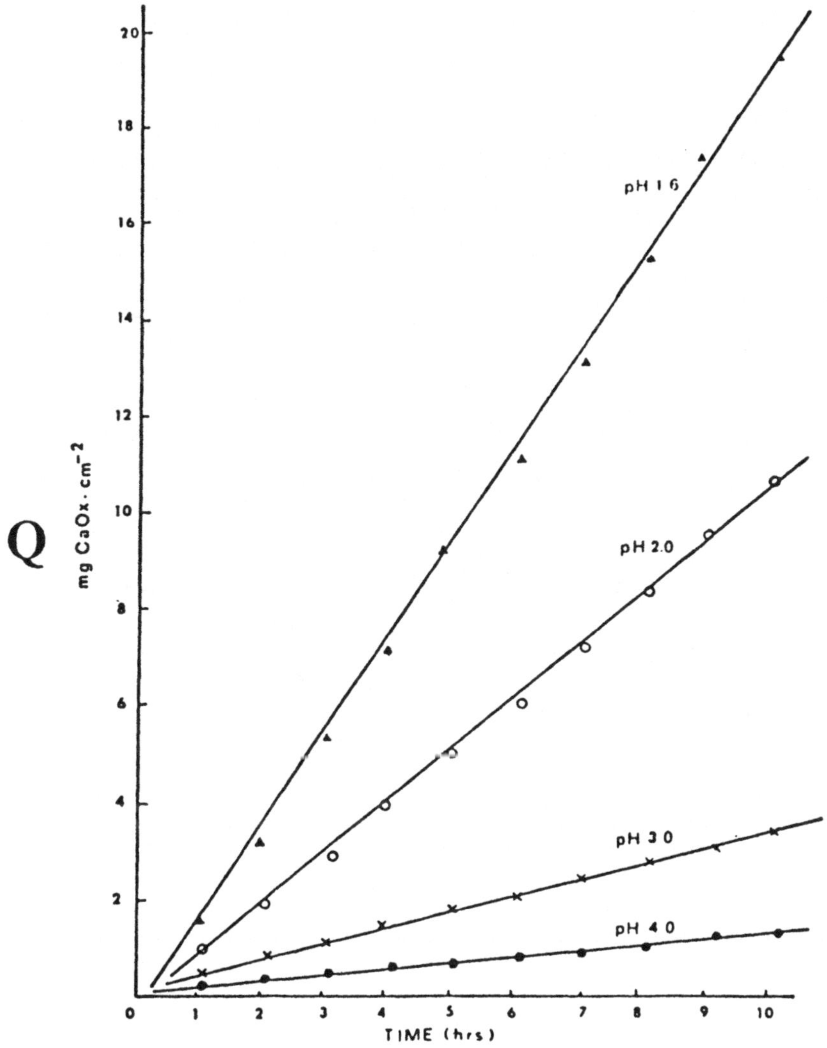

Figure 2. Dissolution of pure CaOx samples into various HCL solutions.

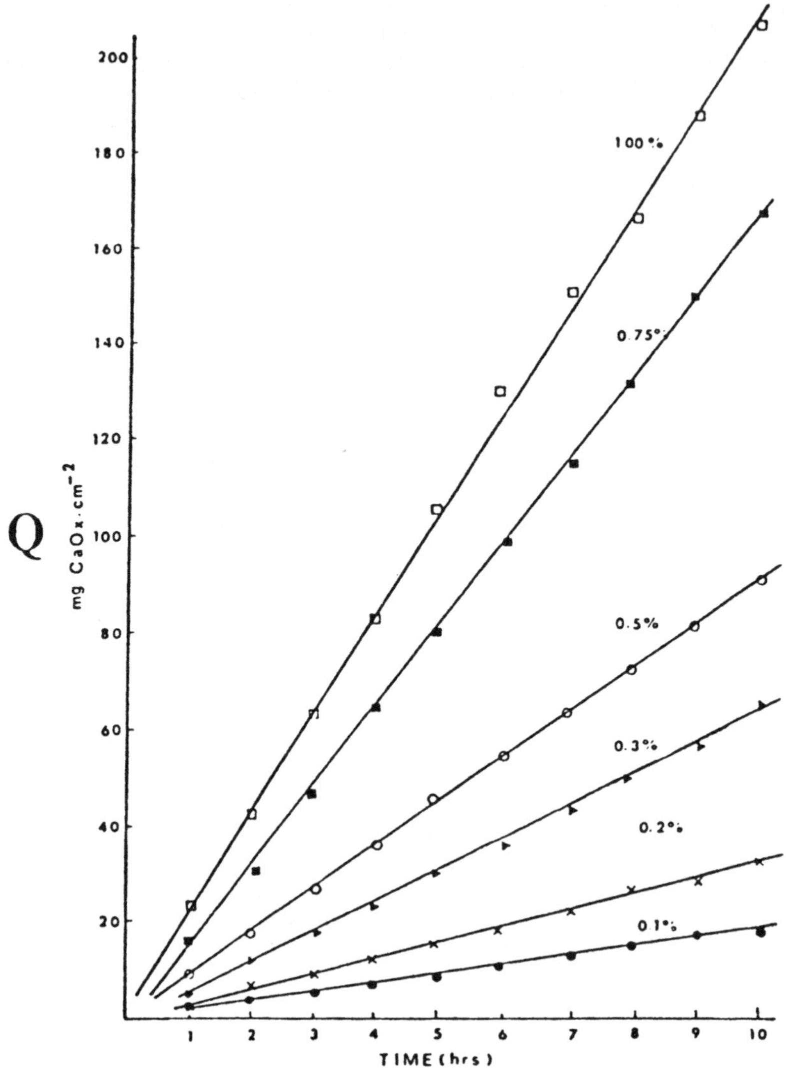

Figure 3. Dissolution of pure CaOx samples into various EDTA solutions.

The release profile of COM from the sectional real calculi in 1% EDTA shown in Figure 4 did not exhibit the same constant rate as a function of time. The dissolution profile shown is a typical plot which was characteristic of other EDTA %'s as well as non-EDTA solutions at various pH's. The dissolution profiles are not zero order or linear with time despite the maintenance of constant surface area, hydrodynamics and sink conditions for the entire experiment. The profiles show a definite parabolic time dependency indicating that the release rate decreases as a function of time.

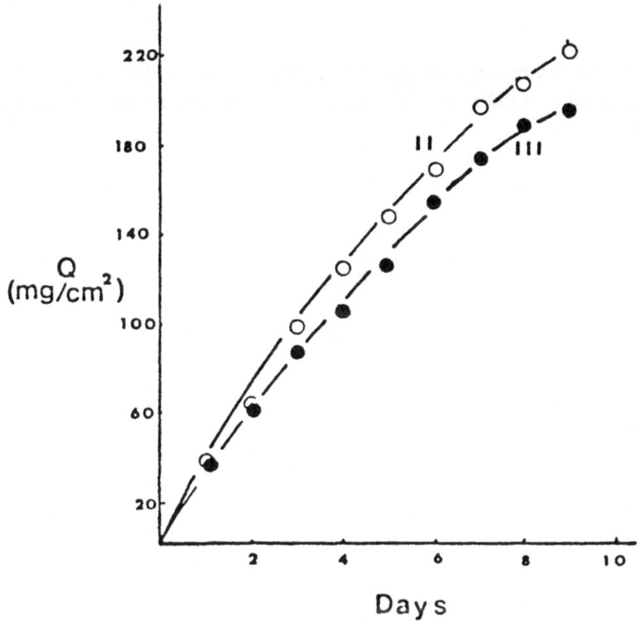

Figure 4. Dissolution profile for renal calculi.

These results demonstrate clearly that pure COM discs follow a simple diffusion-controlled dissolution mechanism which is proportional to the solubility of COM under constant hydrodynamics but that real calculi do not follow this simple mechanism. It can be concluded that the parabolic dissolution profiles of real calculi are not due to any intrinsic properties of COM but due to other diffusional factors that are not present in pure COM systems. These other factors and their elucidation will be discussed in the next two presentations[2,3] in this series.

REFERENCES

1. A. P. Simonelli, S. C. Mehta, and W. I. Higuchi, J. Pharm. Sci. 58:583 (1969).
2. J. Pawelchak, D. R. Flanagan, and A. P. Simonelli, in:"Proceedings of the Fourth International Symposium on Urolithiasis Research," L. H. Smith, B. Finlayson, W. G. Robertson, eds., Plenum Press, New York (in press).
3. J. Pawelchak, D. R. Flanagan, and A. P. Simonelli, in:"Proceedings of the Fourth International Symposium on Urolithiasis Research," L. H. Smith, B. Finlayson, W. G. Robertson, eds., Plenum Press, New York (in press).

ACKNOWLEDGMENT

This work was supported in part by Grants from the National Institutes of Health (AM 18891) and the University of Connecticut Research Foundation.

RATES AND MECHANISMS OF DISSOLUTION OF RENAL CALCULI. II. DEVELOPMENT AND DISCUSSION OF POTENTIAL MODELS FOR DISSOLUTION OF OXALATE CALCULI

John Pawelchak, Douglas R. Flanagan, and
Anthony P. Simonelli
University of Connecticut
School of Pharmacy and Institute of Materials Science
Storrs, Connecticut 06268

In our previous paper[1], we demonstrated that even though pure calcium oxalate followed a simple diffusion-controlled dissolution model that real calculi exhibited a more complex dissolution behavior. In this paper we will elaborate five dissolution models that are possibly applicable to renal calculi dissolution and develop criteria for determining their applicability.

Figures 1-4 depict the first four models. The differential equations describing the rates of calcium oxalate dissolution were derived and integrated to obtain theoretical concentration-time profiles. The complex relationships were greatly simplified by restricting the system to constant sample surface area, constant hydrodynamic and sink conditions; conditions easily achieved experimentally[1]. Each of the first three models (i.e., diffusion layer, shrinking membrane, and constant membrane) predict linear dissolution profiles as a function of time when constant surface area and sink conditions are maintained. The general equations for these systems are Rate of Dissolution = $dQ/dt = SDC_s/L$ and the amount dissolved = $Q = (SDC_s/L)t$ where S is the surface area of the tablet exposed to the solvent, D is the effective diffusion coefficient of calcium oxalate in the respective barrier, C_s is the solubility of calcium oxalate in the respective barrier, L is the thickness of the respective barrier and t is the time elapsed from the start of the experiment.

The final two models (matrix and biphasic) predict more complex time dependencies. The matrix model[2,3] predicting linear behavior when release data is plotted versus the square-root of time or rate is plotted versus reciprocal square root of time according to:

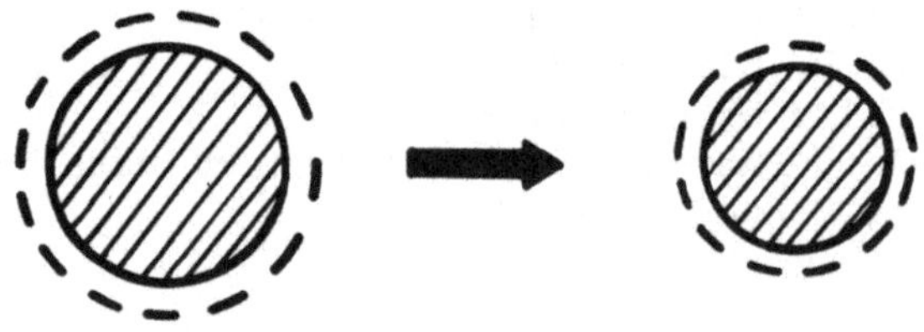

Figure 1. Diffusion Layer Model.

DIFFUSION LAYER BARRIER
UNDISSOLVED PART OF STONE
MEMBRANE BARRIER

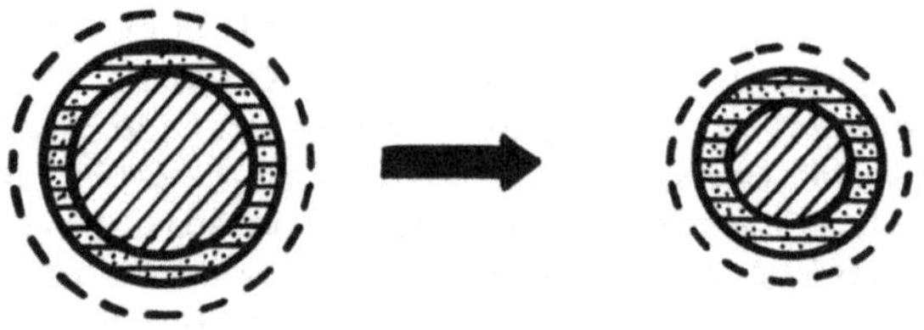

Figure 2. Shrinking Membrane Model.

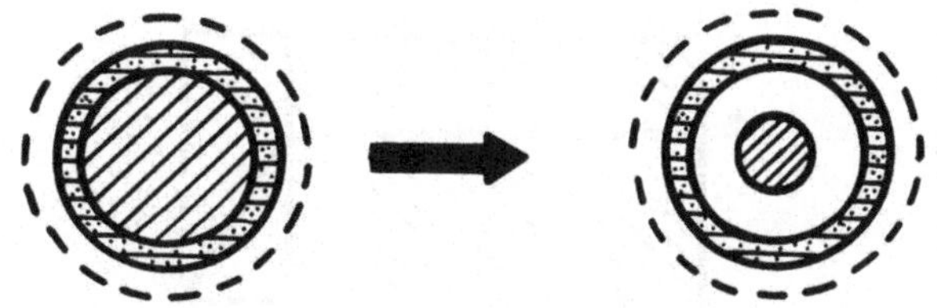

Figure 3. Constant Membrane Model

DIFFUSION LAYER BARRIER
UNDISSOLVED PART OF STONE
MEMBRANE BARRIER
SATURATED CaOx SOLUTION
LEACHED STONE

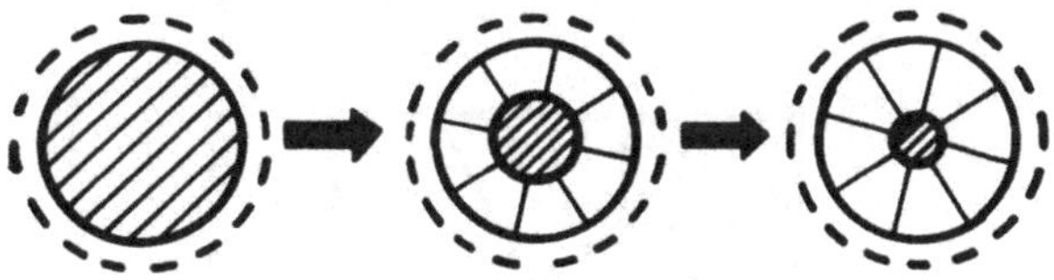

Figure 4. Matrix Model.

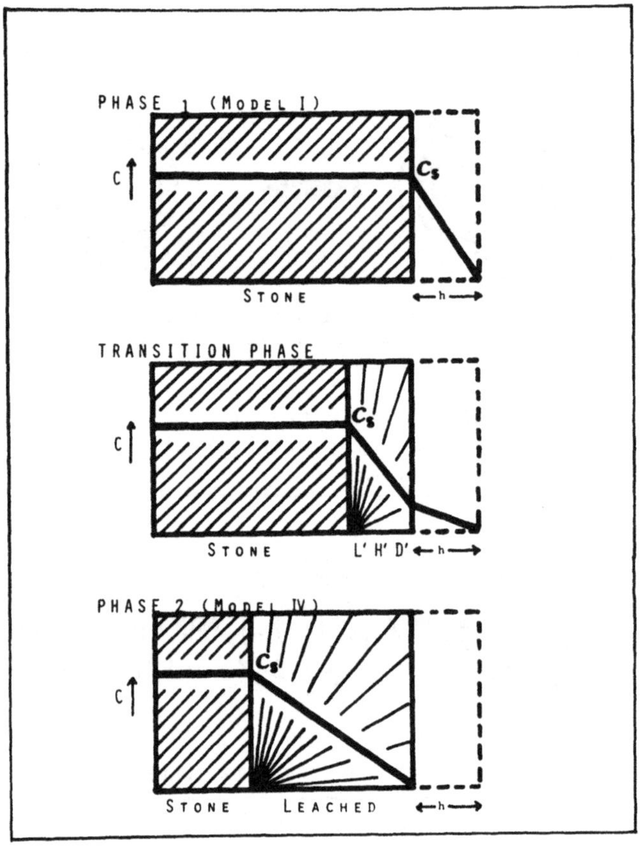

Figure 5. Biphasic Model

$$dQ/dt = K/t^{1/2} \qquad \text{and} \qquad Q = Kt^{1/2}$$

where $K = [(DC_s t/t)(2W-\varepsilon C_s)]^{1/2}$, ε is the porosity of matrix, t is the tortuosity of the matrix, W is the weight of CaOx in stone and the other parameters have been previously defined.

The final model combines the first model and the last model. In this model initially the dissolution rate is diffusion layer controlled but later is matrix barrier controlled. As a result, the biphasic model changes from a linear time dependency to a square-root of time dependency during the dissolution experiment. The applicable rate equation is:

$$Q = \frac{-WL\varepsilon}{\tau} + \left[\left(\frac{LW\varepsilon}{\tau}\right)^2 + \frac{2D_A\varepsilon WC_s t}{\tau}\right]^{1/2}$$

The concentration gradient and transition from Model I to Model IV is shown in Figure 5. It seems clear that the latter two models show the most promise for accounting for the dissolution characteristics of renal calculi when they are compared to the results obtained earlier on real stones. Thus, a matrix or biphasic-diffusion controlled/matrix model gives the time dependency observed in actual experiments. These models will be evaluated in our next paper[4] against data obtained with artificial calculi prepared to simulate the behavior of renal stones.

REFERENCES

1. J. Pawelchak, D. R. Flanagan, and A. P. Simonelli, in:"Proceedings of the Fourth International Symposium on Urolithiasis Research," L. H. Smith, B. Finlayson, and W. G. Robertson, eds., Plenum Press, New York (in press).
2. S. J. Desai, A. P. Simonelli, and W. I. Higuchi, J. Pharm. Sci. 54:1 (1965).
3. F. Sjuib, A. P. Simonelli, and W. I. Higuchi, J. Pharm. Sci. 61:381 (1972).
4. J. Pawelchak, D. R. Flanagan, and A. P. Simonelli, in:"Proceedings of the Fourth International Symposium on Urolithiasis Research," L. H. Smith, B. Finlayson, and W. G. Robertson, eds., Plenum Press, New York (in press).

ACKNOWLEDGMENT

This work was supported in part by Grants from the National Institutes of Health (AM 18891) and the University of Connecticut Research Foundation.

RATES AND MECHANISMS OF DISSOLUTION OF RENAL CALCULI. III. MECHANISMS AND RATES OF DISSOLUTION OF SIMULATED OXALATE CALCULI IN ACID AND EDTA SOLUTIONS

John Pawelchak, Douglas R. Flanagan, and
Anthony P. Simonelli
University of Connecticut
School of Pharmacy and Institute of Materials Science
Storrs, Connecticut 06268

A previous communication[1] showed that dissolution or urinary calculi sections did not exhibit zero-order (i.e., constant) rates under sink conditions. Since pure calcium oxalate discs did exhibit a constant dissolution rate, it was concluded that controlling processes other than the intrinsic solution properties of calcium oxalate must be operative in the dissolution behavior of real calculi. In this paper we intend to compare models described previously[2] with the dissolution behavior of artificial calculi in various media.

Since real calculi contain, in addition to a mineral component, a proteinaceous matrix, it was decided that artificial calculi should be prepared with a similar matrix component to determine its influence on the release properties of such systems. Cross-linked gelatin at 3% levels was selected to simulate the ubiquitous mucoprotein stone matrix and, as will be shown, produced dissolution behavior that closely paralleled that of real stones.

EXPERIMENTAL

Calcium oxalate monohydrate (COM) was prepared by preheating 600 ml of 0.25 m calcium nitrate and 800 ml of 0.3 m oxalic acid to 60°C and then mixing both solutions. The resulting COM precipitate was separated by filtration, washed thoroughly with water and dried at 50°C.

Artificial calculi discs were prepared by mixing COM with a gelatin solution, drying, grinding the resulting mass to a fine powder, and finally cross-linking with 25% glutarladehyde by rapid trituration in a glass mortar. The putty-like mass created during cross-linking was molded into 19 mm discs which were finally hardened and dried by heating overnight at 50°C. The resulting discs contained 3% cross-linked gelatin and had sufficient structured integrity to permit final grinding and shaping to obtain perfectly flat-faced discs.

Dissolution was monitored under sink conditions in a system described previously[1] which yielded constant hydrodynamics. Samples of the dissolution medium were removed at one hour intervals and assayed for calcium by atomic absorption spectrophotometry.

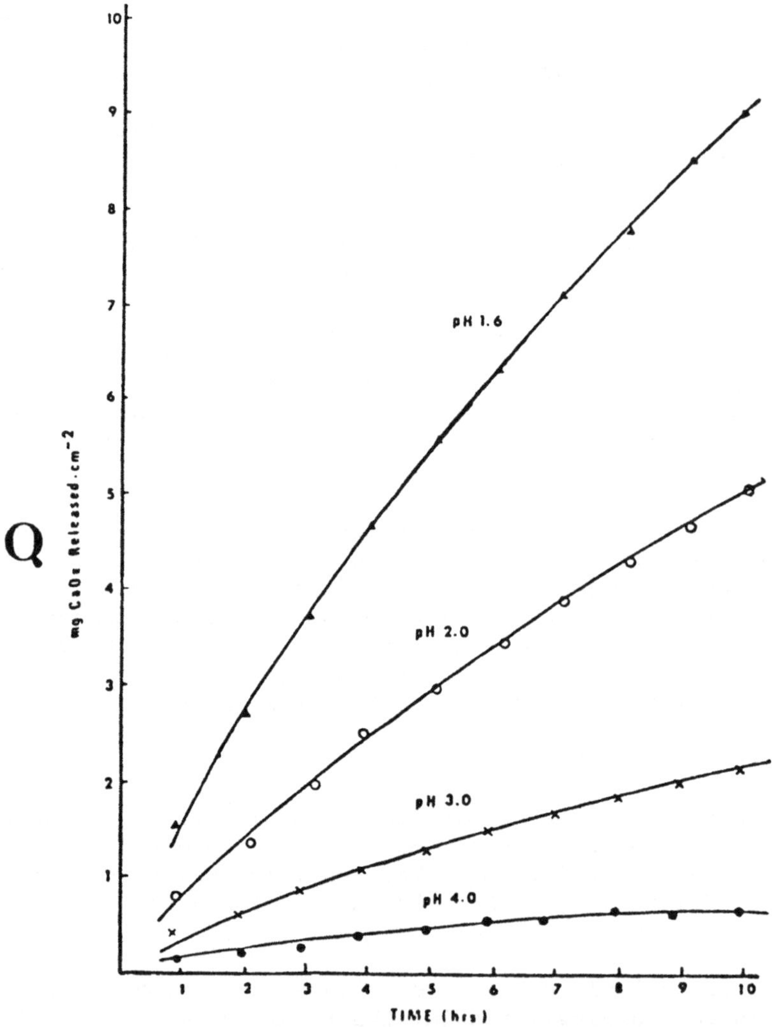

Figure 1. Release of CaOx from artificial calculi into HCl solution.

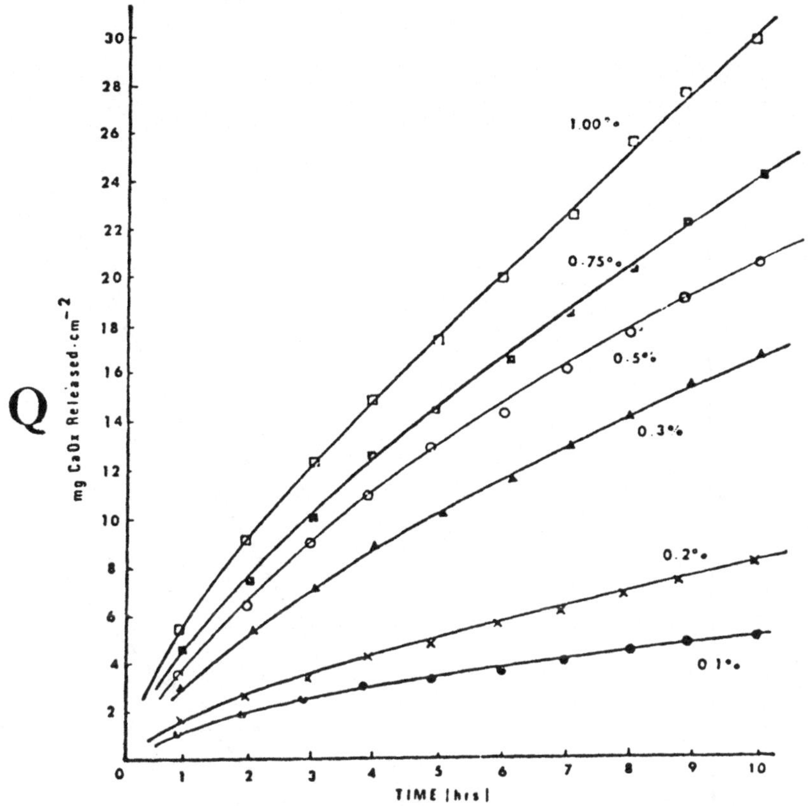

Figure 2. Release of CaOx from artificial calculi into various EDTA solutions.

RESULTS AND DISCUSSION

The dissolution profiles of artificial calculi in various pH media and at various EDTA concentrations are shown in Figure 1 and 2, respectively. In all cases, it can be seen that a parabolic time dependency for COM release is obtained. It is evident that the low level of matrix produces this effect on the release profiles because pure COM discs exhibited both higher and constant release rates in the same media. In addition, the generation of a porous gelatinour layer could be observed visually as dissolution proceeded.

These studies strongly suggest that the matrix presents a dissolution rate-controlling barrier to COM release. Such a dependency on an increasing matrix barrier was described mathematically in our previous paper[1] by the equation:

$$Q = (D_e C_s 2At)^{\frac{1}{2}}$$

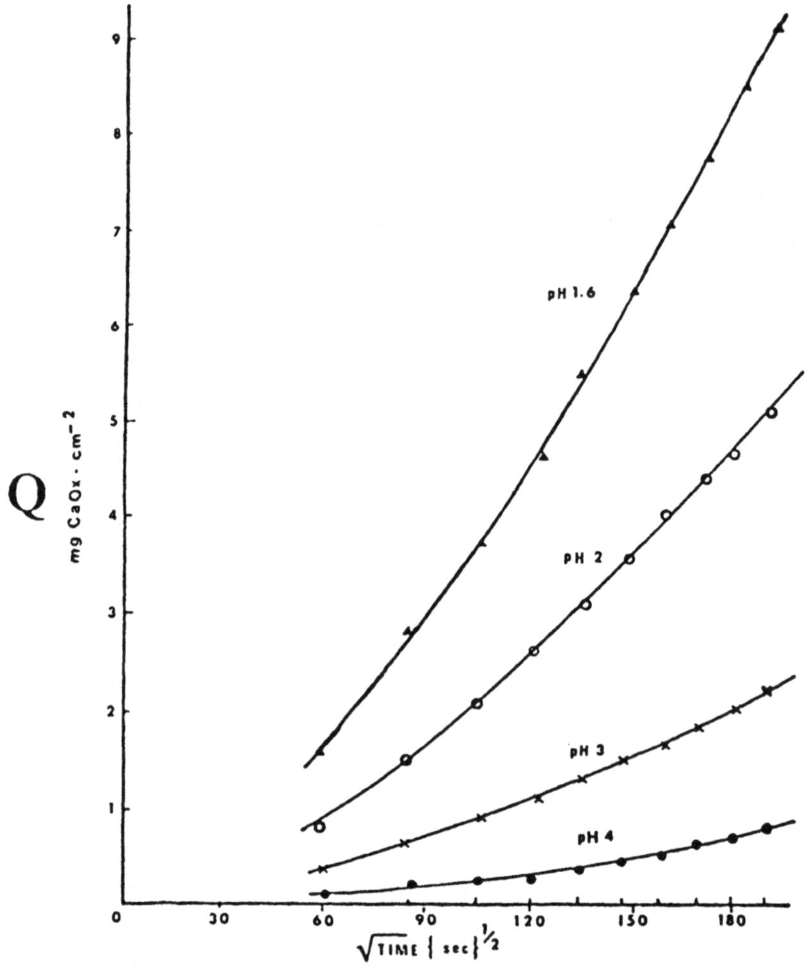

Figure 3. Release of CaOx from artificial calculi into HCl solutions as a function of $(\text{time})^{\frac{1}{2}}$.

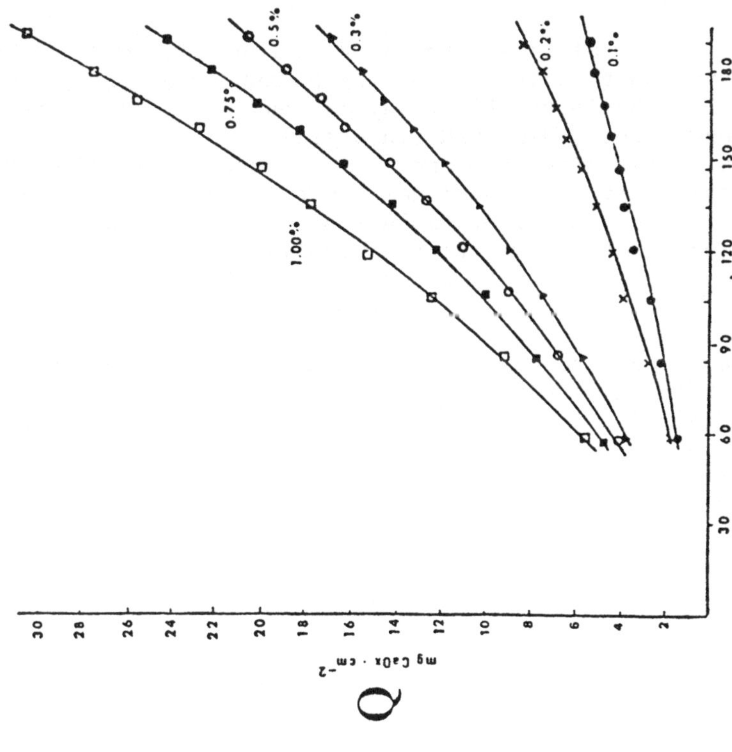

Figure 4. Release of CaOx from artificial calculi into EDTA solutions as a function of (time)½.

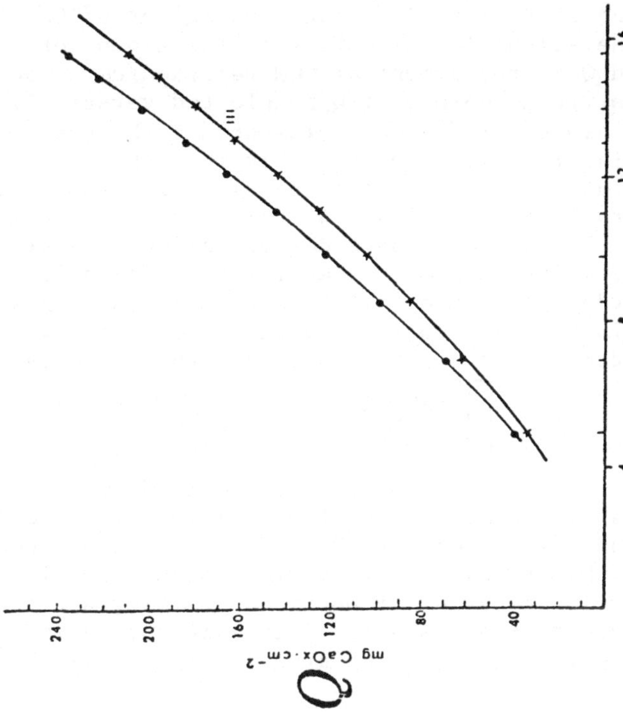

Figure 5. Renal calculi as a function of time½.

where: D_e is the effective diffusion coefficient of COM in the matrix, C_s is the solubility of COM, A is the amount of COM/cm^3 in the disc, and Q is the amount of COM released/cm^2. This equation predicts a linear relationship if Q is plotted versus $t^{\frac{1}{2}}$. Figure 3 and 4 show such plots for the data presented in Figures 1 and 2, and show that non-linearity is observed. Figure 5 shows the equivalent plot from dissolution of real renal calculi which shows the same type of curvature as Figures 3 and 4. Clearly the initial stages of both artificial and real stones do not follow a square-root of time dependency, which indicates that initially dissolution follows a simple zero-order model under sink conditions which gradually turns into matrix barrier control. Such biphasic behavior was previously described[1] and can be depicted mathematically by:

$$Q = \frac{-hAD_e t}{D_a} + \left[\left(\frac{hAD_e}{D_a}\right)^2 + 2D_e AC_s t\right]^{1/2}$$

The symbols are as above with the addition of D_a being the aqueous diffusion coefficient of COM and h being the aqueous diffusion layer thickness. This equation accounts well for the biphasic dissolution behavior of matrix-containing artificial calculi and serves as the basis for future investigations of the dissolution properties of real and artificial calculi.

REFERENCES

1. J. Pawelchak, D. R. Flanagan, and A. P. Simonelli, in:"Proceedings of the Fourth International Symposium on Urolithiasis Research," L. H. Smith, B. Finlayson, and W. G. Robertson, eds., Plenum Press, New York (in press).
2. J. Pawelchak, D. R. Flanagan, and A. P. Simonelli, in:"Proceedings of the Fourth International Symposium on Urolithiasis Research," L. H. Smith, B. Finlayson, and W. G. Robertson, eds., Plenum Press, New York (in press).

ACKNOWLEDGMENTS

This work was supported in part by Grants from the National Institutes of Health (AM 18891) and the University of Connecticut Research Foundation.

IV. INHIBITORS AND PROMOTERS

INHIBITION OF PTH-INDUCED NEPHROCALCINOSIS BY PHOSPHOCITRATE

W. P. Tew, C. D. Malis, A. L. Lehninger,
G. W. Walker, and J. E. Howard
The Johns Hopkins University School of Medicine

Baltimore, Maryland

Earlier studies from this Institution have suggested that phosphocitrate may play an important role in the regulation of physiological calcification[1,2]. It has been proposed as a constituent of normal urine and mitochondrial extracts which can prevent the transformation of amorphous calcium phosphate to crystalline phases.

We have recently reported the organic synthesis of phosphocitrate and documented its powerful inhibitory effect upon hydroxyapatite crystal growth[3]. The effects produced by phosphocitrate in seeded crystal growth assays have shown this compound to be more potent than equal concentrations of either pyrophosphate, ATP, or ethane-1hydroxy-1,1-diphosphonate (EHDP) in reducing the rate and extent of hydroxyapatite crystal growth. As previously demonstrated with other inhibitors of apatite growth, phosphocitrate has a high affinity for hydroxyapatite crystals, and its inhibitory action at low concentrations may be related to a selective absorption onto the active growth sites of the crystals.

The physical effects demonstrated by inhibitors of apatite growth have lead to studies of their use as potential therapeutic agents for pathological forms of calcification. These applications have been based on the assumption that the same physical-chemical relationships of crystal growth and its inhibition, developed through <u>in vitro</u> studies, must hold true in physiological mineralization. The reduction of vitamin D-induced renal calcification in rats by several diphosphonates and pyrophosphate supports this concept[4].

Small doses of phosphocitrate have been found effective in reducing the rate and extent of nephrocalcinosis produced in mice by large doses of parathyroid extract (PTH). The data presented in this report suggest that phosphocitrate functions at the cellular level to prevent the accumulation of calcium phosphate salts within the kidney. Additional studies indicate that long-term administration of phosphocitrate produces minimal effects on bone metabolism.

MATERIALS AND METHODS

Synthesis of Phosphocitrate

Phosphocitrate was synthesized as previously reported by the condensation of o-phenylene phosphorochloridate and triethylcitrate, catalytic removal of the o-phenylene group, and alkaline hydrolysis of the ethyl protecting group[3]. The final product was purified by elution from a Whatman DEAE-23 cellulose column with a gradient triethylamine-bicarbonate buffer (50 mM to 500 mM). The triethylamine salt was converted to the acid form by passage through a Chelex H^+ column and neutralized with NaOH.

Phosphocitrate was assayed by measuring the phosphate and citrate released after treatment with alkaline phosphatase. Phosphate was determined by the method of Bajinski, et al. and citrate by a modification of the enzymatic method of Dagley[3]. The sodium salt of phosphocitrate was used in all experiments.

Animals

Young male swiss mice weighing 15 to 18 grams were obtained from Buckberg Laboratories, Tomkins Cove, NY, and young male CD rats, 50 to 80 g from Charles River, Wilmington, MA. Details of the experimental protocols used including doses of PTH and phosphocitrate are given in the legends of each figure.

The animals were sacrificed under pentobarbitol anesthesia, blood removed from the inferior vena cava for serum calcium measurements and both kidneys removed for determination of tissue calcium content.

Calcium Determinations

Calcium was determined by atomic absorption spectrometry in the serum without deproteination by addition of 10 µl of serum to 1 ml of a lanthanum butanol-HCl medium[5]. For determination of kidney calcium content, mid-coronal sections of the kidneys were weighed, homogenized by sonication in 5 ml of a butanol-HCl-lanthanum medium, and centrifuged to remove insoluble debris. Calcium in the supernatant was determined by atomic absorption spectrophotometry. Calcium determinations were obtained with an Instrumentation Laboratories model 251, atomic absorption spectrophotometer.

Tissue Histology

Representative kidney tissue, sectioned along the medial plane, was examined by light microscopy for the presence of calcium deposits after fixation in methacrane and staining by the von Kossa technique.

Bone History

Comparisons were made of the effects of phosphocitrate and equivalent doses of EHDP on the growth rate and thickness of the epiphyseal plate of the tibia of young male rats (50 to 60 g). Phosphocitrate and EHDP were given as intraperitoneal injections at a dose level of 3.0 μmol/day for 14 days. Tibias were removed, fixed in 10% buffered formalin and decalcified with EDTA. Thin sections were examined by light microscopy for abnormal bone growth within the epiphyseal zone.

Evaluation of the effects of phosphocitrate on the PTH-induced osteoclastic activity in bone was made on tibias from mice given daily injections of 1.0 μmol/phosphocitrate followed by 50 units of PTH for 4 days. These were compared with tibias from a control group receiving only saline and another group given saline and 50 units of PTH. Tissue preparation and light microscopy examination were provided by Dr. H. D. Dorfman, Chief Pathologist, Sinai Hospital, Baltimore, Maryland.

PTH extract was purchased from Eli Lilly. All other chemicals were of the highest purity commercially available.

RESULTS

Effects of Phosphocitrate on Nephrocalcinosis

The effects of phosphocitrate on the nephrocalcinosis produced by excess PTH are shown in Figure 1. In the control group receiving saline and PTH, the calcium content of the kidneys increased from approximately 2 μmol/g tissue to over 50 μmol/g tissue by day 4. In contrast, those mice receiving 1.0 μmol/phosphocitrate prior to PTH showed a significant reduction in the rate and extent of kidney calcification over the same period, so that by day 4 the mean calcium content was less than 25 μmol/g tissue. Such results were qualatively reproducible in numerous experiments as long as the animal weights in the beginning were 15 to 17 g. Smaller mice did not survive the PTH treatment long enough for accurate studies and with large animals (20 to 25 g) the resulting nephrocalcinosis was extremely variable. In identical control experiments, injections of either 1.0 μmol/day of sodium citrate or sodium phosphate, in place of phosphocitrate, did not reduce the nephrocalcinosis produced by PTH.

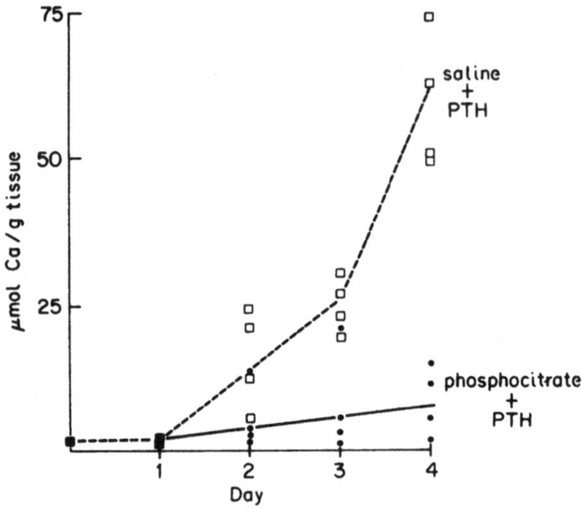

Figure 1. Effects of Phosphocitrate on Nephrocalcinosis: Groups of mice were given daily intraperitoneal injections of either saline or 1.0 µmol of Na^+-phosphocitrate followed one hour later by 50 units of PTH over 4 consecutive days. Four mice from each group were sacrificed 24 hours after the 1st, 2nd, 3rd, and 4th injections and the calcium content of the kidneys determined as described. The data presented are the average Ca levels from paired kidneys for each point.

Dose Response

Inhibition of PTH-induced nephrocalcinosis was observed over a wide range of phosphocitrate doses (Figure 2). In contrast to control animals receiving saline and PTH, there was a marked reduction in the extent of calcium accumulation in the kidneys with phosphocitrate administrations from 0.075 µmol/day to 3.0 µmol/day. These data indicate that the higher doses were more effective in preventing nephrocalcinosis, however even with as little as .075 µmol of phosphocitrate per day the reduction in calcification was significant.

Serum Calcium Levels

As expected, the administration of excess PTH produced a sustained hypercalcemia throughout the experimental period. Serum calcium level rose from a mean of 1.8 mM to a maximum of about 4.0 mM within 2 days after the first PTH injection and was maintained by daily PTH injections. Comparisons of the serum calcium levels of mice given saline-PTH or 1.0 µmol phosphocitrate-PTH showed that phosphocitrate had no measureable effect on the PTH-induced hypercalcemia (Figure 3). Phosphocitrate was similarly ineffective in lowering the hypercalcemia when given in doses between .075 μmol and 3.0 μmol daily for 4 days. Direct measurements of ionized calcium in the serum with a Ca^{2+}-selective electrode showed the Ca^{2+} to be elevated but essentially equal in both the saline-PTH and phosphocitrate-PTH groups.

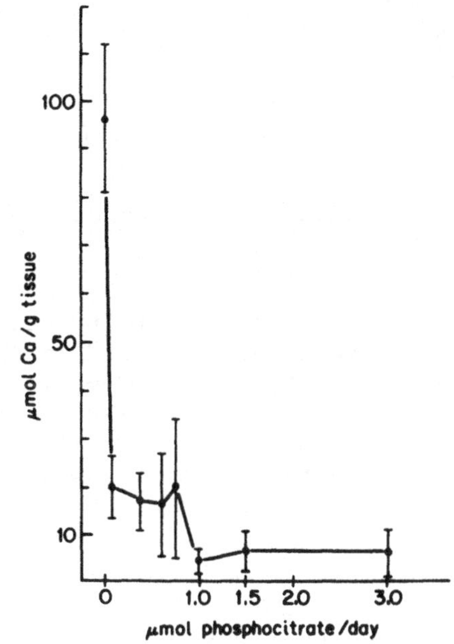

Figure 2. Inhibition of Nephrocalcinosis by Various Doses of Phosphocitrate: Groups of mice were given daily injections of Na^+-phosphocitrate (at doses indicated) followed 1 hour later by 50 units of PTH for 4 days. Twenty-four hours after the last injection, the calcium levels of the kidneys were determined. The values are the means and standard deviations of the kidney calcium levels from 4 mice for each dose of phosphocitrate.

Kidney Histology

Kidney sections containing greater than 25 μmol Ca/g gave positive von Kossa staining. At lower calcium levels the von Kossa stain was negative. By the fourth day of PTH administration, deposits of calcium salts were observed within the cells of the proximal tubules and within the tubular lumen. In contrast, kidney sections from those animals receiving phosphocitrate in addition to PTH were remarkably free from obvious calcium deposits.

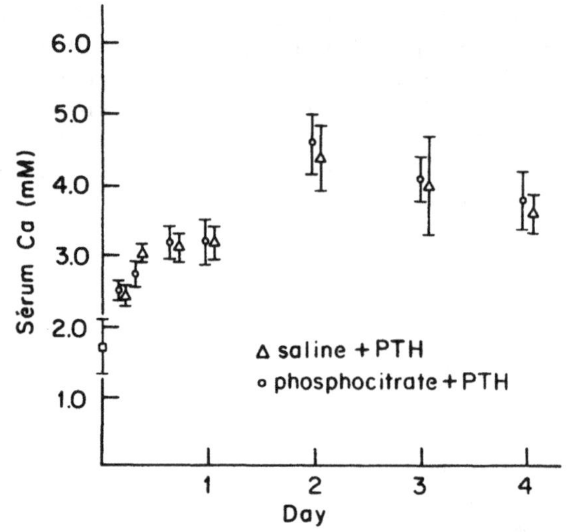

Figure 3. Effect of Phosphocitrate on PTH-Induced Hypercalcemia: Serum calcium levels were measured in the saline-PTH and phosphocitrate-PTH groups from Figure 1. Serum was diluted with a lanthanum-butanol-HCl medium (10 µl serum to 1 ml diluent) and calcium determined by atomic absorption. The data are the means and standard deviations of serum calcium levels from 4 mice for each point.

Effects of Phosphocitrate on Bone Growth

The effects of long-term administration of phosphocitrate on normal bone growth were evaluated in young male rats (50 to 60 g) and compared with equivalent doses of EHDP. Phosphocitrate and EHDP were given as daily intraperitoneal injections of 3.0 µmol for 14 days. Thin sections of the tibias from animals given EHPD showed abnormal bone growth within the epiphyseal zone as previously reported[6]. EHDP produced a significant thickening of the epiphyseal plate and reduced the longitudinal growth rate. Other abnormalities characteristic of impaired mineralization in the trabecular of the metaphysis were also present[6]. In contrast, equivalent doses of phosphocitrate produced only a slight widening of the epiphyseal plate with no evidence of abnormal mineralization of the metaphysis (Figure 4).

The effects of phosphocitrate on the osteoclastic activity produced by PTH administration were also assessed. Undecalcified sections from the tibias of mice administered 1.0 µmol phosphocitrate-PTH and saline-PTH daily for 4 days were compared to qualitatively assess the osteoclastic activity in each group. Comparisons with untreated mice showed as expected, an increase in

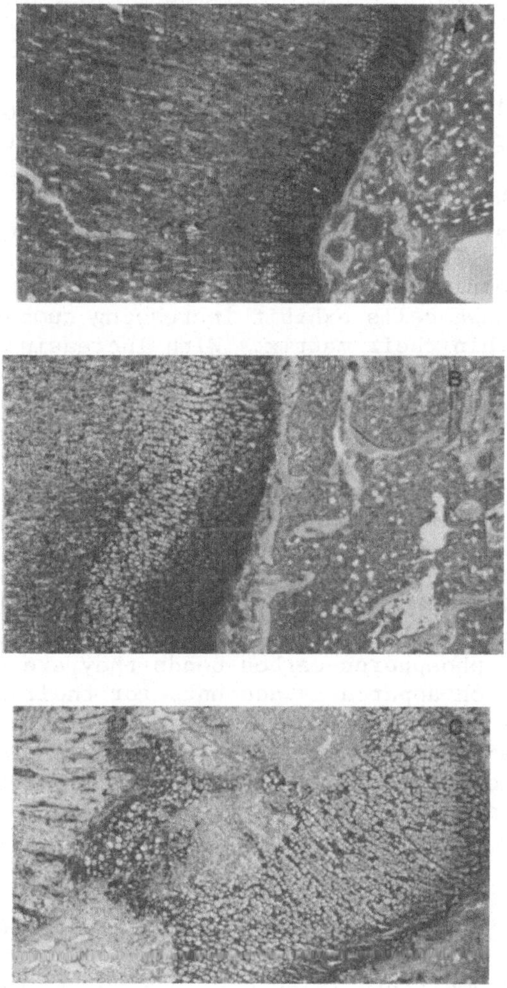

Figure 4. Effects of phosphocitrate on bone growth: Young male rats (50 to 60 g) were given daily intraperitoneal injections of 3.0 μmol of Na^{+}-phosphocitrate or EHDP for 14 days. Tibias were fixed in formalin, decalcified with EDTA, and thin sections of the epiphyseal area examined by light microscopy for evidence of abnormal bone growth. A. control (untreated); B. phosphocitrate; C. EHDP.

bone resorption in the saline-PTH group. The stimulation of osteoclastic activity produced by PTH was unaltered by phosphocitrate.

DISCUSSION

The nephrocalcinosis produced by excess PTH provides a convenient experimental model of soft tissue calcification in which to assay the effects of potential inhibitors of metastatic calcification processes. Such kidney calcification has been well described in many previous investigations[7,8]. Nephrocalcinosis produced by excess PTH is characterized by increasing calcium accumulation within the cells of the proximal tubules. In the initial stages of calcification the mitochondria of these cells exhibit increasing numbers of electron dense deposits within their matrix. With increasing calcium accumulation, apatite-like deposits appear both intracellularly within the mitochondria and the cytoplasm of the tubule cells and extracellularly along the basement membrane of the proximal tubules.

The possible role of crystallization inhibitors in regulating physiological mineralization processes and preventing the deposition of calcium salts within soft tissues has been repeatedly discussed [1,2]. This concept has been supported by the demonstration that synthetic organodiphosphonates are capable of preventing soft tissue calcification in several experimental models[9]. Since these substances contain phosphorus-carbon bonds they are not hydrolyzed by phosphonates which apparently accounts for their profound inhibitory effects in animal models of metastatic calcification. However, their resistence to enzymatic hydrolysis also causes severe inhibitory effects on normal bone calcification[6] which restricts their possible usefulness in inhibiting renal calcification.

Phosphocitrate is even more potent on a molar basis than the diphosphonates in <u>in vitro</u> tests of the inhibition of hydroxyapatite crystallization[3]. In contrast to the diphosphonates, the P-O-C bond of phosphocitrate is susceptable to hydrolysis to citrate and phosphate by purified phosphatase preparation[3]. Since bone is rich in phosphatase activity, phosphocitrate in the doses described here may have little effect on bone metabolism. Our preliminary studies of long-term administration of phosphocitrate to young male rats have shown only slight alterations of normal bone growth or structure. These data suggest however, that any additional effects of phosphocitrate will be considerably less than those produced by EHDP.

The data reported here show that administration of phosphocitrate reduces the rate and extent of nephrocalcinosis induced by excess PTH in laboratory mice, despite the demonstrated hydrolysis of phosphocitrate by purified alkaline and acid phosphatases. Its activity in suppressing such calcification may indicate that significant levels of the compound are maintained in the kidney and/or blood, and suggests either than enzymatic degradation is not significant with intraperitoneal administration of phosphocitrate or that repeated injections maintain sufficient levels to influence renal calcification.

The mechanism by which phosphocitrate functions as an inhibitor of hydroxyapatite growth is currently under investigation. The administration of phosphocitrate in the dose used here had no effect on the elevation of serum calcium produced by excess PTH. Therefore, the observed reduction on total kidney calcium could occur either by restriction of calcium movement from the extracellular fluid into the cell through the plasma membrane or by preventing precipitation and/or crystallization of calcium phosphate within the cell. The latter mechanism is more consistent with the anticalcification activity of phosphocitrate and its high affinity for binding to hydroxyapatite crystals and preventing their further growth[3].

The prevention of nephrocalcinosis by phosphocitrate and its inability to greatly alter normal bone growth suggests that inactivation of phosphocitrate by enzymatic hydrolysis may be less complete in serum and within the kidneys than in areas of bone formation. These differences may reflect local variations in phosphatases concentration, possible differences in substrate specificity of tissue phosphatase, or variations in the isoenzyme composition of alkaline phosphatase in different tissues.

The preliminary data suggests that phosphocitrate may be of potential therapeutic importance for soft tissue calcification without the detrimental side effects of organodiphosphonates.

REFERENCES

1. A. L. Lehninger, in:"Horizons in Biochemistry and Biophysics," Addison-Wesley Publishing Co., Reading, MA (1977).
2. J. E. Howard, Johns Hopkins Med. J. 139:239 (1976).
3. W. P. Tew, C. Mahle, J. Benavides, J. E. Howard, and A. L. Lehninger, Biochem. 19:1983 (1980).
4. H. A. Fleisch, R. G. G. Russell, S. Bisaz, and R. C. Muhlbauer, Europ. J. Clin. Invest. 1:12 (1970).
5. N. Gochman and H. Givelber, Clin. Chem. 16:229 (1970).
6. R. Schenk, W. A. Merz, R. Muhlbauer, R. G. G. Russell, and H. A. Fleisch, Calc. Tiss. Res. 11:196 (1973).
7. A. F. Schneider, E. P. Reaven, and G. Reaven, Endocrin. 67:733 (1960).
8. J. B. Caulfield and P. E. Schrag, Am. J. Pathol. 44:365 (1964).

9. H. Fleisch, R. G. G. Russell, S. Bisaz, P. A. Casey, and R. C. Muhlbauer, Calcif. Tiss. Res. 2:10 (1968).

ACKNOWLEDGMENT

The authors would like to thank Ms. Jane Foard for her expert technical assistance and Drs. Dan McDonald and Brian Scoffield of the Johns Hopkins University Orthopaedic Research Laboratories for preparing the bone tissue and its histologic study.

THE SOURCES OF PHOSPHOCITRATE AND ITS ROLE AS AN INHIBITOR OF CALCIUM PHOSPHATE AND CALCIUM OXALATE CRYSTALLIZATION

G. Williams and J. D. Sallis

Department of Biochemistry, University of Tasmania,

Hobart, Tasmania, Australia

Earlier studies reported by Howard[1] and Lehninger[2] suggested that a substance containing P_i and citrate, and tentatively assigned the structure of phosphocitrate, existed in nature and was a potent inhibitor of hydroxyapatite (HAP) formation. These observations led us to attempt to isolate and characterize phosphocitrate from biological sources with a view to defining a physiological role for this compound in calcification systems.

As an initial step toward achieving this goal, we have recently synthesized and characterized labelled and unlabelled phosphocitrate[3]. During the developmental period, systems for monitoring reactions and identifying phosphocitrate in biological studies were established. Whilst NMR data (^{1}H-NMR, ^{13}C-NMR, ^{31}P-NMR) together with mass spectrometry provide information on the structural nature of a compound, with biological samples it is not always possible to obtain sufficient amounts of pure material for analysis by these methods. Instead, we have found that a range of techniques is more valuable for characterizing phosphocitrate than any single method, and a summary of systems that we are now using is presented in Table 1.

Ion exchange chromatography at neutral pH enables preliminary separation of biological samples with minimal hydrolysis and eliminates phosphocitrate artefact formation. Thin layer chromatography, high voltage electrophoresis, enzymatic and chemical analyses provide versatility for identification. Currently, we are investigating the application of analytical isotachophoresis for identification and quantitation of phosphocitrate as analysis is rapid, and separation of phosphocitrate from interfering ions or compounds appears complete.

Synthetic phosphocitrate has been tested in vitro for its ability to inhibit HAP and calcium oxalate crystal formation. By simultaneous measurement of alkali addition, calcium ion concentration and laser beam light scattering, information on the relative ability of compounds to inhibit the transformation of amorphous calcium phosphate (ACP) into HAP can be assessed. Comparative studies have shown that phosphocitrate is the most potent of many inhibitors tested including ethane-1-hydroxy-1, 1-diphosphonate (EHDP), ATP and pyrophosphate[4,5]. Data derived from this system have proved useful in defining the structural requirements of a compound for inhibition.

More recently, our studies with the system have been extended and light scattering data (Figure 1) used to demonstrate that inhibitors may be classified into two groups, Type I and Type II. Type I are all crystal growth inhibitors and, at lower concentrations result in the formation of highly dispersed HAP suspensions, as indicated by an increase in the turbidity change. At higher concentrations the extent of conversion into HAP is inhibited. In contrast, Type II compounds do not inhibit crystal growth nor alter the turbidity measurements or extent of conversion. Electron microscopic observations have substantiated these conclusions. As examples, Type I (in order of potency) includes phosphocitrate, EHDP, tripolyphosphate, imidodiphosphate and pyrophosphate whereas Type II includes ATP, ADP, phosphonoformate, 2-phosphoglyceric acid, 3-phosphoglyceric acid and citrate. Although such physicochemical studies are well defined in vitro, it is of questionable validity to extrapolate the results to the physiological situation. For example, inhibitors can, under certain conditions, interact synergistically to inhibit HAP formation.

If phosphocitrate is to play an influential role in urolithiasis, it should inhibit calcium oxalate crystallization. We have studied the influence of phosphocitrate on calcium oxalate crystal growth, using both calcium ion monitoring systems and growth of calcium oxalate crystals on glass fibers. With the latter system, 300 μM phosphocitrate inhibits growth of the crystals to an extent of 66 ± 3% (relative to buffer); 1 mM pyrophosphate 49 ± 4%, and 100 μM chondroitin sulphate C 55 ± 7%. As with other inhibitors, crystal morphology changes noticeably in their presence.

With phosphocitrate established as a potent inhibitor of calcification and with the availability of systems for the isolation and detection of the compound, we next turned our attention to possible tissue sources. Rabbit liver and kidney homogenates were acid extracted and, after neutralization, subjected to ion exchange chromatography. Following batch elution of P_i and citrate, a gradient was applied, and fractions revealing the presence of citrate after hydrolysis were found to elute with the same elution volume as

Table 1. Techniques for Identification of Phosphocitrate

System	Details	Comments
1. ion-exchange chromatography	AG1-X8, HCO_3^- , pH7.4 (ref.3)	batch or gradient with definitive separation of P_i,citrate & PC.
2. thin layer chromatography	cellulose; isobutyric/5% NH_3/ methanol (66:40:100) (ref.3)	R_f values; PC (0.20), P_i (0.44), citrate (0.42).
3. high voltage electrophoresis	paper; 0.05M triethanolamine-HCO_3, pH 7.5; 2,000V/2 hr.	distance from origin in cm. PC (23), P_i (32), citrate (25).
4. enzymatic	coupled assay with phosphatase, citrate lyase and malic dehydrogenase; U.V. or fluorimetric (ref.3)	PC sensitivity; 0.5 - 10 ug.
5. chemical analysis	pentabromoacetone derivative (ref.3)	
	benzidine chromaphore (ref.4)	PC sensitivity; 0.5 - 5 ug.
6. isotachophoresis	leading electrolyte; 0.005M HCl-aniline,0.2% HPMC. trailing electrolyte: 0.005M glutamic,0.02% HPMC, conductimetric.	step height in cm. Cl (0), PC (30), citrate (45), P_i (60), glutamate (95). PC sensitivity. pmoles- nmoles.

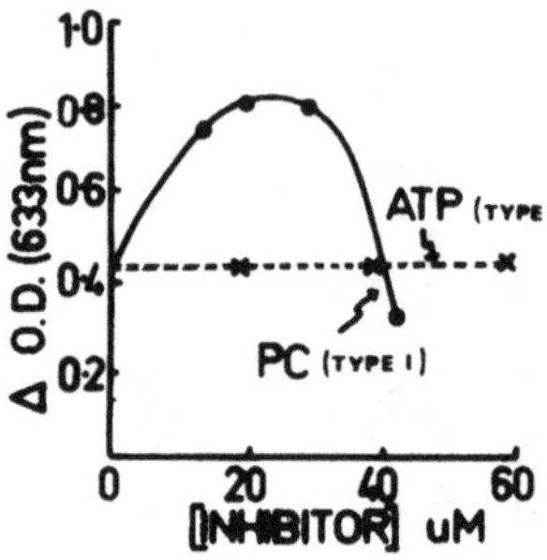

Figure 1. Effect of inhibitor concentration on the magnitude of the turbidity change associated with the transformation of amorphous calcium phosphate to hydroxyapatite.

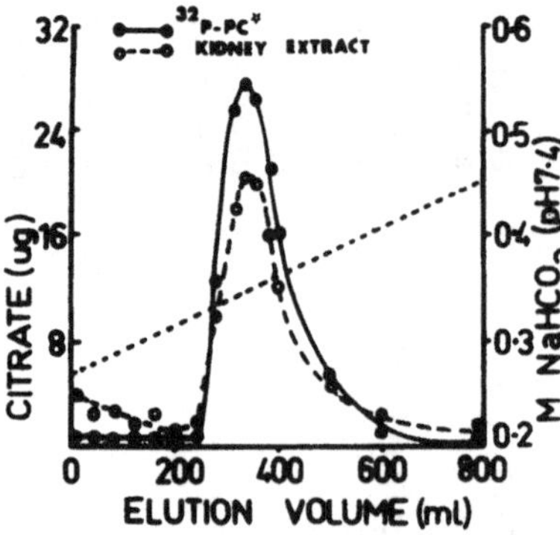

Figure 2. Separation of phosphocitrate from a kidney extract by ion exchange chromatography. Column 10 x 1.5 cm; AG1-X8, HCO_3^-. Batch elution with 0.27M $NaHCO_3$ pH 7.4, then gradient elution as shown above (----). *Radioactivity profile has been superimposed.

synthetic phosphocitrate (Figure 2). We have no evidence that citrate and P_i together lead to phosphocitrate production under these conditions. Enzymatic analysis provided additional evidence that the compound isolated was phosphocitrate for only when the compound was preincubated with a phosphatase was it possible to obtain a reaction with citrate lyase. Although citryl-1-phosphate (i.e. phosphate esterified to a carboxyl group) might meet the enzyme requirements, stability data eliminate the possibility, as this compound, relative to phosphocitrate, is short-lived[3]. In additional experiments, isolated phosphocitrate subjected to thin layer chromatography showed only a single band which co-chromatographed with the reference standard and, when hydrolyzed, gave citrate and P_i.

This demonstration that phosphocitrate does exist in tissues, led us to examine the suggestion[2] that the mitochondria might be an important source of this compound. Mitochondria from rabbit liver, kidney and intestine were found to contain phosphocitrate and, on preliminary estimates, have 1.2, 0.8 and 0.5 nmol phosphocitrate/mg mitochondrial protein respectively. More recent experiments, however, have led us to doubt the validity of the quantitative data as it is now clear that enzymatic hydrolysis is very active in tissues. If a similar situation occurs during isolation of the mitochondria, it might lead to an under-estimation of the true concentration. Further, the status of the mitochondria or indeed the whole animal with regard to calcium and phosphate levels could influence the value obtained. Phosphocitrate has been detected but not yet quantitated in the skeleton and, at present, we have no evidence for its existence in urine. Techniques are being investigated which will allow quantitation of phosphocitrate in bone, where presently, hydroxyapatite avidly binds the compound. In urine, metabolites and salts have so far made investigation of this possible source more difficult.

In order to help define sites of action of phosphocitrate, [^{32}P]-phosphocitrate was injected intravenously into rats and the time course of the accumulation of radioactivity in selected tissues was followed. The results are shown in Figure 3a. After 30 minutes, the majority of the radioactivity was associated with the skeleton (40%) and kidney (15%) whereas liver had only 5% of the initial radioactivity. These results alone, however, do not allow interpretation of the distribution of phosphocitrate in tissue or of its specific binding. To have meaning, the radioactivity must be associated with phosphocitrate and not its hydrolyzed product, P_i. Two approaches have been made to resolve this problem.

In the first instance, [^{32}P]-P_i was injected into rats to determine rates of tissue labelling over the same time period, and to assess the affinity of the label for the skeleton (Figure 3b). Results indicate that only 20% radioactivity from [^{32}P]-P_i was taken up by the skeleton in comparison to 40% when [^{32}P]-phosphocitrate was injected. Kidney shows a similar pattern whereas for liver, the relationship was reversed with minimal radioactivity accumulating after [^{32}P]-phosphocitrate was given.

In the second approach, acid extracts of soft tissue were prepared, the radioactivity associated with the organic and inorganic phosphate determined[7], and the labelled metabolites further resolved and quantitated using high voltage electrophoresis. The organic phosphate to P_i ratio shows that after 30 minutes, 80% of the radioactivity in blood was in the organic phosphate fraction. Electrophoretic patterns (Figures 4 and 5) indicate that this radioactivity was associated with phosphocitrate. By contrast, the kidney has 40% represented as organic phosphates after 5 minutes, and electrophoresis indicates that only 15% of the radioactivity was due to

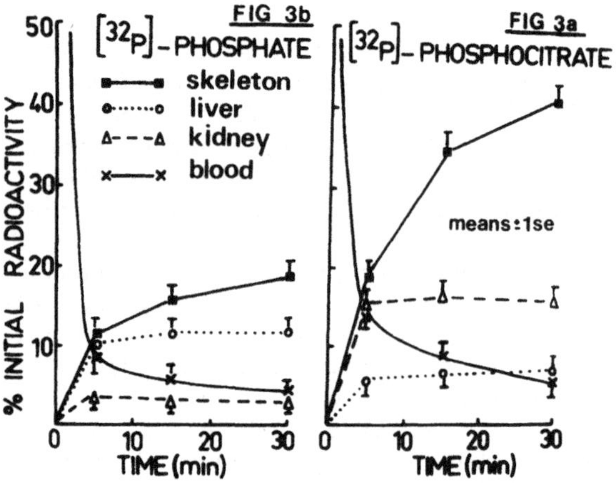

Figure 3. Rate of disappearance of radioactivity in blood and its appearance in tissues following administration of [^{32}P]-P_i or [^{32}P]-phosphocitrate in rats. Female rats (170 g) were injected intravenously with 1 mg of the sodium salts of the labelled compounds. At designated times, samples of blood, bone and soft tissues were taken, oxidized and counted. Values shown are means ± 1 S.E. Total weights were obtained for liver and kidney; skeletal mass was calculated[8] and the total blood volume assessed at 64 ml/kg.

FIG 4: [32P]-PHOSPHOCITRATE

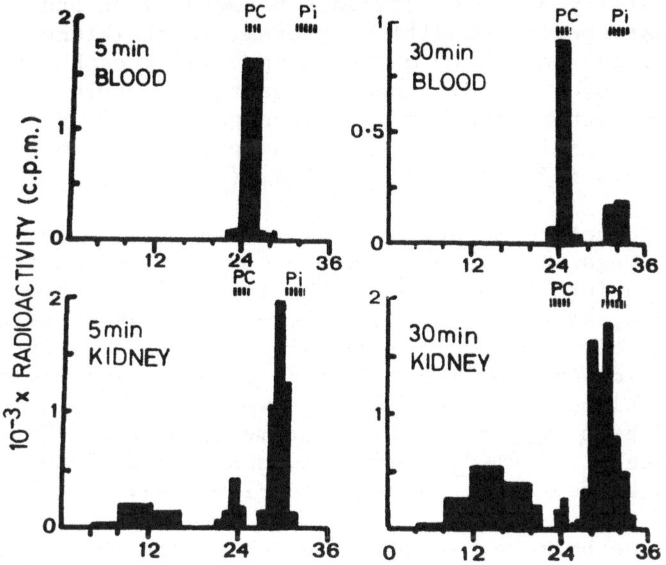

FIG 5: [32P]-Pi

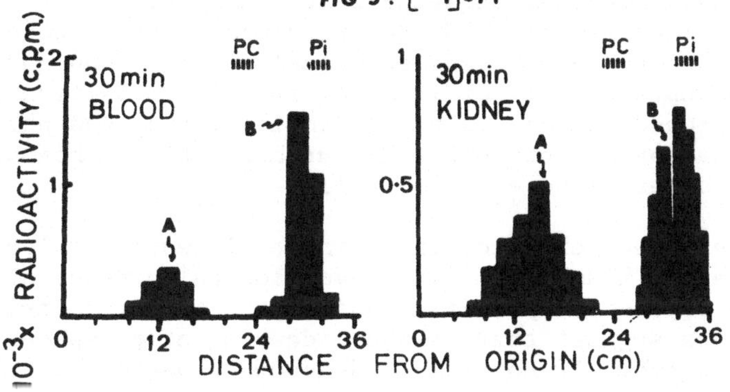

Figures 4 and 5. Radioactive patterns for electrophoresis. Rats were injected intravenously with 1 mg (0.5 μCi) of either [^{32}P]-phosphocitrate (specific activity = 200 μCi/mmol or [^{32}P]-P_i (specific activity = 70 μCi/mmol) and at time intervals, relevant samples were collected, frozen and then extracted with trichloracetic acid. Following neutralization, aliquots were taken for high voltage electrophoresis as described in the text. The dried paper was marked in a grid pattern, then cut, and after acid extraction, radioactivity (▬) associated with the separated compounds was determined. Phosphocitrate and P_i were identified from reference standards (|||||||) treated in an identical manner.

phosphocitrate. Even less (about 5% of phosphocitrate) was found in kidney after 30 minutes, as shown in Figure 4. Because of the contrast in lability of phosphocitrate between blood and kidney, it is possible that special conditions prevail in the kidney for phosphatase action, or that there exists a specific phosphocitrate cleavage enzyme which rapidly inactivates the molecule. It should be noted that no other labelled compounds were detected of the same electrophoretic mobility as authentic phosphocitrate in tissue extracts from rats injected with $[^{32}P]$-P_i (Figure 5).

In order to determine whether (a) phosphocitrate was being metabolized to organic phosphate esters or (b) phosphocitrate was being hydrolyzed into P_i which was then incorporated into organic phosphate esters, samples from the $[^{32}P]$-P_i experiment were subjected to an identical electrophoretic analysis (Figure 5). Liver (not shown here) rapidly metabolized $[^{32}P]$-P_i into several organic phosphates whereas blood and kidney formed two major organic compounds, shown as A and B in Figure 5. In experiments using $[^{32}P]$-phosphocitrate in place of $[^{32}P]$-P_i, both components A and B were discernable in kidney after 30 minutes (Figure 4).

The data, we believe, support the contention that phosphocitrate is hydrolyzed to P_i and citrate before any further metabolism occurs. Due to the avid binding of phosphocitrate in bone, as yet we have been unable to identify the radioactive compound(s) in bone. However, based on the electrophoretic analysis of blood and the relatively low uptake (20%) of $[^{32}P]$-P_i itself, we believe that the radioactivity found in bone is a true indication of phosphocitrate uptake. Once adsorbed onto HAP, the further fate of phosphocitrate is difficult to determine experimentally.

Exogenous phosphocitrate, then, is localized in at least two tissues - bone and kidney, but its physiological potency at least two sites must be dependent upon its stability in the microenvironment. Our in vivo data suggest that at the kidney site, phosphocitrate is rapidly inactivated. If however, endogenous phosphocitrate is strictly compartmentalized within the mitochondria, the lability data from whole tissue may be of limited meaning. Clearly it is important to gain further information regarding the intracellular distribution of phosphocitrate and to elucidate its biological site(s) of synthesis and degradation. The availability of a stable analogue of phosphocitrate capable of resisting enzyme attack would also be valuable. We are currently investigating the synthesis of two such compounds since their biological inertness should permit advantage to be taken, at the kidney site, of the physicochemical properties associated with the parent molecule, phosphocitrate. Because of the possible lability of phosphocitrate in bone, this compound may be more desirable in the treatment of skeletal disorders than an inert analogue.

Whilst, from the data presented here, a physiological role for phosphocitrate in the maintenance of mitochondrial calcium phosphate deposits in the amorphous state is easily envisaged, a much broader role for this molecule in the control of stone formation and other calcifying systems is forseen but has yet to be elucidated.

REFERENCES

1. J. E. Howard, Johns Hopkins Med. J. 139:239 (1976).
2. A. L. Lehninger, Horiz. Biochem. Biophys. 4:1 (1977).
3. G. Williams and J. D. Sallis, Anal. Biochem. 102:365 (1980).
4. G. B. Jones, Anal. Biochem. 21:286 (1967).
5. G. Williams, E. S. Holdsworth and J. D. Sallis, Clin. Exp. Pharm. Physiol. (in press).
6. G. Williams and J. D. Sallis, Biochem. J. 184:181 (1979).
7. S. T. Ohnishi, Anal. Biochem. 86:201 (1978).
8. H. H. Donaldson, Am. J. Anat. 26:237 (1920).

ACKNOWLEDGMENTS

Research grants were made available from the National Health and Medical Research Council of Australia and the University of Tasmania. The technical support of J. Jordan and N. Cliffe-Hickline together with helpful discussions by Professor E. S. Holdsworth is gratefully acknowledged. Personal thanks (J.D.S.) for travel support to Williamsburg.

CHARACTERIZATION OF THE CALCIUM OXALATE CRYSTAL GROWTH INHIBITORS IN HUMAN URINE

E. E. Schrier*, J. L. Rubin*, K. E. Lee, P. G. Werness, and L. H. Smith
*Department of Chemistry, SUNY at Binghamton, Binghamton, New York; and Mayo Clinic, Rochester, Minnesota

Although the concentration of inhibitors of calcium oxalate crystal growth in stone former's urine does not appear to differ from that in normal urine[1] the inhibitors must be characterized in order to better assess their role in stone disease. We have focused on the development of new methods for their separation and purification, concentrating our efforts on the high molecular weight inhibitors.

Development of a Purification Scheme

The development of our general purification scheme was based on a number of preliminary observations which suggested that a significant fraction of the inhibition was associated with charged macromolecules which were precipitated from a 75% (v/v) ethanol solution and which had an appreciable phosphorous content. In addition, preliminary studies on whole urine and urine concentrates showed that the inhibition was susceptible to attack by bovine pancreatic ribonuclease A (RNAase). This information led us to consider the inhibitor substances at least in part as RNA or RNA-like molecules and to proceed with the purification on that basis.

The general procedure for purification was concentration using ultrafiltration, phenol extraction to reduce the protein concentration of the samples, and fractionation on Sephadex G-10 columns. While this procedure did not resolve protein, nucleic acids, and glycosaminoglycans (GAGS), it removed extraneous protein while conserving virtually all of the macromolecular portion of the inhibition of the original urine.

MATERIALS

Urine was obtained from several adult normal male subjects. Where possible it was used fresh; otherwise, it was stored frozen until use. All chemicals were the best grade commercially available. Ultrapure guanidinium chloride was purchased from Becton-Dickenson Diagnostics. Two different preparations of RNAase were utilized in the digestions (Sigma Chemical and Worthington Co.). Both preparations were certified to be protease-free by the manufacturers.

METHODS

Ultrafiltration procedures were carried out at 4°C. An Amicon 2000 apparatus was used in conjunction with either a UM-05 or UM-10 membrane. The urine was prefiltered through Whatman #1 filter paper. A volume of 1.5 to 2.0 liters of urine produced a retentate of 0.15 - 0.20 liters with the process taking five hours using the UM-10 membrane and 3 - 4 days using the UM-05 membrane.

In the phenol-extraction step, 0.15 liters of urine concentrate was mixed with 0.27 liters of 80% redistilled phenol. After one half hour of vigorous stirring, the mixture was centrifuged at 10,000 g at 4°C to break the emulsion. The aqueous phase was separated from the phenol phase with the latter being discarded. 0.300 liters of absolute ethanol and 0.030 liters of 10% potassium acetate in ethanol were added to the aqueous phase. The resulting suspension was centrifuged at 10,000 g. The pellet was redissolved in 0.050 liters double-distilled water.

This solution was applied to a 4.0 x 100 cm Sephadex G-10 column at 4°C. The column was eluted with distilled water. 0.015-liter aliquots were collected using an LKB Red-Rac fraction collector.

Fractions resulting from column chromatography on Sephadex G-10 were analyzed by high performance liquid chromatography (HPLC) using a Waters Instruments Analytical System equipped with fixed-wavelength (254 nm) ultraviolet and refractive index detection. An E-125 Bondagel size exclusion chromatographic column was employed and elution was accomplished with water. The system pressure was 1000 psi at a flow rate of 1 ml/min.

U.v. scans of the fractions were performed using a Cary 14 spectrophotometer specially equipped for high sensitivity.

GAGS were determined by the modified carbazole method of Bitter and Muir[2]. D-Glucuronolactone was used as a standard. A small correction (< 5%) was applied to these results to account for the contribution of RNA-like material to the carbazole color at the wavelength of analysis. The corrected results were multiplied by two to give the concentration of GAGs.

RNA was determined using the modified orcinol procedure of Almog and Shirey[3]. Yeast RNA was used as the standard. A correction was made to account for the contribution of GAGs to the orcinol color at the wavelength of analysis. The GAGs concentration was multiplied by the factor, 0.53, determined from the assay of chondroitin sulfate (CDS). The correction was then subtracted from the orcinol data to give the corrected RNA value. Other possible polymeric ribose-containing species in urine were not removed before analysis.

The analysis for protein was carried out using the modified biuret method of Dorsey et al[4]. There were no corrections applied in this assay.

Two methods were used for the determination of the inhibition of crystallization of calcium oxalate. The spontaneous crystallization assay of Gardner and Doremus[5] was most extensively utilized except that observations of the onset of visible crystal formation were enhanced with the use of a Brinkmann Instruments Fiber Optics Colorimeter. The point of first rise of the absorbance was arbitrarily taken to be the start of spontaneous crystallization. The entire experimental procedure was carried out at 37°C with synthetic urine formulation described previously[5]. The pH was held fixed at 5.8. The initial concentration of $CaCl_2$ in the bath was 3.3×10^{-3} M while that of sodium oxalate was 6.5×10^{-4}M.

In the presence of inhibitors, the induction time preceding the onset of spontaneous crystallization was increased. The difference in time between the onset of spontaneous crystallization in the presence of inhibitors and in their absence was a measure of the effectiveness of the inhibitors. The assay system was calibrated with heparin using the value of the specific inhibition of heparin, 3×10^{-9} M/IU, determined in the seeded growth assay of Meyer and Smith[6]. The calibration curve of induction time versus heparin concentration was linear in the inhibitor concentration region in which the measurements were made.

For some of the studies involving RNAase digestions the seeded growth assay of Meyer and Smith[6] was used. The spontaneous crystallization assays were also used to assay the digested samples. When the assay systems were intercalibrated as described above, the changes observed in the inhibition arising from RNAase digestion were completely consistent between the two assay systems.

The effect of digestion with RNAase was observed on whole urine samples, urine retentates, and purified urine retentates. Some of the conditions were those used originally by Ito and Coe[7]. The concentration of enzyme utilized was 0.3 mg/ml. The pH in these digestions was controlled potentiostatically at 6.8. The usual time for digestion was 18 hours although variations of this procedure were utilized. Sodium azide at 0.01% (w/v) was added to the digestion mixture to retard bacterial growth.

An important feature of these experiments was the use of a zero time control. The experimental control was a mixture containing all components including the enzyme at zero time, i.e., before any digestion had occurred. In this way, effects of components such as the azide or complexing between the enzyme and any of the inhibitor components could be taken into account.

The molecular weight of an inhibitor fraction was determined in 6 M guanidinium chloride using column chromatography on Sepharose CL-6B as described by Ansare and Mage[8]. Purified proteins were used as molecular weight markers. While the use of such markers to measure the molecular weight of only partially proteinaceous material may be questioned, the presence of guanidinium chloride at high ionic strength should produce random coil behavior in all macromolecular species[9].

RESULTS AND DISCUSSION

The yield of inhibitor material in the retentate from ultrafiltration at $4^{o}C$ averaged over several runs was 65 ± 15% of the inhibitor material present in urine. The yield was the same whether a UM-10 membrane (nominal molecular weight cutoff 10,000 daltons) or a UM-05 membrane (cutoff 500 daltons) was used. Whatever the significance of this finding, the presence of aggregates or their formation during ultrafiltration cannot be ruled out. One hundred percent of the inhibition originally present in the starting urine could be accounted for within experimental error (± 10%) by adding the inhibition in the retentate to that measured in the ultrafiltrate.

When the retentate was subjected to phenol extraction and ethanol precipitation as described above, 90% of the inhibitor activity was recovered. In separate experiments, it was shown that ethanol and phenol did not modify the crystallization behavior of calcium oxalate in the spontaneous crystallization assay at the concentrations found in the purified extracts.

Fractionation of the purified extracts on Sephadex G-10 gave two peaks. Conductivity measurements indicated that the first was salt-free while the second contained concentrations of salt averaging 0.35 M. Inhibitor activity measurements with appropriate corrections for the concentration of salt in the second peak indicated that 60% of the activity resides in the salt-free peak while 40% coelutes with the peak containing salt. The experiments to be described were carried out on the salt-free peak.

Since much of the further discussion is involved with u.v. spectroscopic results, it is important to note the fate of any extraneous phenol left over from the phenol extraction step since phenol absorbs u.v. strongly between 250 nm and 290 nm. Phenol was retained by the Sephadex G-10 column and was eluted at the trailing edge of the salt-containing peak. This result and other experiments showed conclusively that there was no phenol contamination of the salt-free peak.

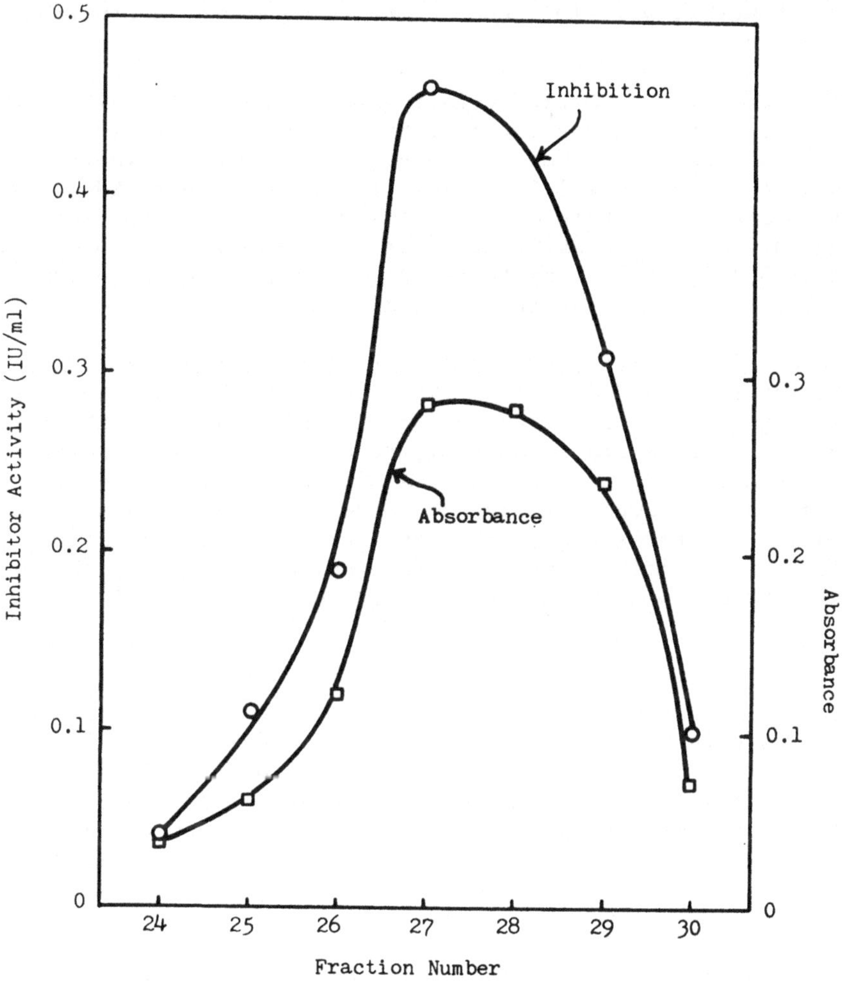

Figure 1. Inhibitor activity and absorbance at 254 nm for fractions from a phenol-extracted and desalted concentrate of urine.

Figure 1 records the distribution of ultraviolet peak absorbances at 254 nm as a function of fraction number for a typical group of fractions eluted in the salt-free peak from the Sephadex G-10 column. These absorbances are determined directly from the HPLC traces for individual fractions. Also plotted are the inhibitor activity values for the various fractions obtained from the spontaneous crystallization assay.

The fractions having the maximum absorbance is also the one with the maximum inhibitor potency. Since GAGs do not absorb u.v. light in this spectral region, they can be ruled out as the u.v. absorbing species. However, proteins and nucleic acids may both contribute to the absorbance at 254 nm.

Some further information relating to the protein-nucleic acid ratio in these samples was obtained by measuring the ratio of the absorbance at 260 nm to that at 280 nm for purified, desalted material. The ratio was 1.5 as against values for pure RNA of 2.5 and for an average protein of 0.5. A simple calculation from these data indicates that the purified materials contain a ratio of 50% protein to 50% RNA. This protein-nucleic acid ratio is in good accord with the results of the chemical analysis.

The chemically-determined concentrations of protein, RNA and RNA-like material, and GAGs from the same group of fractions are shown in Figure 2. The concentration of inhibitors in each of these fractions is given again in this figure to facilitate comparison. The concentrations of protein and RNA are seen to be quite close to each other in the samples while the concentrations of GAGs is somewhat smaller. Interestingly, the total concentration of solutes, e.g., 1.5 ± 0.5 mg/ml in the peak fraction, determined by these chemical methods is confirmed by refractive index analysis using HPLC.

Closer inspection of Figure 2 indicates that the protein peak comes two to three fractions before the peak of inhibitor activity. The GAGs peak is only one fraction away from the fraction containing the maximum inhibitor activity while the peak RNA concentration corresponds exactly with peak inhibition. While not ruling out protein and GAGs as inhibitor constituents, these data support the contribution of RNA-like material to the inhibitory activity.

A detailed analysis of the HPLC data given in Figure 3 further implicates RNA-like material in the inhibition process. Fraction #27 of Figure 2 gives pattern A in HPLC with the maximum absorbance at 254 nm eluting near the void volume of the column, i.e., being retained very slightly if at all. Hydrolysis of this sample at 37°C for 1 hour at pH 13 and return to pH 6 gives pattern B in Figure 3 with the peak absorbance now exhibiting a dramatically longer retention time.

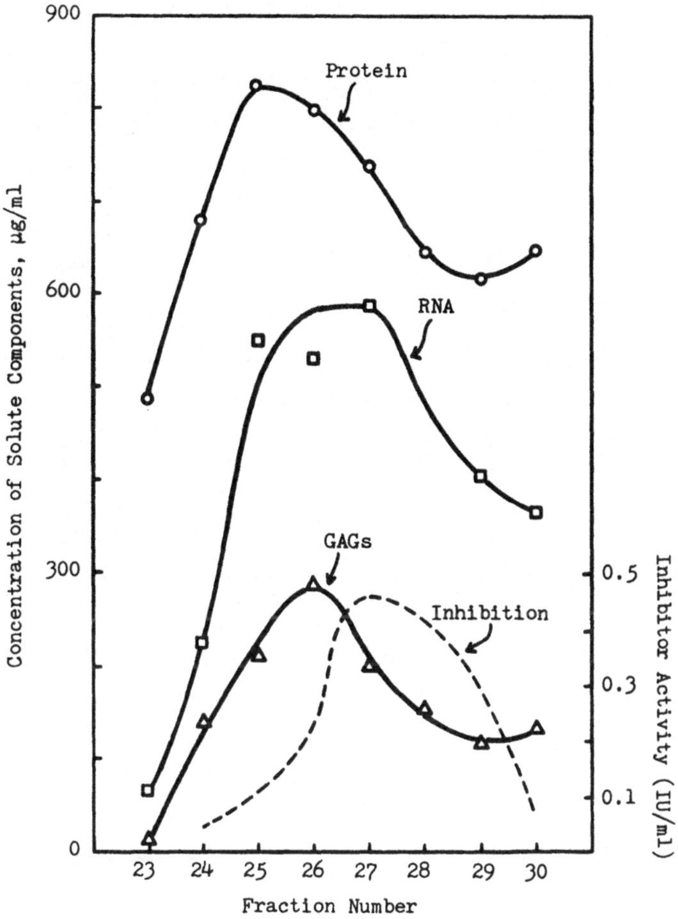

Figure 2. Chemical analysis of the solute components and inhibitor activity of fractions from a phenol-extracted and desalted concentrate of urine.

HPLC patterns for native and alkali-hydrolyzed yeast RNA, chondroitin sulfate (CDS), and bovine serum albumin (BSA), each at a concentration of 1 mg/ml, are given in Figure 3 as C and D (RNA), E and F (CDS), and G and H (BSA). The 1 mg/ml concentration for the model substances was chosen to conform to the 1.5 mg/ml overall solute concentration of fraction #27.

While pattern E, F and G, H show miniscule absorbance for both the native and alkaline hydrolyzed peaks, only the HPLC patterns exhibited by yeast RNA, C and D, are strikingly similar to those exhibited by fraction #27, patterns A and B. A calculation of the concentration of RNA-like material in fraction #27 can be made using

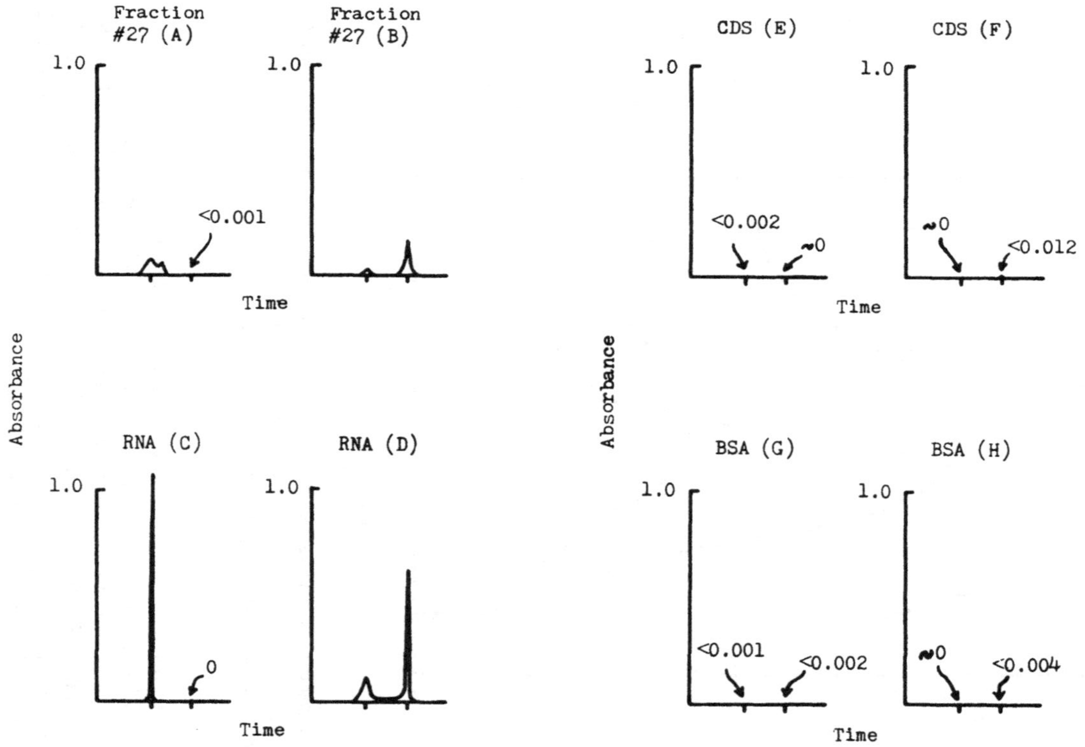

Figure 3. HPLC patterns for untreated and alkaline-hydrolyzed model compounds and a sample fraction. See text for meaning of designations.

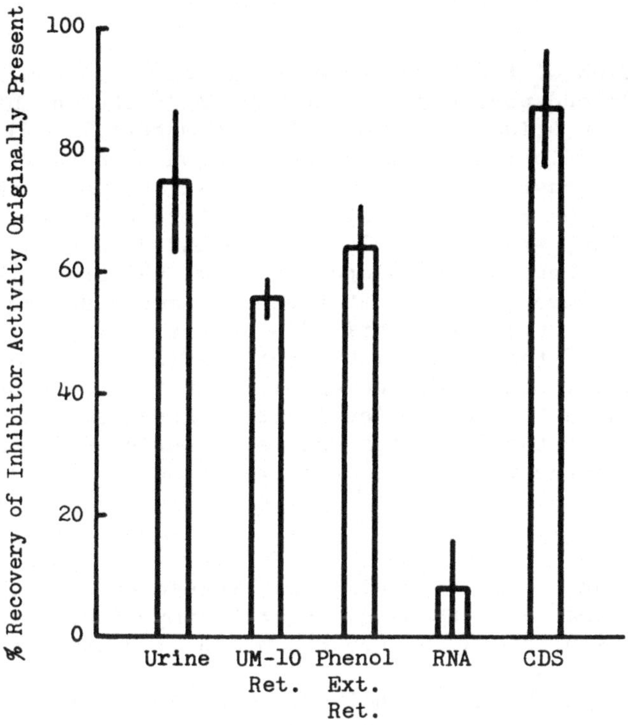

Figure 4. Effect of RNAase digestion on inhibitors of calcium oxalate crystal growth.

the relative areas of these peaks. The value of 0.4 ± 0.1 mg/ml obtained compares favorably with 0.6 ± 0.1 mg/ml from chemical analysis.

The results of the RNAase digestion experiments are shown in Figure 4. RNAase digestion reduces the inhibition of whole urine by 25 ± 12%, of urine retentates by 44 ± 3%, and of material carried through the purification scheme by 36 ± 7%. A slight reduction of the inhibitor activity of RNAase of CDS was noted while the inhibitor activity of yeast RNA was almost totally destroyed.

The average molecular weight of the solutes in the peak fraction as determined by gel exclusion chromatography was 4700 ± 300 daltons. The uncertainty is the average deviation of the mean of two determinations. It must be emphasized that the molecular weight is determined in 6 M guanidinium chloride which dissociates all aggregates.

CONCLUSIONS

Consideration of the data presented leads us to conclude that no less than 20% and possibly as much as 40% of the inhibitor material in normal human urine is RNA or RNA-like material. While this conclusion is based primarily on the digestion studies with RNAase, it is completely consistent with the chemical analysis, the spectroscopic data, and the HPLC results. Our preference is to term the material, RNA-like, since the molecular weight data strongly imply that fragments rather than complete chains of RNA are existent in urine. The likelihood exists that these fragments do not contain a full complement of purine and pyrimidine bases. Finally, the molecular weight of the active inhibitor species is probably higher than is shown here. Charged species will interact with other macromolecules and cause the macromolecules to aggregate. The ultimate characterization of the inhibitor species in urine will require a detailed study of the importance of aggregation.

REFERENCES

1. R. L. Ryall and V. R. Marshall, in:"Proceedings Fourth International Urolithiasis Research Symposium," L. H. Smith, B. Finlayson, and W. G. Robertson, eds., Plenum Press, New York, (in press).
2. T. Bitter and M. H. Muir, Anal. Biochem. 4:330 (1962).
3. R. Almog and T. L. Shirey, Anal. Biochem. 91:130 (1978).
4. T. E. Dorsey, P. W. McDonald, and O. A. Roels, Anal. Biochem. 78:156 (1977).
5. G. L. Gardner and R. H. Doremus, Invest. Urol. 15:478 (1978).
6. J. L. Meyer and L. H. Smith, Invest. Urol. 13:31 (1975).
7. H. Ito and F. L. Coe, Am. J. Physiol. 233:F455 (1977).
8. A. A. Ansari and R. G. Mage, J. Chromatog. 140:98 (1977).
9. W. W. Fish, K. G. Mann, and C. Tanford, J. Biol. Chem. 244:4989 (1969).

ACKNOWLEDGMENT

This work was supported in part by AM 20605 from the National Institutes of Health.

INHIBITORS OF CALCIUM OXALATE AND CALCIUM PHOSPHATE CRYSTAL FORMATION IN URINE - A CRITIQUE AND REAPPRAISAL

P. C. Hallson, G. Alan Rose, and C. T. Samuell

St. Peter's Hospitals and Institute of Urology

London, England

INTRODUCTION

Previous studies of the role of inhibitors of calcium oxalate and calcium phosphate crystal formation in urine have usually been performed either in relatively simple aqueous solutions or by addition of dilute urine samples to solutions supersaturated for calcium oxalate or phosphate[1-4]. These experiments however are open to serious objections: 1) Urine contains macromolecular promoters of crystal formation, probably uromucoids[5], which should be included but have previously been excluded, and 2) the effect of certain inhibitors, notably pyrophosphate, citrate and methylene blue on calcium oxalate and calcium phosphate crystal formation is much less in whole urine than in simple inorganic solutions[6]. Even the studies of whole urine have not been physiological because they relied on addition of calcium and oxalate (or phosphate) to urine and this procedure can lead to abnormal crystal habits[7].

A new test for the ability of a chemical to inhibit crystal formation in whole urine has therefore been devised. It relies upon removal of water from urine at 37°C and stimulates what occurs in the collecting tubules of the kidneys when urine is undergoing concentration.

METHODS

Urine is passed directly into a Dewar flask and maintained at 37°C throughout the procedure which is commenced immediately or as soon as possible (usually within two hours). The sample is divided into two aliquots and the test substance added to one. Both samples are reduced in volume on a vacuum rotary evaporator at pH 5.3 to study calcium oxalate or pH 6.8 (or higher) to study calcium phosphate crystals. In order to increase the certainty of obtaining the oxalate crystals sufficient extra oxalate was added to both samples to raise the final concentration in the evaporated samples by 0.22 mmol/l. It was then found possible to lower the final concentration from 1450 mosmol/l as previously described[7] to 1050 mosmol/l and this procedure gave larger crystals that were easier to count. In studying calcium phosphate crystals the final urine concentration was 1250 mosmol/l and nothing other than the test substance was added. After evaporation the samples were incubated at 37°C either for zero time or for approximately 1 hour or for approximately 3 hours. At the end of this time the samples were centrifuged and the deposit, including the mucoid-like material present, withdrawn and homogenized in a constant volume of urine of approximately 200 μl. Fifty μl was transferred to a microscope slide and a cover slip applied. Crystals were counted using an eye-piece graticule as an aid. To quantitate results chemically all the precipitate was re-centrifuged, washed with pH 7.9 barbitone buffer and dissolved in exactly 1 or 2 ml of 1 M HCl. Calcium was then measured by atomic absorption flame photometry.

The preparation of GAGS was from fresh human urine using precipitation with cetyl-pyridinium chloride, and washing with ethanolic solutions. It contained 440 μmol/l of GAGS as glucuronic acid[8], and also 7.8 mmol/l of uric acid.

RESULTS

1. Calculation of Results

The differences in crystalluria found by combined macroscopic and microscopic inspection in 38 pairs of urine samples were compared with measurements of calcium content of the crystals in each pair of samples. Twenty-five of the pairs contained oxalate crystals and the rest phosphate crystals. These results are shown in Figure 1. In 26 pairs of urine samples where visual inspection had shown that there was no significant difference between the crystals in the two samples comprising the pair, the calcium analysis showed variations of 0-49.2% (mean 13.9%). In 12 cases where a significant change had been noted visually the differences revealed chemically were 1.2-200% (mean 41%). It should be noted that if one takes a 25% change as the dividing line between no change and a significant change, then on vision alone there would have been 3 false negatives out of 20, and 5 false positives out of fourteen, an overall error rate of 18.6%.

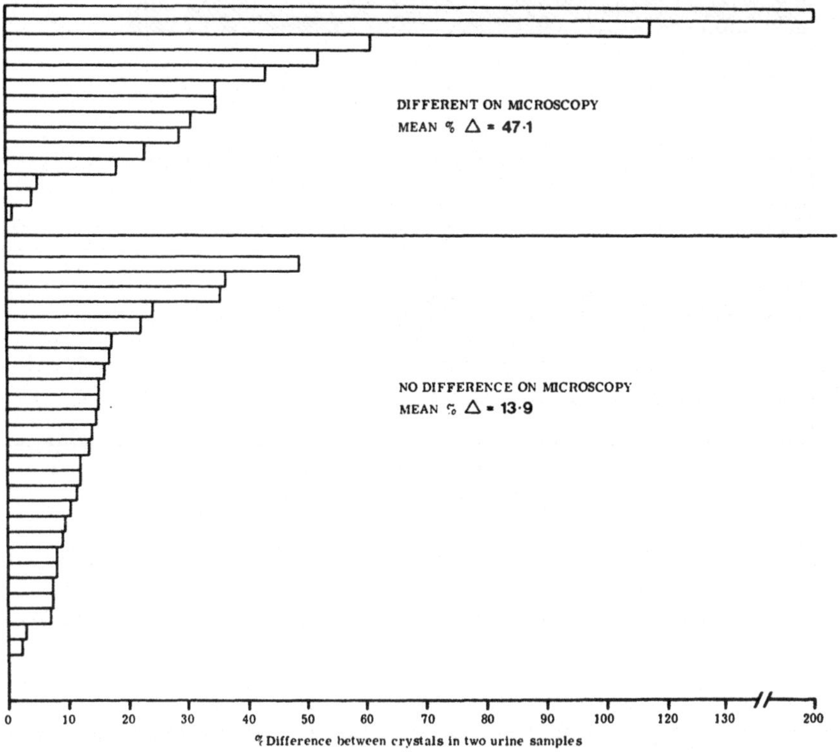

Figure 1. Forty-three pairs of urine samples were studied. After microscopy each pair was reported as showing either similar or dissimilar amounts of crystals. The crystals in each pair of samples were then analyzed chemically for calcium and the actual difference between the two compared with the microscopy report.

2. Effect of EHDP on Oxalate Crystalluria

Twenty samples of urine were evaporated at pH 5.3 with and without addition of the diphosphonate EHDP to yield a final concentration of .062 mmol/l (20 mg/l) and examined for crystals afterwards. The results in Figure 2 show that 45% of the samples with EHDP showed an immediate reduction in crystalluria. When there was up to 1 hour incubation time between evaporation and examination, however, only 19% of the samples with EHDP showed a reduction in crystalluria. The reductions were due principally to the number of crystals seen and not size, although sometimes there was change from envelope to small amorphous crystals.

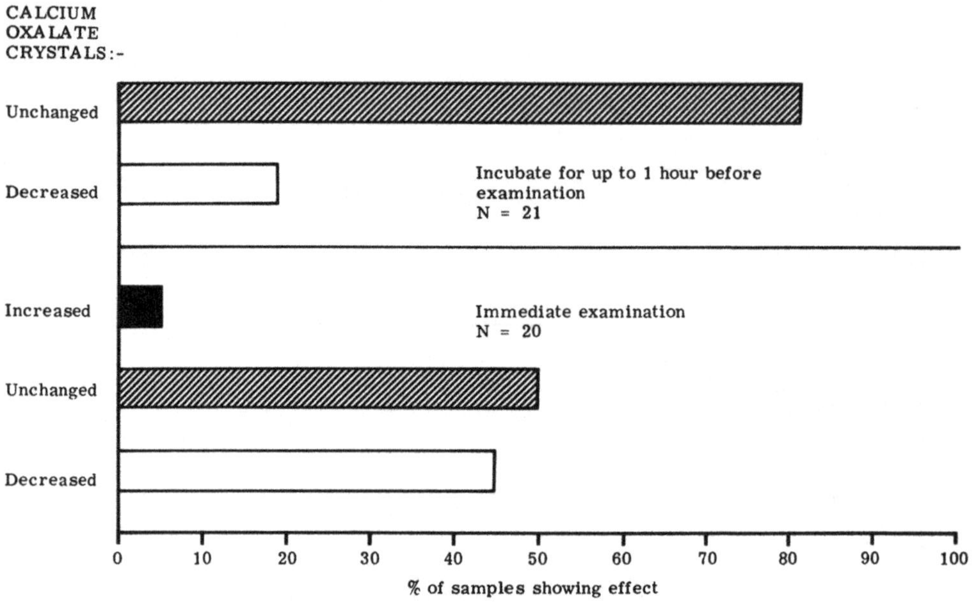

Figure 2. Effect of EHDP when added to normal urine at pH 5.3 before evaporation. The crystals are markedly reduced on immediate examination but much less so after a delay of up to 1 hour.

In 3 cases where EHDP had been added to urine there was high incidence of deformed envelope calcium oxalate crystals as shown in Figures 3 and 4. Normal untreated urine may rarely show an occasional crystal deformed in this way, but their occurrence in such large numbers does not occur in untreated urine.

3. Chondroitin Sulphate

Chondroitin sulphate was added to 20 samples of whole urine to yield a final concentration of 100 mg/l. Nine were examined immediately after evaporation and 11 after a delay of 1 hour at 37°C. Ten ultrafiltrates of urine were also evaporated with and without chondroitin sulphate. In all these experiments urine pH was 5.3. In none of the procedures did the chondroitin sulphate result in any reduction in oxalate crystalluria.

4. GAGS

When the GAGS recovered from normal human urine was added to normal human urine at pH 5.3 in amount sufficient to raise the final concentration by 10 mg/l there was, after evaporation a reduction in oxalate crystalluria in 50% of the samples (see Figure 5).

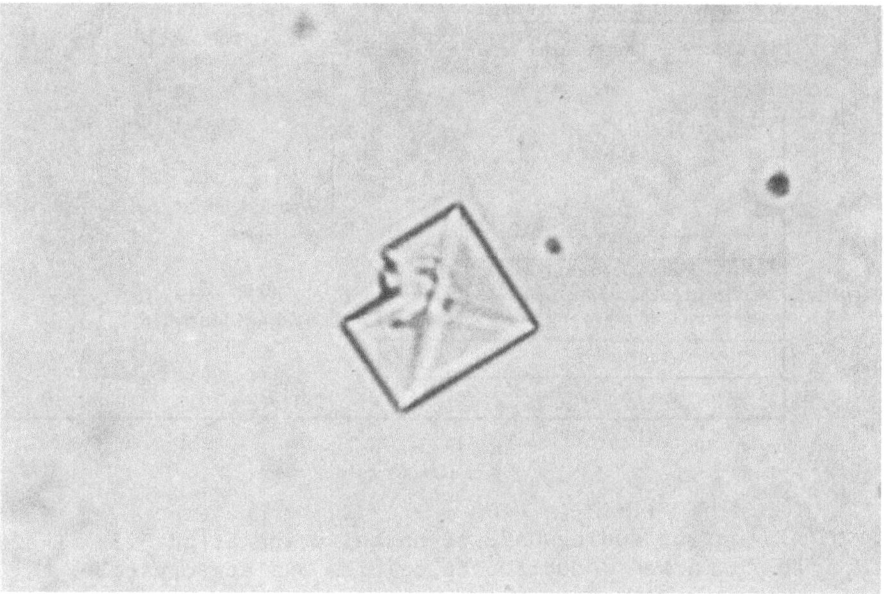

Figure 3. Deformed envelope calcium oxalate crystal obtained after evaporation of urine containing EHDP.

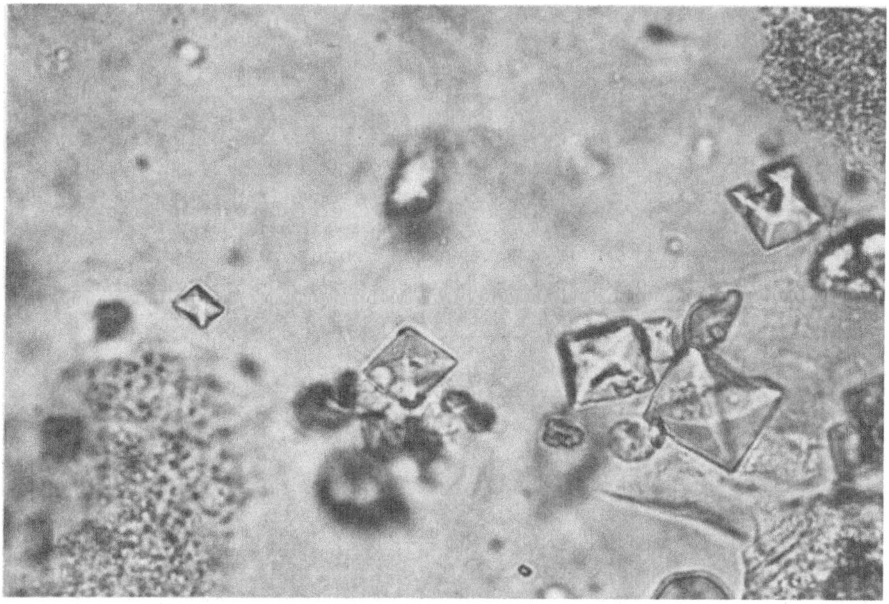

Figure 4. Deformed envelope calcium oxalate crystals obtained after evaporation of urine containing EHDP.

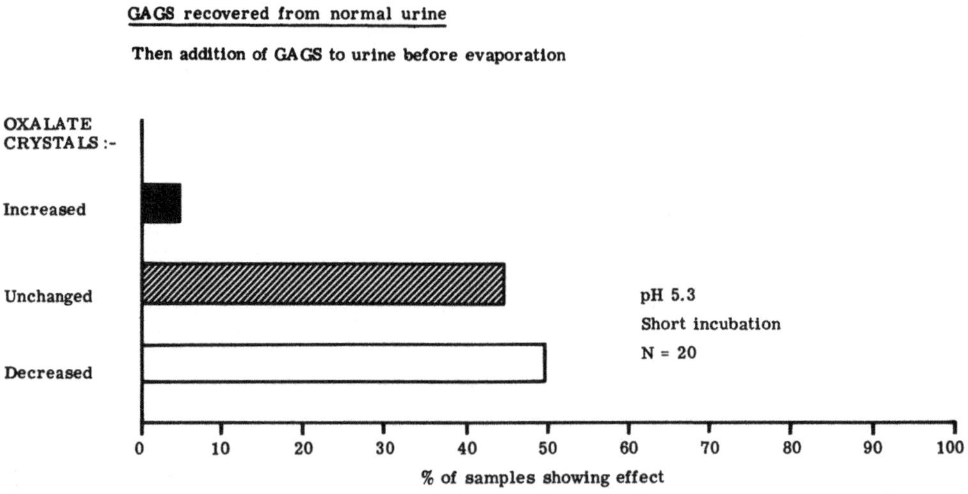

Figure 5. Effect of adding GAGS to normal urine at pH 5.3. There is a marked reduction in calcium oxalate crystals.

5. Methylene Blue

Methylene blue was added to 77 normal samples of urine to yield a final concentration after evaporation of 0.112 mmol/l (40 mg/l). The effects on the crystal formation are shown in Figures 6 and 7. At pH 5.3 there was a reduction in calcium oxalate crystals in 30% of the tests when an incubation time of 1 hour or less was used. However, when the incubation time was extended to 3 hours this reduction was almost entirely abolished. At pH 6.8 there was no effect upon calcium phosphate crystalluria with either incubation time.

6. Pyrophosphate

Sodium pyrophosphate was added to 75 whole urine samples and to 15 ultrafiltrates of urine to raise the final concentration after evaporation by 0.30 mmol/l (80 mg/l). These results have been published at a previous conference[9] and will therefore only be summarized here. At pH 5.3 whole urine samples, regardless of incubation time, showed no change in calcium oxalate crystalluria. There was however a reduction in the calcium oxalate crystals in the ultrafiltrates of urine. At pH 6.8 there was no decrease, but

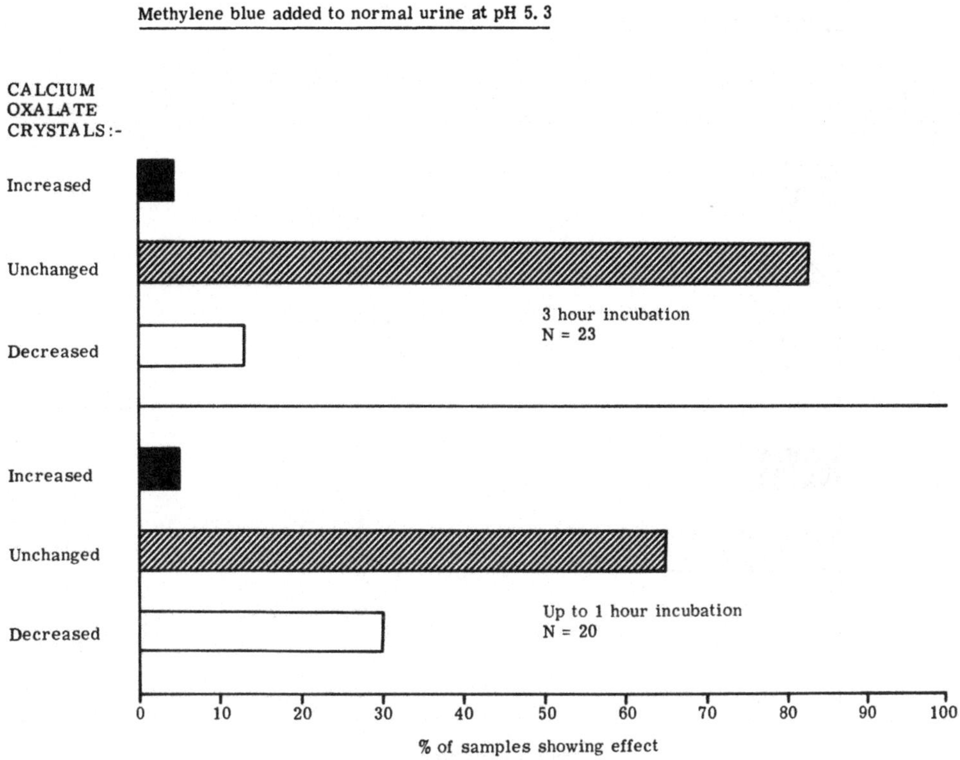

Figure 6. Effect of adding methylene blue to normal urine at pH 5.3. A considerable reduction in calcium oxalate crystals of short incubation is largely abolished after a 3 hour incubation.

rather an increase in calcium phosphate crystalluria in whole urine samples, with no change in the ultrafiltrates of urine.

7. Urate and Xanthine

Sodium biurate was added to 37 samples of normal urine so as to raise the final concentration of urate after evaporation by 4 mmol/l (676 mg/l). Using a 1 hour post-evaporation incubation time calcium oxalate crystalluria at pH 5.3 was unchanged in 32 tests (86.5%), increased in 4 tests (10.8%) and decreased in 1 test (2.7%). These results indicate no significant effect of urate on the calcium oxalate crystals formation.

An equimolar quantity of xanthine was similarly tested. In 25 out of 26 tests there was no change in calcium oxalate crystalluria

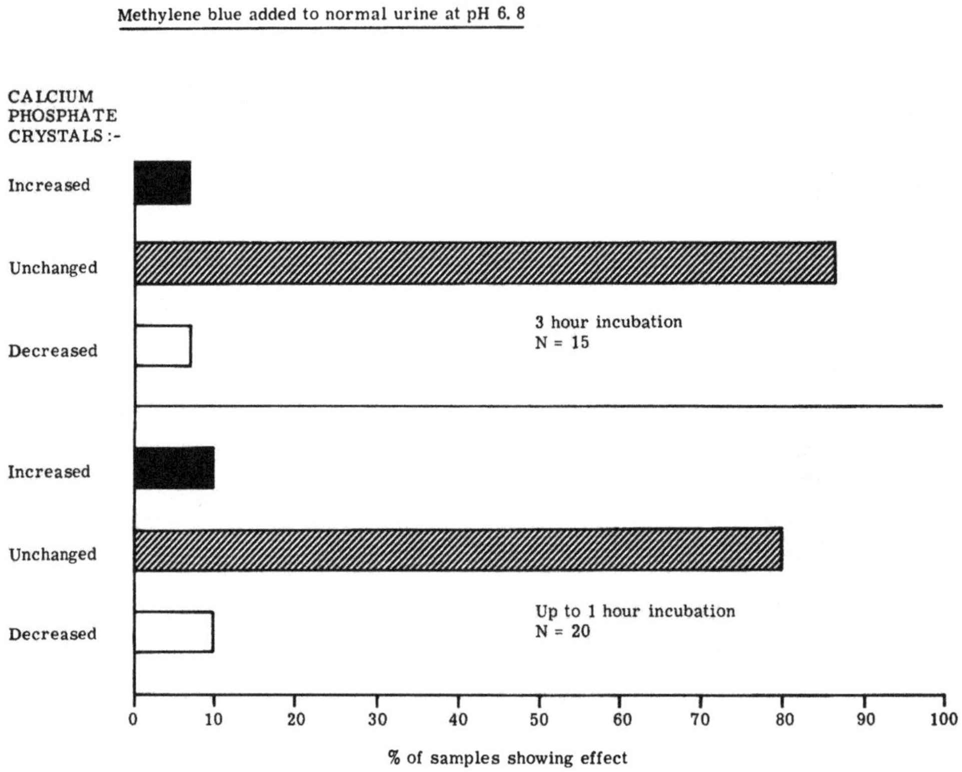

Figure 7. Lack of effect of adding methylene blue to normal urine at pH 6.8 on calcium phosphate crystals.

and the 26th test showed a reduction. These results indicate no significant effect of xanthine.

DISCUSSION

The method described for assessing the potency of inhibitors of crystal formation is novel in providing a simple way of studying whole urine. The principle of the method, normally removal of water from dilute urine, simulates the final concentration of urine in the collecting tubules of the kidney. While this procedure yields calcium oxalate envelope crystals of the type seen in urine samples of stone formers, it was found advantageous to raise slightly the oxalate content of urine. The amount added however was so small that the final oxalate content of the urine remained within normal physiological limits.

The comparison of the assessment of the crystals by visual means showed a sufficiently good correlation with the independently made quantitative chemical findings, for the former alone to be useful in assessing small alterations in crystals. Thus, using a 25% change as the minimum that might be recognized by vision alone, although there might be a number of false negatives, false positives would occur in only 1 in 10 sample pairs. This means that if, as in the present work, 20 urine samples are tested for an inhibitor and more than 2 samples show inhibition then there is evidence that the inhibitor causes 25% or more reduction in crystal volume. The microscopy method is also useful in being able to differentiate between a reduction in crystal volume due to crystal numbers or to crystal size. In fact the changes reported here were thought to be due mostly to crystal numbers.

The disphosphonate EHDP resulted in the marked diminution of crystalluria when the samples were examined by microscopy immediately after evaporation. However, when microscopy examination was delayed for up to 1 hour the reduction in crystalluria was much less. This indicates that EHDP delays rather than prevents oxalate crystalluria in urine, a particularly important observation since only crystalluria within the kidneys or upper urinary tract can result in the upper urinary tract stones with which we are here concerned. Addition of EHDP to normal urine sometimes resulted in another remarkable change, namely the occurrence in large numbers of deformed envelope calcium oxalate crystals. As shown in Figures 3 and 4 they have bits missing and one can speculate that the EHDP is in high concentration on the surface preventing the completion of crystal growth. This could be an important new way of recognizing visually the action of an inhibitor of crystal formation.

It was of interest that although the GAGS recovered from normal human urine show potent inhibition of calcium oxalate crystal formation in whole urine, chondroitin sulphate did not apparently account for this effect. However, it is known that the GAGS made by the technique used contain substances other than chondroitin sulphate and we do not yet know the nature of the active principle in our crude GAGS preparation.

Results with methylene blue are of interest because, as in the case of EHDP, while some evidence of inhibition of calcium oxalate crystalluria was seen with a short incubation time, this inhibition was greatly reduced with longer incubation time, again indicating a delay in crystal formation rather than abolition. No evidence for reduction in calcium phosphate crystalluria by methylene blue could however be found.

Results with pyrophosphate have already been discussed elsewhere[9] but it may be noted here that this substance seemed quite inactive as an inhibitor of calcium phosphate crystals either in whole urine or ultrafiltrates thereof. There is however some evidence of inhibition of calcium oxalate crystal formation in ultrafiltrates of urine, but not in whole urine, again showing the necessity of studying the whole product rather than simple derivatives thereof.

The effect of added urate to urine was studied, not to see if it inhibited crystalluria, but in case it promoted crystalluria as it should do according to certain authors. It is therefore of great interest that no effect could be shown on calcium oxalate crystal formation at pH 5.3. Xanthine was likewise tested because, had an increase of calcium oxalate crystalluria been caused by urate, it would then have become important to know whether xanthine had a similar effect. In the event however, xanthine, like urate, proved not to alter calcium oxalate crystalluria.

SUMMARY

1. Previous tests of the effect of possible inhibitors of crystal formation in urine have suffered from various defects which may have rendered them inapplicable to whole urine. A new test based on rapid removal of water from whole urine has therefore been devised.

2. Methylene blue and the disphosphonate EHDP have been found to delay calcium oxalate crystal formation in whole urine. The potent inhibitor EHDP also led to production of deformed envelope crystals.

3. Pyrophosphate was found to be ineffective on either calcium oxalate or calcium phosphate crystals in whole urine.

4. GAGS extracted from normal human urine was found to be a potent inhibitor of calcium oxalate crystalluria when added to normal urine. A chondroitin sulphate however was inactive.

5. Urate and xanthine were without effect on calcium oxalate crystalluria in whole urine.

REFERENCES

1. W. G. Robertson, M. Peacock, and B. E. C. Nordin, Clin. Chim. Acta. 43:31 (1973).
2. W. G. Robertson, M. Peacock, D. H. Marshall, and B. E. C. Nordin, N. Eng. J. Med. 294:349 (1976).
3. J. H. Baumann, S. Bisaz, H. Fleisch, and M. Walker, Clin. Sci. and Mol. Med. 54:509 (1978).
4. C. Y. C. Pak, K. Holt, and J. E. Zerwekh, Invest. Urol. 17:138 (1979).
5. P. C. Hallson and G. A. Rose, Lancet 1:1000 (1979).

6. S. G. Welshman and M. G. McGeown, Br. J. Urol. 44:677 (1972).
7. P. C. Hallson and G. A. Rose, Br. J. Urol. 50:442 (1978).
8. T. Bitter and H. M. Muir, Analyt. Biochem. 4:330 (1962).

STUDIES ON INHIBITORS AND PROMOTERS OF THE CRYSTALLIZATION OF CALCIUM OXALATE IN URINE AND IN MATRIX FROM CALCIUM OXALATE STONES

D. S. Scurr, C. M. Bridge, and W. G. Robertson

M.R.C. Mineral Metabolism Unit, The General Infirmary

Leeds LS1 3EX, U.K.

Urine contains some potent inhibitors of the crystal growth and/or aggregation of calcium oxalate crystals. The present concensus is that the main ones lie in the macromolecular fraction of urine[1-6]. Only a small fraction of calcium oxalate inhibitory activity appears to be due to small ions[7] such as magnesium, pyrophosphate and citrate. The high molecular weight inhibitors appear to be acidic glycosaminoglycans (GAGS)[1,3,5], acidic peptides[4] or an RNA-like compound[6]. Some workers claim that stone-formers have less net inhibitory activity in their urine than normal subjects[8,9,10].

An alternative hypothesis to account for the observed differences in crystalluria between stone-formers and normals[11] is that they are due not to greater inhibitory activity in normal urine but to the presence of some promoters of crystallization in the urine of stone-formers. This is considered by a few to be "matrix substance A" (a constituent of stone matrix)[12] and by others to be Tamm-Horsfall mucoprotein (uromucoid)[13].

Separation of the Macromolecular Polyanionic Fractions of Urine

Normal urine was treated with cetyl trimethylammonium bromide (CTAB) to separate the high molecular weight polyanions according to the procedure of Scott and Newton[14]. It was further fractionated according to Robertson et al.[15] to produce fractions SR-0 to SR-3a as shown in Table 1. These contain various combinations of acidic GAGS, Tamm-Horsfall mucoprotein (THM) and RNA. The compositions have been analyzed and presented elsewhere[15].

Table 1 also shows the ability of each fraction to inhibit or promote the crystal growth and combined growth and aggregation of calcium oxalate crystals in a high supersaturation system in which spontaneous crystallization occurs[15] and a metastable seeded growth system[7]. In the high supersaturation system the fractions were tested at the same concentrations as in whole urine and in the metastable system at concentrations of 1% of those in the original urine. There is a wide range of responses produced by the various fractions from a weak-moderate degree of promotion of growth and aggregation to strong inhibition. The effects of the fractions were always greater on aggregation than on growth alone.

In one study the promoter fraction (SR-0) and inhibitory fraction (SR-2a) were mixed together in the same proportions as in the original urine. The combination produced strong net inhibition suggesting that the promoter is probably of little significance in whole urine.

Separation of Stone Matrix Fractions

Several calcium oxalate stones (10.01g) were powdered and dissolved in 10% EDTA (pH 8.0) over 48 h. The insoluble residue was separated (36 mg) and the supernatant containing the water-soluble matrix dialysed to remove EDTA and other salts. The remaining non-dialysable fraction was freeze-dried (50.4 mg) and analyzed for alcian blue precipitable material (6.2 mg) and acidic GAGS by the uronic method (2.9 mg). The insoluble residue and the water-soluble fraction were tested at various concentrations for their ability to inhibit or promote crystal growth and the combined growth and aggregation of calcium oxalate.

One of the major problems is deciding what concentration of each fraction is relevant to use. We are in the process of testing each fraction at a number of concentrations and the data in Table 2 represents our preliminary findings. This shows that the insoluble fraction at a concentration of 20 μg/l is a weak promoter of growth and aggregation in the high supersaturation system but is a strong inhibitor of growth and an extremely potent promoter of aggregation in the seeded growth system. The soluble fraction which should contain matrix substance "A" is, on the other hand, always a good inhibitor of both growth and combined growth and aggregation. This confirms the observation that the soluble fraction of stone matrix is a good inhibitor of the crystal growth of calcium oxalate as measured by the rate of decrease of oxalate in solution[16].

Finally, Table 2 shows that when the insoluble and soluble fractions of stone matrix are re-mixed in approximately the same proportions as in the original matrix the net effect is to produce strong inhibition of crystal growth and moderate inhibition of combined growth and aggregation. Further studies are under way to identify these materials.

Table 1. The Effect of the Various Fractions of Urine on the Inhibition or Promotion of Calcium Oxalate Growth and Aggregation *in vitro*

Fraction	Concentration in urine (mg/1)	Composition	High supersaturation system: Inhibition of Crystal Growth (%)	High supersaturation system: Inhibition of Aggregation (%)	Seeded growth system: Inhibition of Crystal Growth (%)	Seeded growth system: Inhibition of Aggregation (%)	Summary
SR-0	9	Insoluble urinary residue	0	-14	0	-5	Weak-moderate promoter of aggregation
SR-1	-	Supernatant after CTAB precipitation containing low MW inhibitors	+10*	+15*	+5	+10	Weak inhibitor of growth and of aggregation
SR-2a	32.4	Soluble Ba salts of GAGS, THM and RNA	+35	+72	+20	+61	Weak-moderate inhibitor of growth, strong inhibitor of aggregation
SR-2b	2.5	Insoluble Ba salts	0	0	0	0	No effect as inhibitor or as promoter
SR-3	7.4	Deproteinized sub-fraction of SR-2a containing GAGS and RNA	+36	+79	+30	+75	Moderate inhibitor of growth, strong inhibitor of aggregation
SR-3a	2.5	Hyaluronidase-treated sub-fraction of SR-3 containing RNA and dermatan sulphate	-	-	+5	+15	Weak-inhibitor of both growth and aggregation
SR-0 + SR-2a	9 32.4	Promoter from SR-0 + inhibitors from SR-2a	+35	+64	+20	+61	Moderate-strong inhibition

* Estimated from combined effects of pyrophosphate, magnesium and citrate.

Table 2. The Effect of Various Fractions of the Matrix from Calcium Oxalate Stones on the Inhibition or Promotion of Calcium Oxalate Crystal Growth and Aggregation *in vitro*

Fraction	% by weight of stone	Composition	Concentration (μg/1)	Inhibition of crystal growth (%)	Inhibition of aggregation (%)	Concentration (μg/1)	Inhibition of crystal growth (%)	Inhibition of aggregation (%)	Summary
M-insoluble	0.36	?	20	-4	-19	20	90	-162	Promoter or aggregation: inhibitor of growth
M-soluble	0.50	Acidic GAGS, THM(?) and MSA (%)	20.2	91	100	20.20	95	100	Inhibitor of both growth and aggregation.
			2.02	0	5	2.00	31	57	
						0.20	9	26	
						0.02	0	12	
M-insoluble + M-soluble		Promoter from M-insoluble + Inhibitor from M-soluble	20 + 20.2	25	28	20 + 20.2	90	53	Moderate-strong inhibition
						20 + 2.02	82	-35	Strong inhibition of growth; moderate promotion of aggregation

REFERENCES

1. W. G. Robertson, C. F. Knowles, and M. Peacock, in:"Urolithiasis Research," H. Fleisch, W. G. Robertson, L. H. Smith and W. Vahlensieck, eds., Plenum Press, New York (1976).
2. W. B. Gill, J. W. Karesh, L. Garsin, and M. J. Roma, Invest. Urol. 15:95 (1977).
3. G. L. Gardner and R. H. Doremus, Invest. Urol. 15:478 (1978).
4. H. Ito and F. L. Coe, Amer. J. Physiol. 233:F455 (1977).
5. J. D. Sallis and M. F. Lumley, Invest. Urol. 16:296 (1979).
6. E. E. Schrier, K. E. Lee, J. L. Rubin, P. G. Werness, and L. H. Smith, in:"Oxalate in Human Biochemistry and Clinical Pathology," G. A. Rose, W. G. Robertson, R. W. E. Watts, eds., Wellcome Foundation, London (1980).
7. W. G. Robertson, M. Peacock, and F. Knowles, in:"Urinary Calculi," L. Cifuentes-Delatte, A. Rapado, and A. Hodgkinson, eds., Karger, Basel (1973).
8. W. G. Robertson, M. Peacock, R. W. Marshall, D. H. Marshall, and B. E. C. Nordin, N. Eng. J. Med. 294:249 (1976).
9. F. L. Coe, H. C. Margolis, L. H. Deutsch, and A. L. Straus, Mineral Electrolyte Metab. 3:268 (1980).
10. A. Ligabue, M. Fini, and W. G. Robertson, Clin. Chim. Acta. 98:39 (1979).
11. W. G. Robertson and M. Peacock, Clin. Sci. 43:499 (1972).
12. W. H. Boyce and J. S. King, Ann. N. Y. Acad. Sci. 104:563 (1963).
13. P. C. Hallson and G. A. Rose, Lancet 1:1000 (1979).
14. J. E. Scott and D. J. Newton, Connect. Tiss. Res. 3:157 (1975).
15. W. G. Robertson, D. S. Curr, and C. M. Bridge, J. Cryst. Growth (in press).
16. J. C. Gjaldbaek and W. G. Robertson, Clin. Chim. Acta (in press).

EFFECT OF DIFFERENT URINARY CONSTITUENTS ON INHIBITING OR ACCELERATING CALCIUM OXALATE CRYSTALLIZATION

B. K. Sur and H. N. Pandey

Department of Biochemistry, G.S.V.M. Medical College,

Kanpur, India

Sutor[1] has described a method for assessing the effect of different compounds on the inhibition or acceleration of crystallization of calcium oxalate. This method was qualitative and did not give sufficiently reproducible values. The assay procedure was made quantitative by measuring calcium and considerably improved to give more reproducible values (details to be communicated elsewhere). Preliminary trials using acetate and phosphate buffers showed that the inhibitory effects of some compounds were dependent on the type of buffer used. Since acetate buffer is unphysiological it was felt that more useful and reliable information could be obtained if our improved method was applied using a phosphate buffer.

MATERIAL AND METHODS

To 50 ml of KH_2PO_4 - NaOH buffer (0.025M) of pH 6.0, $CaCl_2 \cdot 2H_2O$ (0.05M) and Na Oxalate (0.05M) solutions were added by Whatman 3 MM filter paper wicks under an air-tight closed chamber for 16 h. The amount of calcium oxalate crystallized on glass fibers was assayed by measuring calcium using a modification of Trinder's[2] method. The effectiveness of various urinary substances as inhibitors or accelerators of calcium oxalate crystallization was studied by dissolving the test substances individually in the phosphate buffer in concentrations simulating their occurrence in normal urine of low, average and high concentration.

RESULTS

The results of the present study showed that Mg, Na, PPi, glucuronic acid, citric acid, pyruvic acid, vitamin B_6, aspartic acid, threonine and glutamic acid inhibit calcium oxalate crystallization at physiological levels. Histidine, phosphate, glycine, creatinine, urea and taurine had neither inhibiting nor accelerating effects. Uric acid and α-ketoglutaric acid accelerated crystallization of calcium oxalate. The results are summarized in Table 1.

Table 1. Inhibiting or Accelerating Effects of Different Urinary Constituents on Calcium Oxalate Crystallization

Compound	Conc./1	Percent Inhibition	Compound	Conc./1	Percent Inhibition
$MgCl_2,6H_2O$	+ 4.0 mEq	60	Pyruvic acid	+ 55 μM	48
	+ 8.0 mEq	60		+110 μM	62
	+ 16.0 mEq	67		+440 μM	72
				880 μM	76
NaCl	50.0 mEq	55	Aspartic acid	+ 0.4mM	10
	+100.0 mEq	69		+ 0.8mM	44
	+150.0 mEq	69		+ 1.6mM	66
	+200.0 mEq	85		3.2mM	75
Sodium Pyrophosphate	+ 40.0 μM	30	Threonine	+ 0.2mM	42
	+80.0 μM	50		+ 0.4mM	48
				+ 1.0mM	56
				2.0mM	63
Vitamin B_6	+ 0.5 mg	50	Glutamic acid	+ 0.1mM	13
	+ 1.0 mg	57		+ 0.7mM	25
	1.5 mg	71		+ 3.5mM	38
Glucuronic acid	1.3 mM	40	Uric acid*	7.0mM	38
	+ 2.6 mM	47		1.5mM	33
	+ 5.2 mM	60		+ 3.0mM	60
				+ 6.0mM	71
Citrate	+ 1.0 mM	4			
	+ 2.0 mM	4	α-ketoglutaric acid	+ 70 μM	30
	+ 5.0 mM	52		+140 μM	35
	10.0 mM	55		350 μM	42

+Shows physiological limits of concentration of above constituents of urine.
*Acceleration.

DISCUSSION

From a therapeutic point of view it is not enough to know which urinary constituents have potent inhibitory activity. Only those urinary constituents which considerably increase inhibitory activity as their concentrations are increased from the lower to upper limits of normal excretion, have potential therapeutic value. A urinary constituent such as Mg, which has strong inhibitory activity, may prove of little therapeutic value as its inhibitory effect cannot be increased by augmenting its concentration in urine. Thus at 4.0 mEq/l Mg induced 60% inhibition, at 16 mEq/l the inhibition was only 67%. Thus by increasing dietary intake of Mg and thereby increasing its urinary excretion there would not be any further inhibition of calcium oxalate crystallization.

Our results showed inhibition by Mg and vitamin B_6 and acceleration by uric acid. Sutor found neither inhibition nor acceleration with these compounds. While she found phosphate had an inhibitory effect, we did not find any such effect. In the present experiments NaCl inhibited calcium oxalate crystallization while Sutor reported acceleration by this compound. These gross differences in results are probably attributable to the different buffer systems used.

It is possible that other urinary constituents may alter the inhibiting or accelerating effects observed in the present experiments. The studies reported here are, therefore, being repeated using a synthetic normal urine containing all the constituents investigated in the present study. Citric acid, aspartic acid, glutamic acid, pyrophosphate and pyruvic acid significantly increased inhibition as their concentrations increased from the lower to upper limit of normal. Feeding phosphate increases urinary pyrophosphate[3]. The use of dietary phosphate in the reduction of stone recurrence rate is well documented[4,5]. Dietary phosphate supplementation completely abolishes calcium oxalate crystalluria[6]. Although ingestion of citric acid does not increase urinary citrate[7], alkalinization of urine does[8,9]. This may provide another useful means of inhibiting calcium oxalate crystallization. The usefulness of the inhibition by aspartic acid appears doubtful as patients with idiopathic renal calculi already have an increased urinary aspartate[10]. It is interesting to note that matrix of renal calculi contains 50% aspartic and glutamic acid[11].

REFERENCES

1. D. J. Sutor, Br. J. Urol. 41:171 (1969).
2. P. Trinder, Analyst 85:889 (1960).
3. H. Fleisch, S. Bisaz, and A. D. Care, Lancet 1:1065 (1964).
4. L. H. Smith, W. C. Thomas, Jr., and C. D. Arnaud, in:"Urinary Calculi," L. Cifuentes-Delatte, A. Rapado, and A. Hodgkinson, eds., Karger, Basel (1973).
5. B. E. C. Nordin, H. Barry, L. Bulusu, and R. Speed, in: "Urinary Calculi," L. Cifuentes-Delatte, A. Rapado, and A. Hodgkinson, eds., Karger, Basel (1973).

6. A. Valyasevi, S. Dhanmitta, and R. Van Reen, Am. J. Clin. Nutr. 26:1207 (1973).
7. T. Thunberg, Physiol. Rev. 33:1 (1953).
8. R. N. Class and A. H. Smith, J. Biol. Chem. 151:363 (1943).
9. M. A. Crawford, M. S. Milne, and B. H. Scribner, J. Physiol. 149:413 (1959).
10. W. C. Thomas, M. H. Malagodi, and O. M. Rennert, in:"Proceedings Fourth International Urolithiasis Research Symposium," L. H. Smith, B. Finlayson, and W. G. Robertson, eds., Plenum Press, New York (in press).
11. A. R. Spector, A. Gray, and E. L. Prien, Jr., Invest. Urol. 13:387 (1976).

THE EFFECT OF NORMAL AND STONE-FORMING URINE ON THE GROWTH AND AGGREGATION OF CALCIUM OXALATE CRYSTALS IN RELATION TO URINARY GLYCOSAMINOGLYCAN AND URATE CONCENTRATIONS

R. L. Ryall and V. R. Marshall

Urology Unit, Department of Surgery, Flinders Medical Center, Bedford Park, South Australia 5042, Australia

INTRODUCTION

The factors which play a determinant role in urinary stone formation can be broadly classified into two main categories - those affecting the supersaturation of the urine with respect to the precipitating salt, and those which influence the ability of the urine to inhibit crystal nucleation, growth and aggregation. The supersaturation of urine with calcium oxalate is principally a function of calcium and oxalate excretion[1] and urinary pH, while inhibitory activity has been attributed to the presence of pyrophosphate and glycosaminoglycans (GAGS)[2]. For some years uric acid has been implicated in calcium oxalate stone formation[3] by virtue of its effect on calcium oxalate solubility[4] and the capability of its sodium salt of inducing heterogeneous nucleation of calcium oxalate[5]. More recently[2] it has been proposed that uric acid can indirectly predispose to calcium oxalate stone formation by interacting with urinary GAGS, thereby reducing their inhibitory capacity. Although it is widely accepted that urine can strongly inhibit crystal growth and aggregation, the significant reduction[6] of this activity in urine from stone-formers compared with normal subjects has not been confirmed[7].

Thus the aims of this study were threefold: 1) to determine whether a group of stone-formers could be distinguished from a group of normal subjects on the basis of daily excretion of calcium, oxalate, uric acid and GAGS, and 24-hour urinary pH and volume; 2) to resolve whether urine from the same groups differed in their ability to inhibit crystal growth and aggregation in vitro; and 3) to ascertain whether this inhibitory activity could be related to the urinary concentration of GAGS, and more particularly to the ratio of GAGS/uric acid concentration.

MATERIALS AND METHODS

Measurement of Inhibitory Activity

The method used was essentially that of Robertson and Peacock[6] with N-morpholinoethanesulphonic acid (MES) substituted for sodium cacodylate. A TA II Coulter Counter fitted with a 70 μm orifice tube was used to measure crystal growth and aggregation: crystal growth was expressed as the increase in total crystal volume (ΔV) and crystal aggregation as the decrease in total crystal number (ΔN). A parallel incubation containing 5×10^{-6}M pyrophosphate was included in each experiment to provide values for zero time crystal volume and number, since both growth and aggregation are completely inhibited under these conditions[8]. The time courses of crystal growth in a control incubation and in the presence of a urine at a concentration of 1% are shown in Figure 1a. While this concentration of urine was found to inhibit growth to a marked degree, it was not possible to quantify this effect from data expressed in this form. The same results are shown in Figure 1b expressed as T/ΔV versus T, where T is incubation time. This plot transforms the data shown in Figure 1a to a linear form and allows the calculation of the y-intercept at zero time. It can be seen that the reciprocal of this intercept is a measure of the initial reaction rate. The activity of an inhibitor can therefore be quantified in terms of its effect on the initial reaction rate in relation to a control as follows:

$$\text{Inhibition of growth (Ig)} = 100 - 100\left[\frac{\Delta V/T \text{ inhibitor}}{\Delta V/T \text{ control}}\right] \%$$

Calculation of the y-intercept involved unweighted robust regression analysis[9] and was performed on the Dec10 computer of the Flinders University. The time course of crystal aggregation was also non-linear (Figure 1b) and the data were similarly transformed to linear form by plotting T/ΔN against T. The calculation of the effect of an inhibitor on crystal aggregation (Ia) was then performed in an analogous manner to that of Ig, by substituting ΔN for ΔV.

Urine Specimens

Twenty-four hour urine specimens were collected without preservative and kept refrigerated for the duration of the collection. They were processed for crystal growth and aggregation experiments within three hours of completion of the collection. Spot urines consisted either of the first specimen passed after completion of the 24-hour collection or of the first urine sample passed upon waking during the 24-hour co-lection. In the latter

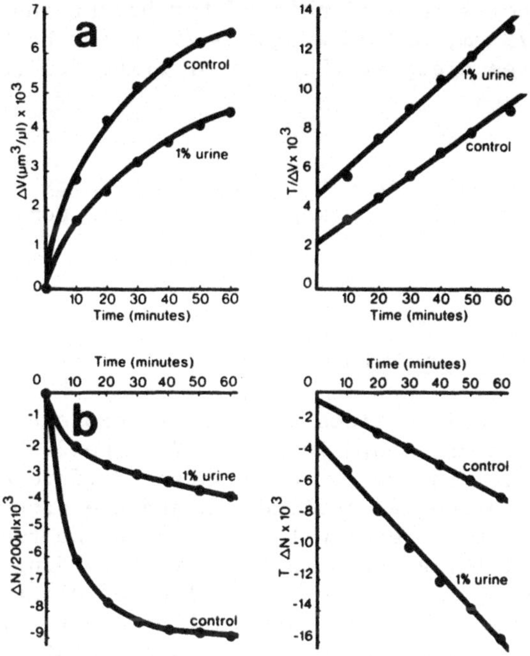

Figure 1. (a) The time course of crystal growth and its transformation to linear form.
(b) The time course of crystal aggregation and its transformation to linear form.

case the waking sample was collected separately and then a 24-hour specimen was obtained by mixing the waking sample with the remainder of the collection in proportion to their respective volumes. After measurement of volume and pH the urine was spun at 8000 x g in a Beckman J-21B centrifuge for 10 minutes, filtered through a 0.44 μm Millipore filter and then used in the incubations at a final concentration of 1% v/v. Calcium, uric acid and creatinine were measured using a standard Technicon SMA Auto Analyser system. Osmolality was measured by freezing point depression. Oxalate was determined using the technique of Farrington and Chalmers[10] and GAGS by the method of Blumenkrantz and Asboe-Hansen[11].

Subjects

Stone-formers consisted of male patients who had formed at least one stone composed of pure calcium oxalate or calcium oxalate in combination with other components such as phosphate and magnesium. Normal subjects were male members of the hospital staff who had never shown any evidence of renal stone. Although the ages of the two groups differed (median normal age = 32 years; median stone-former age = 48 years), they were well matched for height and weight (median height = 175 cm, median weight = 75 kg for both groups). All subjects were on free diets at the time of urine collection.

Statistics

Statistics were calculated using the University of Pittsburgh SPSS-10, Release 7.01 (1977) package on the Dec10 computer of the Flinders University.

RESULTS

Twenty-Four Hour Excretion Data

The 24-hour excretion values of calcium, oxalate, uric acid and GAGS for all subjects are shown in Figure 2. The 24-hour urinary volume and pH are also included. No apparent difference was found between the values for normal individuals and the stone-formers as a whole. The large overlap between the values in the two groups was not reduced by subdividing the stone-formers according to whether they had formed one or more stones. The lack of discrimination between the two groups, which is obvious from Figure 2, was confirmed by performing a Mann-Whitney U test on each group of data. In each case the median value is indicated.

Inhibition of Growth and Aggregation

Figure 3 shows the values of Ig and Ia obtained from the 24-hour and spot urine specimens for all subjects. Once again the stone-formers were classified according to whether they had formed one or more stones. Although no difference between normal and stone-forming urines could be detected with respect to their ability to inhibit crystal growth and aggregation (Mann-Whitney U test), there was an obvious difference between the levels of inhibition of growth and of aggregation for each group of subjects. Overall, urine inhibited crystal aggregation more strongly than it did crystal growth. The mean ± 1SD level of Ig and Ia for normal subjects was 50.6±21.0% and 72.0±22.0% respectively. The corresponding values for the stone-formers were 45.1±21.4% and 72.7±15.0%.

Inhibition of Growth and Aggregation in Relation to Urinary GAGS and Uric Acid Concentration

Since there was no detectable difference between normal and stone-forming urines on the basis of 24 hour GAGS and uric acid excretion, or on the basis of GAGS and uric acid concentration, all values from both groups were combined for this study. Despite the scatter of points, there was a significant correlation between Ig and GAGS concentration (Figure 4a, $n = 121$, $r = 0.2218$, $p < 0.01$).

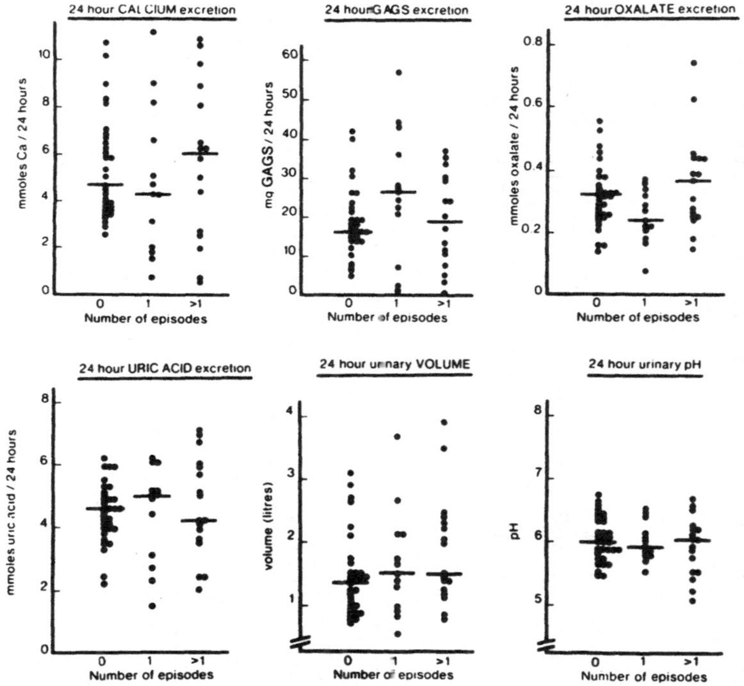

Figure 2. 24-hour urinary parameters in normals (0 episodes) and stone-formers (1, > 1 episode).

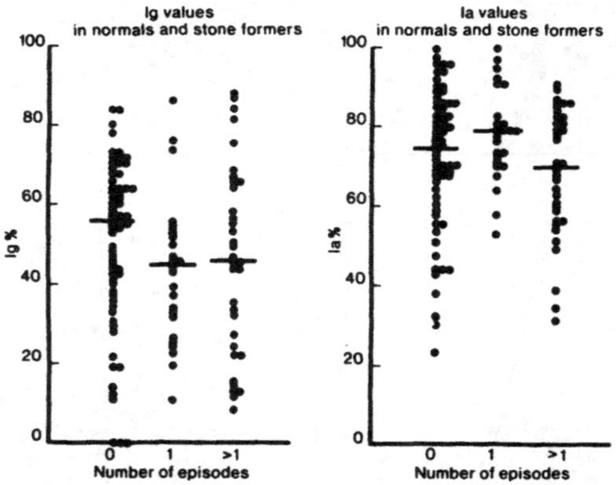

Figure 3. Inhibition of growth (Ig) and and aggregation (Ia) in urine from normals (0episodes) and stone-formers (1, > 1 episode).

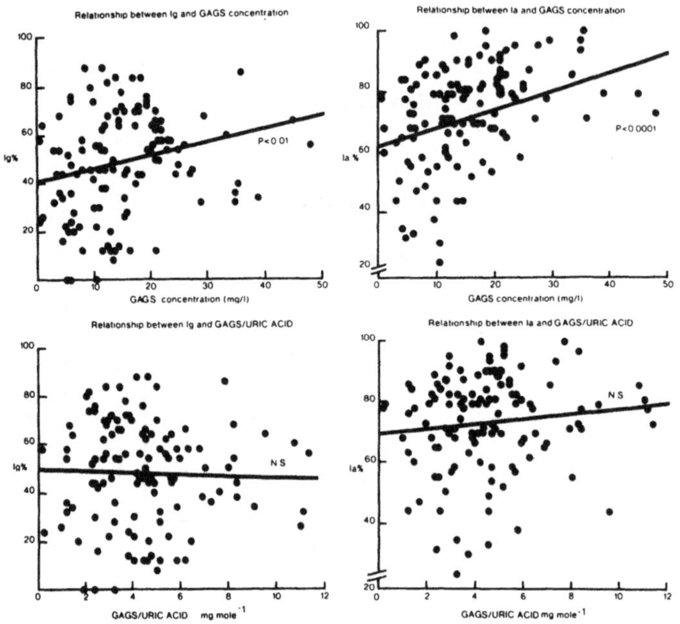

Figure 4. Inhibition of growth (Ig) and aggregation (Ia) in relation to GAGS concentration and the ratio of GAGS concentration to uric acid concentration.

Ia and GAGS concentration were more strongly correlated (Figure 4b, $n = 121$, $r = 0.4644$, $p < 0.0001$). However, when Ig and Ia were plotted against the ratio of GAGS to uric acid concentration (Figures 4c, 4d) then no correlation could be demonstrated.

DISCUSSION

A number of factors are presumed to contribute to the formation of calcium urinary stones, yet the treatment of calcium nephrolithiasis is traditionally based on 24-hour excretion data[12]. The parameters measured in the present investigation were selected because a previous study[13] reported a significant difference between their 24-hour values in urine from normal subjects and from recurrent stone-formers. However, we were unable to detect any differences in the daily excretion rates of calcium, oxalate, uric acid and GAGS, or in the 24-hour volume and pH of urines from normal volunteers and stone-formers in our series. This was in spite of the fact that a large proportion of the stone-formers (57%) had formed at least two stones. Thus, the prediction of a patient's likelihood of suffering further stone episodes remains very much an unsolved problem in our institution.

One notable observation regarding the 24-hour excretion data was that the daily excretion rate of uric acid in our normal subjects (4.5 ± 0.9 mmoles) was higher than the level quoted for recurrent stone-formers (3.4±0.1 mmoles) in the Leeds series[13], and we did not observe the tendency of stone-formers to excrete higher than normal levels of uric acid than has been reported for other studies[3,13].

Despite a report by Robertson and Peacock[6] that the ability of urine from stone-formers to inhibit calcium oxalate crystal growth and aggregation in an in vitro system was significantly less than that of normal urine, a more recent study[7] was unable to confirm this difference. The same method of calculation of inhibitory activity was used in both these studies and it has since been shown[14] that such a method produces inhibitory indices which cannot be interpreted unequivocally. However, the effects of urine on growth and aggregation were measured separately in the present investigation and were based on an estimate of the retardation of the initial reaction rate, rather than on readings taken at one arbitrarily selected time point. Despite the improved method for measuring inhibitory activity, it was not possible to detect any differences in inhibitory activity with respect to growth and aggregation between urine from stone-formers and normals. One interesting finding that emerged was that urine was a more efficient inhibitor of crystal aggregation than of crystal growth. This would support the proposal[2] that the principal portion of urinary inhibitory activity lies with the GAGS, which we have also shown[8] to be more potent inhibitors of aggregation than of growth. Furthermore, GAGS are present in 1% urine in sufficient quantities to account almost entirely for the effect of 1% urine on crystal aggregation[8].

Although we found a significant correlation between the inhibition of growth and urinary GAGS concentration, there was a stronger relationship between the inhibition of aggregation and GAGS concentration. In view of the greater effect of GAGS on aggregation than on growth, this finding was not unexpected. Though it has been proposed[2] that the inhibitory activity of urine in this in vitro system is more strongly dependent on the ratio of GAGS concentration to urate concentration, we obtained no evidence to support this. No correlation of Ig or Ia with GAGS/uric acid was found. In fact, both Ig and Ia were found to correlate well with uric acid concentration, a consequence presumably of the fact that Ig, Ia, GAGS and uric acid were all proportional to creatinine concentration. Since the concentration of GAGS and uric acid increased equally in proportion to overall urine concentration, the absence of a relationship between Ig, Ia and GAGS/uric acid was not surprising. These results demonstrate that in this experimental system, the inhibitory potency of GAGS is not diminished by their binding to uric acid. This is in accord with the observation of Laurent[15] that increasing concentrations of chondroitin sulphate actually lessened the solubility of sodium urate. Such a relationship between GAGS and uric acid would have important implications with regard to their involvement in calcium nephrolithiasis by reinforcing the proposed role of urate in heterogeneous nucleation.

REFERENCES

1. H. Fleisch, Kid. Int. 13:361 (1978).
2. W. G. Robertson, F. Knowles, and M. Peacock, in:"Urolithiasis Research," H. Fleisch, W. G. Robertson, L. H. Smith, and W. Vahlensieck, eds., Plenum Press, New York/London (1976).
3. F. L. Coe, Kid. Int. 13:418 (1978).
4. W. G. Robertson, M. Peacock, and B. E. C. Nordin, Clin. Sci. 40:365 (1971).
5. F. L. Coe, R. L. Lawton, R. B. Goldstein, and V. Tembe, Proc. Soc. Exp. Biol. Med. 149:926 (1975).
6. W. G. Robertson and M. Peacock, Clin. Sci. 43:499 (1972).
7. J. M. Baumann, S. Bisaz, R. Felix, H. Fleisch, U. Ganz, and R. G. G. Russel, Clin. Sci. Mol. Med. 53:141 (1977).
8. R. L. Ryall and V. R. Marshall. These proceedings.
9. N. A. C. Cressie and D. D. Keightley, J. Steroid Biochem. 11:1173 (1979).
10. C. J. Farrington and A. H. Chalmers, Clin. Chem. 25:1993 (1979).
11. N. Blumenkrantz and G. Asboe-Hansen, Anal. Biochem. 54:484 (1973).
12. D. V. Weber, F. L. Coe, J. H. Parks, M. S. L. Dunn, and V. Tembe, Ann. Int. Med. 90:180 (1979).
13. W. G. Robertson, M. Peacock, P. J. Heyburn, D. H. Marshall, and P. B. Clark, Br. J. Urol. 50:449 (1978).
14. R. L. Ryall, R. G. Ryall, and V. R. Marshall, in:"Proceedings International Urinary Stone Conference, Perth," J. G. Brockis and B. Finlayson, eds., PSG Publishing Company, Littleton, Connecticut (in press).
15. T. C. Laurent, Nature 202:1334 (1964).

ACKNOWLEDGEMENTS

The authors wish to acknowledge the expert technical assistance of Miss Ruth Harnett and the invaluable advice of Drs. D. Keightley and R. G. Ryall with regard to computing and statistics. We would like to thank Mrs. Leigh Sinton who performed the oxalate analyses. This work was supported by Grant No. AKF G23/80 from the Australian Kidney Foundation.

URINARY GLYCOSAMINOGLYCAN EXCRETION IN PATIENTS WITH UROLITHIASIS

John D. Sallis*, K.-H. Bichler, S. Korn, and A. Haußmann

*Department of Biochemistry, University of Tasmania, Australia, and Department of Urology, University of Tubingen, West Germany

Present evidence based on the physicochemical properties and distribution of glycosaminoglycans suggest that these compounds may play an important role in urolithiasis. Although the organic matrix of stones is not known to contain appreciable amounts of glycosaminoglycans[1], it has been suggested that glycosaminoglycans and, in particular, the degree of sulphation of the molecules, may be a regulating factor in the initiation or development of calculi[2]. Both natural and commercially prepared glycosaminoglycans in vitro have been shown to be powerful inhibitors of calcium oxalate crystal formation and growth[3,4]. Urine contains several types of glycosaminoglycans, the predominant class being chondroitin sulphates A and C. Undoubtedly, the so called inhibitory power of urine is to some degree associated with these polyanionic substances[4]. The true potential of the compounds however, may be subject to modification by some other urinary components, for example, urates[5].

Alterations in the excretion patterns of glycosaminoglycans are notable in diseases of connective tissue and the skeleton[6]. In urolithiasis, there is conflicting evidence regarding the level of glycosaminoglycans present in the urine of stone-formers compared to the concentrations found in healthy persons[2,5]. With the present studies, we have attempted to define and compare the amounts of glycosaminoglycans excreted daily by stone-formers and normals and to see if there is any correlation with regard to the nature of the stone material, the tissue site of lodgement of the stone, and the concentration of glycosaminoglycans in the urine.

MATERIALS AND METHODS

Daily collections of urine (24 hour specimen) were made from 33 healthy staff volunteers and 77 patients presenting with stones. Aside from routine clinical biochemical analyses, the concentrations of the following urinary constituents were determined: oxalate (enzymatic, Hallson and Rose[7]); uromucoid (Bichler et al.[8]); citrate (Knappwost and Gerlach[9]); glycosaminoglycans (uronic acid, Blumenkrantz and Asboe-Hansen[10]) and in a limited series, B-mirco-globulin by radioimmunoassay. Following surgery, the composition of calculi was determined by polarization microscopy.

RESULTS AND DISCUSSION

As can be seen from Table 1 there was a significant decrease in the amounts of glycosaminoglycans excreted in patients with staghorn calculi compared to the other stone-former groups and the controls. We have observed that over a period of 7 days, the daily excretion patterns for glycosaminoglycans in normals and stone-formers remains essentially constant. Citrate concentrations were lower than normal in all the stone-former groups as were the uro-mucoid levels, the latter result probably reflecting the extent of tubular damage and a reduced capacity for uromucoid synthesis[11]. Limited data, not shown here, were obtained on the concentration of B-microglobulin from the urine of staghorn-calculi patients. The levels found were near the upper limit of the normal range with a few even higher, again a finding consistent with obstruction or tubular damage. A comparison of the data between patients with renal pelvic calculi and those with ureter stones revealed no significant variations. Hyperoxaluria was not observed in any of the groups studied.

Table 1. Concentration of Some Constituents in Urine From Normals and Stone-Formers Presenting with Stones at a Particular Site

		Parameters Measured (mg/24 hr. urine)			
No. Patients Observed	Location of Calculi	GAG	Citrate	Oxalate	Uromucoid
30	none	5.84±1.84	*450±186	26.1± 9.6	*65.3±17.7
31	renal pelvic calculi	5.20±2.20	334±158	25.7±11.5	40.8±19.4
23	ureter	5.08±2.85	315±214	25.7±16.3	41.1±21.3
20	staghorn calculi	*2.55±1.44	265±139	34.2±20.0	31.0±17.1

* Significantly different at $p < 0.05$.

An attempt was made to correlate urinary glycosaminoglycan concentration with the composition of the stone material. As shown in Table 2, there appeared to be a trend toward a reduced amount of glycosaminoglycan excreted by patients whose calculi contained struvite. A closer statistical examination of the data, however, revealed that a greater number of patients would need to be sampled in order to demonstrate a difference significant at the 0.05 level.

Table 2. Calculi Identified and Urine Glycosaminoglycan Concentration

No. Patients	Calculi Type	GAG (Uronic acid, mg/day)
10	weddellite-whellite	5.4 ± 2.3
22	struvite-apatite	4.0 ± 2.7
12	struvite-weddellite	4.2 ± 2.3
11	uric acid	5.0 ± 2.7

A simple quantitative relationship between glycosaminoglycan excretion and calculi production was not evident. Further, the results suggest that routine measurement of glycosaminoglycans would have little diagnostic value except perhaps as an additional guide for patients with staghorn calculi. The fact that total glycosaminoglycan excretion did not alter from the normal in other stone-former groups does not in itself prove that there is no change in the amount of the individual glycosaminoglycans excreted. Further, it may well be that the degree of sulphation or change in structure of the components could have taken place and would not have been detected by the method of assay. A detailed biochemical investigation of these parameters might well be more revealing of a role for glycosaminoglycans in urolithiasis.

REFERENCES

1. W. H. Boyce and F. K. Garvey, J. Urol. 76:213 (1956).
2. W. O. Foye, H. S. Hong, C. M. Kim, and E. L. Prien, Sr., Invest. Urol. 14:33 (1976).
3. W. G. Robertson, M. Peacock, and B. E. C. Nordin, Clin. Chim. Acta. 43:31 (1973).
4. J. D. Sallis and M. E. Lumley, Invest. Urol. 16:296 (1979).
5. W. G. Robertson, M. Peacock, P. J. Heyburn, D. H. Marshall, and P. B. Clark. Br. J. Urol. 50:449 (1978).
6. D. Kaplan, Am. J. Med. 47:721 (1969).
7. P. C. Hallson and G. A. Rose, Clin. Chim. Acta. 52:29 (1974).
8. K.-H. Bichler, H. Haupt, G. Uhlemann, and H. G. Schwick, Urol. Res. 1:50 (1973).

9. A. Knappwost and S. Gerlach, in:"Pathogenese und Klinik der Harnsteine," V. G. Gasser and W. Vahlensieck, eds., D. Steinkoff-Verlag, Darmstadt (1977).
10. N. Blumenkrantz and G. Asboe-Hansen, Anal. Biochem. 54:484 (1973).
11. K.-H. Bichler, C. Kirchner, and V. Ideler, Br. J. Urol. 47:733 (1976).

INHIBITION OF CALCIUM OXALATE CRYSTAL GROWTH IN PATIENTS WITH UROLITHIASIS

Hans-Göran Tiselius and Lasse Larsson

Department of Urology and Department of Clinical Chemistry
University Hospital
S-581 85 Linköping, Sweden

It is now generally accepted that the formation of calcium oxalate stones occurs in urine which is supersaturated with respect to calcium oxalate[1]. Formation, growth and aggregation of calcium oxalate crystals are modified by urinary inhibitors. Information on the activity of these inhibitors are of importance when estimating the risk of renal stone formation[2].

METHODS

Urine was collected during 24 hours in plastic bottles without preservative. Samples were obtained from 129 normal men with an age of 43 ± 10 years (mean ± SD) and 84 male patients with calcium oxalate stone disease, age 46 ± 11 years. During the study all subjects remained on their ordinary diet. The urine samples were immediately brought to the laboratory after the collection was completed and the samples were kept frozen at -20°C until analyzed.

The inhibition of calcium-oxalate crystal growth was estimated by measuring the decrease in ^{14}C-oxalate remaining in solution following addition of seed-crystals to a crystallization system containing calcium chloride and sodium oxalate in a metastable state. The composition of the system was mainly as described by Robertson et al.[3].

Before urine was added to the crystallization system, each sample was heated to 37°C, carefully mixed and filtered through a Millipore filter (0.22 µm) and finally diluted in order to contain 5 µmol of creatinine per ml. One ml. of this urine solution was added to the crystallization system for determination of inhibitory activity.

An inhibition index (I) was calculated in the following way:

$$I = 1 - \frac{k_i}{k_c}$$

where k_i is the rate in the system containing urine, and k_c the rate constant in a control system containing saline[4]. For each urine sample an inhibition index was calculated as the mean of 4 different determinations during the first two hours.

RESULTS

Figure 1 demonstrates the frequency distribution of inhibition indices from 129 normal men and 84 male patients with calcium oxalate stone disease. The mean inhibition index (± SD) for normal men was 0.57 ± 0.06 and for male patients with calcium oxalate stone disease 0.54 ± 0.08 ($p < 0.005$).

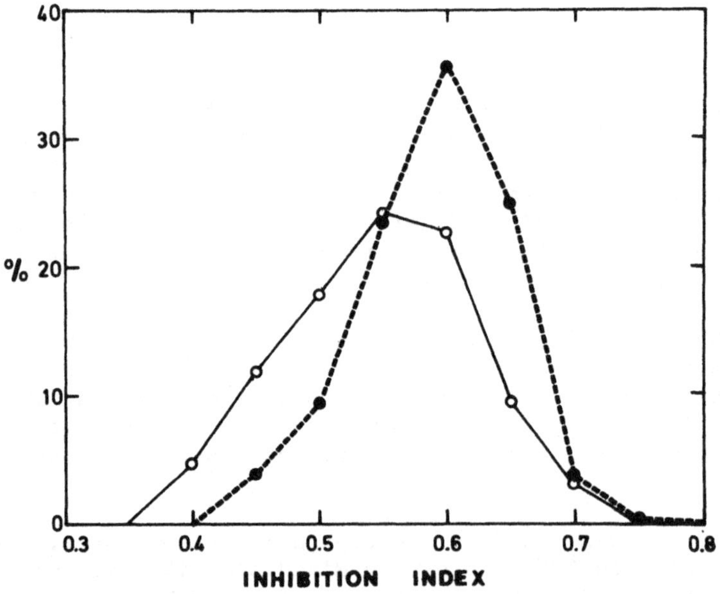

Figure 1. Frequency distribution curves of inhibition indices from 129 normal men and 84 male patients with calcium oxalate stone disease.

There was a considerable variation of the inhibition index during the day from 0.32 to 0.58 in a normal man and from 0.46 to 0.66 in a normal woman.

In order to obtain information on the effect of pH on the inhibition of calcium oxalate crystal growth, pH of the crystallization system was varied between pH 4.0 to 8.0. The result obtained with 4 different urine samples is demonstrated in Figure 2, where an increase in the inhibiting activity in the pH-interval 5.5 to 8.0 can be observed. A similar increase in inhibiting activity in this pH-interval was obtained for pyrophosphate and citrate but not for condroitin sulphate. When urinary pH differs from 6.0, (the normal pH of the crystallization system) it is evident that it might be difficult to draw conclusions from the inhibition index obtained. From a number of urine samples we have, therefore, calculated correction factors to be used for correction of the inhibition index to a value which would more appropriately correspond to the current urine pH. In Figure 3 the inhibition index at different times during the day, before and after such a correction, is demonstrated.

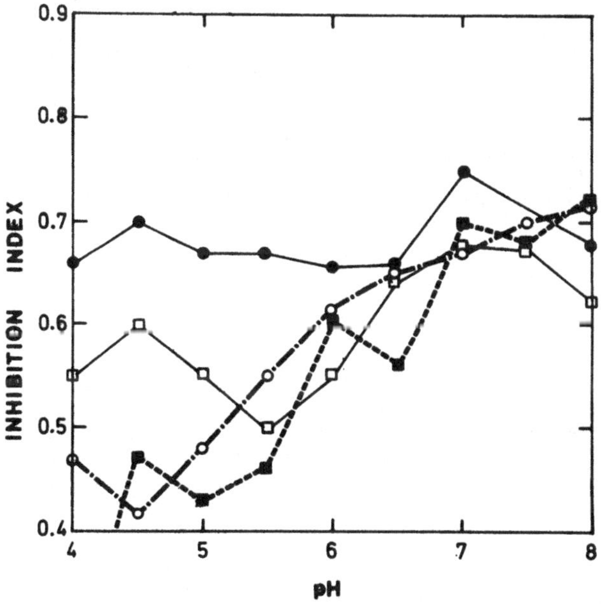

Figure 2. Effect of pH on the inhibiting properties of urine from four patients with calcium oxalate stone disease.

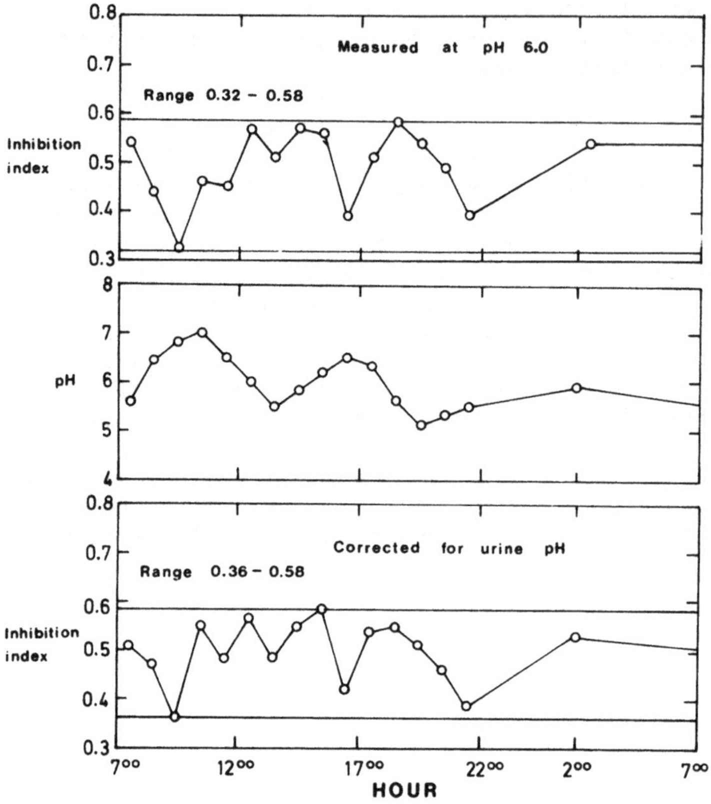

Figure 3. Variation of inhibition index before and after correction with respect to pH in urine, as obtained from pH measurement at the collection time.

In a previous investigation[5] we have demonstrated that the quotient $\frac{\text{calcium x oxalate}}{\text{magnesium}}$ is higher in stone formers than in normal subjects. This is demonstrated for these patients in Figure 4. The difference between the groups is statistically significant ($p < 0.01$).

Since urinary calcium, oxalate, magnesium, citrate and inhibition are considered to be important for calcium oxalate stone formation, these factors were combined in a risk quotient:

$$\frac{\text{calcium x oxalate}}{\text{magnesium x citrate x inhibition}}$$

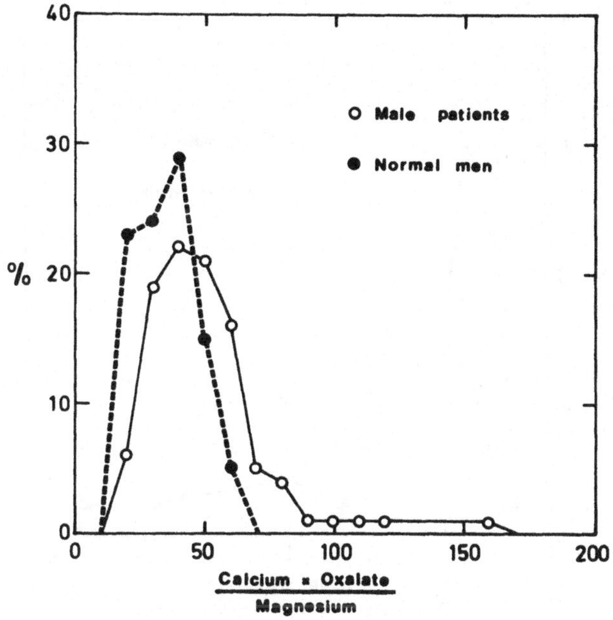

Figure 4. Frequency distribution curves of the calcium x oxalate/ magnesium quotient in normal subjects and patients with calcium oxalate stone disease.

The frequency distribution curves of this risk quotient for normal subjects and patients with urolithiasis are shown in Figure 5. The difference between the two groups was statistically significant ($p < 0.005$).

The calcium oxalate risk quotient was analyzed at different times during the day and meal related peaks were observed. This risk quotient was also corrected for pH of the urine samples and a slightly different pattern was obtained. However, when urinary pH does not differ very much from 6.0, such a correction seems unnecessary since the difference between the two patterns of risk quotients during the day was of minor degree.

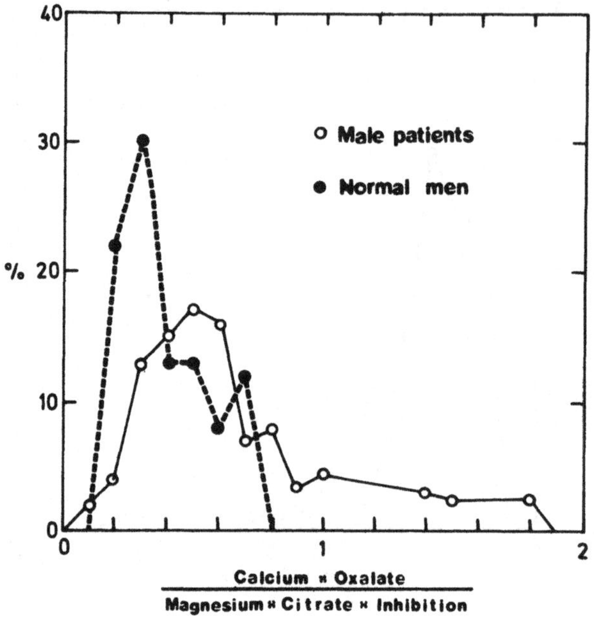

Figure 5. Frequency distribution curves of risk quotients (for explanation see text) in normal subjects and patients with calcium oxalate stone disease.

CONCLUSIONS

1. The inhibition index was significantly lower in male patients with calcium oxalate stone disease as compared to normal men.

2. There was a considerable variation of the inhibition index during the day.

3. In the pH-interval 5.5 to 8.0, the inhibition of calcium oxalate crystal growth increased and if urine pH differs much from the pH in the crystallization system, the inhibition index should be appraised in relation to the current urine pH.

4. The suggested risk quotient for calcium oxalate stone formation:

$$\frac{\text{calcium x oxalate}}{\text{magnesium x citrate x inhibition}}$$

appears to separate stone formers and normal subjects fairly well and might be useful in the evaluation of patients with urolithiasis.

REFERENCES

1. W. G. Robertson, M. Peacock, R. W. Marshall, D. H. Marshall, and B. E. C. Nordin, NEJM 294:249 (1976).
2. H. Fleisch, Kid. Int. 13:361 (1978).
3. W. G. Robertson, M. Peacock, and B. E. C. Nordin, Clin. Chim. Acta. 43:31 (1973).
4. E. J. Will, O. L. M. Bijvoet, and H. van der Linden, in: "Urolithiasis Research," H. Fleisch, W. G. Robertson, L. H. Smith, W. Vahlensieck, eds., Plenum Press, New York (1976).
5. H.-G. Tiselius, L. E. Almgard, L. Larsson, and B. Sörbo, Eur. Urol. 4:241 (1978).

THE EFFECT OF URINE AND OTHER INHIBITORS ON THE GROWTH AND AGGREGATION OF CALCIUM OXALATE CRYSTALS IN VITRO

Rosemary L. Ryall and Villis R. Marshall

Urology Unit, Department of Surgery, Flinders Medical Centre, Bedford Park, South Australia 5042

INTRODUCTION

Crystal growth and aggregation are generally regarded as important steps in the formation of renal stones, but no previous study has examined the effects of urine or its components on these two processes by measuring them as separate phenomena. Using a modification[1] of the Coulter Counter technique[2] it has been possible to measure crystal growth and aggregation independently even when they are occurring simultaneously. In this study we have quantified the effect of various inhibitors found in urine over a range of concentrations spanning those which would be anticipated in urine diluted to 1%. These results have then been compared with the mean level of inhibition of growth and of aggregation observed for 66 urine specimens (1% v/v) from normal males in an attempt to identify those urinary constituents most likely to be responsible for that inhibition.

METHODS

The experimental technique, preparation of urine samples, calculation of Ig (inhibition of growth) and Ia (inhibition of aggregation) are described in detail elsewhere[3]. All chemicals were of analytical grade except the chondroitin sulphate (sodium salt, type A; Sigma Chemical Co.) and the heparin (sodium salt; a gift from David Bull Laboratories, Australia).

RESULTS

The inhibitory effects of urine, pyrophosphate, citrate, Mg^{2+}, heparin and chondroitin sulphate on growth and aggregation were measured and the results are shown in Figure 1. The effect of urine is illustrated by the shaded area in each graph which delineates the range of inhibition of growth (Ig = 50.6±21% - mean ± S.D.) or aggregation (Ia = 72.0 ± 17.8%) produced by 66 specimens of 1% urine from males with no history of stone disease. The small cross-hatched bands indicate the concentration of each inhibitor which would be expected in urine diluted to 1% v/v. These were based on values reported for undiluted urine as follows: pyrophosphate, 10^{-5}-10^{-4} moles/litre[4]; citrate, 1.5 - 4.8 x 10^{-3} moles/litre[5]; magnesium, 1.5 - 5.8 x 10^{-3} moles/litre[5] and glycosaminoglycans, 7.6 - 21.6 mg/litre[3].

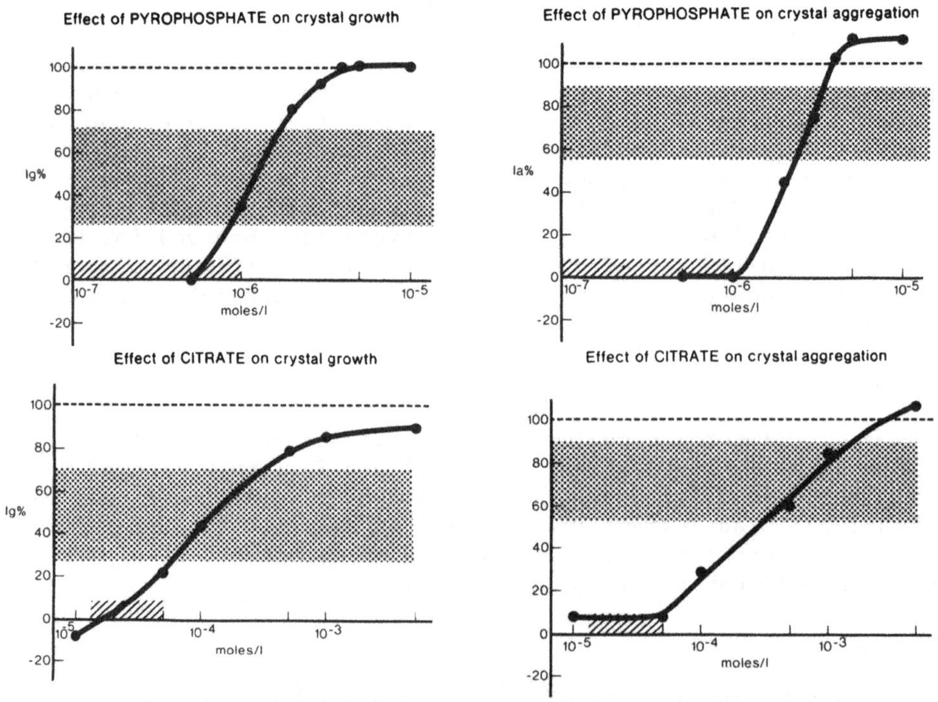

Figure 1. The effect of urine and various inhibitors on crystal growth and aggregation.

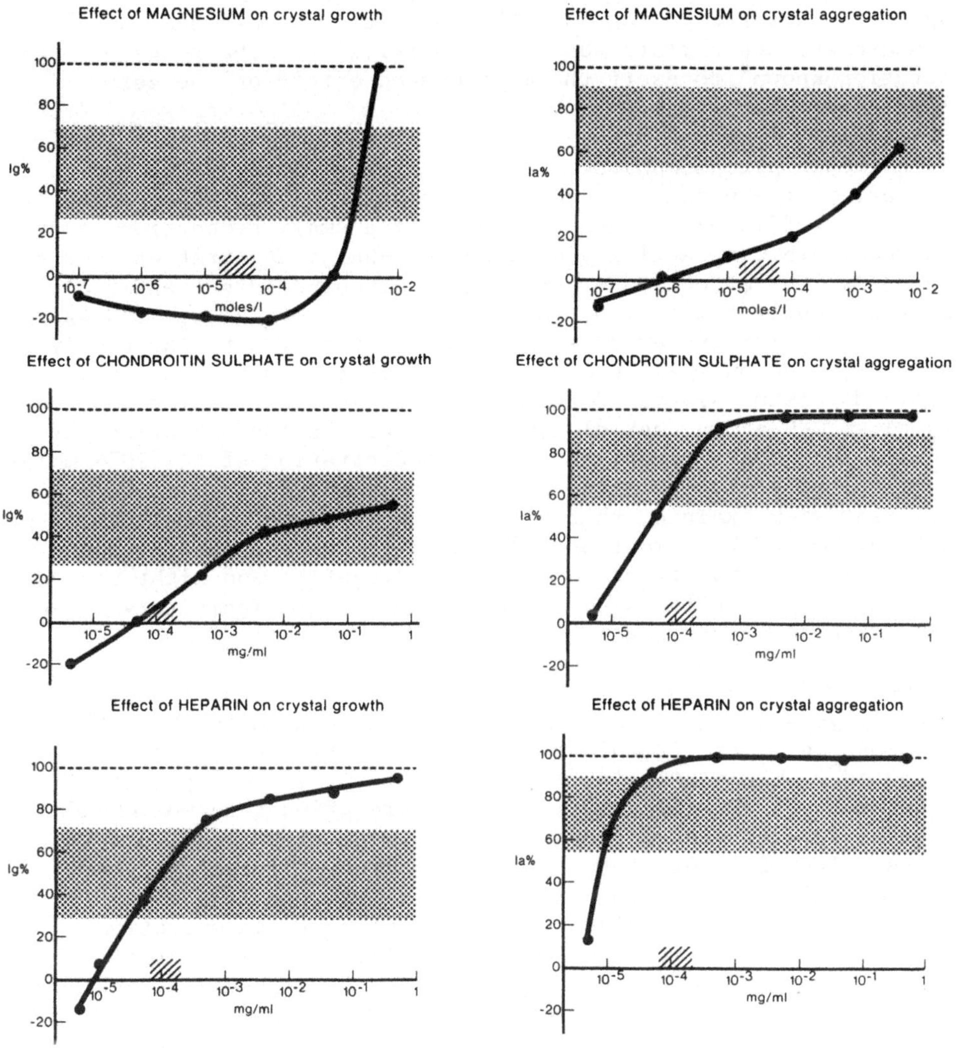

Figure 1. Continued.

DISCUSSION

The most notable feature of the results presented in Figure 1 is the finding that all substances tested, including urine, affected crystal growth and aggregation to differing degrees. These findings were not unexpected in view of the fact that crystal growth and aggregation are governed by different factors[6], growth being affected by absorption of inhibitor molecules on to specific crystal growth sites, and aggregation being influenced by molecules which alter the zeta potential of the crystal surface. In this last respect it is worth noting that the inhibition of aggregation by pyrophosphate and citrate was most sensitive over the range of concentration known[6] to exert the most marked effect on the zeta potential of whewellite.

Although pyrophosphate strongly inhibited both growth and aggregation, its potency at concentrations likely to be found in 1% urine, was sufficient to account for only a small proportion of the observed inhibitory activity of urine at that concentration. On the same basis, its effect on crystal aggregation would be negligible. Similarly, while citrate was shown to inhibit both growth and aggregation to significant extents, it would be expected to exert only a small influence on these processes at concentrations found in 1% urine. Magnesium displayed the unexpected ability to promote crystal growth above control levels between the concentrations of 10^{-7} and 10^{-4} moles/liter. But at a concentration of 5×10^{-3} moles/liter it completely inhibited growth, presumably as a consequence of complexing with oxalate, thereby lowering the supersaturation of the solution. Over the same range of concentrations magnesium showed a steadily increasing effect on crystal aggregation and might be expected to account for a small proportion of the inhibitory effect of 1% urine on crystal aggregation.

Chondroitin sulphate is the principal constituent of human urinary glycosaminoglycans[7], the class of compounds to which the major portion of the inhibitory activity of urine has been attributed[8]. While heparin was found to be a far more potent inhibitor both of crystal growth and of aggregation than was chondroitin sulphate, its virtual absence from human urine[7] precludes its responsibility for any of the known inhibitory effects of urine. Despite the fact that chondroitin sulphate was the less effective of these two glycosaminoglycans, its activity at concentrations likely to be present in 1% urine was sufficient to account almost completely for the observed effect of urine on crystal aggregation. By comparison, chondroitin sulphate was a relatively poor inhibitor of crystal growth, its activity being similar to that of pyrophosphate over the appropriate concentration ranges.

Whilst the inhibitory activity of urine on crystal aggregation could be attributed almost entirely to the presence of chondroitin sulphate, no other single compound tested could account for the effect of urine on crystal growth. It must therefore be concluded that the observed effect of 1% urine on crystal growth in this *in vitro* system is due either to the presence of an untested, more potent inhibitor, or more probably, is a result of the additive or synergistic effects of known inhibitors. Although chondroitin sulphate was a most effective inhibitor of crystal aggregation, and would appear to be responsible for most of the inhibitory activity of 1% urine, it did not produce disaggregation, even at concentrations many times those expected in whole urine. We have frequently observed crystal disaggregation in the presence of 10% urine. This finding highlights the problem of extrapolating from results obtained in the presence of diluted urine to conditions existing in whole urine. Nonetheless, the results reported in this study provide a guide as to the relative inhibitory efficacy of certain urinary components and indicate their comparative effects on crystal growth and on crystal aggregation. This in vitro system should now allow preliminary studies on the competitive or synergistic effects of known urinary constituents.

REFERENCES

1. R. L. Ryall and V. R. Marshall, in:"Urinary Calculi, Proceedings of the International Urinary Stone Conference, 1979," J. G. Brockis and B. Finlayson, eds., PSG Publication Co., Inc., Littleton, MA (1980) (in press).
2. W. G. Robertson and M. Peacock, Clin. Sci. 43:499 (1972).
3. R. L. Ryall and V. R. Marshall, in:"Proceedings Fourth International Urolithiasis Research Symposium," L. H. Smith, B. Finlayson and W. G. Robertson, eds., Plenum Press, New York (in press).
4. H. Fleisch, Kid. Int. 13:361 (1978).
5. D. J. Sutor, J. M. Percival, and K. A. J. Piper, Br. J. Urol. 51:1 (1979).
6. B. Finlayson, Kid. Int. 13:344 (1978).
7. J. M. Goldberg and E. Cotlier, Clin. Chim. Acta. 41:19 (1972).
8. W. G. Robertson, F. Knowles, and M. Peacock, in:"Urolithiasis Research," H. Fleisch, W. G. Robertson, L. H. Smith, and W. Vahlensieck, eds., Plenum Press, New York/London (1976).

ACKNOWLEDGMENTS

The authors wish to acknowledge the expert technical assistance of Miss Ruth Harnett and the receipt of Grant No. AKF G23/80 from the Australian Kidney Foundation.

IDENTIFICATION OF A SMALL MOLECULAR WEIGHT INHIBITOR OF THE OXALATE PRECIPITATION

B. Pinto and J. Pujol

Servicio de Analisis Clinicos, Hospital Juan XXIII,

Tarragona, Catalunya, Spain

After removal of mucoproteins from urine, a high level of promoter activity of calcium oxalate precipitation was found in the remaining supernatant. This observation may be explained by the presence of an inhibitor in whole urine which was removed during the purification process. This paper attempts to describe some of the characteristics of this inhibitor.

EXPERIMENTAL PROCEDURE

Inhibitory Activity Assay

The incubation solution consisted of 38 µmol of potassium phosphate buffer (pH 5.8), 5.5 µmol calcium chloride, 0.45 µmol oxalic acid, 40 x 10^3 cpm ^{14}C-oxalic acid and increasing concentrations of the sample to be tested to give a final volume of 1 ml. Assays were performed in triplicate. The mixtures were incubated at room temperature for 24 h. The calcium oxalate precipitates were separated by centrifugation at 10,000 rpm on a Sorvall RC-2B centrifuge for 15 min. They were dissolved in 0.5 ml 2M NaOH and counted in 10 ml of 0.2% PPO (2,5-diphenyl-oxazole) 0.02% POPOP (1,4 bis (2-5-phenyl-oxazolyl)benzene) in dioxane. The vials were counted for 10 min in a scintillation counter (Table 1).

Sample Preparation

Urine from normal individuals was thoroughly dialyzed against distilled water and the dialysate evaporated to dryness in a flash evaporator at 45°C. The residue was dissolved in the minimum amount of water.

Table 1. The Inhibitory Activity in
0.1 ml of Dialysate Residue from 5 l of Urine

Sample	^{14}C-oxalate precipitate cpm
Blanks	8,692
In the presence of 0.1 ml dialysate residue	1,314

Electrofocusing

The dialysate from 5 liters of normal urine was dissolved in 110 ml of water and the sample added to an LKB 8100 electrofocusing column. It was developed at room temperature for 48 h in the pH range 3 to 7. Fractions of 1.5 ml were collected. Inhibitory activity against calcium oxalate precipitation was tested in alternate fractions. (The results are shown in Figure 1.)

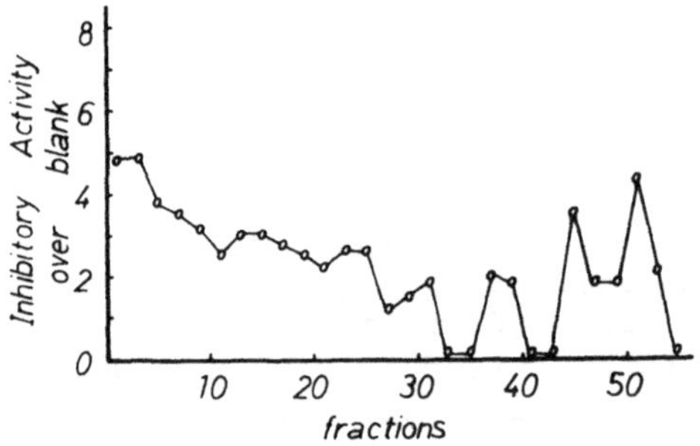

Figure 1. Typical profile of inhibition of calcium oxalate precipitation after electrofocusing.

Physicochemical properties

Five ml of the dialysate were extracted with 150 ml of ether followed by evaporation. No inhibitory activity was detected in the ether extract. No change in the inhibitory activity was detected when the dialysate residue was treated with pyrophosphatase.

Comment

Little can be deduced about the physicochemical characteristics of this inhibitory material. It is a small molecule since it is present in the dialysate from normal urine. It is not either pyrophosphate or a lipid molecule. In the electrofocusing studies the inhibitory activity was displaced towards the initial fractions.

THE EFFECT OF SOME URINARY CONSTITUENTS ON THE *IN VITRO* NUCLEATION AND GROWTH KINETICS OF CALCIUM OXALATE

A. Rodgers and J. Garside*

Department of Medical Biochemistry, Medical School, University of Cape Town, Republic of South Africa; and *Department of Chemical and Biochemical Engineering, University College, London

INTRODUCTION

The *in vitro* crystallization of calcium oxalate has been investigated by many workers in the field of renal stone disease with a view to providing some insight into the cause as well as the possible treatment of the disorder[1-4]. Using different techniques and under a variety of conditions, nucleation, growth and aggregation characteristics of this compound have been examined. In particular, the inhibitory effect of several compounds has received a lot of attention[5-10]. These studies however have all been limited to static, supersaturated systems and have failed to produce definitive nucleation and growth kinetics. Today the role of inhibitors is recognized as being an important factor in the genesis of renal calculi and recent studies have accordingly been directed towards quantitizing this inhibitory power. In attaining accurate quantitative crystallization kinetics, two important approaches have been utilized. The first employs the use of a continuous crystallizer system and the second involves particle size distribution analysis using a Coulter counter. Finlayson[11] was the first to describe the usefulness of a continuous crystallizer as a simple urinary tract model while Robertson and Peacock[4] determined the size distribution of calcium oxalate crystalluria in normal and stone forming patients. Miller, Randolph and Drach combined these ideas and have determined the crystallization kinetics of calcium oxalate in simulated urine[12] and have also measured the inhibition of calcium oxalate crystallization by pyrophosphate and methylene blue[13].

The experiments reported in the present study were undertaken to determine quantitative nucleation and growth kinetics of calcium oxalate in an artificial urine and to examine the effect of varying the composition of the latter. Measurements of this kind can provide useful data for defining the inhibitory role of individual urinary constituents.

EXPERIMENTAL

A schematic diagram of the continuous crystallizer system and reaction chamber is presented in figures 1a and 1b respectively. (A detailed description of the apparatus and its operation is to be presented elsewhere)[14]. Calcium chloride and sodium oxalate solutions containing various combinations of urinary constituents were pumped into the reaction vessel. The concentration of the constituents in the feed solutions, when present, are shown in Table one and correspond to the concentration of that component in a synthetic urine[15]. In order to prevent the formation of crystals other than calcium oxalate, magnesium sulphate was included in the calcium chloride feed but excluded from the sodium oxalate supply while the sodium phosphates were included with the sodium oxalate but excluded from the calcium chloride stream. The pH of all solutions were adjusted to lie in the range 5.6 - 6.2. The reaction chamber volume was kept constant by the automatic valve but flow rates into the vessel were varied, thereby permitting experiments to be carried out at different levels of supersaturation. The steady state size distribution was determined by withdrawing aliquots of suspended particles from the crystallizer and transferring to azide free ISOTON II solution for measurement using a model TA Coulter counter. Analytical grade reagents were used throughout and all experiments were conducted at 37°C. After each experiment, the product formed was identified by the x-ray powder diffraction method.

Table 1. Composition of Feed Solutions (g/l)

Feed Solution 1	Feed Solution 2
7.56 $Na_2SO_4.10H_2O$	7.56 $Na_2SO_4.10H_2O$
3.18 NH_4Cl	3.18 NH_4Cl
8.31 KCl	8.31 KCl
9.25 NaCl	9.25 NaCl
0.80 $Na_3C_6H_5O_7.2H_2O$	0.80 $Na_3C_6H_5O_7.2H_2O$
4.00 $MgSO_4.7H_2O$	2.93 $Na_2HPO_4.12H_2O$
2.94 $CaCl_2$	9.32 $NaH_2PO_4.2H_2O$
	0.80 $Na_2C_2O_4$

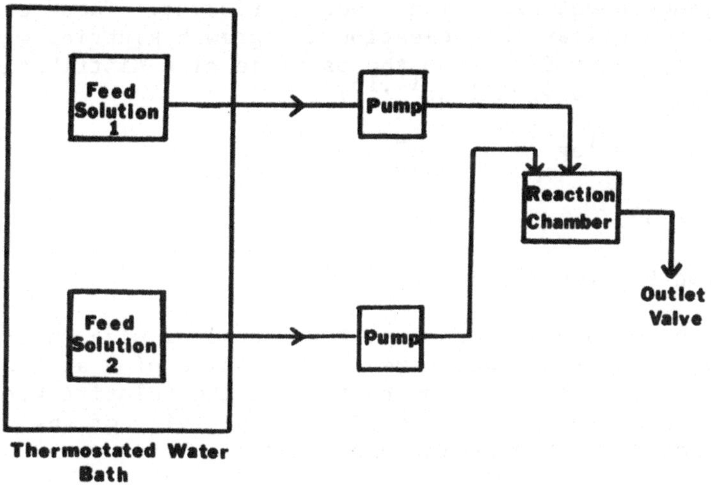

Figure 1(a): Flow diagram of continuous crystallizer.

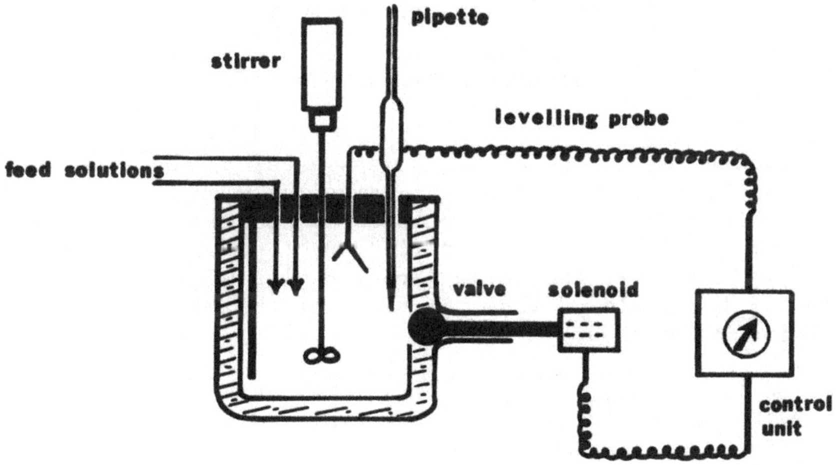

Figure 1(b): Continuous crystallizer reaction chamber.

RESULTS

Five independent experiments were performed. These are listed in Table 2. Quantitative nucleation and growth kinetics were simultaneously determined from the particle size distributions by application of three equations[14,16]:

(1) $\log n = \log n^o - \dfrac{L}{2{,}303 G\,\tau}$

(2) $B = n^o G$

(3) $\log B = \log K + i \log G$

where n is the population density, L the crystal size, G the crystal growth rate, τ the residence time, n^o the value of n at L=O, B the nucleation rate, K the rate constant and i the relative kinetic order. i is a measure of the relative sensitivity of the nucleation and growth rates to changes in supersaturation.

Table 2. Calcium Oxalate Kinetics Experiments

1. In artificial urine
2. From pure components
3. In presence of sodium citrate only
4. In presence of Mg^{2+}, SO_4^{2-}, Na^+, PO_4^{3-} and citrate ions
5. In presence of artificial urine without citrate

The growth rate at a particular τ was calculated from the slope of the straight line obtained by plotting log n vs L. The corresponding nucleation rate was calculated by substituting the value of the intercept, n^o, in equation (2). By conducting experiments at different values of τ, the variation of B with G was determined and the value of i calculated from the slope of the log B vs log G graph as suggested by equation (3).

In the first experiment, an artificial urine, identical to that used by Miller et al.[12] (Table 1) was employed as the crystallization medium. Size distributions were obtained at four different residence times and a plot of log n vs L at τ = 7.1 mm is shown in Figure 2. Figure 3 compares the log B vs log G plot for this experiment with that obtained by Miller et al.[12] and shows good agreement, despite the higher growth rates (~2X) in the present work, thereby lending confidence to our results.

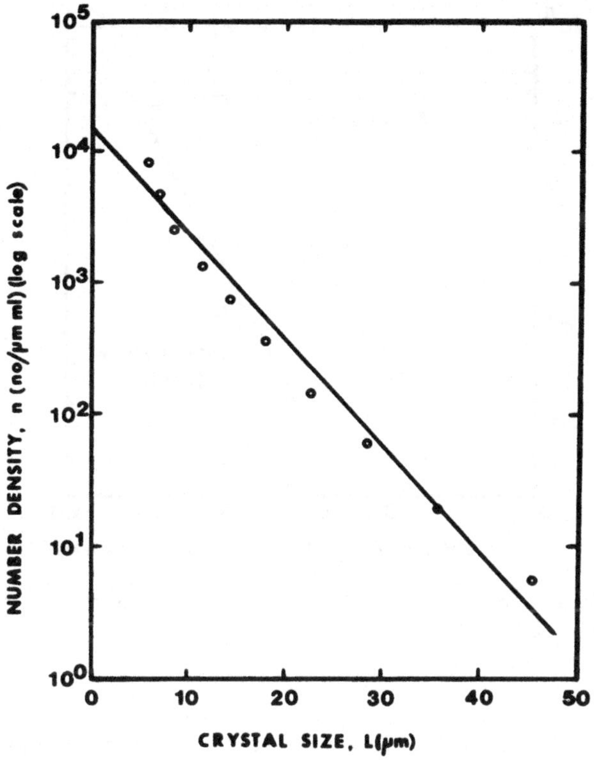

Figure 2. Population density plot for calcium oxalate crystallization in artificial urine.

The product obtained was a mixture of approximately equal proportions of calcium oxalate dihydrate (COD) and trihydrate (COT). Miller et al.[12] however report the formation of COD only.

In order to obtain kinetic data on the inhibitory effect of citrate, the latter was omitted from the artificial urine and the experiment repeated. Figure 4 shows that elimination of citrate resulted in an increased value of i and small increases in the values of G and B for the same residence time. Thus the presence of citrate in artificial urine inhibits the growth and also reduces (to some extent) the nucleation rate of calcium oxalate. The product obtained was COT only.

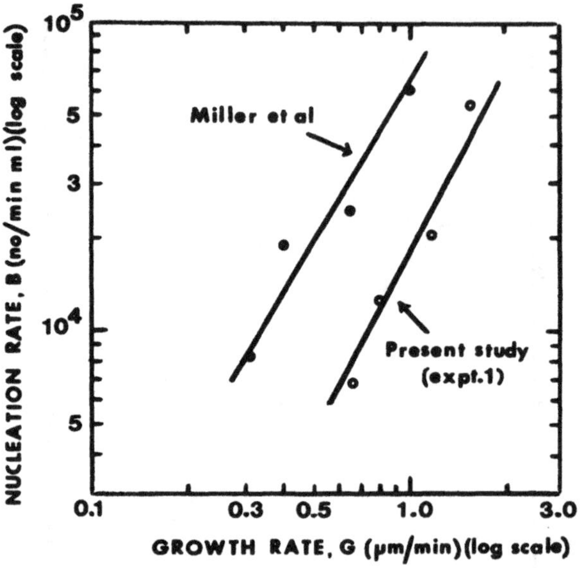

Figure 3. Nucleation and growth kinetics for present study and Miller et al.[12]

By determining the kinetics of calcium oxalate crystallization from pure components only (experiment 2) and then introducing sodium citrate (experiment 3), it was possible to further characterize the inhibitory role of citrate. The kinetic plots of these two experiments are presented in figure 5 and show that the presence of citrate resulted in higher growth rates while nucleation rates are an order of magnitude lower.

The products formed were calcium oxalate monohydrate (COM, experiment 2) and COT with a small trace of COD (experiment 3).

The final experiment of the series was conducted in a medium containing sodium citrate plus magnesium sulphate and the two sodium phosphates. This combination of components permitted examination of the influen-e of citrate on the kinetics, in the presence of various other ions. In figure 6 the kinetics of this run are plotted as well as those for experiments 1 (artificial urine) and 3 (pure components and sodium citrate). Comparison of the present experiment with experiment 3 shows that the addition of the three compounds $MgSO_4$, Na_2HPO_4 and NaH_2PO_4 induced several changes, all of which brought the system closer to that of artificial urine. Allowing for experimental scatter of the points, there is in fact no difference in the kinetics of the present run with that of the artificial urine.

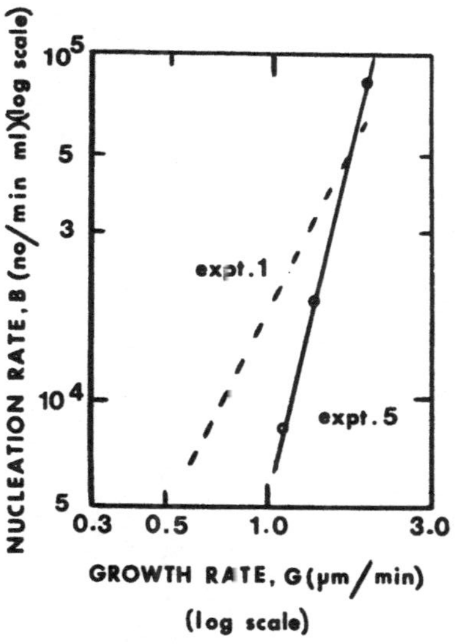

Figure 4. Nucleation and growth kinetics of calcium oxalate in artificial urine (expt. 1) and in artificial urine less citrate (expt. 5).

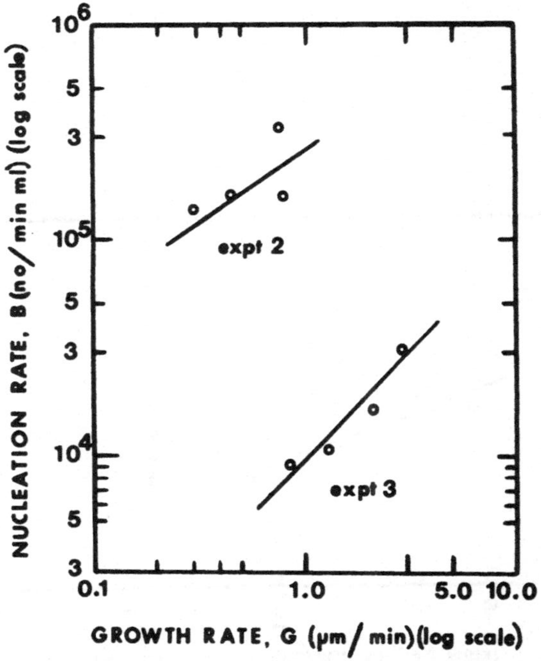

Figure 5. Nucleation and growth kinetics of calcium oxalate from calcium chloride and sodium oxalate solutions (expt. 2) and in presence of sodium citrate (expt. 3).

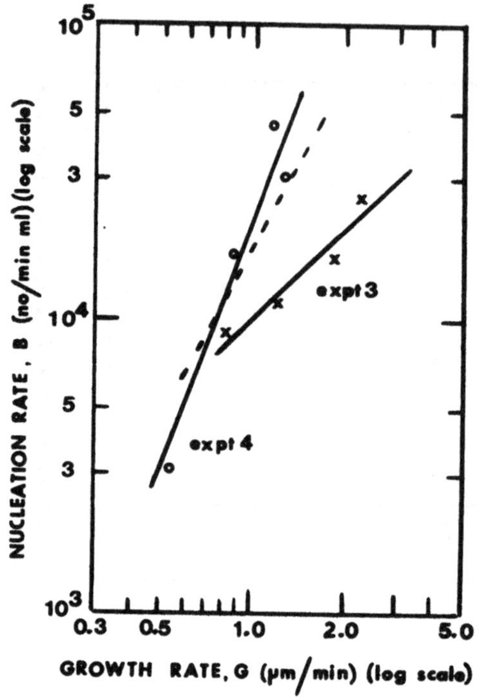

Figure 6. Nucleation and growth kinetics of calcium oxalate in artificial urine (expt. 1), in pure components plus citrate (expt. 3) and in the presence of various ions (expt. 4).

DISCUSSION

Although citrate has long been recognized as an inhibitor of calcium oxalate formation, some doubt exists as to whether it (and some other inhibitors) exert their influence by inhibiting nucleation or growth mechanisms or both. Comparison of experiments 5 and 1 shows that introduction of citrate to an artificial urine system results in a retardation of both nucleation and growth rates. On the other hand the presence of citrate in the simpler pure component system (comparison of experiments 2 and 3), while again inhibiting the rate of nucleation, this time produced higher growth rates. This suggests that citrate possibly exerts its influence by inhibiting nucleation and that inhibition of growth rate is dependent on the presence (or absence) of other ions. The lower value of i obtained in experiment 1 indicates that the presence of citrate reduces the relative sensitivity of B and G to changes in supersaturation.

It is of some interest to note that Leskovar et al.[17] have reported that one of the most significant differences between recurrent stone formers and healthy controls was a clearly reduced urinary citrate level in stone patients. They conducted quantitative _in vitro_ experiments by the Coulter-counter-size distribution analyzer measuring technique and have shown that citric acid strongly inhibited the precipitation and growth of calcium oxalate.

Comparison of the kinetics obtained in the artificial urine (experiment 1) and the solution of $MgSO_4$, Na_2HPO_4, NaH_2PO_4 and sodium citrate (experiment 4) shows them to be the same. It is therefore concluded that these components _together_ determine the crystallization kinetics of calcium oxalate in artificial urine and that the other urinary components, Na_2SO_4, NH_4Cl, KCl and NaCl, while increasing the ionic strength, appears not to affect the overall kinetics. Magnesium, like citrate, has long been known as a calcium oxalate inhibitor and it is thus perhaps not surprising to find these substances playing a key role in the determination of calcium oxalate crystallization kinetics.

It is a well established fact that the most common form of calcium oxalate found in urinary calculi is the monohydrate[18]. The dihydrate occurs in much lower concentrations and usually on the outside surface while the trihydrate has been detected only once[18]. Robertson and Peacock[4] on the other hand have shown that while most normal persons have COM crystalluria, patients with recu-rent idiopathic stone disease who are between episodes have _COD_ crystalluria under the same conditions of urinary concentration - yet these patients form _COM_ stones. On the basis of this and other evidence, Tomazic and Nancollas[19] have postulated that during the formation of COM renal calculi, precursor phases consisting of the higher, less stable hydrates may play an important role. In the present study, COT was formed in four of the five experiments. This is in agreement with the observation of Gardner and Doremus[20] that COT is the major product formed in simulated urine solutions and tends to lend support to the precursor postulate of Tomazic and Nancollas. Further experimentation should provide further insight into this mechanism.

REFERENCES

1. D. J. Sutor, Br. J. Urol. 41:171 (1969).
2. D. Fraser, R. Russell, O. Pohler, W. Robertson, and H. Fleisch, Clin. Sci. 42:197 (1972).

3. C. E. Dent and D. J. Sutor, Lancet 775 (1971).
4. W. Robertson and M. Peacock, Clin. Sci. 43:499 (1972).
5. D. Sutor and S. Wooley, Br. J. Urol. 42:296 (1970).
6. S. Welshman and M. McGeown, Br. J. Urol. 44:677 (1972).
7. W. Robertson, M. Peacock, and B. Nordin, Clin. Chim. Acta. 43:31 (1973).
8. D. J. Sutor, in:"Urinary Calculi: Recent Advances in Aetiology, Stone Structure and Treatment," L. Cifuentes-Delatte, A. Rapado, and A. Hodgkinson, eds., S. Karger, Basel (1973).
9. J. Meyer and L. H. Smith, Invest. Urol. 13:31 (1975).
10. J. Meyer and L. H. Smith, Invest. Urol. 13:36 (1975).
11. B. Finlayson, Invest. Urol. 9:258 (1972).
12. J. Miller, A. Randolph, and G. Drach, J. Urol. 117:342 (1977).
13. G. Drach, A. Randolph, and J. Miller, J. Urol. 119:99 (1978).
14. A. Rodgers and J. Garside, Br. J. Urol. (submitted for publication)
15. L. Isaacson, Invest. Urol. 5:406 (1968).
16. A. Randolph and M. Larson, in:"Theory of Particulate Processes," Academic Press, New York (1971).
17. P. Leskovar, R. Hartung, M. Simmel, R. Algayer, and M. Hropot, in:"Proceedings Fourth International Urolithiasis Research Symposium," L. H. Smith, B. Finlayson, W. G. Robertson, eds., Plenum Press, New York (in press).
18. D. J. Sutor, S. E. Wooley, and J. J. Illingworth, Br. J. Urol. 46:393 (1974).
19. B. Tomazic and G. Nancollas, Invest. Urol. 16:329 (1979).
20. G. Gardner and R. Doremus, Invest. Urol. 15:478 (1978).

ACKNOWLEDGMENTS

We would like to thank Dr. D. J. Sutor for her helpful advice and the use of the x-ray equipment. One of us (A.R.) would like to thank the South African C.S.I.R. and the University of Cape Town for the award of post-doctorate research bursaries and overseas travel grants.

ISOLATION OF A URINARY MUCOPROTEIN CAPABLE TO PRECIPITATE OXALATE

B. Pinto, J. L. Paternain and J. Bernshtam

Laboratorio de Exploraciónes Metabólicas

Barcelona, Catalunya, Spain

Mucoproteins are components of urinary stones. Some authors had suggested that these components promote stone formation[1,2]. We have shown the promoting effect of the stone mucoproteins on oxalate precipitation[3]. The calcium concentration appears to play an important role in the mineral-mucoprotein interaction[4]. This paper presents evidence on the isolation and some of the physicochemical properties of a mucoprotein from stone former urine. The material binds calcium and phosphate and promotes oxalate precipitation.

EXPERIMENTAL PROCEDURE

The promoting of precipitation activity of urinary mucoprotein was tested in polypropylene tubes containing a final volume of 1 ml: 5 μmoles of phosphate buffer (pH 7.5), 5 μmoles of oxalic acid, ten μmoles of calcium chloride, 40 x 10^3 cpm of ^{14}C-oxalic acid (U) and increasing concentrations of the mucoprotein preparation to show linear kinetics. In blanks the mucoprotein was left out. After 1 hour incubation, the precipitates were separated by high speed centrifugation and the precipitates dissolved in 0.1 M NaOH and the radioactivity counted (Table 1).

Urinary mucoprotein was purified from 5 liters of uninfected urine from stone formers. The urine was concentrated to 250 ml in a flash evaporator and thoroughly dialyzed. The concentrated urine was twice supersaturated with ammonium sulfate. The combined precipitates were dialyzed against 2.5 mM EDTA (pH 7.5) and the EDTA was removed by re-dialysis against Tris-buffer (pH 7.5).

Table 1. Typical Results of the Mucoprotein Activity on Oxalate Precipitation

Type of Sample	^{14}C-oxalate precipitated
	cpm
Blanks	8,562
Purified mucoprotein 3 ng	21,314

The dialysand was made up to 0.1 M concentration with calcium chloride and sodium phosphate buffer (pH 7.5). The resulting calcium phosphate was harvested by centrifugation. Then the precipitate was dissolved by dialysis against EDTA and Tris-buffer (pH 7.5). Further purification of this dialysand performed on a preparative electrofocusing column on a 2.5 to 5 pH gradient range (Table 2).

PHYSICOCHEMICAL PROPERTIES

The mucoprotein material in the final dialysand contained hexoses, hexosamines, hexuronic and sialic acids (Table 3). The aminoacid composition indicated the presence of glycine and glutamic acid as main components (Table 4). The isoelectric point was obtained at pH 2.8. The molecular weight was of 51,200 daltons. The mucoprotein binds calcium and phosphate in such a way that any trace of calcium or phosphate in the water induced the material to aggregate by forming small flakes or precipitates. To avoid aggregation it was necessary to use 0.5 M EDTA (pH 7.4).

Table 3. Composition of the Precipitating Material

Fourteen mg of protein from the purified material were incubated with phosphate and calcium chloride. The precipitate was dissolved with NaOH followed by the determination of protein, hexoses hexosamines, hexuronic and sialic acids.

Component	mg
Protein	5.04
Hexoses	0.80
Hexosamines	0.25
Hexuronic acid	0.03
Sialic acid	0.02

Table 2. Purification Procedure

Purification Step	Volume	Specific activity Oxalate Precipitated	Total activity	Yield	Purification
	ml	µmoles/mg protein	µmoles	%	Fold
Concentrated urine	124	10.79	8,027	100	--
Ammonium sulfate Precipitation	219	119.88	131,268	1635	11.11
Calcium phosphate Precipitation	60	1,848.00	266,112	3315	171.26
Electrofocusing	2.4	45,670.58	186,333	2321	4,232.00

Table 4. Aminoacid Composition of the Mucoprotein Material

Type	Percentage	Specific Amount nmoles/mg Protein
Aspartic A.	9.31	227.58
Threonine	5.77	141.22
Serine	9.23	225.57
Glutamic A.	12.23	298.95
Proline	3.31	80.99
Glycine	31.38	766.91
Alanine	8.95	218.87
Cysteine	0.12	2.92
Valine	4.38	107.24
Methionine	3.08	75.39
Isoleucine	1.65	40.37
Leucine	4.75	116.25
Tyrosine	0.42	10.41
Phenilalanine	0.54	13.21
Histidine	0.37	9.25
Lysine	2.41	63.88
Arginine	1.81	44.39

COMMENT

The mucoprotein material herein described binds phosphate and calcium and promotes the precipitation of oxalate. Therefore, this material is a heterogeneous nucleating factor of some of the urinary minerals.

The purification procedure indicated a yield higher than the starting activity possibly due to the presence of a small molecular weight inhibitor that it is removed through the purification process.

REFERENCES

1. W. H. Boyce and M. Swanson, J. Clin. Invest. 34:1581 (1955).
2. W. H. Boyce and J. Stanton-King, Ann. N. Y. Acad. Sci. 104:563 (1963).

3. B. Pinto, in:"Urinary Calculi," L. Cifuentes, A. Rapado, and A. Hodgkinson, ed., Karger, Basel (1973).
4. J. Bernshtam and B. Pinto, in:"Urolithiasis Research," H. Fleisch, W. G. Robertson, L. H. Smith, and W. Vahlensieck, eds., Plenum Press, New York and London (1976).

THE INHIBITORY EFFECT OF POLYMERIC CARBOXYLIC AMINO-ACIDS AND URINE ON CALCIUM OXALATE CRYSTALLIZATION

Nissim Garti, Francoise Tibika,
Sara Sarig, and Shaul Perlberg*
Casali Institute of Applied Chemistry, School of Applied Science and Technology, The Hebrew University of Jerusalem, Jerusalem, Israel.
*Department of Urology, Hadassah-Medical School, The Hebrew University of Jerusalem, Jerusalem, Israel.

INTRODUCTION

The "organic matrix" which precipitates out with almost every stone is believed, by some investigators, to contain the compounds involved in renal stone formation. It has been shown that up to 50% of the protein in the matrix is a combination of glutamic and aspartic acids[1].

According to one of the hypotheses kidney stone formation may be caused by a deficiency of inhibitors that usually are present in normal supersaturated urine. Many such inhibitors have been reported[2-7] but none of those were found in a sufficient concentration in human urine to prevent calcium oxalate formation at the concentrations involved[7].

In some recent works an inhibitory effect in aqueous seeded solutions by polymeric peptides and proteins[6,8-10] as well as polyglutamic and aspartic acids[10] has been reported. Nakagawa[10] isolated four polypeptides from normal urine and showed an inhibitory effect of those compounds on mimic urine.

The present study evaluates the effect of polymeric carboxylic-amino acids such as polyglutamic and polyaspartic acids together with other polymers on the retardation of precipitation of calcium oxalate and compares it to the effects of normal and pathological urine.

The main idea behind this work is to evaluate the retardation effect of several polymeric amino-acids and derivatives on the nucleation and crystallization processes of calcium oxalate in mimic urine and to compare them to the retardation effect noticed previously[10] on the crystal growth of calcium oxalate.

EXPERIMENTAL

Materials

Mimic urine was prepared on the basis of compounds present in normal urine according to the Ciba Geigy Scientific Tables Documenta. One liter of solution contains 20g urea, 2.27g Na_2SO_4, 4.84g KCl, 5.00g NaCl, 2.18g NaH_2PO_4 and 0.55g $CaCl_2$. All the materials were BDH A.R. The water was triple distilled.

Creatinine, hypuric acid, ammonium chloride were not included since in preliminary studies it was found that they have no significant effect on calcium oxalate precipitation. Magnesium ions were excluded to prevent any potential interference to the electrode. Ionic strength of the mimic urine was determined at the beginning of each experiment.

Calcium chloride solutions (BDH A.R.) were used to adjust ionic strength and calcium concentrations. Sodium oxalate solutions were prepared prior to every measurement (Baker's C.P.) in $1 \cdot 10^{-3}$ to $2 \cdot 10^{-3}$M concentration.

Procedure

The calcium ion concentration was measured continuously by 93200 P Orion Calcium specific electrode mounted in PBS-710 El-Hama modified digital pH/mv meter, using double junction reference electrode (Orion Model 90-02). Calibration of the electrodes was done prior to every experiment by stock calcium chloride solutions.

The additives (poly-amino acids or urine) were added to the mimic urine and equilibrated prior to the addition of the oxalate solution.

The calcium oxalate was filtered and centrifuged out (17000 rpm) and analyzed by x-ray technique (Philips diffractometer with Cu radiation and Ni filter); differential thermoanalysis (Mettler Thermoanalyzer) and scanning electronic microscope (Joel SEM Model JSM 35).

Possible poisoning effect of the electrodes by PGA has been ruled out since in a control experiment, in which the calcium ions were mixed with the retardant for several hours, there was no change in the calcium concentration measurements.

RESULTS

Mimic urine solution of 10^{-3} M Ca^{++} concentration was mixed with equimolar oxalate solution and the calcium ion concentration (activity) was followed. From Figure 1 it can be seen that there is no delay time (except for up to 45 sec. due to electrode equilibration) and after 30 minutes the calcium ion concentration reaches a plateau corresponding to calculated K_{sp} value for the given ionic strength ($1.8 \cdot 10^{-4}$M).

In a similar experiment 100 ppm of PGA-I or PAsA-I were added to the mimic urine. From Figure 1 it is clear that the drop in the calcium ion concentration is retarded markedly and the curve is practically composed of two parts. In the first minutes there is only moderate or no decrease in the calcium concentration related to induction time which is in good agreement with Crawford's[9] results. The second part of the curve represents faster decrease but still slow in comparison to the control reaction. Same types of curves are obtained with 100 ppm of PAsA. It is significant that all curves reach the same concentration after 22-26 hours.

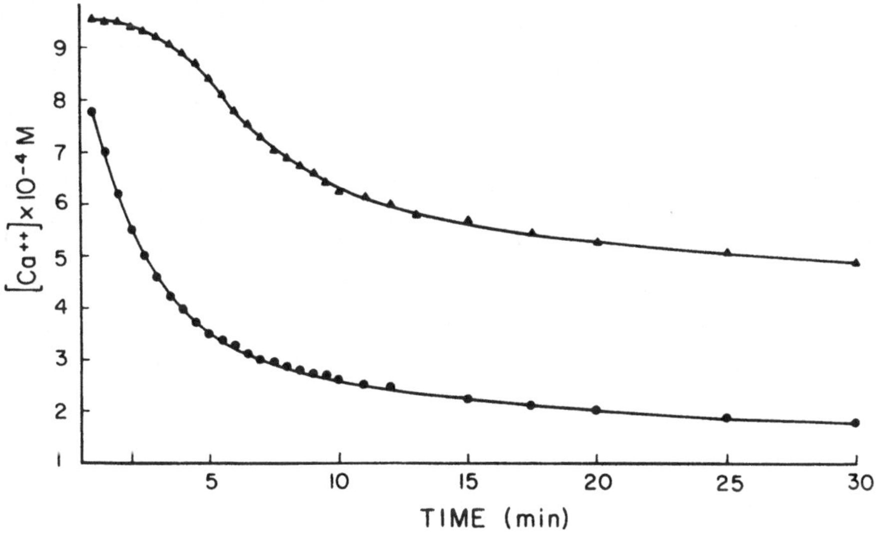

Figure 1. The decrease in calcium ion concentration with time in mimic urine containing no inhibitor (o) and 100 ppm PGA (Δ).

The effect of the chain-length and number of repeatable glutamic acid units has been examined and is summarized in Table 1. Glutamic or aspartic acid (monomer) and glutamyl-glutamic acid (dimer) had no retardation effect when added in higher concentrations (on monomer concentration basis). When the free carboxylic group on the polymer had been blocked by benzyl ester radical the inhibitory effect disappeared completely.

Three other polymers with free carboxylic or sulfonic groups were examined and found to inhibit the calcium precipitation in a similar way to the PGA (Table 1). On the other hand, when regular protein such as albumin or polymers such as polyethylenglycol or polyoxyethylene were used no retardation effect was observed (Table 1).

Table 1. Effects of Various Retardants on Calcium Oxalate Crystal Nucleation and Growth in Mimic Urine. (Calcium Concentration 10^{-3}M and oxalate 10^{-3}M)

Additive	Mol. Wt. (Avg.)	Conc. (ppm)	$t_{1/2}$ (min.)	$\frac{C_t}{C_o}$**
None (control)	--	--	3.0	1
PGA (Type I)	7000	100	25.0	0.379
		50	17.0	0.440
		25	11.0	0.449
		5	5.5	0.524
PGA (Type III)	70,000	100	20.0	0.423
PAsA (Type I)	9,000	100	19.5	0.431
		50	17.0	0.440
		25	11.0	0.478
PAS*	~50,000	100	--	0.379
PAA*	90,000	100	--	0.354
CMC	--	100	15.0	0.379
Sodium heparin	--	100	--	0.390
Glutamic acid (monomer)	147	100	--	0.916
Glutamyl-glutamic acid	276	100	--	0.980
Poly-Benzyl-asparate	14,000	100	--	0.970
Albumin	--	500	--	1.050
Polyoxyethylene	300,000	500	--	0.990

* Calcium ion concentration $2\cdot10^{-3}$

** C_t - Calcium ion concentration after 15 min. in the presence of an additive; Co - calcium ion concentration in a control experiment.

The effect of normal and pathological urine on the precipitation of calcium oxalate from mimic urine has been studied by adding 5-10% of fresh urine to the examined solution. While the normal urine retards the calcium precipitation, the addition of 10% of pathological urine does not show any significant retardation effect (Figure 2). The experiments have been carried out on 20 pathological urines. More than 35 normal urines have been examined.

The results of the present study are based on a continuous measurement of the calcium ion concentration remaining in the solution during the nucleation and crystal growth of the calcium precipitate and thus permits possible estimation of the effect of the retardants on the nucleation process as well as on the crystal growth.

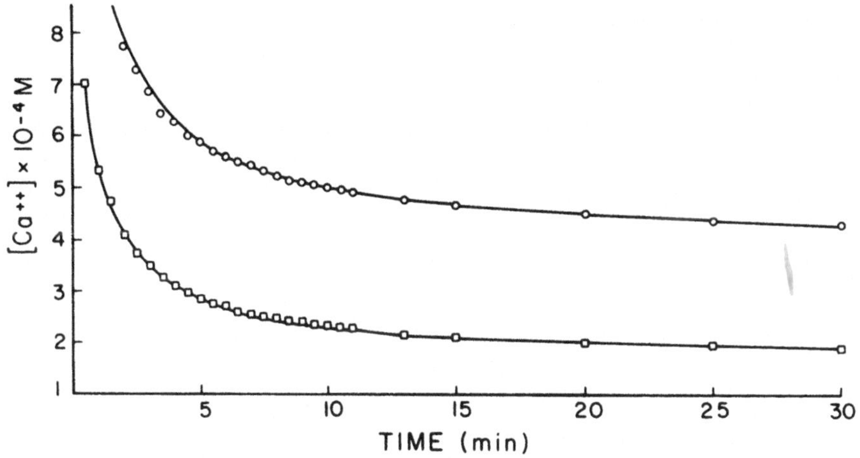

Figure 2. The decrease in Ca^{++} concentration with time in mimic urine containing 10% of normal (o) and pathological (□) urine.

REFERENCES

1. A. R. Spector, A. Gray, and E. L. Prien, Jr., Invest. Urol. 13:387 (1976).
2. A. M. Lewis, W. C. Thomas, Jr., and A. A. Tomt, Clin. Sci. 30:389 (1966).
3. J. S. Elliot and E. Eusebio, Invest. Urol. Res. 16:145 (1972).
4. H. Fleisch and S. Bisaz, Am. J. Physiol. 203:671 (1962).
5. J. L. Meyer and L. H. Smith, Invest. Urol. 13:36 (1975).
6. J. L. Meyer, J. T. McCall, and L. H. Smith, Calc. Tiss. Res. 15:287 (1974).
7. S. G. Welshman and M. G. McGeown, Br. J. Urol. 44:677 (1972).
8. W. B. Gill, J. W. Karesh, L. Garsin, and M. J. Roma, Invest. Urol. 15:95 (1977).

9. J. W. Crawford, E. P. Crematy, and A. E. Alexander, Aust. J. Chem. 81:1067 (1968).
10. Y. Nakagawa, E. T. Kaiser, and F. L. Coe, Biochem. Biophy. Res. Comm. 84:1038 (1978).

INHIBITED PRECIPITATION AND GROWTH OF Ca-OXALATE CRYSTALS IN THE PRESENCE OF THE ALKALINE SALTS OF SOME POLYHYDROXYCARBOXYLIC ACIDS

R. Hartung, P. Leskovar, R. Allgayer, H. Schneider, O. Bender, E. Wellnhofer, and M. Simmel
Urologische Klinik und Poliklinik Rechts der Isar der Technischen Universität Munchen
Munchen, Germany

INTRODUCTION

About 70-90% of renal calculi are composed of poorly soluble salts of calcium and magnesium. Among them 65-75% are calcium oxalate stones (whewellite and weddellite) and the remaining 15-25% are calcium phosphate stones (apatite, brushite, whitlockite and monetite) or magnesium-ammonium-phosphate (struvite) and magnesium phosphate (newberyte and bobierrite) calculi. Only uric acid, uric acid-dihydrate, ammonium urate and sometimes cystine concrements can be dissolved perorally. The chemolitholysis of the calcium and magnesium urinary calculi is still an unresolved problem.

Therefore, we endeavored to develop a relatively rapid method for screening new substances that would be able to inhibit the nucleation and growth of calcium oxalate and phosphate crystals and to disaggregate or partially dissolve preformed calcium oxalate crystals and disintegrated renal calculi. This quantitative method has been described previously[1,2]. Among the screened substances, the polyhydroxymonocarboxylic acids and their Na-salts (galacturonate, glucuronate) as well as the polyhydroxydicarboxylic acids and their Na-salts (galactarate, glucarate) attracted our attention because of their surprising inhibitory effect on growing Ca-oxalate crystals. In addition, they showed a disaggregating and dissolving activity on preformed oxalate and phosphate crystals as well as on predesintegrated native stones. They are of special interest because they are untoxic and occur regularly or occasionally in urine. One of them, the glucuronic acid is an obligate, quantitatively important constituent of urine. As it is known, the glucuronic acid, synthetized in the liver, is actively involved in the detoxication process.

MATERIALS AND METHODS

The following reagents were used: D-Glucuronic acid (C. Roth/ Karlsruhe, Art. 3771); calcium chloride-2-hydrate (Merck/Darmstadt, Art. 2382); di-Na-oxalate (Merck, Art. 6557); sodium chloride (Merck, Art. 6404); sodium hydroxide (Merck, Art. 9956); calcium oxalate (equimolar: $CaCl_2 \cdot 2H_2O$ (Merck, 2382)+$Na_2C_2O_4$ (Merck 6557); hydroxylapatite (Merck, Art. 11490).

The following instruments were used: Coulter counter ZF (capillary: 100 µm; aspiration volume: 500 µl; attenuation: 1, aperture: 128; treshold: 5; treshold factor: 28, 30; calibration latex: E.14 with D = 12, 6 µm, V = 1047 m^3, peak at 37%, channelyzer (size distribution analyzer) P 128 (count mode: manometer; count range: 64, 256, 2048), Präzisions-pH-meter E510; impulsomat E 473; dosimat E 535.

In this paper, only the simplified histograms, representing the absolute number and volume of crystals of a definite diameter before and after treatment by the test substance are presented. The comparison of the crystal size distribution in the absence of test-substance (blank), in the presence of citrate (reference), and in the presence of the tested substance gives however an unequivocal information about the inhibitory and disaggregating efficacy of the examined substance.

In the one type of the graphs, the absolute numbers of crystals in the nine particular size classes are depicted. In the other graph type with the integrated size-classes, both the absolute number and the absolute volume of crystals are demonstrated. The limited space allows to show here only two of the graphs that have been presented as poster; the first one demonstrates the high inhibitory activity of D-glucuronate (20 mM) on crystals, growing out of a model solution, containing 4 mmoles/l Ca^{2+}, 0.8 mmoles/l oxalate and 1.5 mg/10 ml Ca-oxalate seed crystals. The second graph shows the chemolytic effect of the 20 mM D-glucuronate on hydroxylapatite crystals. The direct comparison of the crystal number (volume) in the presence (hatched columns) and absence of D-glucuronate gives evidence of the efficacy of the tested substance.

RESULTS

Sodium salts of both, the polyhydroxymono- as well as of polyhydroxydicarboxylic acids are highly effective in the inhibition of the precipitation and growth of Ca-oxalate crystals out of saturated solutions (with and without seed crystals added). They not only inhibit crystal growth but also bring in solution the added Ca-oxalate seed crystals. In addition, they are able to dissolve partially the crystalline material of native phosphate calculi.

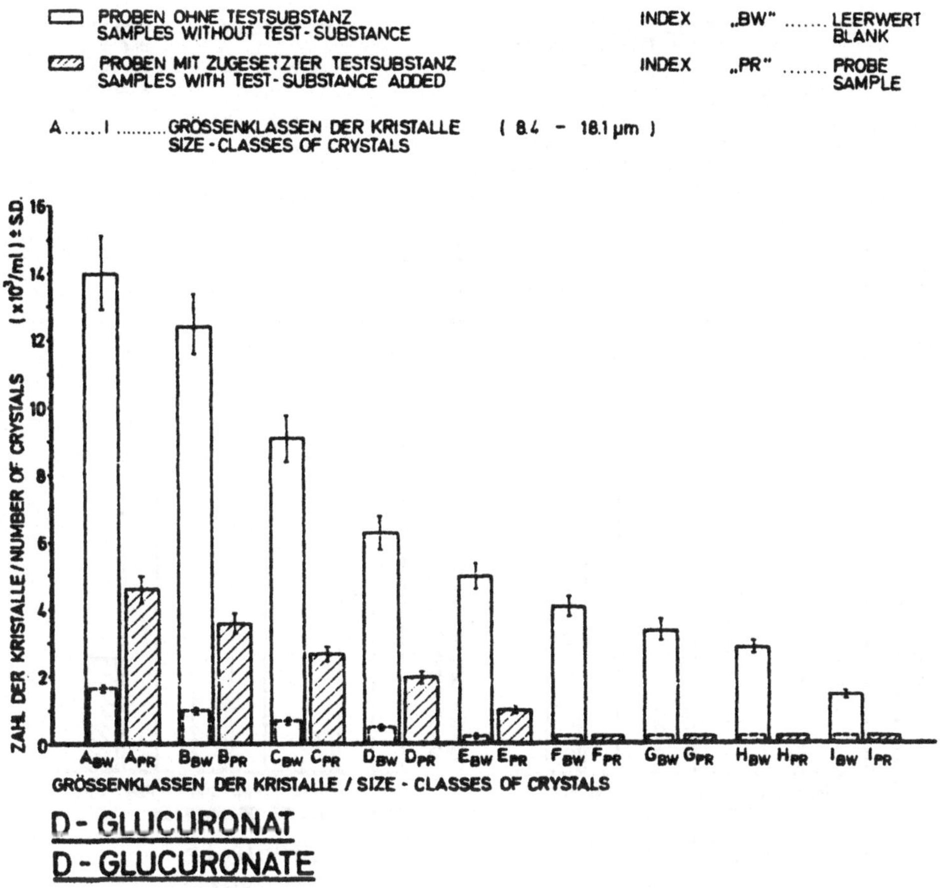

Figure 1. In this graph, the strong inhibition of Ca-oxalate crystal growth in the presence of D-glucuronate (2.10^{-2} mol/l) is demonstrated (pH 6.0; t = 48 h; T = 20°C).

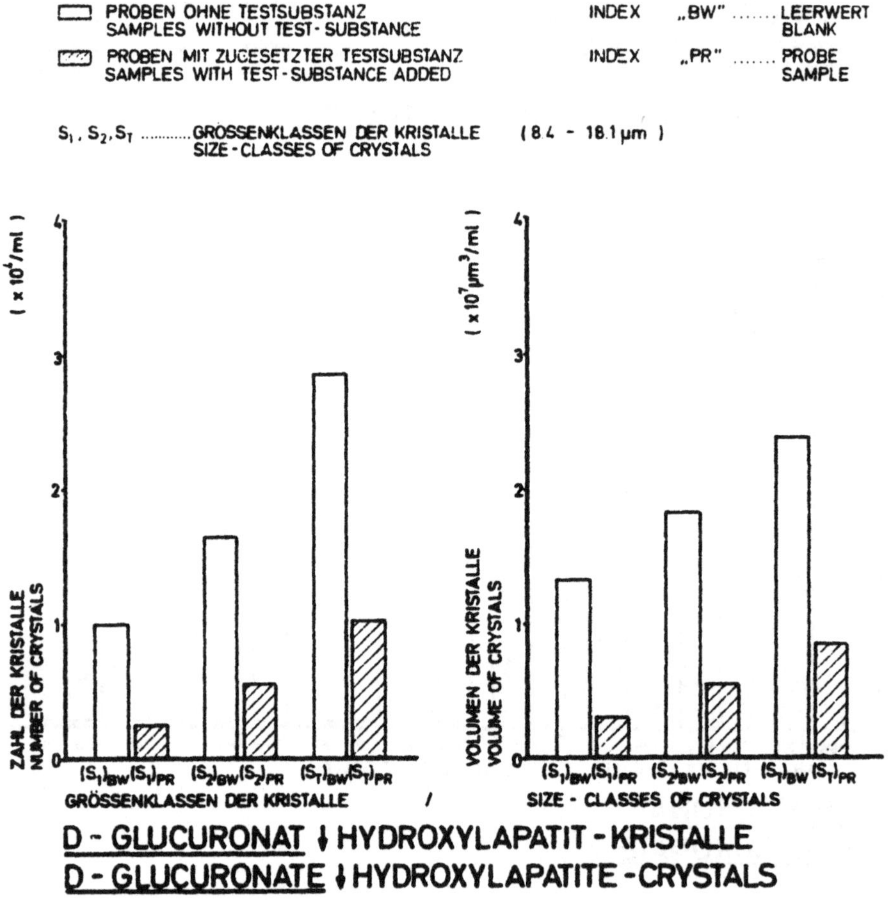

Figure 2. D-glucuronate acts litholytically on hydroxylapatite - crystals (C = 2.1^{-2} mol/l; pH 6.0; t = 48 h; T = 20°C).

Under the chosen experimental conditions (2.10^{-2} mol/l respectively 1/10 of the saturation concentration) their efficacy is comparable with that of citrate.

CONCLUSION

This class of substances could be of special interest because of the possible role in the inhibitory activity of urine. Especially the urinary glucoronic acid, originating from the detoxication of foreign substances in the liver, could as a regular urine constituent represent one of urinary inhibitors, unperceived until today.

REFERENCES

1. P. Leskovar, Akt. Nephrol./Wiss. Inform. Fres. Stift. 1:149 (1979).
2. P. Leskovar, R. Allgayer, and A. Siebert, Akt. Nephrol./Wiss. Inform. Fres. Stift. 2:329 (1979).

ACKNOWLEDGMENT

The authors would like to thank Mrs. D. Scherm, Mr. K.-L. Schade, Mrs. H. Richter and Mr. M. Gottinger (München) for their kind technical assistance.

INTERACTION OF DYES WITH INORGANIC CONSTITUENTS OF KIDNEY STONES

Bart van't Riet and Charles E. O'Rear*

VCU/Medical College of Virginia, Box 581 MCV Station, Richmond, VA 23298; *Department of Forensic Sciences, George Washington University, Washington, D.C. 20052

Inhibitory effect of dyes on formation and growth of urinary calculi has been shown for methylene blue *in vivo*, not only in animals[1], but also in clinical studies[2,3]. Because the mechanism of action is not certain, our purpose was to study the interaction of a variety of dyes with crystals which can be present in urinary calculi. Generally the assumption is made that dyes are absorbed on the surface of crystals, reaching a saturation value, probably a monolayer of dye on certain faces of the crystals, and no more dye is absorbed with further increase of the dye concentration in solution. This assumption was tested for 6 dyes in adsorption studies on calcium oxalate monohydrate, calcium hydrogen phosphate, and on magnesium ammonium phosphate hexahydrate. The crystals were prepared by standard precipitation procedures, and air dried. In the dye solutions an excess of one of the crystal ions was also used in order to evaluate competition of dye ions with these crystal ions for sites on the surface. Generally 0.01M excess of either a positive or negative ion, and an equivalent aqueous dye solution were used. Excess of CA^{++} precipitated Wool Violet 4BN, and therefore this combination was eliminated.

In the tests 1 gram of crystals was shaken with 5 ml of dye solution of various concentrations for a period of 15 minutes. Samples of the original dye solution and the dye solution remaining after adsorption were measured by spectrophotometer (Beckman Model B) after appropriate dilutions.

The samples were shaken for an additional 15 minutes to check for slow uptake into the interior of the crystals. The results are tabulated in Table 1, and illustrations of adsorption curves are given in Figures 1 and 2.

Table 1

Salt → / Dye ↓	$CaC_2O_4.H_2O$	$CaHPO_4$	$MgNH_4PO_4.6H_2O$
Methylene blue cationic	No adsorption under any conditions	Surface saturation at 0.05% in 0.01 MCa or equiv.; at 0.02% in 0.01M PO_4	Surface saturation at 0.01% in all solutions
Methyl Green 0.0 cationic	Surface saturation at 0.03% in 0.01MCa or equivalent; at 0.2% in $0.01MC_2O_4^{=}$	Mixed crystals	Mixed crystals
Wool Violet 4BN anionic	Surface saturation at 0.01%; excess of Ca^{++} precipitates dye	Mixed crystals	Surface saturation at 0.03%
Ponceau 3R anionic	Mixed crystals	Mixed crystals	No adsorption under any conditions
Alphazurin A anionic	Mixed crystals	Mixed crystals	Surface saturation at 0.08%
Alphazurin 2G anionic	Mixed crystals (slow)	Surface saturation at 0.04%	Surface saturation at 0.02%

DISCUSSION

The phenomenon of surface saturation of dye on crystals is less frequent than mixed crystal formation in this set of experiments. The most dye in surface saturation is adsorbed from solutions which contain the crystal ion of opposite charge compared to the dye ion. This fact suggests an exchange mechanism, in which the dye ion replaces a crystal ion in the surface. Additional dye can be adsorbed as an electrically neutral species when the dye is combined with the crystal counter ion which is available in excess.

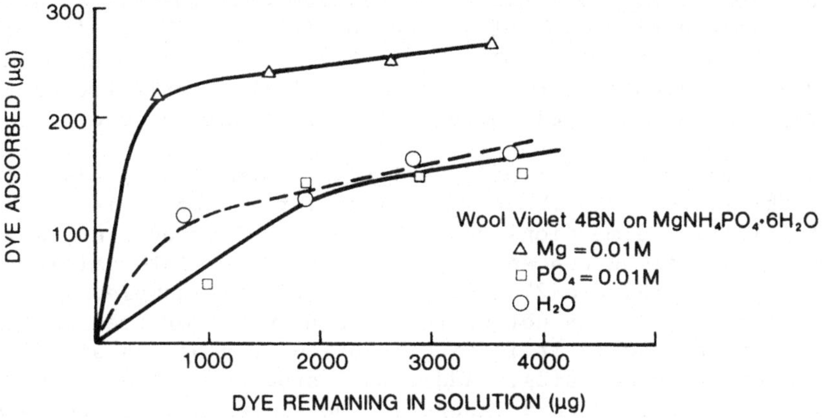

Figure 1. Example of surface saturation.

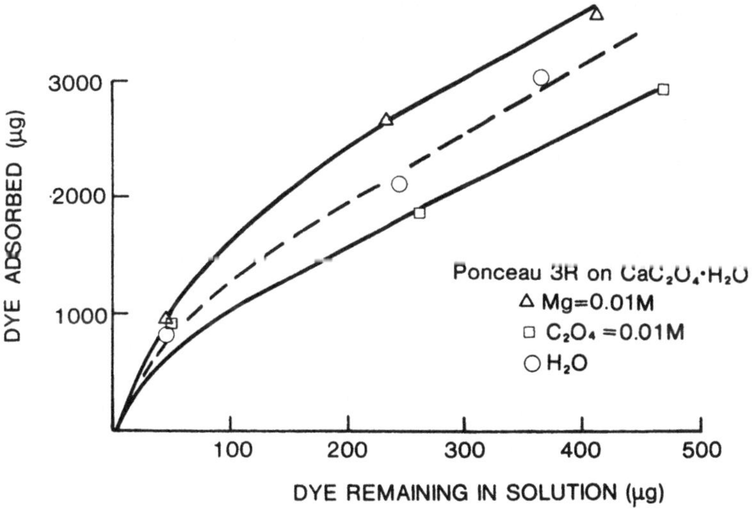

Figure 2. Example of mixed crystal formation.

Two instances of complete absence of adsorption were encountered. The more significant one is methylene blue on calcium oxalate monohydrate. . Combined with the requirement of co-administrating vitamin C for in vivo inhibition of calcium oxalithiasis by methylene blue, a simple explanation of its action is impossible. The organic matrix and lower oxidation states of the dye must be considered in any suggested mechanism, e.g. a reversal of the matrix from a glue to a calcium oxalate repelling entity when it absorbs dye.

The mixed crystal (or solid solution) formation is significant in urolithiasis because the composition of the deposit is changed, including lattice dimensions and other physical properties, e.g. hardness. The strong concentration of Ponceau 3R into calcium oxalate crystals (Figure 2) is the most striking example. Unfortunately the dye is not excreted in urine after oral administration, but its use in irrigating solutions can have a significant effect on existing deposits. Additional studies will be required to establish whether such a change in the composition of the deposit is beneficial in therapy.

REFERENCES

1. B. van't Riet, C. E. O'Rear, and M. J. V. Smith, Invest. Urol. 16:201 (1978).
2. W. H. Boyce, W. M. McKinney, T. L. Long, and G. W. Drach, J. Urol. 97:783 (1967).
3. M. J. V. Smith, Urol. 6:676 (1975).

V. MATRIX

URINARY CALCIUM BINDING PROTEINS AND RENAL CALCULI

Martin I. Resnick, Carl W. Gammon, Michael B. Sorrell, and William H. Boyce
Department of Surgery, Section of Urology
Bowman Gray School of Medicine
Winston-Salem, North Carolina

All urinary stones are in part composed of proteinaceous organic matrix, however, there has been much debate as to the importance of this material in urinary stone formation[1-4]. It has been suggested that matrix has an active role in stone formation and may act as a binding or cementing material that is necessary for crystal aggregation and growth. Others believe that this material plays only a passive role in stone formation and represents adsorption of non-specific urinary proteins onto a growing crystal. Vitamin D has been suggested as having a role in active stone formation and interestingly Vitamin D sensitive intestinal and renal calcium binding proteins have been identified in several biologic systems[5-7]. One investigator has identified an electrophoretically homogeneous calcium binding protein which is present in both normal and pathological urine[8] but to date no investigations have been made to study the presence of calcium binding proteins in a group of active stone formers. The present investigation was designed to determine if excretion of this substance(s) was related to urinary stone formation.

MATERIAL AND METHODS

Twenty-four hour urine specimens were obtained from active calcium oxalate, inactive calcium oxalate, active uric acid and active cystine stone-formers. The activity of stone disease was classified as defined by Smith[9]. To insure patient uniformity, all patients were maintained on a 150 mg. calcium, 100 mEq sodium diet two days before and during the period of collection[10,11]. Urine specimens were also obtained from a group of non-stone forming controls who neither had a prior history or family history of urinary calculus disease. All patients had routine urine cultures and active calcium stone formers underwent a calcium fast and load test to identify any metabolic abnormalities predisposing to stone formation. During the period of collection, each 24-hour specimen was refrigerated at 4°C and following completion, an aliquot assayed for calcium, phosphorus, uric acid and creatinine. Normal values for our laboratory have been reported previously[11].

The entire remaining urine specimen was ultrafiltrated at 4°C utilizing an Amicon Cell Model 2000 (Amicon Corporation, Lexington, Mass.) fitted with a Diaflo XM-50 membrane (Molecular weight cutoff - 50,000 daltons) under nitrogen at 40 psi. The complete ultrafiltrate was re-ultrafiltered utilizing the same cell, under the same conditions, but with a Diaflow UM-2 membrane (Molecular weight cutoff - 1,000 daltons) and concentrated to 200 ml. The specimen was then placed in a smaller stirred cell (Amicon Corporation Standard Cell - Model 202) with a Diaflo UM-2 membrane and further concentrated to 25 ml. The concentrated specimen was separated by gel filtration chromatography utilizing Sephadex superfine G-75 (2.5 x 90 cm column) at 4°c. The elution buffer was 0.01M ammonium bicarbonate with 0.02% sodium azide. The flow rate was maintained at 30 ml per hour. The eluant was monitored for protein content (at 280 nm) and individual 15 ml fractions were collected during the separation.

Each fraction was analyzed for calcium binding activity utilizing the chelex resin binding assay[12,13]. This assay consists of a competition for added radioactively labeled calcium between soluble calcium binding protein in the supernatant and Chelex, an insoluble cation exchange resin which is easily separated from solution by centrifugation. Chelex-100 (Bio-Rad, Rockville Centre, New York) was washed several times in buffer (0.04M Tris-HCL, pH 7.4) and diluted in the same buffer so that 0.2 ml of resin suspension contained 0.05 to 0.1 ml of packed resin. Aliquots of 1.0 ml were taken from each fraction obtained from the chromatography column and combined with 0.2 ml of Chelex resin suspension and 0.1 ml ^{45}Ca solution (approximately 10,000 c.p.m. in 0.1M Tris-HCl Buffer, pH 7.5 calcium chloride, New England Nuclear, Boston, Mass.) agitated for five minutes and centrifuged. Into 7.0 ml scintillation vials containing 5.0 ml Bray's solution 0.2 ml aliquots of the supernatant were pipetted and ^{45}Ca radioactivity measured with a Perkin-Elmer liquid scintillation counter. A control sample consisted of 1.2 ml of Tris-HCl buffer and 0.1 ml of ^{45}Ca solution. Blank control samples consisted of 1.0 ml Tris-HCl buffer, 0.12 ml of Chelex suspension and 0.1 ml ^{45}Ca solution. Calcium binding activity was expressed as:

$$\text{S/R Net} = \frac{\%\ 45\ \text{Ca in test supernatant}}{\%\ 45\ \text{Ca in test resin}} - \frac{\%\ 45\ \text{Ca in blank supernatant}}{\%\ 45\ \text{Ca in blank resin}}$$

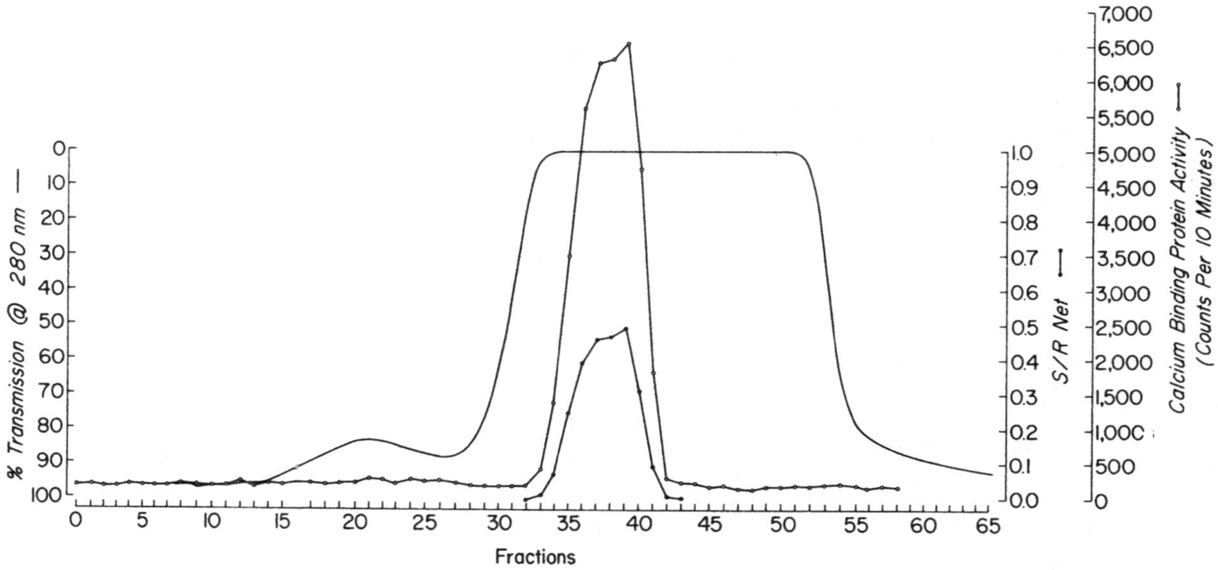

Figure 1. Superfine G-75 Sephadex chromatography of concentrated 24-hour urine specimen from active calcium oxalate stone former. Elution profile of protein and calcium binding activity is indicated. Total S/R Net is computed as outlined in text.

A. Active calcium oxalate stone former.

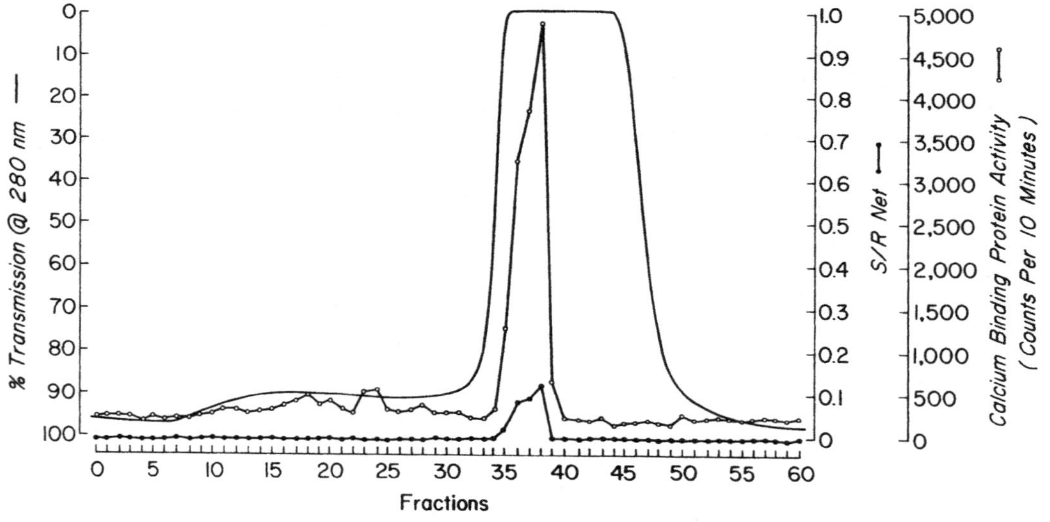

Figure 1. Superfine G-75 Sephadex chromatography of concentrated 24-hour urine specimen from active calcium oxalate stone former. Elution profile of protein and calcium binding activity is indicated. Total S/R Net is computed as outlined in text.

B. Inactive calcium oxalate stone former.

The rationale for expressing calcium binding activity as S/R Net has been previously reported[12,14]. By performing a concentration series binding affinity, the binding capacity and the total amount of calcium binding activity present in the urine can then be calculated. Utilizing S/R Net as a measurement for each fraction, the elution pattern for each concentrated urine specimen was plotted on standard graph paper and the total area representing calcium-binding protein activity was expressed as total S/R Net (Figures 1A and B). The expression of calcium binding protein activity in this manner allowed for the calculation of the total calcium binding activity present in a total 24-hour urine specimen. It was then possible to make comparisons between individual patients and groups of patients.

Molecular weight determinations of the calcium binding fraction were made by prior calibration of the column utilizing known proteins (Ovalbumin-MW 46,000, Myoglobulin MW 17,000, Cytochrome C MW 12,300 and Insulin MW 5,700).

RESULTS

A total of 44 patients were evaluated: 27 active calcium oxalate stone-formers (18 males, 9 females); 7 inactive calcium oxalate stone formers (4 males, 3 females); 2 active male uric acid stone formers; 1 active female cystine stone former and 7 non-stone forming controls (5 males, 2 females). All patients had negative urine cultures and normal corrected creatinine clearances. Metabolic evaluation of the 27 active calcium oxalate stone formers revealed: absorptive hypercalciuria 10; renal hypercalciuria 2; hyperuricosuria six; absorptive hypercalciuria and hyperuricosuria 5; hyperoxaluria 1 and no abnormalities 3. Both uric acid stone formers were hyperuricosuric and the cystine stone former had homozygous cystinuria confirmed by quantitative amino acid analysis. One male control patient was hypercalciuric.

Mean urinary S/R Net for each group studied was 1164.6 for active calcium oxalate stone formers; 1079.5 for non-stone forming controls; 480.2 for uric acid stone formers; and 614.9 for one cystine stone former (Figure 2). Total urinary calcium binding protein activity was significantly greater in the active calcium oxalate stone formers when compared with either inactive calcium oxalate stone formers ($p < 0.005$) or non-stone forming controls ($p < 0.025$). (One tailed Mann-Whitney Test)[15]. Based on the elution pattern of the calcium binding substance(s) the molecular weight was estimated to be approximately 26,000 daltons.

The number of uric acid and cystine stone formers was too small to make meaningful comparisons. No correlation was noted between calcium binding activity and patient age, sex or type of metabolic abnormality uncovered in the active calcium oxalate stone formers. Ten of the 27 active calcium oxalate stone formers had variable degrees of calyceal calcification but calcium binding activity in this group did not differ significantly from those patients free of such calcification.

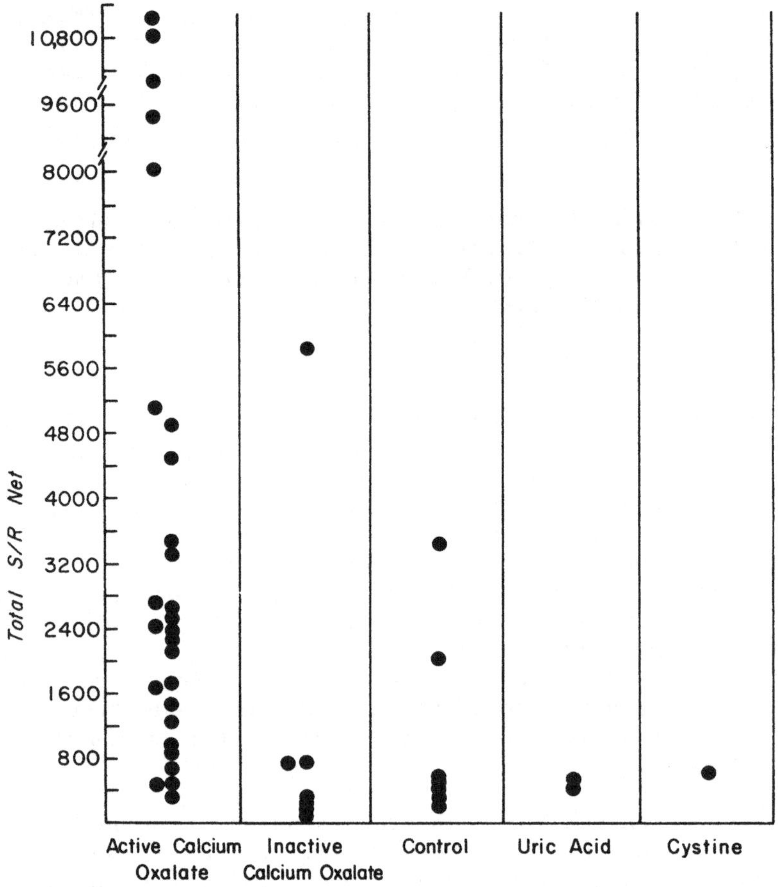

Figure 2. Total S/R Net. Total urinary calcium binding protein activity was significantly greater in the active calcium oxalate stone formers when compared with either inactive calcium oxalate stone formers ($p < 0.005$) or non-stone forming controls ($p < 0.025$).

Of the three patients in the control and inactive stone forming groups having elevated urinary calcium binding protein activity, one control patient had hypercalciuria but no abnormalities were noted in the other two. Comparison of the amount of urinary calcium binding protein activity and degree of calciuria showed no significant correlation (r = 0.1032). (Figure 3)

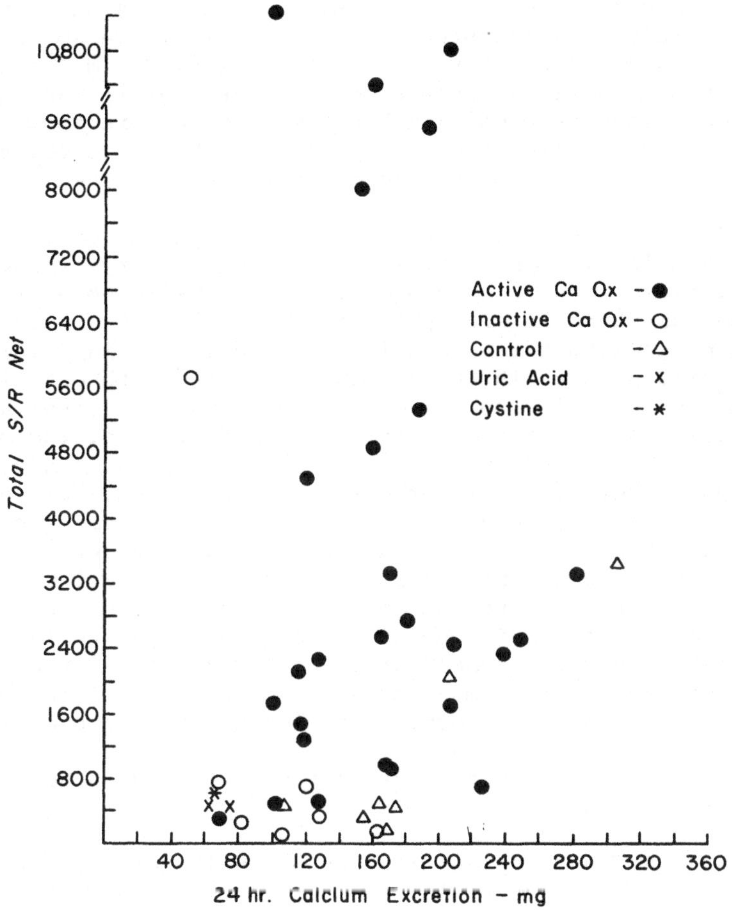

Figure 3. Relationship between Total S/R Net and 24-hour calcium excretion for individual patients and patient groups. No significant correlation noted (r = 0.1032).

DISCUSSION

Vitamin D sensitive calcium binding proteins were first identified in the intestine of chicks by Wasserman and Associates in 1966[16]. Further studies of this material revealed its molecular weight to be 24,000 daltons and it was found to influence the intestinal absorption of calcium[17,18]. Studies by other investigators revealed calcium binding proteins to be present in different organs of several species and the molecular weight of these substances was found to be either 28,000 daltons or 10,000 daltons[6]. It is of interest that antisera against chick intestinal calcium binding protein cross-reacts immunologically with the rat and human kidney and rat and bovine brain, however, antisera against other intestinal calcium binding proteins (pig, bovine) are species specific and no cross reactivity has been observed. Major questions regarding these substances relate to the fact that it has not been clearly established that calcium binding proteins are required for Vitamin-D induced calcium transport and that the exact cellular location of the protein has not been clearly established[19].

Of related interest are the studies of Lian and Associates who measured urinary stone matrix content and urinary excretion of γ-carboxyglutamic acid (Gla) containing proteins in both stone forming and non-stone forming patients[20,21]. Gla is a calcium binding amino acid that is found in four blood-clotting proteins and in the proteins present in the matrix associated with ectopic calcification[22,23,24]. The number of Gla residues/1000 total amino acid residues was high in the matrix obtained from calcium oxalate and hydroxyapatite stones while the matrix from pure magnesium ammonium phosphate, uric acid or cystine stones had little or no Gla content. The Gla containing stone protein also differed from the Gla containing bone protein and prothrobin fragments. Patients with a history of recurrent calcium oxalate urinary calculi were found to excrete from 30 to 50% more free and protein-bound Gla in the urine than normal individuals. These investigators suggest that the presence of this amino acid in the protein matrix of calcium containing urinary calculi may serve as a specific calcium buffering or nucleating substance. Whether the calcium binding protein identified in the present study also contains a higher percentage of Gla than non-calcium binding urinary proteins is unknown but deserves further study.

The findings in the present study of an increase in urinary calcium binding protein activity in active calcium oxalate stone formers suggests that this material may have some role in calcium oxalate urinary stone formation. Low levels in inactive calcium oxalate stone formers also suggests that excretion of these substances may be related to stone activity. The specificity of activity in calcium oxalate stone formers is further suggested by the presence of low levels of activity in the few uric acid and cystine stone formers studied. Only one previous study attempted measurement of calcium binding proteins in human urine[8]. The protein identified was electrophoretically homogenous, of slow $alpha_2$ mobility and had a molecular weight of approximately 50,000 daltons. Interestingly, elevated activity was noted in one patient with idiopathic hypercalciuria but patients with malignant reticulosis with hypercalcemia, nephrocalcinosis, chronic pyelonephritis and hyperparathyroidism had seemingly normal activity. These determinations were qualitative and were based on degree of staining rather than any quantitative measurement. The present study demonstrated increased activity in patients with active calcium oxalate stone disease and no correlation was noted between degree of activity and amount of calcium excretion. Further studies are planned to measure the response of calcium binding activity to calcium deprivation and load.

What role calcium binding substances have in urinary stone formation is unknown. One can speculate that these materials allow for high local concentrations of calcium so that formation products are exceeded and nucleation is initiated. With growth of a stone or nucleation by another material, adsorption of these substances onto the surface of the crystal could enhance growth and possible crystal aggregation. These materials may also influence the transport of calcium across the membrane of renal tubular cells. Activating proteins affecting 3', 5' monophosphate (cyclic AMP) have been identified that influence calcium transport across red blood cell membranes[25].

It is important to point out that a similar argument can be made for the protecting role of these materials in both inhibiting nucleation and retarding crystal growth and aggregation. It is quite possible that calcium binding materials may serve either as inhibitors or promoters of nucleation or crystal growth depending upon ambient conditions; for example, specific ionic activity which may influence cross linkages between such molecules or molecular configuration. It is only through further investigations as to the structure and properties of these materials, their origin, their effect on crystal nucleation and growth and their role in the handling of calcium by the kidney will the true role of these materials in urinary stone disease be fully elucidated.

REFERENCES

1. W. H. Boyce, Am. J. Med. 45:673 (1968).
2. J. J. Leal and B. Finlayson, Invest. Urol. 27:278 (1977).
3. C. W. Vermuelen and E. S. Lyons, Am. J. Med. 45:684 (1968).
4. M. I. Resnick, in:"Idiopathic Urinary Bladder Stone Disease," Fogarty International Center Proceedings No. 37, DHEW Publication No. (NIH) 77-1063 (1977).
5. C. L. Hermsdorf and F. Bronne, Biochimica et Biophysica Acta 379:53 (1976).
6. C. H. Wasserman and J. J. Feher, in:"Calcium Binding Proteins and Calcium Function," R. A. Corradino, C. H. Wasserman, E. Carafoli, R. H. Kretsinger, D. H. Mac Lennan, and F. L. Siegel, ed. North-Holland Press, New York (1977).

7. R. H. Wasserman, C. S. Fullmer, and A. N. Taylor, in:"Vitamin D," D. E. M. Lawson, ed., Academic Press, New York (1978).
8. F. Lingarde, J. Malmquist, L. Tejler, and O. Bettervaoi, IRCS Med. Sci. 2:1004 (1974).
9. L. H. Smith, Urol. Clin. N. Am. 1:241 (1974).
10. G. W. Pitts and M. I. Resnick, Urol. Clin. N. Am. 7:45 (1979).
11. W. H. Boyce and M. I. Resnick, J. Urol. 121:706 (1979).
12. C. H. Wasserman, R. A. Corradino, and A. N. J. Taylor, J. Biol. Chem. 243:3979 (1968).
13. T. Freund and F. Bonner, Am. J. Physiol. 228:861 (1975).
14. R. L. Morrissey and D. F. Rath, Proc. Soc. Exper. Biol. Med. 145:699 (1974).
15. J. H. Zar, in:"Biostatistical Analysis," Prentice-Hall, Inc., Englewood Cliffs, New Jersey (1974).
16. R. H. Wasserman and A. N. Taylor, Science 152:793 (1966).
17. R. H. Wasserman, A. N. Taylor, and C. S. Fulmer, Biochem. Soc. Spec. Publ. 3:55 (1975).
18. R. L. Morrissey and R. H. Wasserman, Am. J. Physiol. 220:1509 (1971).
19. H. F. DeLuca, in:"Vitamin D Metabolism and Function," Springer-Verlag, Berlin (1979).
20. J. B. Lian, M. J. Glimcher, and P. M. Gallop, R. H. Wasserman, R. A. Corradino, C. Carfoli, R. H. Kretsinger, D. A. MacLennan, F. L. Siege, eds., North Holland, New York (1977).
21. J. B. Lian, M. Skinner, M. J. Glimcher, and P. M. Gallop, Biochem. Biophys. Res. Commun. 73:349 (1976).
22. J. B. Lian, M. Skinner, M. J. Glimcher, and P. M. Gallop, J. Clin. Invest. 59:115 (1977).
23. G. L. Nelsestuen and J. W. Suttie, Proc. Nat. Acad. Sci. 70: 3366 (1973).
24. P. A. Price, A. S. Otsuka, J. W. Posev, J. Prestaponis, and N. Raman, Proc. Nat. Acad. Sci. 73:1447 (1976).
25. F. L. Larsen and F. F. Vincenzi, Science 204:306 (1979).

ACKNOWLEDGMENT

This work was supported by Grant Number AM 20066 from the National Institute of Arthritis, Metabolic and Digestive Diseases, National Institutes of Health.

EXCRETION OF TAMM-HORSFALL URINARY GLYCOPROTEIN (UROMUCOID) IN RENAL CALCIUM STONE FORMERS

B. Wikström and J. Wieslander

Department of Internal Medicine, University Hospital, Uppsala and Department of Nephrology, University Hospital, Lund, Sweden

INTRODUCTION

Tamm-Horsfall protein (TH) is a high molecular weight glycoprotein which is excreted in substantial amounts in normal human urine[1]. TH has been suggested as a possible pathophysiological factor in nephrolithiasis being discussed as a component of the stones[2]. The purpose of this study was to quantitate TH excretion in stone formers and to study its relationship to renal acidification capacity and urine concentrating ability.

SUBJECTS AND METHODS

Patients

Seventy-four consecutive renal calcium stone formers (58 males, 16 females) with a mean age of 46 years (range 22-72). All patients had normal serum creatinine values.

Controls

Ninety-nine healthy subjects (61 males, 38 females). Mean age 44 years (range 15-81).

Renal acidification capacity

Short time (3-5 hours) ammonium chloride loading test[3] was performed in 57 stone formers. Forty-four of them had a normal urinary acidification (no RTA). In 13 patients renal tubular acidosis (RTA) of the incomplete forms were disclosed (9 patients had incomplete proximal RTA and 4 patients incomplete distal RTA).

Urine concentrating ability was determined in 62 patients as morning urine osmolality after a night's water restriction.

Assay of Tamm-Horsfall protein

Urinary TH was determined with a method based on quantitative electroimmunoassay[4].

RESULTS

We found no correlation of TH excretion to sex, age or urine volume in controls.

Stone formers had a reduced excretion of TH compared to controls. Patients with impaired renal acidification exhibited the lowest TH (Table I). A diminished TH excretion during the morning was found in the patients with low urine osmolality (Table II).

Table I. Urinary excretion of Tamm-Horsfall protein in healthy subjects and stone formers with normal urinary acidification (no RTA) and renal tubular acidosis (RTA) of the incomplete forms.

	Controls	Stone formers		
		All	no RTA	RTA
Urinary Tamm-Horsfall protein ($mg/24h/m^2$ BS) (mean value ± SD)	30.3±12.9	19.7±13.2[a]	21.3±13.7[a]	14.0±9.9[a,b]
n	99	57	44	13

a = $p < 0.001$ compared to controls
b = $p < 0.05$ compared to noRTA

There was also a relationship between TH excretion and the clinical stone disease to the extent that patients who had experienced several stone episodes had a lower TH excretion (Table III). Furthermore, an acid urine seemed to reduce the excretion of TH although the reduction was not clearly significant (Table IV).

Table II. Urinary excretion of Tamm-Horsfall protein in relation to urine concentrating ability in stone formers (n = 62).

	Urine Osmolality (mosmol/kg)		
	> 800	600-800	< 600
Urinary Tamm-Horsfall protein ($mg/24h/m^2$ BS) (mean value ± SD)	22.6±9.1	20.9±13.2	15.1±9.2[a]
n	23	25	14

a = $p < 0.05$ compared to stone formers with urine osmolality >800 mosmol/kg.

Table III. Urinary excretion of Tamm-Horsfall protein in relation to the number of stone episodes experienced by calcium stone patients (n = 63).

	1 stone episode	2-10 stone episodes	10 stone episodes
Urinary Tamm-Horsfall protein ($mg/24h/m^2$BS) (mean value ± SD)	25.4±7.7	21.2±12.4	16.1±9.6[a]
n	12	28	23

a = $p < 0.01$ compared to stone formers with one stone episode

Table IV. Hourly excretion of Tamm-Horsfall protein in stone formers (n=15) before and during acute acidosis produced by a load of ammonium chloride (17 g). Mean base deficit and urine pH during the acidosis was 9.1±2.4 (SD) mM and 5.17±0.90 (SD) mM respectively.

Urinary Tamm-Horsfall protein ($mg/hour/m^2$ BS)			
Before acidosis	During acidosis	t^b	p
1.74 ± 0.74[a]	1.39 ± 0.44[a]	1.79	$0.1>p>0.05$

a = mean value ± SD; b = paired t-test

DISCUSSION

It is known that TH is localized at the surface membranes of distal renal tubular cells. The pathophysiology of TH has recently been extensively reviewed[1]. However, there is limited knowledge of the urinary excretion of the protein in pathological conditions.

As a possible factor of importance in renal stone formation, interest has been focused on the role of TH as a constituent of concrements[2]. One would then expect larger amounts of TH in urine from stone formers, compared to stone-free subjects, but we found the contrary.

On the other hand TH could be regarded as a marker for specific tubular cell functions such as urine acidification and concentrating ability[5]. Tubular dysfunctions were recently observed to exist in a high frequency in stone formers[6]. The findings in the present study suggests an association of diminished TH excretion to impaired tubular function.

It is notable that immunologic responses to tubular cells have been demonstrated in patients with RTA[7]. The immunologic reaction may be directed to TH protein thus causing a reduced urinary excretion of the glycoprotein.

Variations in urinary concentration of hydrogen ions and electrolytes cause different physico-chemical states of TH[8] and may thus influence the urinary excretion pattern of TH. This may be one explanation to the lower TH excretion during acute acidosis in our stone formers.

CONCLUSIONS

Urinary 24 hour excretion of Tamm-Horsfall protein was decreased in patients with calcium stones. The lowest excretion was seen in stone formers with incomplete RTA, urinary concentration disability or a heavy stone formation. Tubular function defects have been shown to be associated with calcium stone disease. The findings in this study suggest that low urinary Tamm-Horsfall protein may indicate such tubular defects.

REFERENCES

1. J. R. Hoyer and M. W. Seiler, Kid. Int. 16:279 (1979).
2. A. M. S. Grant, L. R. J. Baker and A. Neuberger, Clin. Sci. 44:377 (1973).
3. U. Backman, B. G. Danielson, and M. Sohtell, Scand. J. Urol. Nephrol. Suppl. 35:33 (1976).

4. J. Wieslander, P. Bygren, and D. Heinegard, Clin. Chim. Acta. 78:391 (1977).
5. R. A. Lewis, R. H. Schwarz, and E. A. Schenk, Lab. Invest. 26:728 (1972).
6. U. Backman, B. G. Danielson, G. Johansson, S. Ljunghall, and B. Wikström, Nephron 25:96 (1980).
7. I. Chanarin, G. Loewi, A. S. Tavill, S. P. Swain, and E. Tidmarsh, Lancet 2:317 (1974).
8. E. G. McQueen and G. B. Engle, J. Clin. Pathol. 19:392 (1966).

PROTEOLYTIC ACTIVITY AND ORGANIC SUBSTANCES IN URINE

H.-J. Schneider and R.-H. Börner

Clinic of Urology, Friedrich - Schiller - University,

Jena, Lessingstraße 1, German Democratic Republic

INTRODUCTION

Reports on the influence of organic substances on the formation and growth of stones are often contradictory. Several urinary proteins, which are not present in the urine of normal persons, however, have been identified in stone-forming urine[1].

The protein composition of stones, in turn, depends on their crystalline composition[2-5]. This implies that there must be a selective process in the incorporation of urinary proteins into the forming stone. Furthermore, there is always non-specific adsorption of urinary mucoproteins onto the crystal surface[6] and some specific mechanisms must be taken into consideration[7]. Proteins found in stones have mean molecular weights of about 40,000 daltons. Any change in this pattern of molecular weight distribution, e.g. due to changes in the proteolytic activity of the urine, should act on the mechanisms already mentioned.

To investigate these relationships, we studied the excretion pattern of organic substances in the urines of Ca-oxalate stone formers and normal persons by means of gel permeation chromatography (GPC) and correlated the results obtained with the respective protease and enzyme inhibiting activities ("inhibitory concentration"). The experimental design is shown in Figure 1.

MATERIAL AND METHODS

Urines from patients with recurrent Ca-oxalate urolithiasis (n = 22, age 20 - 65 years) were analyzed. They did not receive any drugs two weeks before analysis. The control group (normal group)

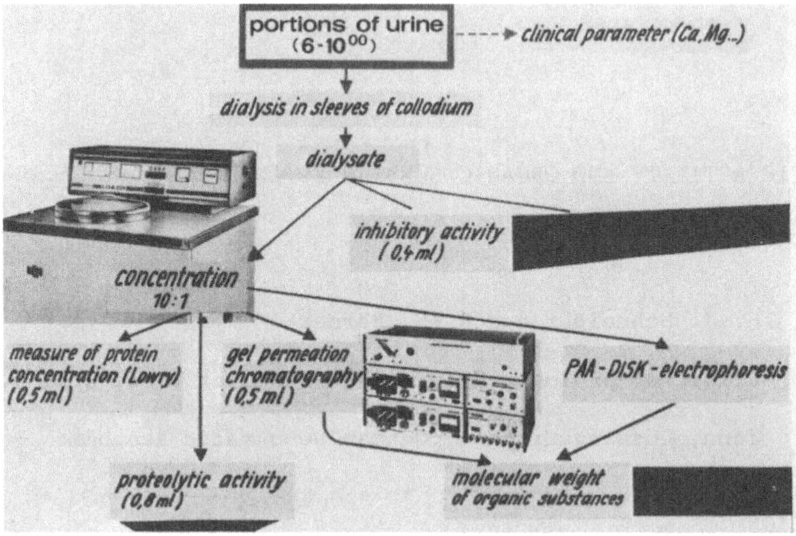

Figure 1. Scheme of experiments to study proteolytic activity and organic substances in urine.

consisted of members of staff and students (n = 10, age 20 - 50) with clinical and clinical-chemical findings within the normal range.

Normally, the determination of proteolytic activity (PA) in the urine cannot be performed without separating the respective enzyme inhibitors because the existing enzyme inhibitor complex does not affect the substrate. This involves much analytical work. For instance the sample must be first passed through a Sephadex gel column to which a synthetically prepared enzyme inhibitor must be bound. The enzyme-enzyme inhibitor complex must be measured. Using protamine sulfate (clupeine sulfate from herring sperm) as a substrate offers a more elegant method because it is affected even in the presence of a high excess of inhibitors. With this technique, quantitative determination of proteolytic degradation in urine is relatively simple.

The determination of enzyme inhibitor activity (AC = inhibitor activity = capacity of trypsin adhesion) is based on the fact that trypsin is rapidly bound by the inhibitors in the urine.

The total antitryptic activity can be calculated from the difference between the activities of the trypsin added to the urine and the remaining enzyme activity after incubation.

GPC is a special form of liquid chromatography which is excellently suited for fractionating high molecular compounds. In our GPC investigations we assumed that high molecular weight proteins mainly occur in urine when the glomerular permeability is impaired. If tubular function is impaired, the low molecular proteins normally filtered are not sufficiently reabsorbed and appear increasingly in urine.

RESULTS

Figure 2 shows the molecular weight distribution of organic substances in the urines of normal persons. This shows that low molecular substances occur having molecular weights of less than 10,000, possibly suggesting some "normal" proteolysis. This contrasts with the results in recurrent Ca oxalate stone formers where the maximum is shifted towards higher molecular weights. Since the possibility of glomerular damage cannot be excluded in this group, we cannot conclude definitely that there is reduced proteolysis in stone-forming urine. The determination of proteolytic activity and inhibitor activity, however, should distinguish between these possibilities (Table 1).

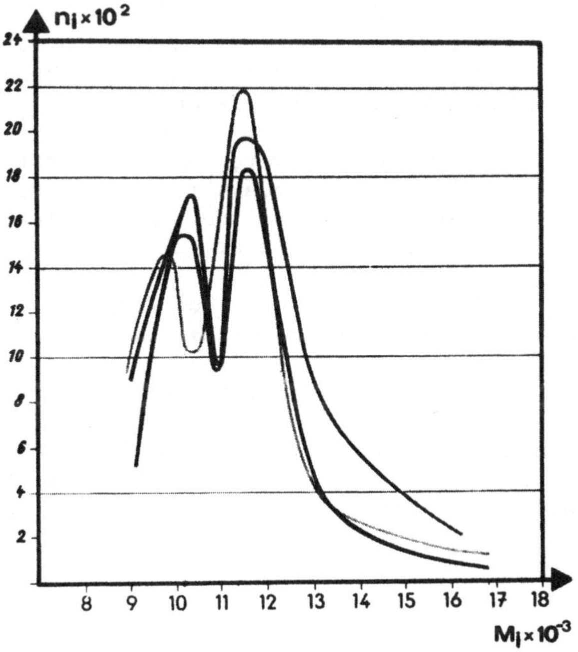

Figure 2. Differential relative molecular weight distribution of organic substances in urines of normal persons.

Table 1. Proteolytic and Antiproteolytic Activities in Urine from Normals and Recurrent Ca-Oxalate Stone-Formers

	Proteolytic activity (PA) nmol Prot/min/ml	Capacity of trypsin adhesion (AC) µg/0.2 ml/Urin
Controls	0.458 ± 0.161	2.64 ± 2.92
Oxalate Stone Formers	0.547 ± 0.386	4.54 ± 2.89

Compared with normals, Ca oxalate stone formers had a slightly increased proteolytic activity. Apparently this increased protease activity cannot be effective because the enzyme binding capacity is simultaneously increased. This relationship between proteolytic and antiproteolytic activities becomes evident on regression analysis. The linear equations found show that in normals a higher proteolytic activity is present, i.e. it can contribute to the formation of a low molecular protective colloid system because the binding capacity is not high. The error of the estimation is between 10 and 20%, taking into account the natural biological range of variation, the methodological error of about 20% and a fairly low probable error due to diuresis which was neglected in this analysis.

In Ca oxalate stone formers, however, increased protease activity is prevented by the simultaneously increased enzyme inhibitor concentration. This partly explains the shift in the maximum of the mean molecular weight towards higher values.

From this we have introduced the quotient PA/AC related to the total protein content as an index of potential proteolysis in urine. In normal persons the index is 10 times higher than in recurrent Ca oxalate stone formers. In conjunction with other urinary variables this quotient should help to provide a suitable index of the tendency to crystallization in urine. The difference in the dependence of protease activity on the correlated binding capacity and the molecular weight distribution of organic substances in the urine of normal persons and Ca oxalate stone formers might be taken into account in future programs of stone prevention.

REFERENCES

1. W. H. Boyce, Am. J. Med. 45:673 (1968).
2. W. Flach, H. Feist, and A. Hesse, in:"V Jenaer Harnsteinsymposium," (1977).

3. W. O. Foye, H. S. Hong, C. M. Kim, and E. L. Prien, Invest. Urol. 14:33 (1976).
4. R. H. Borner, H. Feist, and H.-J. Schneider, (in preparation).
5. A. R. Spector and E. L. Prien, Invest. Urol. 13:387 (1976).
6. C. W. Vermeulen and E. S. Lyon, Am. J. Med. 45:684 (1968).
7. J. J. Leal and B. Finlayson, Invest. Urol. 27:278 (1977).

MECHANISM OF THE HETEROGENEOUS NUCLEATION BY A URINARY MUCOPROTEIN

B. Pinto, J. Bernshtam, and J. L. Paternain

Laboratorio de Exploraciones Metabolicas

Barcelona, Catalunya, Spain

Previous studies have reported[1] the isolation of a mucoprotein of 51,200 daltons molecular weight. Its aminoacid composition is mainly glycine and glutamic acid. The carbohydrate accounts for 30% of its structure. It has hexoses, hexosamines and small amounts of hexuronic and sialic acids.

The physicochemical properties of this protein does not suggest similarity to either uromucoid[2] or matrix protein A from urinary stones[3]. This report describes a study on the mechanism of reaction of this mucoprotein with the precipitated calcium stone salts, as well as the aggregation of the mucoprotein with itself.

Experimental Procedure

The experimental procedure attempts to study the behavior of the mucoprotein towards the minerals (calcium, phosphate and oxalate) by studying the reactions in the sol state, and the transformation from sol to gel and viceversa.

A. Reactions Occurring in the Sol State

Phosphate and oxalate binding by the mucoprotein and modulation of the binding by calcium was investigated.

Phosphate binding was investigated in the presence of Tris-HCl buffer (pH 7.5), 0.87 μg of protein from purified mucoprotein preparation[1] was mixed with various amounts of (^{32}P) labeled phosphate. The free and bound phosphate was estimated after filtration of the mixture through a Millipore filter. The mucoprotein binding of phosphate at pH 7.4 follows a sigmoid shaped curve.

Oxalate binding was investigated by similar methods. The effect of calcium on the oxalate and phosphate binding was tested by adding two µmoles of calcium chloride to the 1 ml final volume assay system. Oxalate was bound quite poorly by the mucoprotein. However the oxalate binding increased in the presence of calcium and phosphate. Calcium was the limiting step of the reaction. In the presence of calcium excess, the oxalate bound by the mucoprotein had a good correlation with the oxalate added.

B. Reactions Occurring in the Gel State and Sol Gel Transformations

The formation of aggregates was investigated by testing the calcium and phosphate effects using stepwise gradient columns from 70 to 0% sucrose concentration. Several factors controlling the aggregates formation were tested by preparing these columns in the presence of calcium or phosphate plus calcium.

In the presence of calcium plus phosphate three major aggregates were formed. The heaviest was eluted from the sucrose calcium within the first fractions. These aggregates were visible as small flakes (Figure 1).

The aggregates eluted with the second radioactive peak (II) were smaller in size and they were eluted within the 10 - 20 fractions. The third peak (III) appeared within the 50% sucrose concentration zone. The fifth peak (V) did not migrate beyond the buffer region. In the presence of calcium alone, peak-I did not appear. However, a fourth peak (IV) was present in the last portion of the 25% sucrose concentration solution. Peaks-I and II were not present when the sample contained phosphate in addition to the mucoprotein. The calcium phosphate without mucoprotein did not move at all.

COMMENT

The mucoprotein herein investigated exists as two reversible states: sol and gel. The sol - gel transformation is controlled by the calcium and phosphate concentration.

In the sol state a limited amount of mucoprotein units interact with oxalate through phosphate bridges. Phosphate units are also bound to calcium oxalate chains. Calcium is the limiting step of the reactions.

The elementary mucoprotein units are assembled through calcium and phosphate bridges. As the mucoprotein polymer grows it is transformed to the gel state. (Figure 2).

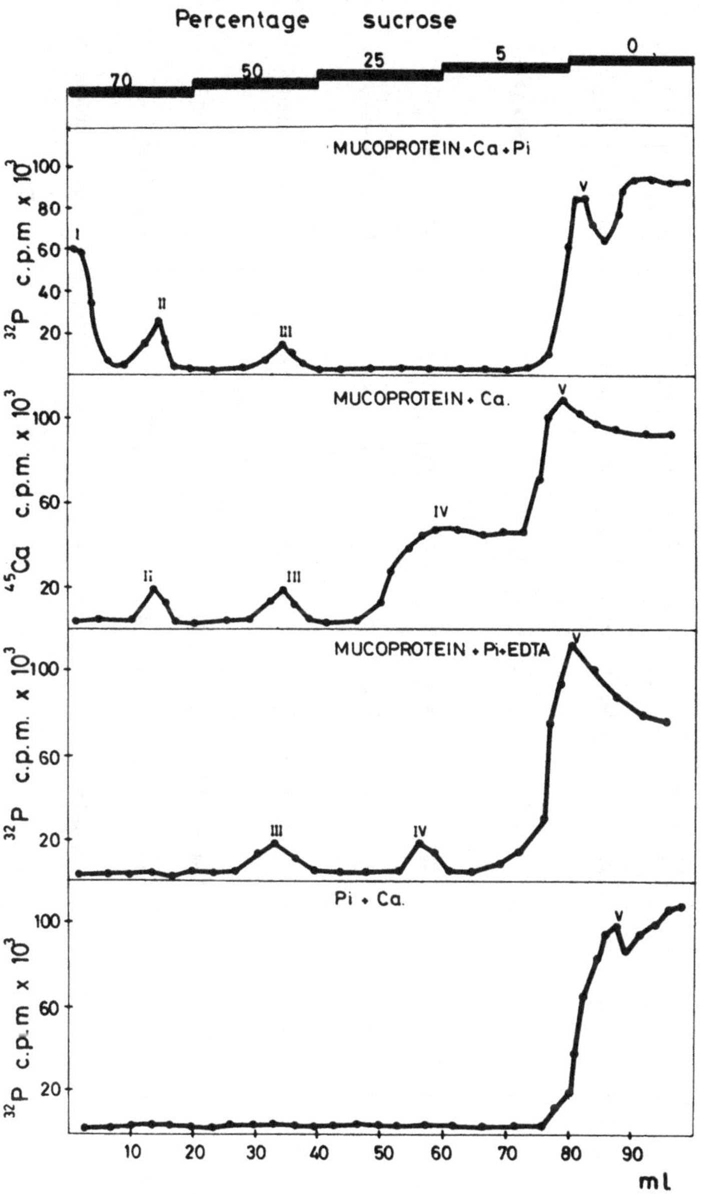

Figure 1. Sol-gel Mucoprotein Transformation. Mucoprotein (1.8 mg) were incubates in the presence of 10 mM calcium chloride, or calcium plus phosphate or phosphate plus EDTA. Samples were layered on sucrose columns of 0, 5, 25, 50 and 70% sucrose concentrations. After 2 hours, 1 ml fractions were collected and the radioactivity from alternate fractions was counted. ^{32}Pi was used as tracer but it was replaced with ^{45}Ca in one column in which the effect of calcium alone was tested. In another column mucoprotein was omitted in the sample.

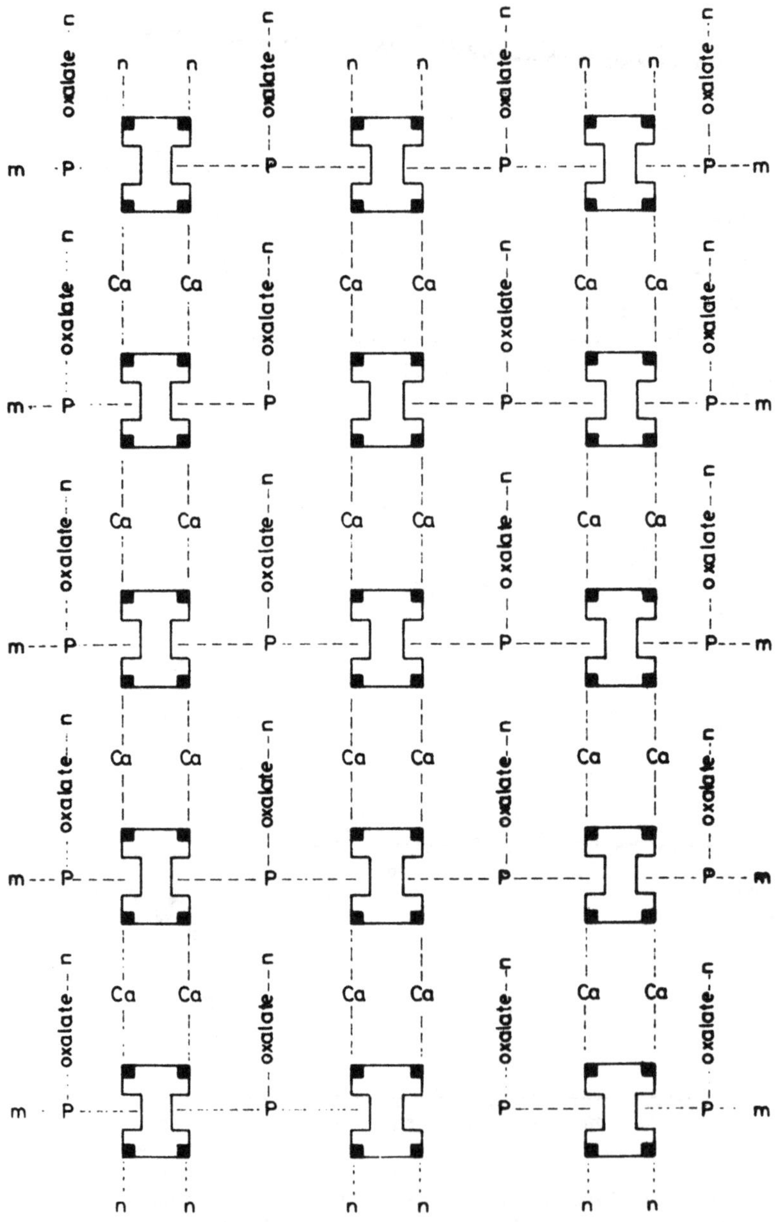

Figure 2. Proposed Structure of the Heterogeneous Nucleus. n number of elementary units are attached through calcium sites. m number of these units are joined through phosphate sites and n number of oxalate molecules are bound to phosphate through calcium.

REFERENCES

1. B. Pinto, J. L. Paternain, and J. Bernshtam, in:"Proceedings Fourth International Urolithiasis Research Symposium," L. H. Smith, B. Finlayson, and W. G. Robertson, eds., Plenum Press, New York (in press).
2. W. H. Boyce and M. Swanson, J. Clin. Invest. 34:1581 (1955).
3. W. H. Boyce, in:"Proteins in Normal and Pathological Urine," Y. Manuel, J. P. Revillard, and H. Betuel, eds., S. Karger, Basel/New York (1970).

NEPHROLITHIASIS IN DIALYSED PATIENTS - EVIDENCE FOR A PECULIAR TYPE OF MATRIX STONES WITH Ca-OXALATE INCLUSIONS

J. Bommer, E. Ritz, R. Waldherr, and W. Tschöppe

Medizinische Universitätsklinik Heidelberg, Bergheimer Straße 58, D-6900 Heidelberg, Germany - FRT and Pathologisches Institut der Universität Heidelberg, Berliner Straße, D-6900 Heidelberg - FRG

Recently it has been recognized by Bommer[1] and Caralps[2] that nephrolithiasis may arise de novo in patients on maintenance hemodialysis. Such stones were shown to consist of a protein matrix with amyloid-like microfibrillar ultrastructure. The organic phase consisted primarily of protein with little carbohydrate or lipid. A small admixture of inorganic material (whewellite) or ammonium-hydrogen-urate was found; the amount of which varied from 15-50% of dry weight in the study of Bommer[1]. The present study was designed (1) to further characterize the natural history of this type of nephrolithiasis, and (2) to further analyse the composition of the stones.

CLINICAL OBSERVATIONS

Out of 137 patients on maintenance hemodialysis, 11 patients passed stones. None of the patients had a history of nephrolithiasis, papillary necrosis, urinary tract infection, urotuberculosis and none had a metabolic disorder predisposing to stone formation. A total of 123 stones were observed, varying in size from 0.5-8 mm (diameter). The median number of stones per patient was 8 with a range from 1-50. Stones were passed asymptomatically or after an acute renal colic with unilateral hydronephrosis (computer tomogram).

AUTOPSY FINDINGS

Ten patients with terminal renal failure (2 prior to hemodialysis, 8 after varying periods of hemodialysis) were studied at autopsy. In 6 patients, matrix stones were found which were located within small cysts found in the renal medulla and cortex.

URINE ANALYSIS

Twenty-four hour urine collections (under exclusion of air) in stone patients gave the following results: pH 5.0-6.0, urinary Ca 0.48-0.91 mmol/l, urinary Pi 4.1-12.6 mmol/l, urinary oxalate (isotachophoresis) 0.23-1.8 mmol/l and urinary uric acid 1.0-2.3 mmol/l.

STONE ANALYSIS

The stones obtained in vivo and the stones recovered at autopsy were analyzed by light microscopy (ultrathin sections), under polarised light and with transmission electron microscopy. Immunofluorescence studies of cryostat cut sections were carried out with nonspecific rabbit antihuman IgA, IgG, IgM, fibrinogen, Tamm-Horsfall protein, albumin and complement components. As described previously by Bommer[1], all stones that were passed spontaneously and all stones that were recovered at autopsy exhibited a peculiar texture with concentris lame-lae of alternating density. The material demonstrated pronounced affinity for congo red and was anisotropic under polarised light (green birefringence). Transmission electron microscopy revealed more or less tightly packed interwoven, non-branching microfibrils. The density of fiber packing was high in the zones which appeared as dark lamellae under light microscopy and was less dense in the interspace between. The same type of texture and ultrastructure was observed in the concrements recovered from the renal cysts observed at autopsy. Furthermore, in some casts were observed which exhibited similar lamellar texture and microfibrillar ultrastructure (Figure 1). These observations are compatible with the notion that the matrix stones arise by slow intermittent growth within dilated renal tubules or cysts.

Analysis with immunofluorescence showed negative staining for complement components, immunoglobulins and mostly negative staining for fibrinogen and albumin. The dense innermost core of the matrix stones usually exhibited faint staining for Tamm-Horsfall protein, whereas the peripheral parts of the stones were consistently negative. This finding is in agreement with chemical analyses, previously reported by Bommer[1], which showed very low carbohydrate content, and argues against a major admixture of native Tamm-Horsfall protein.

Whereas previous analyses with scanning electron mircoscopy had revealed the presence of whewellite in only a minority of the stones, systematic serial sectioning of stones obtained in vivo and at autopsy usually showed the presence of some oxalate microcrystals in the dense lamellae of the matrix core.

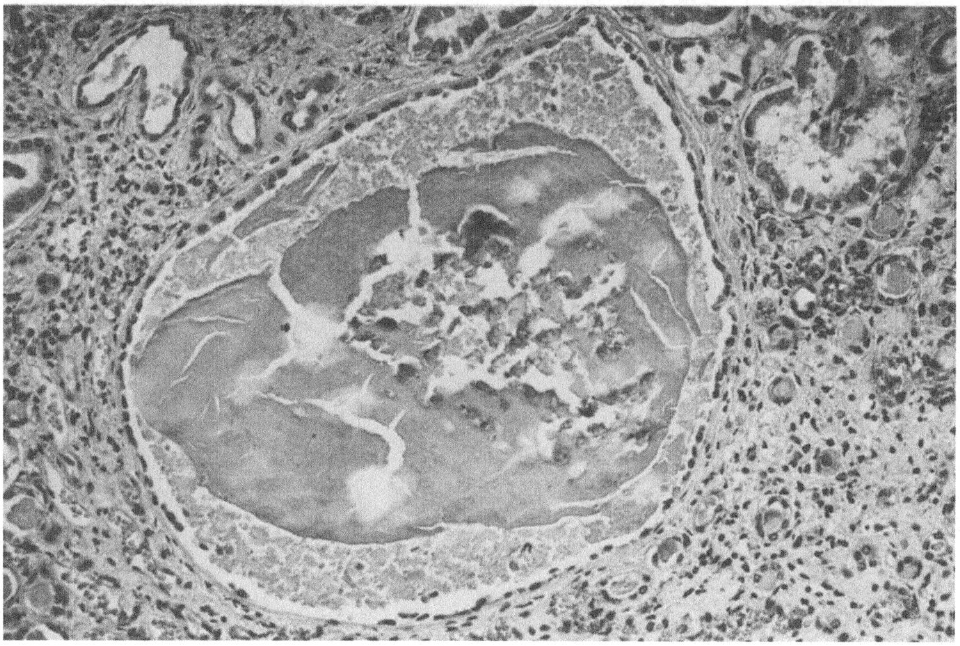

Figure 1. Formation of cysts with lamellar texture in dilated nephrons of a patient on maintenance hemodialysis.

SUMMARY

De novo renal stone formation is relatively common in dialysed patients. The dialysis procedure does not seem to be a prerequisite since analogous material was also found in kidneys of uremic patients prior to dialysis. The common location in cysts and dilated tubules, and the similarity in structure to casts, suggest that the amyloid-like protein matrix material arises from protein rich stagnant urine. This process appears to be an extension of what commonly occurs in cast formation. It differs from ordinary cast formation by the virtual absence of Tamm-Horsfall protein. The concomitant presence of some oxalate is consistent with the observation that oxalate concentration is rather high in the urine of patients with oliguric terminal renal failure.

REFERENCES

1. J. Bommer, E. Ritz, W. Tschöpe, R. Waldherr, and M. Gebhardt, Kid. Int. 16:722 (1979).
2. A. Caralps, J. Andreu, A. Brulles, J. Lloveras, J. Masramon, J. M. Gil-Vernet, M. Fernandez Conde, and M. T. Vidal, (abstract), Min. Electrol. Metab. 2:213 (1979).

THE CHEMICAL COMPOSITION OF A NON-CRYSTALLINE FELINE KIDNEY STONE

U. M. Cowgill

Department of Biological Sciences, University of Pittsburgh, Pittsburgh, Pennsylvania 15260

INTRODUCTION

This study concerns a peculiar kidney concretion that was produced by a 17+ year old female Burmese cat. The outward appearance of this stone, its hardness and gross inhomogeneity suggested that its chemical and mineralogical composition might be unusual and thus it was decided to carry out as complete a study as the 61.2 mg weight permitted.

MATERIALS AND METHODS

Cat's Background

For the whole of this cat's life she lived on a high protein diet in a medium hardwater region. Eight months prior to her death she suffered a respiratory infection. She was treated with 10 mg per day of cephalexin ($C_{16}H_{17}N_3O_4S$) for 5 days. After an interval of 2 days the dosage was repeated for 5 more days. One gram was administered over a period of 6 months. Shortly before her death she was vaccinated with panleukopenia, calici and rhinotracheitis viruses.

Her necropsy report indicates atrophy of the right kidney with stones in the pelvis and hilum. The architectural pattern suggests the possibility of a highly decomposed included epithelial cyst. The left kidney was hydronephrotic. Both kidneys revealed tubules in the renal cortex to be dilated and filled with eosinophilic colloid. The cause of death was kidney failure.

Table 1. The Chemical Composition of a Feline Kidney Stone

Element	mg kg^{-1}	Element	mg kg^{-1}	Element	mg kg^{-1}
Na	215	Hg	0.112	Mo	4.1
K	776	Al	134	Cl	330
Li	9.6	Ga	0.1	Br	22
Rb	10	B	34	Fe	214
Cu	19	Si	25	Mn	26
Ag	0.043	Sn	0.042	Co	0.212
Be	0.085	Pb	22	Ni	1.8
Ca	2667	P	421		
Mg	3100	Bi	0.066		%
Sr	11	V	0.042	C	48.95
Zn	29	S	23356	H	6.20
Cd	0.065	Cr	2.5	N	13.87

Mineral Matter		7.06%
H_2O ignition loss		92.79%
Amino Acids	59.47	
Cholesterol	0.84	
Phthalates	0.02	
Water	32.31	
Subtotal	92.64	
Grand Total		99.85%

Calculated molecular weight 43819

Calculated formula $C_{152}H_{235}N_{39}O_{46}S$

Table 2. Results of Organic Analysis of a Feline Kidney Stone

Amino Acids %

Corrected for H_2O loss

Aspartic acid	6.39	Methionine	0.79
Threonine	2.55	Isoleucine	0.86
Serine	2.83	Leucine	8.62
Glutamic acid	4.90	Tyrosine	0.73
Proline	2.32	Phenylalanine	5.82
Glycine	2.07	Histidine	4.37
Alanine	5.07	Lysine	2.76
Cystine	1.12	Arginine	2.37
Valine	5.76	Cysteic acid and Taurine	0.14
	Total	59.47	

Mass Spectrometry

Cholesterol	0.84%	Phthalates	0.02%

Gas Chromatography

No clear cut evidence for simple carbohydrates or for polymers derived from them in acid hydrolysate followed by derivatization to trimethylsilyl compounds[4]. Alkaline extraction revealed no detectable simple carbohydrates.

Infrared Spectroscopy

Strong amide I	1650 cm^{-1}	Amide II	1490 cm^{-1}
Carbonyl stretch		C-N stretch	
		lower position than normal	
Broad band	3650 cm^{-1} - 3180 cm^{-1}		
Amid A?			
Amid B?			

Comment: Lower frequency of amide II may reflect some metal-amine interaction.

Description of Stone

The stone was 7.2 mm in diameter and weighed 0.06124 g. It had no nucleus. The external color was dark brown to black. The internal portion contained light brown to yellow striations, interrupted by an occasional white speck. Mohs' scale of hardness was 6-7. The stone was insoluble in a variety of acids, alkalis and organic solvents. Solubility occurred only with 6NHCl, 100°C under 5μ vacuum for 24 h. Water loss was 32.31%. Petrographic microscope analysis of a small sample revealed the presence of orthorhombic sulfur, calcite and hydroxylapatite.

Analytical Techniques

Various portions of the stone were examined by x-ray diffraction[1], x-ray fluorescence[2], optical emission spectroscopy[3], carbon, hydrogen and nitrogen analyses, amino acid analysis, gas chromatography, mass spectrometer analysis and infrared analysis.

RESULTS

The results are shown in Tables 1 and 2 and Figure 1. The diffractogram shows only two diffuse peaks, one at 9.65 Å and the other at 4.65 Å. This pattern is certainly reminiscent of polypeptide chains[5] and bears similarities to the polymer polystyrene[6], to elastin[7] as well as beta-keratin[8].

CONCLUDING COMMENTS

This stone bears some similarity to those produced by patients on maintenance hemodialysis[9]. Possible sequence of events that produced this feline stone are as follows: cephalexin is a known nephrotoxin and some ctas develop hypersensitive reactions such as eosinophilia to this drug; pathological study suggested the probable presence of an epithelial inclusion cyst in the kidney, and were this the case, the squamous epithelial lining would have elaborated keratin. The infrared results, the diffractogram, and the wet analyses all strongly suggest the presence of a fibrous protein possibly keratin.

REFERENCES

1. U. M. Cowgill, Arch. Hydrobiol. 79:36 (1977).
2. U. M. Cowgill, Appl. Spectrosc. 27:5 (1973).
3. U. M. Cowgill, Dev. Appl. Spectrosc. 10:331 (1972).
4. C. C. Sweeley, R. Bentley, M. Makita, and W. W. Wells, J. Am. Chem. Soc. 85:2497 (1963).
5. J. T. Edsall and J. Wyman, in:"Biophysical Chemistry," Academic Press, New York (1958).

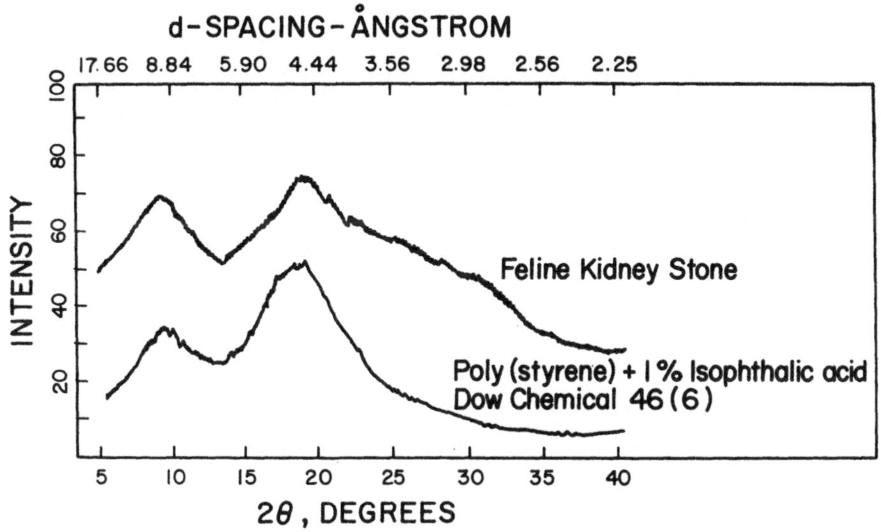

Figure 1. Diffractogram of a feline kidney stone and a pattern of poly(styrene) + 1% isophthalic acid (Dow Chemical Co. No. 46 (6)) added for comparison. Instrumental specifications are: scale factor 5000, time constant 2, 1° beam slit, scanning rate 2° 2 theta min^{-1}, chart speed 1 cm min^{-1}, final scale prior to reduction is 5° 2 theta per 2.54 cm.

6. J. W. Turley, in:"X-ray Diffraction Patterns of Polymers," The Dow Chemical Company, Midland (1965).
7. A. Serafini-Gracassini, F. M. Field, and B. Delf, in:"Elastin and Elastic Tissues," L. B. Sandberg, W. R. Gray, and C. Franzblau, eds., Plenum Press, New York (1977).
8. R. D. B. Fraser and T. P. MacRae, in:"Conformation in fibrous protein and related synthetic polypeptides," Academic Press, New York (1973).
9. J. Bommer, E. Ritz, W. Tschope, R. Waldherr, and M. Gebhardt, Kid. Int. 16:722 (1979).

ACKNOWLEDGMENTS

The author wants to thank the following people for their invaluable assistance in this study: Dr. David Morrow and Professor G. E. Hutchison (Yale University); Dr. M. J. Zagraniski (Wallingford, Ct); Dr. William Brown (Carnegie-Mellon University); Dr. R. Bentley, Dr. I. Campbell, Dr. F. Miller and Dr. I. R. McManus (University of Pittsburgh); Ms. D. Johnston (Langley Library, University of Pittsburgh); and Ms. M. Volk (Mellon Institute Library).

VI. RENAL AND GASTROINTESTINAL PHYSIOLOGY

THE EFFECTS OF CHLOROTHIAZIDE ON SODIUM, CALCIUM, AND MAGNESIUM TRANSPORT IN THE NEPHRON OF THE THYROPARATHYROIDECTOMIZED HAMSTER

John H. Dirks, Gary A. Quamme, and Norman L. M. Wong

Department of Medicine, W. Koerner Acute Care Unit,
University of British Columbia
Vancouver, British Columbia, Canada

The chronic administration of thiazide diuretics results in a marked reduction in urinary calcium excretion which has proved to be of major benefit to patients with recurrent renal calculi[1]. The acute administration of thiazide diuretics results in a smaller increase in urinary calcium than sodium excretion[1,2]. A number of renal and extrarenal factors have been implicated in explaining the chronic hypocalciuric action. First, thiazide diuretics have been shown in micropuncture studies to cause an increased sodium delivery from the distal tubule with little change in calcium delivery, implying a selective inhibition of distal sodium transport and possibly an increase in distal calcium reabsorption[3]. Second, thiazides may lead to depletion of extracellular fluid volume resulting in an enhanced proximal reabsorption of sodium and calcium and a reduced delivery of both ions to the more distal nephron segments where thiazides primarily inhibit sodium reabsorption. Urinary sodium excretion then returns to a control value while calcium excretion falls below control levels. Third, hypocalciuria may not readily develop in hypoparathyroid patients following thiazide administration and a role for parathyroid hormone has been implicated in the hypocalciuric action of thiazides[4,5]. A number of recent reports are relevant to these observations. Most important, Costanza and Windhager have demonstrated a direct effect of chlorothiazide on calcium transport in micropuncture studies of the distal tubule of the rat[6]. Thus, thiazides would appear to decrease sodium transport and increase calcium reabsorption in the distal convoluted tubule. Further evidence indicates that the acute dissociation of sodium from calcium reabsorption with chlorothiazide is independent of circulating parathyroid hormone implying different cellular mechanisms of these two agents on distal tubular function[7].

The effect of thiazide diuretics on urinary magnesium excretion is unclear[2]. Acute administration of chlorothiazide produces either no[2,7] or only modest increases in urinary magnesium excretion[8]. The effect of thiazides on segmental nephron reabsorption of magnesium romains Lo be evaluated. The present studies were directed at assessing the effects of chlorothiazide on calcium and magnesium reabsorption in the proximal and distal tubule. The golden hamster was used because of its unique, marked dependence on parathyroid hormone for renal calcium and magnesium conservation[9]. Acute removal of the parathyroid glands results in an increase in fractional urinary calcium excretion from 3% to 18% and in urinary magnesium excretion from 5% to 19%[10]. Thus, the effect of chlorothiazide on calcium and magnesium transport may be greater in magnitude and be more readily observed in the thyroparathyroidectomized hamster. The present micropuncture experiments demonstrate a direct enhancing effect on chlorothiazide in increasing calcium transport in the distal tubule while reducing sodium reabsorption and leaving magnesium transport unaffected.

METHODS

Clearance and recollection micropuncture experiments were performed by standard techniques on 21 hamsters. All animals were acutely thyroparathyroidectomized at least two hours prior to experimentation. Proximal and distal tubules were identified by injection of small amounts of 4% FD & C green dye into the jugular vein. The experiment consisted of a control phase of two consecutive thirty minute clearance periods during which tubular fluid was collected from late proximal and distal nephrons. Subsequently a priming dose of chlorothiazide (20 mg/kg body weight) followed by a sustaining infusion (20 mg/kg/hr) was administered for thirty minutes. The chlorothiazide (Merck Sharp & Dohme, Montreal as Hydrodiuril) was dissolved and administered in Ringer's solution. A second phase was undertaken which included clearance periods and recollection micropuncture from the same tubules.

Inulin concentrations in urine as determined by the method of Fuhr et al.[11] and in plasma and tubule fluid by the microfluorometric method of Vurek and Pegram[12]. Urine and plasma samples were analyzed for sodium and potassium by flame photometry (Corning 450, Corning Scientific Instruments Co., Medfield, MA, USA), and calcium and magnesium by atomic absorption spectrophotometry (Jarrell-Ash 850, Fisher Scientific Co., Montreal, Canada). Phosphate was determined by the colorimetric method of Chen et al.[13]. Tubule fluid Na, Cl, K, Mg, Ca and phosphorus were quantitated by electron microprobe analysis (Camebax, Cameca Instruments Inc., Stamford, CN, USA). Plasma ultrafiltrates were prepared using Amicon Centriflo ultrafiltration cones (Amicon Co., Lexington, MA, USA)[7].

RESULTS AND DISCUSSION

The urinary excretion data in control and chlorothiazide treatment phases in thyroparathyroidectomized hamsters is summarized in Table 1. Plasma sodium, calcium and magnesium concentrations were 150 mEq/l, 3.8 mEq/l, and 1.9 mEq/l respectively, and remained constant throughout the experiment. Glomerular filtration rate was 0.49 ml/min/100 gm body weight during the control periods and fell by 25% to 0.38 ml/min/100 gm body weight following chlorothiazide administration. This was presumably due to the diuretic per se as the GFR remained stable in a separate set of hamsters which served as time-controls. Urinary electrolyte excretion also remained constant in time-control hamsters. Fractional excretion rates in the thyroparathyroidectomized hamsters were 1%, 23% and 19% for sodium, calcium and magnesium respectively. Acute administration of chlorothiazide resulted in a significant increase in urinary sodium excretion from 1 to 3.4% and a significant fall in calcium excretion from 23 to 18% with no change in magnesium excretion (19 vs 18%).

Table 1. Effect of Chlorothiazide on Urinary Excretion in Thyroparathyroidectomized Hamsters

	GFR ml/min	FE_{H_2O} %	FE_{Na} %	FE_{Ca} %	FE_{Mg} %
Control	0.47±0.07	2.6±0.2	1.0±0.1	23±3	19±1
Chlorothiazide	0.33±0.06†	3.9±0.3	3.4±0.6†	18±2	20±1

FE is the fraction of the respective filtered H_2O and electrolyte appearing in the urine.

† significance ($p<0.01$) compared to control phase.

Table 2 gives the mean micropuncture data observed at the late proximal sampling site. Water reabsorption decreased about 10% following chlorothiazide as indicated by the significant fall in tubular fluid to plasma (TF/P) inulin ratio. The TF/P sodium, TF/UF calcium and TF/UF magnesium ratios remained constant; thus

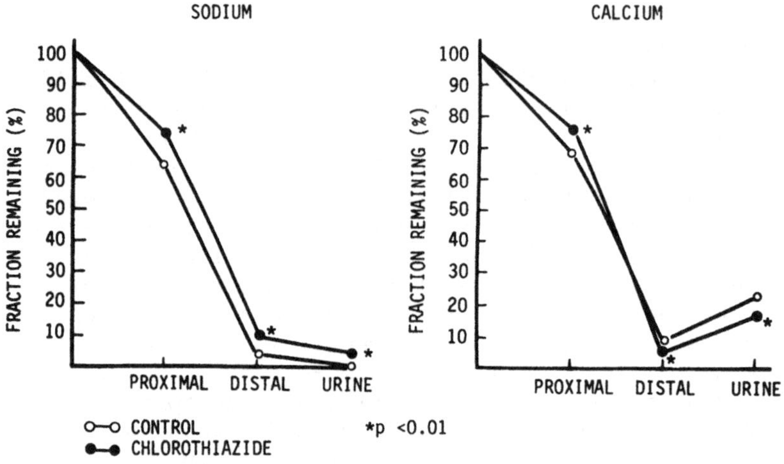

Figure 1. Effect of chlorothiazide on the fraction of sodium and calcium remaining along the nephron of thyroparathyroid-ectimized hamsters (see text for discussion).

there was a proportional decrease of about 10% in proximal reabsorption of each electrolyte which was delivered more distally. It is likely that these effects occur in the proximal tubule as a result of carbonic anhydrase inhibition by chlorothiazide[14]. The parallel relationship between calcium - magnesium reabsorption and sodium reabsorption in the proximal tubule was not disturbed with chlorothiazide.

Table 3 summarizes the effects of chlorothiazide on distal tubule function. TF/P sodium concentration ratio rose significantly (0.24 to 0.44) while TF/UF calcium concentration ratio fell (0.58 to 0.38) in the distal tubular fluid indicating a marked dissociation of sodium and calcium reabsorption. Overall fractional sodium reabsorption was inhibited by 6% while fractional calcium reabsorption was increased by 3%. Delivery of sodium and calcium to the distal tubule from the proximal tubule were high following chlorothiazide despite the significant fall in glomerular filtration rate; thus absolute reabsorption of calcium was significantly enhanced compared to control values. Chlorothiazide did not alter distal magnesium reabsorption as the fraction remaining at the distal tubule and final urine was unchanged. Figure 1 summarizes the effect of chlorothiazide on the fraction of filtered sodium and calcium remaining

Table 2. Effect of Chlorothiazide on Electrolyte Reabsorption in the Proximal Tubule

	TF/P_{In}	TF/P_{Na}	RF_{Na} %	TF/UF_{Ca} %	RF_{Ca} %	TF/UF_{Mg}	RF_{Mg} %
Control	1.73 ±0.13	1.02 ±0.01	65 ±4	1.20 ±0.07	68 ±3	1.38 ±0.09	78 ±4
Chlorothiazide	1.46† ±0.07	1.00 ±0.01	75* ±3	1.13 ±0.06	75* ±4	1.28 ±0.05	85† ±2

RF is the fraction of filtered load remaining at the late proximal sampling site.

* $p<0.05$ compared to control phase.

† $p<0.01$ compared to control phase.

at the various sampling sites. Difference in fractional calcium remaining in the early distal tubule and the urine suggest marked nephron heterogeneity for calcium reabsorption with less reabsorption in deeper nephrons.

In summary, the present study has demonstrated that chlorothiazide inhibits net sodium reabsorption and enhances net calcium reabsorption in the distal tubule reflecting marked dissociation of the sodium and calcium transport systems. This may be via distinctive effects on separate transport processes or through a common mechanism involving changes in luminal permeability and potential difference[15]. However, Costanza and Windhager, were unable to demonstrate a change in transepithelial potential difference with chlorothiazide[6]. The hypocalciuric effect of chlorothiazide occurred in the absence of circulating parathyroid hormone, confirming our previous studies. PTH would further increase the hypocalciuric effect presumably through a different mechanism. These experiments support the thesis that a direct enhancement of calcium reabsorption is a necessary component of the hypocalciuria of thiazide therapy which would be accentuated further by associated overall volume depletion due to the naturesis and by action of parathyroid hormone.

Table 3. Effect of Chlorothiazide on Electrolyte Reabsorption Within the Superficial Distal Tubule

	TF/P_{In}	TF/P_{Na}	RF_{Na} %	TF/UF_{Ca} %	RF_{Ca} %	TF/UF_{Mg}	RF_{Mg} %
Control	6.00 ±0.39	0.24 ±0.03	4.0 ±0.8	0.58 ±0.05	10.2 ±1.1	1.02 ±0.11	11.8 ±1.6
Chlorothiazide	5.01 ±0.45	0.44† ±0.04	10.0† ±1.4	0.38† ±0.06	7.6* ±1.2	0.83 ±0.10	9.9 ±1.4

RF is the fraction of filtered load remaining at the distal sampling site.

* $p<0.05$ compared to control phase.

† $p<0.01$ compared to control phase.

REFERENCES

1. E. R. Yendt, R. J. A. Gagne, and M. Cohanim, Am. J. Med. Sci. 251:449 (1966).
2. S. G. Massry, and J. W. Coburn, Nephron 10:66 (1973).
3. B. R. Edwards, P. C. Baer, R. A. L. Sutton, and J. H. Dirks, J. Clin. Invest. 52:2418 (1973).
4. A. S. Brickman, S. G. Massry, and J. W. Coburn, J. Clin. Invest. 51:945 (1972).
5. A. M. Parfitt, J. Clin. Invest. 51:1879 (1972).
6. L. S. Costanzo, and E. E. Winghager, Am. J. Physiol. 235:492 (1978).
7. G. A. Quamme, N. L. M. Wong, R. A. L. Sutton, and J. H. Dirks, Am. J. Physiol. 229:200 (1975).
8. G. Eknoyan, W. N. Suki, and M. Martinez-Maldonado, J. Lab. Clin. Med. 76:257 (1970).
9. D. M. Biddulph, P. F. Hirsch, C. W. Cooper, and P. L. Munson, Endocrinology 87:1346 (1970).
10. M. A. Burnatowska, C. A. Harris, R. A. L. Sutton, and J. H. Dirks, Am. J. Physiol. 233:514 (1977).
11. J. J. Fuhr, J. J. Kaczmarczyk, and C. D. Kruttgen, Klin. Wochenschr. 33:729 (1955).

12. G. G. Vurek, and S. E. Pegram, Anal. Biochem. 16:409 (1966).
13. P. S. Chen, Jr., T. Y. Toribara, and H. Warner, Anal. Chem. 28:1756 (1956).
14. K. H. Beyer, and J. E. Baer, Pharmacol. Rev. 13:517 (1961).
15. M. Walser, in:"Renal Pharmacology," J. W. Fischer, ed., Appleton-Century-Crafats, New York (1971).

ACKNOWLEDGMENT

This study was supported by grants from the Medical Research Council of Canada (MT-1915) to Dr. Dirks and from the British Columbia Health Care Research Foundation to Drs. Wong and Quamme.

INDOMETHACIN LOWERS URINARY CALCIUM EXCRETION IN NORMAL VOLUNTEERS AND NORMOCALCIURIC STONE-FORMERS

W. C. Carter, III, P. V. Halushka, D. Jones, B. Roof, S. N. Rous, and M. Spector

Departments of Urology, Pharmacology, Medicine and Biological and Physical Sciences, Medical University of South Carolina, Charleston, South Carolina

INTRODUCTION

Indomethacin, a non-steroidal anti-inflammatory agent, has been shown to alter calcium metabolism in patients with metastatic carcinoma. This study was designed to determine the effects of indomethacin on urinary calcium excretion in 20 normal volunteers and 8 patients with urolithiasis.

MATERIALS AND METHODS

The subjects were admitted to a metabolic unit and given a constant diet containing either 10, 109, or 259 mEq of sodium, 800 mg of calcium, 80 mEq of potassium, and 100 grams of protein per day. Serum and urinary calcium, sodium, and creatinine, and urinary cyclic AMP were measured during a control period (6 days), an indomethacin treatment period, (3 days of indomethacin, 75 mg per day; followed by 3 days of indomethacin, 150 mg per day), and a post-treatment period (4 days). Daily aliquots of the first voided a.m. urine were passed through a millipore filter into a negative pressure flask, and the filters were air dried and examined by light and scanning microscopy.

RESULTS

In normal volunteers on the 109 mEq sodium diet, indomethacin decreased urinary calcium excretion from 192 ± 28 mg/24 h to 166 ± 26 mg/24 h (N=9), ($p<.005$) on the first day of indomethacin treatment, and to 176 ± 27 mg/24 h ($p<.02$) for the entire 6 day indomethacin treatment period. Urinary sodium decreased from 101

± 5 mEq/24 h to 64 ± 5 mEq/24 h ($p<.001$) on the first day of indomethacin treatment and mean urinary sodium excretion for the entire treatment period was 86 ± 5 mEq/24 h (N.S.). Serum calcium was not significantly changed by indomethacin. On the 10 mEq sodium diet indomethacin decreased urinary calcium from 172 ± 29 mg/24 h to 152 ± 28 mg/24 h (N=8), ($p<.005$) on the first day of indomethacin treatment and to 153 ± 28 mg/24 h ($p<.02$) for the entire 6 day indomethacin treatment period. Urinary sodium excretion decreased from 3.3 ± 0.7 mg/24 h to 1.4 ± 0.3 mEq/24 h ($p<.05$) on the first day of indomethacin treatment, and mean sodium excretion for the entire treatment period was 2.0 ± 0.4 mEq/24 h (N.S.). In contrast, on the 259 mEq sodium diet, there was no significant change in the 24 hour urinary excretion of calcium during the indomethacin treatment period (N=9). Twenty-four hour urinary excretion of sodium, however, decreased from 247 ± 8 mEq/24 h to 203 ± 12 mEq/24 h (N=9), ($p<.025$), on the first day of indomethacin treatment. Serum calcium decreased from 9.6 ± 0.1 mg/dl to 9.4 ± 0.1 mg/dl ($p<.02$). In all three protocol groups, (10, 109, and 259 mEq sodium diets) indomethacin had no discernible effect on the amount of crystalluria during the treatment period. As would be expected, the amount of crystalluria in these normal volunteers with no history of stone disease was minimal. In normocalciuric (<300 mg urinary calcium per day), stone-formers on a 109 mEq sodium diet, indomethacin decreased urinary calcium excretion from 229 ± 27 mg/24 h to 175 ± 74 mg/24 h ($p<.05$) on the first day of indomethacin treatment and remained depressed during the entire indomethacin treatment period (188 ± 29 mg/24 h, $p<.005$), (N=5). Urinary sodium excretion decreased from 128 ± 17 mEq/24 h to 76 ± 23 mEq/24 h ($p<.02$) on the first day of indomethacin treatment, but the mean for the entire treatment period was unchanged (103 ± 9 mEq/24 h). In hypercalciuric (>300 mg urinary calcium per day) stone formers, indomethacin produced no significant change in 24 hour urinary excretion of calcium or sodium (N=3). Although the amount of crystalluria seen in the stone-formers was greater than observed in the normal volunteers, indomethacin had no effect on the excretion of calcium crystals during the treatment period. Indomethacin did not significantly alter endogenous creatinine clearance or urinary cyclic AMP in the stone formers or in the normal volunteers on any of the 3 sodium diets.

SUMMARY AND CONCLUSIONS

In summary, indomethacin decreased urinary calcium excretion in normal subjects on a normal or low sodium diet but not on a high sodium diet. Also, indomethacin decreased urinary calcium excretion in normocalciuric but not in hypercalciuric stone formers. We conclude that indomethacin decreases urinary calcium excretion by an as yet unknown mechanism that may be independent of changes in urinary sodium excretion. Furthermore, there may be an inherent difference between normocalciuric and hypercalciuric stone formers that can be unmasked by administration with indomethacin.

ON THE MECHANISM OF ACTION OF $1,25(OH)_2D_3$ IN THE INTESTINE

Howard Rasmussen, Olivier Fontaine, Toshio Matsumoto,
and David B. P. Goodman
Department of Internal Medicine
Yale University
New Haven, CT 06510, U.S.A.

One of the major effects of 1,25 dihydroxyvitamin D_3 on the small intestine is that of increasing the transcellular transport of calcium across the mucosal cells[1,2]. Physiological data indicate that a major cellular site of action of this hormone is at the luminal or brush border membrane where it increases the rate of entry of calcium into the cell[3]. In an effort to gain an insight into the biochemical and molecular basis of this specific cellular effect of $1,25(OH)_2D_3$, we have developed a method for preparing small osmotically-intact membrane vesicles from the brush border membranes of chick duodenal mucosal cells[4].

Using these vesicles, we demonstrated that, as predicted, the rate of calcium uptake into vesicles from D-deficient chicks was slower than that into vesicles from chicks treated several hours previously with $1,25(OH)_2D_3$[5]. In both types of vesicles, calcium uptake was a passive process which displayed saturation kinetics indicating that it was carrier-mediated, presumably by a transmembrane protein. The effect of $1,25(OH)_2D_3$ treatment was that of increasing the V_{max} of the process without altering the apparent K_m nor the calcium-binding to the membrane. Such a result indicates that $1,25(OH)_2D_3$ caused either an increase in the number of calcium carriers, or an increase in the rate of turnover of a fixed number of carriers.

Although the first alternative appeared the more attractive, the work of Bikle and associates[6] had shown that the effect of $1,25(OH)_2D_3$ on transcellular calcium transport in the chick duodenum was expressed even in a chick pretreated with cycloheximide, an inhibitor of protein synthesis. We repeated these experiments and obtained similar results. In addition, we found that even when chicks were pretreated with a dose of cycloheximide sufficient to cause an inhibition of the incorporation of labeled amino acids into brush border membrane proteins, there was nevertheless an increase in the calcium permeability of the membrane after $1,25(OH)_2D_3$ administration[7].

This result indicated that de novo synthesis of new membrane protein was not the mechanism by which $1,25(OH)_2D_3$ acted. One of several alternatives was considered, either: 1) a protein already existing in the cytoplasm was incorporated into the membrane after $1,25(OH)_2D_3$ treatment; 2) a covalent modification of a preexisting membrane protein, e.g., phosphorylation, was responsible for the change in calcium permeability; or 3) the hormone had a primary effect upon the lipid rather than the protein structure of the membrane.

At present there is no evidence to support either of the first two possibilities, but considerable evidence in support of the third. The first evidence suggesting that lipids might play a role in regulating calcium transport in the intestine was the demonstration by Adams, Wong and Norman[8] that the polyene antibiotic, filipin, stimulated calcium transport in the intestine when added to the solution bathing the luminal surface of the mucosal cells.

These experiments led us to examine the effect of filipin on calcium transport in the isolated membrane vesicles. We found that addition of filipin to vesicles from D-deficient animals led to an increase in rate of calcium entry, but had no effect on this rate in vesicles from $1,25(OH)_2D_3$-treated animals[5].

Our further work has followed two different lines of investigation: 1) a study of the effect of $1,25(OH)_2D_3$ on lipid metabolism in the intestinal mucosal cell and brush border membrane; and 2) an evaluation of the effect of agents that alter the fluidity of membrane lipids upon calcium transport in the two types of vesicles.

The first type of study has led to the following discoveries: 1) after $1,25(OH)_2D_3$ treatment there is an increase in the phosphatidylcholine (PC) and a decrease in the phosphatidylethanolamine (PE) content of the brush border membrane (unpublished); 2) the changes in PC and PE content are due to changes in the rates of synthesis of these two phospholipids (unpublished); 3) there is a close correlation between the change in PC/PE ratio and the change in calcium transport; 4) the fatty acid composition of the PC fraction of the brush border membrane is altered so that the weight percentage of polyunsaturated fatty acids increases; and 5) this change in the fatty acid composition of the PC fraction is caused by an activation of a deacylation-reacylation cycle in the BBM catalyzed by phospholipase A_2 and lysophosphatidylcholine acyltransferase[9] (and unpublished). Furthermore, the change in the PC/PE is observed in cycloheximide pretreated animals. These results are all consistent with the hypothesis that the primary effect of $1,25(OH)_2D_3$ on the brush border membrane is to induce a change in its PC content, and in the fatty acid content of this PC. Furthermore, these changes in lipid structure appear to be responsible for the changes in the behavior of the calcium transport system in the membrane. This hypothesis would mean that primary changes in lipid structure would determine the behavior of specific membrane proteins. We have suggested that this type of regulation be designated liponomic control of membrane and cell function to indicate that lipids are responsible for directing the function of the protein.

In an effort to obtain independent evidence for liponomic regulation of calcium transport in brush border membranes, we have examined the effects of methyl cis-vaccenic acid (M-CVA) and methyl trans-vaccenic acid (M-TVA) on calcium uptake into vesicles from D-deficient and from $1,25(OH)_2D_3$ treated chicks. Work by others[10,11] had shown that CVA acted to increase and TVA to decrease membrane fluidity. However, because the free fatty acids bind calcium, we employed the methyl esters of these fatty acids[12]. Incubation of membrane vesicles from D-deficient chicks with methyl CVA caused an increase in rate of calcium uptake into these vesicles so that they now behaved like the vesicles from the +D animal. However, M-CVA had no effect on calcium uptake into vesicles from $1,25(OH)_2D_3$-treated chicks. Conversely, M-TVA caused a decrease in rate of calcium transport into vesicles from $1,25(OH)_2D_3$-treated chicks, but not in those from D-deficient controls, i.e., it appeared to convert a +D into a -D vesicle in terms of calcium permeability.

These results supplemented those from the lipid turnover studies and showed that by altering the fluidity of the brush border membrane lipids one can switch the calcium transport system into either a -D or +D configuration. The effect is specific for the calcium transport system because addition of M-CVA and M-TVA to the vesicles had no effect upon Na^+-dependent glucose transport.

Our present evidence indicates that a primary biochemical effect of $1,25(OH)_2D_3$ in the intestinal mucosal cell is to alter the lipid composition of the brush border membrane. The evidence is also consistent with the hypothesis that this biochemical change is responsible for the change in rate of calcium transport across this membrane. Aside from its intrinsic interest to the problem of $1,25(OH)_2D_3$ action, this model of hormone action has far reaching implications. It is likely that other hormones exert their cellular effects by altering membrane lipid structure and thereby altering membrane protein function. Such liponomic control of membrane protein function is likely to be an important means by which the metabolic activities of cells are regulated.

REFERENCES

1. Y. Tanaka, H. F. DeLuca, J. Omdahl, and M. F. Holick, Proc. Nat. Acad. Sci. USA 68:1286 (1971).
2. M. R. Haussler, J. E. Zerwekh, R. H. Hesse, E. Rizzardo, and M. M. Pechet, Proc. Nat. Acad. Sci. USA 70:2248 (1973).
3. M. J. Melancon, Jr., and H. F. DeLuca, Biochem. 9:1658 (1970).
4. E. E. Max, D. B. P. Goodman, and H. Rasmussen, Biochem. Biophys. Acta. 511:224 (1978).
5. H. Rasmussen, O. Fontaine, E. E. Max, and D. B. P. Goodman, J. Biol. Chem. 254:2993 (1979).
6. D. D. Bikle, D. T. Zolock, R. L. Morrissey, and R. H. Herman, J. Biol. Chem. 253:484 (1978).
7. O. Fontaine, T. Matsumoto, M. Simionescu, H. Rasmussen, and D. B. P. Goodman, in:"Vitamin D. Basic Research and Its Clinical Application," A. W. Norman, ed., Walter de Gruyter, Berlin-New York (1979).
8. T. H. Adams, R. G. Wong, and A. W. Norman, J. Biol. Chem. 245:4432 (1970).
9. P. J. A. O'Doherty, Lipids 14:75 (1979).
10. P. F. Pilch, P. A. Thompson, and M. P. Czech, Proc. Nat. Acad. Sci. USA 77:915 (1980).
11. J. Orly, and M. Schramm, Proc. Nat. Acad. Sci. USA 72:3433 (1975).
12. O. Fontaine, T. Matsumoto, D. B. P. Goodman, and H. Rasmussen, (in press).

ACKNOWLEDGMENT

This work was supported by grant AM-19813 from the National Institute of Health of the United States Public Health Service.

The authors wish to thank Ms. Anita See for helpful secretarial and administration assistance.

LOW PHOSPHATE DIET IN RATS:

A MODEL FOR CALCIUM OXALATE UROLITHIASIS

P. G. Werness, F. G. Knox, and L. H. Smith

Mayo Clinic

Rochester, Minnesota 55901

Rats fed low phosphate diet show a marked hypercalciuria. We have shown previously that one week of low phosphate diet in rats results in urine highly supersaturated with respect to calcium oxalate with large amounts of calcium oxalate crystalluria, predominantly calcium oxalate dihydrate[1]. We have extended these studies to ten months and examined kidney tissue to evaluate the suitability of rats fed low phosphate diet as a long-term model for calcium oxalate urolithiasis.

Two groups of 12 male Sprague-Dawley rats, 150-200 g body weight, were placed on diets based on ICN Nutritional Biochemicals Low Phosphorus Diet. The base diet contains less than 0.07% phosphorus and is synthetic and oxalate free. The diet for the first group (NP) was a normal phosphate diet consisting of the base diet supplemented with a neutral mixture of sodium and potassium phosphate to 0.7% phosphorus and with oxalic acid (90 mg oxalate per μg body weight) to normal levels. The diet for the second group (LP) was a low phosphate diet consisting of the base diet supplemented with sodium and potassium chloride and oxalic acid to the same levels of sodium, potassium and oxalate as the normal phosphate diet. Rats were housed in stainless steel metabolism cages and for each group two 24-hour urines were collected under toluene after 6 months on their respective diets. Each urine was analyzed for sodium, potassium, calcium, magnesium, citrate, phosphorus, chloride, sulfate, oxalate, creatinine, protein, ammonia, uric acid, and pH. These values were used as inputs to an iterative computer program which takes into account ionic strength, pH and complexation to calculate free ion activities and activity products. Both groups of rats were judged to have normal kidney function based on their ability to concentrate urine when deprived of water.

Differences between the normal and low phosphate groups are shown in Table 1. A supersaturation (S.S.) of zero indicates a urine which is saturated, negative numbers indicate a urine which is undersaturated and positive numbers indicate a supersaturated urine, that is, a urine that can promote crystal and stone growth. Rats fed low phosphate diet have urine highly supersaturated with respect to calcium oxalate and are at risk for stone formation. Figure 1 shows typical crystals separated from the urine of rats fed low phosphate diet. Crystals were obtained in separate experiments by vacuum filtration of 2 ml freshly voided urine through a 0.22 μ Nuclepore filter[2]. These crystals are calcium oxalate dihydrate and are the most common crystals seen in rats fed low phosphate diet. Rats fed the normal phosphate diet rarely had crystals in their urine.

Table 1.

Urine Values (S.E.)	NP	LP	P
n	11	10	
Total Ca, mM	0.36 (.02)	17 (2.)	<.001
Free Ca, mM	0.09 (.01)	13 (1.)	<.001
Total PO_4, mM	37 (4.)	0.27 (0.02)	<.001
Free PO_4, mM	26 (2.)	0.087 (.007)	<.001
Total C_2O_4, mM	1.0 (.1)	0.31 (.03)	<.001
Free C_2O_4, mM	0.63 (.06)	0.058 (.006)	<.001
$CaHPO_4$ S.S.	-0.09 (.11)	-0.57 (.05)	<.005
CaC_2O_4 S.S.	0.34 (.18)	16 (2.)	<.001

The rats were sacrificed after 10 months on their respective diets and the kidneys examined for evidence of calcification and stones by light microscopy, petrographic microscopy, and scanning electron microscopy with energy dispersive x-ray analysis and single element napping. No calcium deposits were found in the renal medulla or papilla and kidney tissue calcium and oxalate concentrations were not different in the two groups. The only deposits of calcium observed were microstones of calcium oxalate found in the pelvis of the kidney in 6 out of 10 rats fed low phosphate diet. No stones were observed in the rats fed normal phosphate diet. Figure two is a scanning electron micrograph of a typical calcium oxalate microstone from rats fed low phosphate diet for 10 months. The horizontal line at the bottom of the figure represents 100 μm. Figure 3 shows a higher magnification view of the interior crystalline structure of the microstone. The horizontal bar represents 10 μm.

Rats chronically fed low phosphate diet show several features seen in some human stone forming patients. They have normal kidney

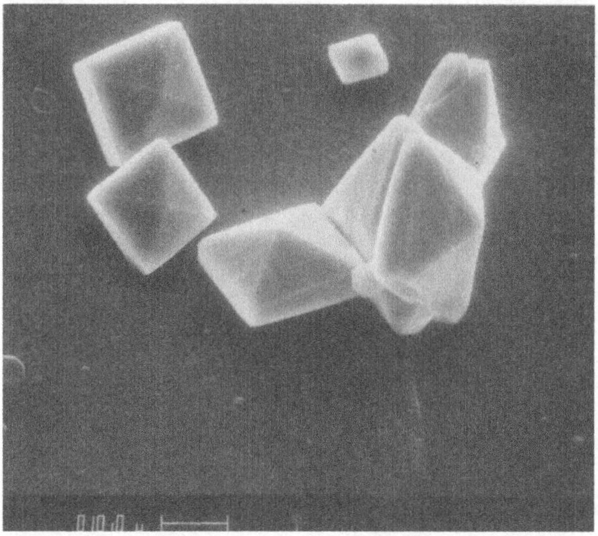

Figure 1. Calcium oxalate dihydrate crystalluria.

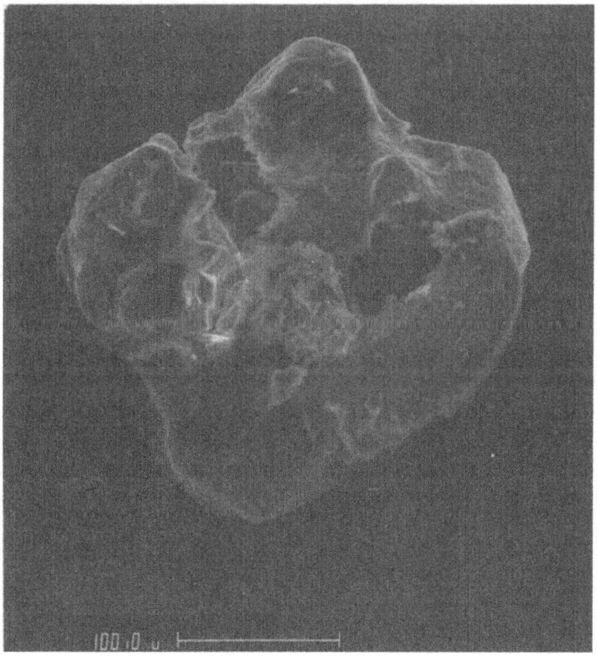

Figure 2. Calcium oxalate microstone.

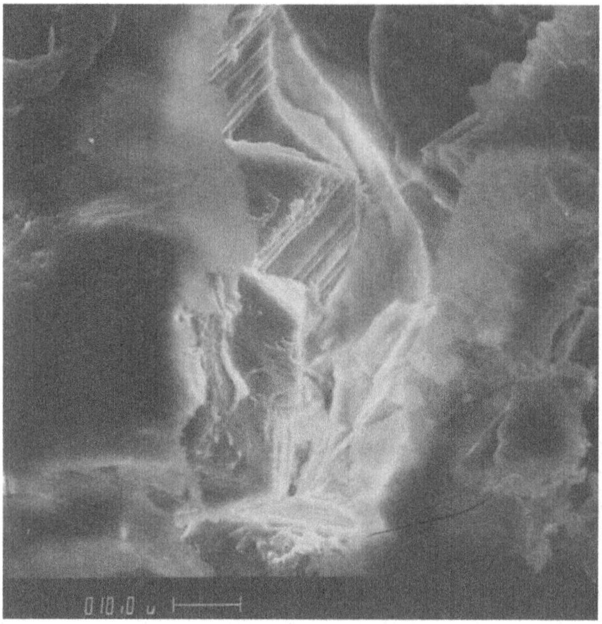

Figure 3. Calcium oxalate microstone, detail.

function, hypercalciuria, no parenchymal calcification, and calcium oxalate crystalluria. Rats fed low phosphate diet may serve as a useful model for the study of calcium oxalate urolithiasis. Urolithiasis in humans is a chronic condition, and an attractive feature of the low phosphate model is that it is well tolerated by rats; and, unlike many other models of stone formation, is suitable for long term studies. Since only 60% of the rats form stones, the model can be used to study the effects of dietary factors, drugs, and other maneuvers which either prevent or promote stone formation.

REFERENCES

1. P. G. Werness, P. H. Lee, T. J. Berndt, F. G. Knox, and L. H. Smith, Clin. Res. 27:710A (1979).
2. C. J. Van Den Berg, T. M. Cahill, and L. H. Smith, in: "Urolithiasis Research," H. Fleisch, W. G. Robertson, L. H. Smith, and W. Vahlensieck, eds., Plenum Press, New York (1976).

ACKNOWLEDGMENTS

This investigation was supported in part by research grant AM 20605 from the National Institutes of Health, Public Health Service and by a grant from the Calorie Control Council.

INTRACELLULAR MECHANISMS UNDERLYING THE PHOSPHATURIC RESPONSE TO PARATHYROID HORMONE IN THE HAMSTER

Theresa Berndt, Stanislaw Czekalski, Marcine Onsgard,
Anek Hoppe and Franklyn G. Knox
Department of Physiology and Biophysics
Mayo Clinic and Foundation
Rochester, MN 55901

INTRODUCTION

We previously reported the lack of a significant phosphaturic effect of parathyroid hormone (PTH) in the fasted hamster[1]. This response was in marked contrast to the fed hamster which is normally responsive to the phosphaturic effect of PTH[2-4]. The refractoriness to the phosphaturic effect of PTH in the fasted hamster was abolished by ammonium chloride infusions[1,3]. Additional studies showed that the ammonium ion itself, rather than the acute acidemia, is responsible for the restoration of the phosphaturic response to PTH[5]. In the present studies we evaluated the role of fasting induced changes in renal ammoniagenesis and metabolism in the resistance to the phosphaturic effect of PTH.

METHODS

To evaluate the effect of overnight fasting on urinary ammonia excretion, metabolic studies were performed in intact fed (n = 6) and fasted (n = 6) hamsters. A control 24 hour urine collection was obtained under oil in all animals and food was removed from one group of hamsters and urine collected from both groups of animals the next day.

To assess changes in renal metabolism during fasting, fed (n = 3) and fasted (n = 3) hamsters were anesthetized and their kidneys removed and snap frozen for determination of nicotine-adenine dinucleotide (NAD) levels in the renal cortical tissue.

In subsequent clearance studies we evaluated the effect of nicotinamide pretreatment, known to increase renal NAD levels,[6,7,8] on the resistance to the phosphaturic effect of PTH (33 U/kg + 1 U/kg/min) in the fasted hamster (n = 6). Clearance studies were performed on male hamsters weighing 80 - 135 grams and maintained on standard rat diet containing 0.9% phosphorus which was withheld sixteen hours before the experiment. Nicotinamide (1 g/kg, i.p.) was administered two hours before anesthesia. Hamsters were anesthetized with Inactin (100 mg/kg) and thyroparathyroidectomized (TPTX) two hours before clearance studies. Blood pCO_2 was maintained in the normocapnic range during the course of the experiment.

The analytical techniques for calcium, phosphate, sodium and inulin determination have been previously described[1]. Creatinine was measured by the Jaffe reaction and titratable acidity and ammonia in the urine were measured immediately after urine collection by the method of Siggard-Andersen[9].

Acidic and alkaline extracts of snap frozen cortical tissue for the determination of oxidized (NAD^+) and reduced (NADH) form of nicotine-adenine dinucleotide were prepared by the methods described by Klingenberg[10]. The results are presented as means ± 1 SE. Statistical comparison was made using Student's t-test for paired data.

RESULTS

The effect of overnight fasting on urinary phosphate, ammonia and titratable acidity are shown in Table 1. A period of 16 hour fasting significantly decreased phosphate, ammonia and titratable excretion.

Renal cortical NAD levels in the fed and fasted state are shown in Table 2. Overnight fasting in the hamster resulted in a significant decrease in the NAD^+/NADH ratio.

Nicotinamide pretreatment increased the NAD^+/NADH ratio to 9.0 ±5 in the renal cortical tissue and elevated basal fractional excretion of phosphate from 19±2 to 39±3% (FE_p). Following the addition of PTH, FE_p was 44±3%. Blood pressure, glomerular filtration rate and acid-base status remained stable throughout the experiment. Fractional excretion of sodium (FE_{Na}) was unchanged. Fractional excretion of calcium FE_{Ca} decreased from 19±5 to 8±1% following PTH. Plasma phosphate and calcium both increased slightly but significantly after PTH from 0.8±.08 to 1.1±0.1 mM and from 0.7±.04 to 1.1±.07 mM respectively.

Table 1. Effect of Fasting on Urinary Phosphate and Ammonia Excretions in Hamsters

Values are expressed in μmoles/mg creatinine mean ± 1 SE

	ANIMAL GROUP	CONTROL DAY	FAST DAY	P
Phosphate	Control	306±14	397±16	NS
	Fast	288±11	165±8	<0.001
Ammonia	Control	141±10	172±14	NS
	Fast	134±14	94±11	<0.05
Titratable Acidity	Control	116±11	171±15	<0.02
	Fast	105±7	-2±9	<0.001

Control animals received food on both the control and fast day, whereas fasting animals received food only on the control day.

Table 2. Renal Cortical NAD^+/NADH Levels in the Hamster

	NAD^+ (nmol/g wet weight)	NADH (nmol/g wet weight)	NAD^+/NADH ratio
FED (n = 3)	689.6 ±31.3	131.3 ±33.7	6.3 ±2.0
FASTED, 16 h (n = 3)	584.0* ±15.7	247.9* ±18.3	2.4* ±0.2

*p<0.05; significantly different from fed state.

DISCUSSION

Fasted hamsters show a blunted phosphaturic response to PTH as compared to fed hamsters and other species[1-5]. The hypocalciuric effect of PTH remains in all groups. Thus, the resistance to the effect of PTH is specific for phosphate transport.

As we previously reported[1], ammonium chloride infusions significantly enhanced the phosphaturic response to PTH in the fasted hamster. This effect was not due to acute extracellular acidosis since metabolic acidosis, achieved by hydrochloric acid infusion did not enhance the responsiveness[5]. Ammonium bicarbonate, on the other hand, which does not cause extracellular acidosis, enhanced the phosphaturic response to PTH[5].

Phosphate depletion induced by fasting may be another factor responsible for the resistance to the phosphaturic effect of PTH. Harris and Seely reported that phosphate infusions restored the phosphaturic effect of PTH in fasted hamsters[3]. In earlier balance studies we compared the effect of fasting and low phosphate diet in hamsters[11]. In the first 24 hours there was a fall in phosphate and hydrogen ion excretions and an increase in calcium and magnesium excretions in both groups. Although the pattern of response was similar between the two groups, the decreases in phosphate and hydrogen ion excretions and increases in calcium and magnesium excretions were significantly greater in the low phosphate group. Further, the changes in electrolyte excretion were transient in the fasting group, whereas they persisted in the low phosphate group. Thus, the baseline fractional excretion of phosphate was considerably higher in the fasted hamsters than in hamsters on a low phosphorus diet.

Rats fed a low phosphate diet are resistant to the phosphaturic effect of PTH, suggesting a resemblance between the fasted hamster and the phosphate depleted rat[12]. Beck[13] reported that the phosphaturic response to PTH could be partially restored in the phosphate depleted rat by administration of NH_4Cl in the drinking water for two days, again suggesting a similarity between fasted hamsters and phosphate depleted rats and a possible role of ammonium salts in the mediation of this phenomenon. Mechanisms other than simply phosphate depletion are probably operative in fasting; however, a role for intracellular phosphate depletion remains a consideration.

Borer, et al.[14], reported that by 8 hours of fast in the hamster, blood metabolites are indicative of mobilization of body fat. The mobilization of free fatty acids and their diversion to ketogenesis result in high levels of free fatty acids and ketones in the blood, while glucose levels were not significantly altered. Harris and Seely concluded that the decrease in circulating insulin levels presumably present in the fasting hamster are probably not responsible for the resistance to the phosphaturic effect of PTH[3]. It has also been reported from both in vivo[15] and in vitro[16] studies that high levels of ketones inhibit ammoniagenesis. In our balance studies, urinary ammonia excretion was reduced by one day of fasting, and in our clearance studies, responsiveness to PTH in the fasted hamster was enhanced by ammonium infusion, perhaps by replacing ammonia that had been suppressed by elevated ketone levels. The mechanism whereby ammonium may be affecting the phosphaturic response to PTH in the fasted hamster remains unknown. The initial steps in the cellular action of PTH in the kidney, stimulation of adenylate cyclase, an accumulation of cAMP in the renal cortex, and activation of protein kinase, were intact in the fasted hamster[1]. Therefore, ammonium is most likely acting upon a PTH-sensitive phosphate transport step subsequent to cAMP generation and protein kinase activation.

The studies of Lemieux et al.[17] have demonstrated that the inhibition of ammoniagenesis is mediated by increases in the oxidation of free fatty acids and ketone bodies within the tricarboxylic acid cycle of the mitochondria and subsequent decrease in the NAD^+/NADH ratio within the renal tubular cell. Our finding of decreased renal cortical NAD^+ and increased NADH levels in the fasted compared to the fed hamsters supports the hypothesis that the increases in oxidation of free fatty acids and ketone bodies decreases the NAD^+/NADH ratio in the renal cortex.

The administration of nicotinamide, a metabolic precursor of NAD, increased the NAD^+/NADH ratio in the renal cortex of the fasted hamster and markedly increased basal FE_p. Kempson et al. have proposed a role for NAD^+ as an intracellular mediator in the regulation of phosphate transport[18]. Additional studies in our laboratory have demonstrated a restoration of the phosphaturic response to PTH in rats fed a low phosphorus diet after nicotinamide treatment[19], implicating a role for NAD^+ as an intracellular mediator in the hormonal regulation of phosphate.

We conclude that the mechanism for the restoration of the phosphaturic response to PTH may be linked to changes in ammoniagenesis, is reversible by either ammonium ion infusion or nicotinamide administration, and is regulated by NAD^+/NADH levels within the kidney.

REFERENCES

1. F. G. Knox, J. Preiss, J. K. Kim, and T. P. Dousa, J. Clin. Invcot. 59:675 (1977).
2. M. A. Burnatowska, C. A. Harris, R. A. L. Sutton, and J. H. Dirks, Am. J. Physiol. 233:F514 (1977).
3. C. A. Harris and J. F. Seely, Am. J. Physiol. 237:F175 (1979).
4. C. A. Harris, M. A. Burnatowska, J. F. Seely, R. A. L. Sutton, G. A. Quamme, and J. H. Dirks, Am. J. Physiol. 236:F342 (1979).
5. A. Hoppe, F. M. Destro, and F. G. Knox, Am. J. Physiol. (in press - 1980).
6. R. L. Blake and E. Kun, Methods Enzymol. 18:113 (1971).
7. N. O. Kaplan, A. Goldin, S. R. Humphreys, M. M. Ciotti, and F. E. Stolzenbach, J. Biol. Chem. 219:287 (1956).
8. H. G. Preuss, J. Lab. Clin. Med. 72:370 (1968).

9. O. Siggaard-Andersen, Ann. N. Y. Acad. of Sci. 133:41 (1966).
10. H. Klingenberg, in:"Methods of Enzyme Analysis," H. U. Bergmeyer, ed., Academic Press, New York, 2nd Edition, 4:2045 (1974).
11. A. Hoppe, J. L. Ziegler, and F. G. Knox, The Physiologist 21:56 (1978).
12. T. H. Steele, J. A. Underwood, B. A. Stromberg, and C. A. Larmore, J. Clin. Invest. 58:1461 (1976).
13. N. Beck, Clin. Res. 27:408A (1979).
14. K. T. Borer, N. Rowland, A. Mirow, R. C. Borer, and R. P. Kelch, Am. J. Physiol. 236:E103 (1979).
15. G. Lemieux, P. Viney, P. Robitaille, G. E. Plante, Y. Lussier, and P. Martin, J. Clin. Invest. 50:1781 (1971).
16. D. M. Roxe, G. E. Schreiner, and H. G. Preuss, Am. J. Physiol. 225:908 (1979).
17. G. Lemieux, G. Baverel, P. Viney, and A. Gougoux, Am. J. Physiol. 237:F7 (1979).
18. T. P. Dousa, S. A. Kempson, and L. Y. Ou, Am. Soc. for Pharmacol. and Exp. Ther. August, 1980 (abstract).
19. T. J. Berndt, F. G. Knox, S. A. Kempson, and T. P. Dousa, Am. Soc. for Pharmacol. and Exp. Ther. August, 1980 (abstract).

ACKNOWLEDGMENT

This work was supported by grants AM 19715 and AM 20605 from the National Institutes of Health.

ROLE OF NICOTINAMIDE ADENINE DINUCLEOTIDE (NAD) IN CONTROL OF PROXIMAL RENAL TUBULAR PHOSPHATE TRANSPORT

Thomas P. Dousa and Stephen A. Kempson

Mayo Clinic and Foundation

Rochester, MN 55901

The molecular mechanism whereby the rate of phosphate (Pi) is transported across the wall of the proximal tubule in response to hormones and metabolic or nutritional stimuli is not yet fully clarified. In recent years it became increasingly evident that the Na^+ gradient-dependent entry of Pi from the tubular lumen across luminal brush border membranes (BBM) of proximal tubules is important and perhaps a quantitatively limiting step in Pi reabsorption in proximal tubules[1].

While investigating the effects of inhibitors of alkaline phosphatase (AP) on the BBM transport processes[1], we recently observed that NAD inhibits specifically the Na^+-dependent BBM uptake of Pi[2]. *In vitro* addition of NAD, in both the oxidized form (NAD^+) and the reduced form (NADH), to BBM vesicles isolated from rat renal cortex caused a dose-dependent decrease in Na^+-dependent BBM uptake of ^{32}Pi[2]. Na^+-independent BBM uptake of Pi, Na^+-dependent as well as Na^+-independent uptake of D-glucose, or BBM uptake of $^{22}Na^+$ was not influenced by NAD. Nicotinamide (NiAm), a structural component of NAD[3], when added to BBM *in vitro*, did not inhibit BBM uptake to ^{32}Pi. We also observed that [^3H]-NAD binds on BBM and that this binding is not dependent on the presence of Na^+ gradient[4]. Head-inactivated BBM membranes did not bind NAD at all. This suggests that the interaction of NAD with BBM is not a simple uptake as that of amino acids, sugars or ions. These observations suggested to us that NAD, a nucleotide known mainly as a co-enzyme of dehydrogenase and which is abundant in cell cytoplasm[3], may regulate the BBM transport of Pi.

Subsequently we studied how changing NAD renal levels *in vivo* influences renal Pi excretion ($U_{Pi}V$) and BBM uptake of Pi. Rats were stabilized on a low Pi diet (0.07%) and then injected intraperitoneally with NiAm[4,5]. At the end of the experiments part of the kidney cortex was taken for preparation of BBM (for transport measurements) and another aliquot of renal cortex for determination of nucleotides. We found that an Na^+-dependent uptake of ^{32}Pi in BBM prepared from NiAm-treated rats was significantly decreased, but uptake of [^3H]-D-glucose and $^{22}Na^+$ was not changed[4,5]. Injection of NiAm elicited marked increase in renal cortical content of NAD^+, increase in the tissue NAD^+/NADH ratio but the levels of ATP or cyclic AMP were not changed[4,5]. BBM uptake of Pi was inversely correlated to the NAD^+ level and to NAD^+/NADH ratio in renal cortex. Injection of NiAm elicited a huge increase in $U_{Pi}V$ but no increase in urine flow or in urinary excretions of creatinine, K^+, Na^+ or Ca^+[4,5]. Increase in $U_{Pi}V$ after NiAm injection was inversely correlated with decrease in BBM uptake of Pi but not with other BBM transport processes[4,5]. Similar response to NiAm injection, in terms of BBM transport of Pi, renal cortical NAD^+ and increase in $U_{Pi}V$, was observed in normal rats and thyroparathyroidectomized (TPTX) rats.

Let us consider how NAD can serve as an intracellular modulator (inhibitor) of the Na^+-dependent transport of Pi in proximal tubules under physiological conditions (Figure 1). Considering which metabolic processes in the cell could change the levels of NAD^+ we deduced that gluconeogenesis (GNG) is most likely to change the NAD^+/NADH ratio in cytoplasm adjacent to BBM. It is most likely that only NAD^+ may serve as a BBM-regulating factor, since NADH is tightly bound on cellular proteins[3]. Free NAD^+ is much more abundant in cytoplasm than NADH[6].

In our recent experiments on the cortical slices we found that increase in the rate of GNG is accompanied by an increase in NAD^+, and that inhibition of GNG by specific inhibitors causes in parallel a decrease in NAD^+[7]. This provides direct evidence that the rate of GNG is associated with changes in NAD^+ content in kidney cortex. Considering which physiologic stimuli may influence GNG, and consequently NAD^+ and Pi transport, it is of note that parathyroid hormone (PTH) has been shown to stimulate the rate of renal GNG[8] as well as to inhibit BBM uptake of Pi[9]. In our recent experiments, in collaboration with Dr. F. G. Knox, we have observed that infusion of PTH to TPTX rats caused an increase in NAD^+/NADH ratio in renal cortex, along with increase $U_{Pi}V$[10].

Renal GNG is altered by various metabolic stimuli (Figure 1). Starvation[11], metabolic acidosis or administration of glucocorticoids [12] which are known stimuli of renal GNG may also increase $U_{Pi}V$. In our recent experiments, we observed that fasting[12] or glucocorticoids [13] caused phosphaturia and decrease in BBM uptake of Pi, suggesting that these phosphaturic responses are mediated by increased GNG and an increased NAD^+/NADH ratio. On the other hand, feeding a low Pi diet[14] or unilateral ureteral obstruction (UUO)[15] are known to

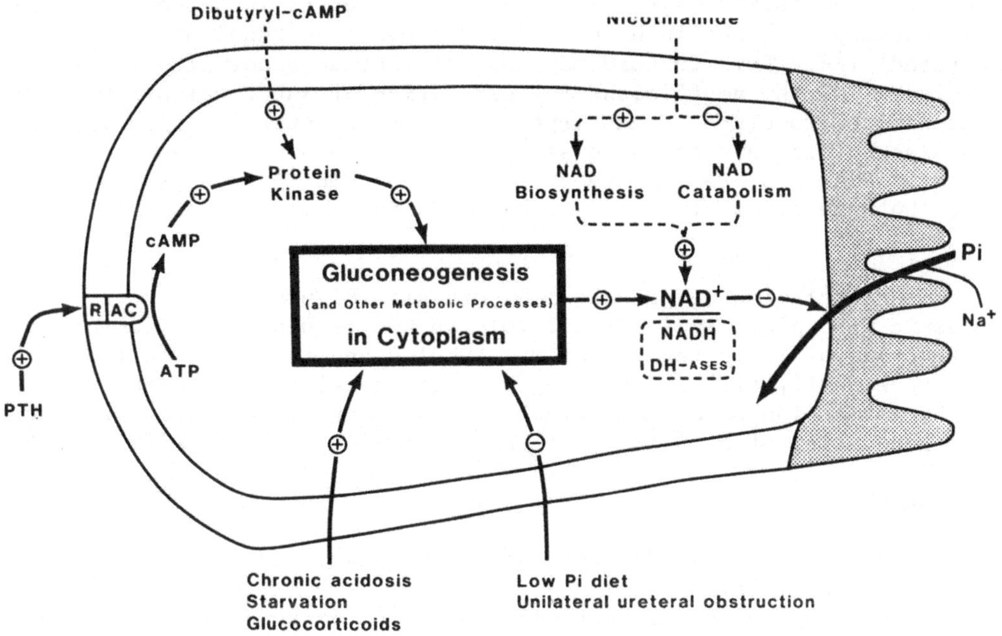

Figure 1. Outline of the proposed hypothesis on the role of cytoplasmic NAD^+ in regulation of Pi transport across BBM of the proximal tubule in response to various physiologic (⟶) or pharmacologic (----➤) phosphaturic stimuli. R, receptor for PTH; AC, adenylate cyclase; DH-ases, cytoplasmic dehydrogenases using NAD^+/NADH as co-enzyme system. ⊕ denotes increase or stimulation, ⊖ denotes decrease or inhibition. The prevailing form in cytoplasm is free NAD^+ since less NADH is present and NADH is bound tightly to DH-ases (denoted by interrupted circle). Increased cytoplasmic gluconeogenesis (GNG) causes an increase in NAD^+ and consequent inhibition of Na^+-dependent Pi uptake across the BBM from the tubular lumen. GNG may be enhanced by metabolic stimuli such as starvation and chronic acidosis by NH_4Cl loading or glucocorticoids; GNG may be depressed by low Pi diet or by unilateral ureteral obstruction. PTH *via* an increase in cAMP, by activation of protein kinase also enhances the rate of GNG and increases NAD^+/NADH ratio. Nicotinamide (NiAm) administration increases NAD by enhancing biosynthesis and by inhibiting NAD^+ breakdown, thereby bypasses all previous cellular steps which influence the NAD^+ level. Increased NAD^+ thus inhibits Pi transport across BBM regardless of the status of preceding cell metabolic and regulatory systems.

result in decreased $U_{Pi}V$, (in a large part due to increase in tubular Pi reabsorption) and in both of these conditions renal GNG is blunted[14,15]. This feature may suggest that an abnormally low rate of renal GNG is insufficient for generation of NAD^+, which results in uninhibited tubular Pi reabsorption. Such an interpretation may be consistent with our recent observation which shows that administration of NiAm restores the renal response to PTH in rats fed low Pi diet both in terms of increased $U_{Pi}V$ and increase in the $NAD^+/NADH$ ratio[10].

In conclusion we propose a hypothesis (Figure 1) that cytoplasmic NAD^+ plays an important role in the regulation of luminal BBM uptake of Pi in renal proximal tubules and that some (although not necessarily all) stimuli may regulate renal tubular handling of Pi by its action on GNG (or other metabolic processes) which increase the generation of NAD^+ in cytoplasm of proximal tubule cells.

REFERENCES

1. T. P. Dousa, S. A. Kempson, and S. V. Shah, Adv. Exp. Med. Biol. 128:69 (1980).
2. S. A. Kempson, D. M. Heublein, and T. P. Dousa, Clin. Res. 28:452A (1980).
3. A. White, P. Handler, E. L. Smith, R. L. Hill, and I. R. Lehman, in:"Principles of Biochemistry," McGraw-Hill Book Company, New York (1978).
4. S. A. Kempson, S.-Y. L. Ou, and T. P. Dousa, Kid. Int. 18:in press (1980).
5. S. A. Kempson, S.-Y. L. Ou, and T. P. Dousa, Clin. Res. 28:in press (1980).
6. R. Kirsten and E. Kirsten, Am. J. Physiol. 223:229 (1972).
7. S.-Y. L. Ou, S. A. Kempson, and T. P. Dousa, Clin. Res. 28:in press (1980).
8. H. Rasmussen, D. B. P. Goodman, N. Friedmann, N. E. Allen, and K. Kurokawa, in:"Handbook of Physiology," G. D. Aurbach, ed., American Physiology Society, Washington, D. C. (1976).
9. C. Evers, H. Murer, and R. Kinne, Biochem. J. 172:49 (1978).
10. T. J. Berndt, F. G. Knox, and T. P. Dousa, Kid. Int. 18:in press (1980).
11. S. A. Kempson, S. V. Shah, P. G. Werness, T. Berndt, P. H. Lee, L. H. Smith, F. G. Knox, and T. P. Dousa, Kid. Int. 18:36 (1980).
12. C. I. Pogson, I. D. Longshaw, A. Roobol, S. A. Smith, and G. A. O. Alleyne, in:"Gluconeogenesis: Its Regulation in Mammalian Species," R. W. Hanson and M. A. Mehlman, eds., John Wiley and Sons, New York (1976).
13. S. T. Turner, G. Colon-Otero, S. A. Kempson, and T. P. Dousa, Clin. Res. 29:in press (1981).

14. W. J. Kreusser, C. Descoeudres, Y. Oda, S. G. Massry, and K. Kurokawa, Mineral Electrolyte Metab. 3:312 (1980).
15. H. Nito, C. Descoeudres, K. Kurokawa, and S. G. Massry, J. Lab. Clin. Med. 91:60 (1978).

ACKNOWLEDGMENTS

This work was supported by USPHS grants AM 16105 and AM 19715, grant-in-aid and stipend from the Minnesota Heart Association and by the Mayo Foundation. We thank Ms. Bonnie Becker for excellent secretarial assistance.

THE INCIDENCE OF NEPHROCALCINOSIS AND THE URINARY EXCRETION OF CITRATE AND CALCIUM IN PATIENTS WITH NON-AZOTEMIC TYPE 4 RENAL TUBULAR ACIDOSIS

Elisabeth McSherry, Jay Gates, and Maria Pialaet

Department of Pediatrics and Medicine
University of California San Francisco
San Francisco, CA

INTRODUCTION

In infants and children with type 1 renal tubular acidosis (RTA) after chronic acidosis, short stature, stunting (height < 2.5 SD from mean for age- and sex- matched normals) and nephrocalcinosis occur [1-12]. Nephrocalcinosis is invariable by age 4 years in children with type I RTA who are maintained on low-dose alkali therapy (< 3 mEq/kg/d) since infancy[1-6]. Recently we have shown that nephrocalcinosis has not occurred over observation periods of 10-20 years in 7 children with type 1 RTA in whom sustained correction of acidosis with high dose alkali therapy (5-14 mEq/kg/d) was maintained since infancy[7-9]. In these children, we demonstrated that urinary excretion of citrate rose to normal values; whereas on low-dose alkali, < 3 mEq/kg/d, it remained subnormal[7-9]. Citrate is a chelator and complexor of urinary calcium and also, acts as an inhibitor of urinary crystal formation[13,14].

In children with non-azotemic, "early childhood," type 4 RTA, after chronic untreated acidosis, we reported height stunting occurred similar to that seen in children with type 1 RTA during low-dose alkali therapy or without treatment[15,16]. As in children with type 1 RTA, in children with type 4 RTA, the height stunting was reversible with sustained correction of acidosis with high-dose alkali therapy alone[15,16]. In the study reported here we evaluated the occurrence of nephrocalcinosis and nephrolithiasis in children with non-azotemic type 4 RTA after chronic acidosis had obtained of sufficient severity to result in short-stature or stunting. We also studied the effect of acidosis and its sustained correction on the urinary excretion of calcium and citrate in these children with non-azotemic type 4 RTA. Azotemia is known to reduce urinary citrate excretion[17,18]; these subjects represent a unique patient group in which to study the pathophysiologic characteristics of the renal tubular defect of type 4 RTA unassociated with the secondary effects of azotemia.

METHODS

Patient Group

Fourteen patients (9 boys and 5 girls), age 2 months to 4 years, were studied on the Pediatric Clinical Research Ward. Each had the findings of non-azotemic type 4 RTA: serum creatinine 0.8 mg%, and $K+ >4.8$ mEq/L, arterial plasma $[HCO_3^-]$ <21 mEq/L (child) <19 mEq/L (infant), hyperchloremia and, during acidosis, a urine pH of <6.0. Additionally in five children, a fixed, low fractional urinary excretion of K+ over a wide range of serum [K+] and $[HCO_3^-]p$ was demonstrated[7-9].

Five patients (4 boys and 1 girl) were members of 4 families in which the type 4 RTA defect occurred in 2 or more same-sexed members.

PROCEDURES

Radiologic Evaluation

All 14 children were radiographically evaluated with conical views of the kidneys, initially after longterm acidosis and again, at least 2-6 years after the longterm administration of alkali therapy.

Urinary Excretion of Citrate and Calcium

All studies were performed on the Pediatric Clinical Research Ward under metabolic conditions with diets of fixed intake of the minimal daily requirements of electrolytes, Ca, P, Mg, and of normal calories and protein content. In each patient, urinary excretion of calcium and citrate was measured when correction of acidosis was sustained with high-dose alkali therapy and during spontaneous or partially treated acidosis.

Correction of acidosis was considered sustained if the early morning fasting arterialized plasma bicarbonate concentration was 19-23 mEq/liter in infants; 24-28 mEq/liter in children. Blood was sampled before breakfast, and at least 4 hours after the last dose of alkali, for blood gases, total CO_2 content, and the concentrations of sodium, potassium, chloride, calcium, phosphorus, magnesium, creatinine and alkaline phosphatase.

Girls

In controlled metabolic studies of 5 girls during spontaneous acidosis (of >6 days <6 months) (5 studies) and during sustained correction of acidosis with alkali therapy (4 studies), urinary calcium, citrate and net base excretion as well as plasma bicarbonate and serum potassium concentrations were measured.

Boys

In controlled metabolic studies of 9 boys during spontaneous acidosis (9 studies) and during sustained correction of acidosis with alkali therapy (5 studies) measurements were made as for the girls.

Total Group

The findings in 23 studies of the 14 patients were compared with findings under similar study conditions in a group of children with non-azotemic type 1 RTA and a group of normal children in whom acidosis was induced by the experimental administration of 0.1 - 0.2 g/kg/d (=2-4 mEq/kg/d) NH_4Cl.

Laboratory determinations were done as previously described[5]. Urine citrate was determined by the citrate lyase method[19]. This method was further tested in our laboratory by measuring serial recoveries of known amounts of added citrate in urines from patients with type 1, 2, and 4 RTA and with uremia, and was found to be reliable and replicable.

Informed Consent

Both parents of each child studied were informed of the purpose, character and risks of the studies, specifically that during 24 hour urine collections with adhesive collection bags, adhesive burns could occur in infants and children not yet potty-trained. The investigators offered to assume continuing responsibility for the management of the child's illness, whether or not the patients gave consent for any of the studies proposed.

RESULTS

In Patients With Non-Azotemic Type 4 RTA

Radiologic Evaluation. In none of the 14 children aged 2 months to 4 years at the time of initial diagnosis of non-azotemic type 4 RTA was nephrocalcinosis or nephrolithiasis observed.

Over 1 to 10 years of observation in each of the 14 children, with a minimum of 1 year and maximum of 4 years of sustained alkali therapy, neither nephrocalcinosis nor nephrolithiasis was demonstrable.

In 5 patients with documented untreated or partially-treated acidosis until 2 to 4 years of age, urinary tract calcification was not radiologically demonstrable at initiation of corrective alkali therapy and has not become demonstrable at the patients current ages of 3-6 years.

Urinary Excretion of Citrate and Calcium.

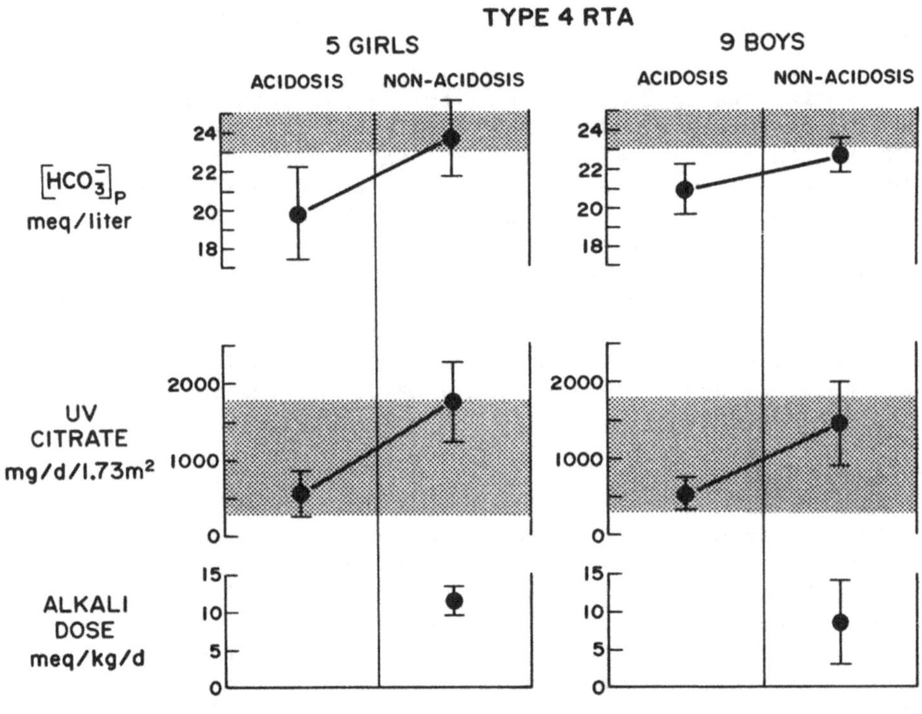

Figure 1. The relationship of urinary citrate excretion to plasma bicarbonate concentration in children with non-azotemic type 4 RTA: girls (left) and boys (right). Shaded areas represent the mean ± 2.5 SD for sex- and age- matched normal children. Normal values for U cit V derived[18,20,21,26-29].

Girls. In 5 studies, after chronic acidosis, urinary excretion of citrate was 559 ± 307 mg/d/1.73 M^2, calcium 1.5 ± 1.2 mg/kg/d. After sustained correction of acidosis with alkali therapy alone urinary excretion of citrate was 1742 ± 532 and calcium 1.9 ± 1.7.

Boys. In 9 studies during chronic acidosis, urinary excretion of citrate was 529 ± 196 mg/d/1.73 M^2, calcium 1.5 ± 1.2 mg/kg/d. After sustained correction of acidosis with alkali therapy alone urinary excretion of citrate was 1432 ± 550 and calcium 1.0 ± 0.2.

Total Group. In 14 patients, in 14 studies during chronic acidosis, mean urinary excretion of citrate was 540 ± 230 mg/d/1.73 M^2, calcium 1.7 ± 1.1 mg/kg/d. After sustained correction of acidosis with alkali therapy alone mean urinary excretion of citrate was 1572 ± 532, calcium 1.5 ± 1.3.

Compared to Other Subjects

These values for urinary excretion of calcium and citrate during acidosis in 4 normal children were 119 ± 72 mg/d/1.73 M^2 and 6.2 ± 3.0 mg/kg/d respectively; and in 4 children with type 1 RTA 192 ± 150 and 3.9 ± 2.0, respectively.

The urinary excretion of citrate was ~3-4 fold greater during acidosis in the children with type 4 RTA compared to the other 2 groups. During sustained correction of acidosis for the 4 normal children, citrate was 1051 ± 160 and calcium was 3.3 ± 1.8; and for the 4 children with type 1 RTA, 726 ± 460 mg/d/1.73 M^2 and calcium was 2.1 ± 1.1 mg/kg/d. During sustained correction of acidosis mean urinary citrate excretion for the patients with type 4 RTA was twice that of patients with type 1 RTA although both groups received approximately 9.5 mEq/kg alkali per day and had comparable urinary net base excretion (6 mEq/kg/d); and 1.5 times that of the normal children. During sustained correction of acidosis, urinary excretion of citrate rose at least 3 fold higher than the baseline value observed during acidosis in each of the 2 patient groups, as well as in the group of normal subjects receiving no alkali.

The Relationship of Serum Potassium Concentration to Urinary Citrate Excretion in Type 4 RTA Patients

During acidosis, the 12 children with type 4 RTA in whom $[HCO_3^-]$ was 22 mEq/L, serum K+ concentration did not positively correlate with urinary excretion of citrate; nor did it in studies of the 7 patients in whom sustained correction of acidosis $[HCO_3^-]p$ was >22.5.

In Comparison to 2 Control Groups: Type 1 RTA and Normal Children

Plasma $[HCO_3^-]$ did not differ significantly between the 3 subject groups during acidosis or after its correction. During sustained correction of acidosis the dose of alkali therapy and the magnitude of urinary net base excretion did not differ in the 2 groups of patients with either type 1 or 4 non-azotemic RTA. During acidosis, urinary excretion of calcium rose significantly in patients with type 1 RTA and in normal subjects: the urinary excretion of calcium during acidosis was significantly higher, ($p<0.02$) and ($p<.005$) respectively, in these 2 groups compared to that of patients with type 4 RTA. In the patients with type 4 RTA, urine calcium excretion was normal. During sustained correction of acidosis urinary calcium excretion was normal in all 3 subjects and no significant difference was present between any of the 3 groups.

DISCUSSION

The results of the present study indicate that radiologically demonstrable nephrocalcinosis and nephrolithiasis did not occur over 2-10 years observation in 14 children with non-azotemic type 4 RTA[15,16,20]. In 5 patients with type 4 RTA, despite chronic untreated acidosis documented for 2-4 years duration, radiologically demonstrable nephrocalcinosis did not occur. These findings are in direct contrast with observations in children with type 1 RTA given low-dose alkali (<3 mEq/kg/d) since infancy in whom nephrocalcinosis is invariable by age 4 years[1-6].

A predictable finding during acidosis, perhaps beneficial in the prevention of nephrocalcinosis in children with type 4 RTA, was that the urinary excretion of calcium did not rise and was significantly lower than that seen in acidotic children with type 1 RTA or in acidotic normal children[20].

A second predictable finding during acidosis, also of possible benefit in the prevention of nephrocalcinosis in the 14 children with non-azotemic type 4 RTA, was that the urinary excretion of citrate was above the lower limits of that characteristic for non-acidotic normal children[26]. This finding is in distinct contrast to findings in normal children experimentally-rendered acidotic with NH_4Cl[6,20,21], or in children with type 1 RTA[7-9,28]. In both groups citrate fell 2 fold to <200 during acidosis. During sustained correction of acidosis with alkali therapy alone, the urinary excretion of citrate in children with type 4 RTA rose 2 to 3 fold; at comparable values of plasma bicarbonate and serum potassium concentration, it was 1-2 fold higher than that observed in non-acidotic normal children or in children with type 1 RTA with sustained correction of acidosis who had equivalent daily alkali doses and magnitudes of urinary excretion of net base to the patients with type 4 RTA.

During acidosis in normal adults citrate is completely reabsorbed by the proximal and distal convoluted tubules and none appears in the urine[26-28]. During non-acidosis citrate is absorbed in large part but some is excreted in the urine[29,30].

Besides acidosis[31,32], a second factor known to reduce the excretion of citrate in the urine of non-azotemic subjects is hypokalemia[34-38]. In this study, serum potassium concentration did not correlate with urinary citrate excretion during acidosis or non-acidosis, within any of the 3 groups of subjects: patients with type 4 RTA and type 1 RTA or normals. Between the 3 groups, during acidosis serum K+ was higher, but not significantly, in patients with type 4 RTA than the other 2 groups. During sustained correction of acidosis no significant difference in serum K+ concentration between the 3 groups of patients was observed, yet the mean urinary excretion of citrate in the patients with type 4 RTA was 2-3 fold that of the other 2 groups.

In reported cases of proximal type 2 RTA and the Fanconi syndrome, a complex of multiple reabsorption dysfunctions of the proximal renal tubule, urinary citrate excretion is very high during untreated acidosis as well as during correction of acidosis[39-41]. Unlike the findings in non-azotemic children with type 4 RTA, in non-azotemic children with type 2 RTA and the Fanconi syndrome, massive hypercalciuria is also present before and after correction of acidosis[39-42]; yet, in these children with type 2 RTA, as in children with type 4 RTA, radiologically demonstrable nephrocalcinosis and nephrolithiasis do not occur[20,22,39,42].

From our study, we conclude that during acidosis the urinary excretion of citrate in non-azotemic children with type 4 RTA is higher than that seen in acidotic normal children. In these children with non-azotemic type 4 RTA as well as reported children with type 2 RTA, nephrocalcinosis and nephrolithiasis did not occur despite chronic acidosis of sufficient severity to cause height stunting (and in the latter group massive hypercalciuria). These two groups of children with types 2 and 4 RTA may be protected from nephrocalcinosis in part because of the abnormally high urinary excretion of citrate which occurs during acidosis. Our study provides the first evidence during acidosis that in a group of patients with non-azotemic type 4 RTA, renal tubular reabsorption of citrate is impaired.

REFERENCES

1. A. J. Greenberg, H. McNamara, and W. W. McCrory, J. Pediatr. 69:610 (1966).
2. R. H. Palmer and D. Cornfeld, Clin. Pediatr. 12:140 (1973).
3. J. Rodriguez-Soriano, A. Vallo, and M. Garcia-Fuentes, J. Pediatr. 86:524 (1975).
4. E. P. Leumann and B. Skinmann, Pediatr. Res. 9:676 (1975).

5. E. McSherry and R. C. Morris, Jr., J. Clin. Invest. 61:509 (1978).
6. E. McSherry and M. Pokroy, Clin. Res. 26:470A (1978).
7. A. M. Butler, J. L. Wilson, and S. Farber, J. Pediatr. 8:489 (1936).
8. F. Albright, W. V. Consolazio, F. S. Coombs, H. W. Sulkowith, and J. H. Talbott, Bull. Johns Hopkins Hosp. 66:7 (1940).
9. R. E. Cooke and C. R. Kleeman, Yale J. Biol. Med. 23:199 (1950).
10. G. L. Foss, C. B. Perry, and F. J. Y. Wood, Q. J. Med. 98: 185 (1956).
11. Y. K. Seedat, S. Afr. Med. J. 38:606 (1964).
12. P. Royer, in:"Nephrology," J. Hamburger, G. Richet, J. Crosnier, J. L. Funck-Brentano, B. Antoine, H. Ducrot, J. P. Mery, and H. DeMontera, ed., W. B. Saunders Company, Philadelphia (1968).
13. J. L. Meyer and L. H. Smith, Invest. Urol. 13:36 (1975).
14. S. Bisaz, R. Felix, and W. F. Neuman, Min. Electr. Metab. 1:74 (1978).
15. E. McSherry, and J. Gates, VIIth International Congress of Nephrology, Montreal, Canada, (abstract) (1978).
16. E. McSherry, Kid. Int. (in press 1981).
17. Recommended Daily Dietary Allowances - Food and Nutrition Board National Research Council, National Academy of Sciences 8th Edition, Washington, D.C. (1974).
18. A. Hodgkinson, Clin. Sci. 23:203 (1962).
19. H. Moellering, and Gruber, W., Anal. Biochem. 17:369 (1966).
20. E. McSherry, J. Gates, and M. Pialaet, in:"Proceedings IV International Symposium on Urolithiasis Research" (in press).
21. M. E. Norman, N. J. Feldman, and R. M. Cohn, J. Pediatr. 92:394 (1978).
22. J. B. Brenner, D. Spring, E. McSherry, and A. Sebastian, Radiology (in press).
23. R. C. Morris, Jr., A. Sebastian, and E. McSherry, in:"Proceedings VII International Congress of Nephrology," Karger, Basel (1978).
24. E. McSherry, in:"Textbook of Pediatrics", 17th Edition (in press).
25. E. McSherry, in:"Proceedings V International Congress of Pediatric Nephrology" (in press).
26. E. Clarke, B. M. Evans, I. MacIntyre, and M. D. Milne, Clin. Sci. 14:421 (1955).
27. E. E. Gordon, and S. Sheps, NEJM 256:1215 (1957).
28. W. Boothby and M. Adams, Am. J. Physio. 107:471 (1934).
29. J. S. Elliott and M. E. Ribeiro, Invest. Urol. 10:102 (1972).
30. H. E. Harrison, Am. J. Med. 20:1 (1956).
31. R. E. Dedmon and O. Wrong, Clin. Sci. 22:19 (1962).
32. E. K. Brodwall, A. Oyri, and K. Skaland, Acta. Med. Scand. 186:161 (1969).
33. E. K. Brodwall, L. Westlie, and E. Myhre, Acta. Med. Scand. 192:137 (1972).
34. M. A. Crawford, M. D. Milne, and B. H. Scribner, J. Physiol. 149:413 (1959).

35. E. Clarke and B. M. Evans, Clin. Sci. 14:421 (1955).
36. S. Adler, B. Anderson, and B. Zett, Kid. Int. 6:92 (1974).
37. P. Fourman and J. R. Robinson, Lancet 2:656 (1953).
38. B. M. Evans, I. MacIntyre, and C. R. MacPherson, Clin. Sci. 16:53 (1957).
39. E. DeToni, Jr., and S. Nordio, Arch. Dis. Child. 34:371 (1959).
40. M. D. Milne, S. W. Stanbury, A. E. Tomson, Quart. J. Med. 21:61 (1952).
41. C. E. Dent and M. Friedman, Arch. Dis. Child. 39:240 (1964).
42. H. A. Bloomer, J. J. Canary, and L. H. Kyle, Am. J. Med. 33:141 (1962).

ACKNOWLEDGMENTS

We wish to thank Tess Jones and Michael Wong for their help in the preparation of this manuscript.

This work was supported by National Foundation Grant 6-198 and National Institutes of Health Grants AM-21771, AM-21605, and RR-00079.

URINARY CITRATE EXCRETION AND ACIDIFICATION DEFECTS IN RENAL CALCIUM STONE FORMERS

B. Wikström, U. Backman, B. G. Danielson,
B. Fellström, G. Johansson, and S. Ljunghall
Department of Internal Medicine
University Hospital
S-750 14 Uppsala, Sweden

INTRODUCTION

A characteristic clinical picture in patients with complete distal (classic) renal tubular acidosis (RTA) includes nephrocalcinosis or nephrolithiasis[1]. These patients also have a low urinary citrate which may be of significance for their stone formation.

The purpose of this study was to investigate if hypocitraturia was a common feature of stone formers with the incomplete forms of proximal and distal RTA.

SUBJECTS AND METHODS

Patients

One hundred sixty-four consecutive patients (117 males, 47 females) with recurrent calcium stones. Mean age was 42 years (range 18 - 69).

Controls

Two hundred apparently healthy subjects (121 males, 79 females). Mean age was 43 years (range 15 - 81).

Citrate

Citrate was assayed by an enzymatic method using citrate lyase[2].

Renal Acidification Capacity

Renal acidification capacity was evaluated with a short (3-5 hours) ammonium chloride load[3,4]. Typical curves of the incomplete forms of proximal and distal RTA are shown in Figure 1.

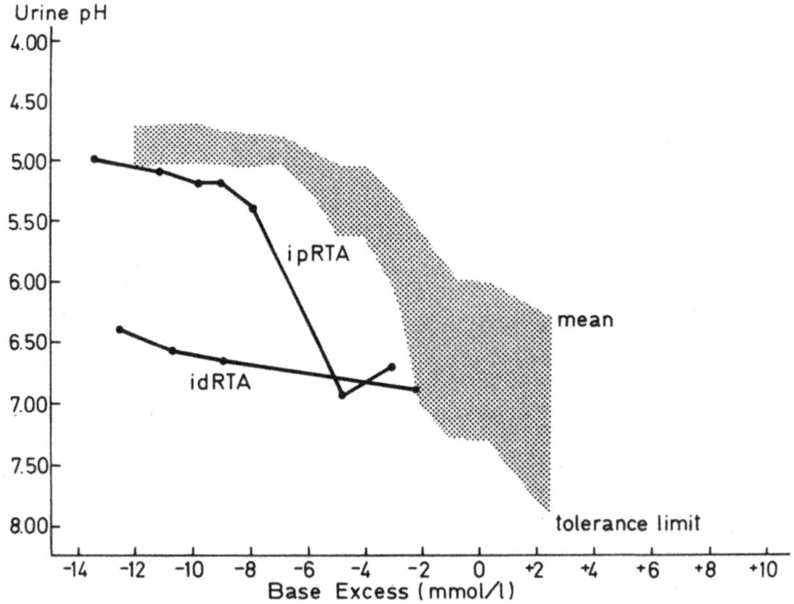

Figure 1. Typical curves of urinary acidification for stone formers with incomplete proximal renal tubular acidosis (ipRTA) and incomplete distal renal tubular acidosis (idRTA). Urine pH is plotted versus base excess after an oral ammonium chloride load (17 g).

RESULTS

The acidification ability in this series of stone formers was distributed as shown in Table 1. No case of complete RTA was disclosed. Stone formers had reduced excretion of citrate compared to controls. The lowest excretion was seen in patients with incomplete distal RTA (see Table 1).

Table 1. 24 Hour Urinary Excretion of Citrate in Controls and Renal Calcium Stone Formers (n=164) Grouped According to Renal Acidification Capacity

	Controls	NoRTA	ipRTA	idRTA
Mean value (mmol/24h)	3.26	2.45[a]	2.18[a]	1.53[a,b,c]
SD (mmol/24h)	1.28	1.18	1.18	1.12
n	200	107	39	18

No RTA: normal renal acidification capacity
ipRTA: incomplete proximal renal tubular acidosis
idRTA: incomplete distal renal tubular acidosis
a $p < 0.001$ compared to controls
b $p < 0.01$ compared to no RTA
c $p < 0.05$ compared to ipRTA

Citrate excretion in patients with incomplete proximal RTA was in the same order as in stone formers without acidification defects.

Urinary citrate in controls was not related to sex or age and sex- and age-matching did not change the difference in urinary citrate between the groups as shown for controls and incomplete distal RTA in Figure 2.

In RTA patients there was no correlation between the urinary citrate and either of blood standard bicarbonate, urinary calcium and β_2-microglobulin or maximal excretion of titratable acid, ammonium ions and phosphate after acid load.

DISCUSSION

In contrast to the picture of complete RTA nephrocalcinosis is not a common finding in our patients with incomplete RTA. However, patients with the incomplete acidification defects often exhibit a severe form of stone disease[5]. One contributing factor to their stone forming propensity may be hypocitraturia as suggested in this study. Only case reports or small patient series concerning citrate excretion in incomplete RTA have been published where hypocitraturia has been noted[6].

Citrate is a potent inhibitor of the precipitation of calcium salts _in vitro_[7]. However, there is limited information about renal citrate handling and the sources of urinary citrate[8]. A reduced urinary citrate excretion in stone formers (where incomplete RTA obviously was not excluded) compared to controls has been reported[9] thus supporting earlier suggestions of an association of stone formation to low urinary citrate. The sex difference which has been noted previously[9] was not confirmed in our study.

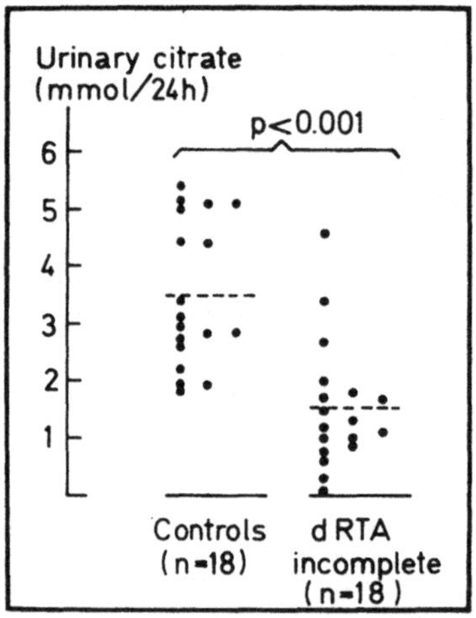

Figure 2. Individual values for urinary citrate in stone formers with distal renal tubular acidosis and controls matched for sex and age.

CONCLUSIONS

Our renal calcium stone formers had a reduced urinary citrate excretion. Stone patients with incomplete distal renal tubular acidosis exhibited marked hypocitraturia. The low urinary citrate may favor stone formation. This suggestion is supported by our previous findings of a severe clinical picture of stone disease in patients with incomplete RTA.

REFERENCES

1. A. Sebastian, E. McSherry, and R. C. Morris, in:"The Kidney," B. M. Brenner and and F. C. Rector, eds., Saunders, Philadelphia (1976).
2. S. G. Welshman and H. Mc Cambridge, Clin. Chim. Acta. 46:243 (1973).
3. U. Backman, B. G. Danielson, and M. Sohtell, Scand. J. Urol. Nephrol. Suppl. 35:33 (1976).
4. U. Backman, B. G. Danielson, and M. Sohtell, Scand. J. Urol. Nephrol. Suppl. 35:49 (1976).
5. U. Backman, B. G. Danielson, G. Johansson, S. Ljunghall, and B. Wikström, Nephron 25:96 (1980).
6. M. E. Norman, N. I. Feldman, R. M. Cohn, K. S. Roth, and D. K. McCurdy, J. Pediatr. 92:394 (1978).
7. H. Fleisch, Kid. Int. 13:361 (1978).
8. J. J. Cohen, and M. Barac-Nieto, in:"Handbook of Physiology," J. Orloff and R. W. Berliner, eds., American Physiology Society, Washington (1973).
9. S. G. Welshman, and M. G. McGeown, Br. J. Urol. 48:7 (1976).

INFLUENCE OF CHANGES IN CALCIUM METABOLISM ON RENAL HANDLING OF OXALATE IN RATS

H. Osswald, J. A. Haas, R. M. Meyer-Hentschel, and R. Hautmann
Department of Pharmacology, RWTH, Aachen, West Germany;

and Department of Physiology, Mayo Clinic, Rochester, MN

Clearance and micropuncture studies on the renal handling of oxalate in rats have led to conflicting results. There is wide agreement that oxalate is excreted into the urine 1.1 to 1.4 fold in excess of the filtered load[1-4]. In micropuncture studies in Sprague-Dawley rats, Weinman et al[1] found not addition of oxalate to the filtered amount in the proximal tubule. However, Hautmann and Osswald[2] did not find oxalate secretion in the superficial proximal tubule of rats. In another study by Greger et al[3], proximal tubular secretion of oxalate was found in Wistar rats. Since different experimental protocols (infused amount of saline and ^{14}C oxalate) and different rat strains were used in the above cited studies, it was the aim of the present investigation to identify factors that can influence the renal handling of oxalate. In addition, the importance of calcium in controlling oxalate fluxes across the tubular epithelium was studied, to test the hypothesis that calcium in the tubular fluid might trap the oxalate ion.

In a first experimental series, the effect of extracellular volume expansion (ECVE) was studied in parathyroidectomized (PTX) Sprague-Dawley and Wistar rats. In the second series, oxalate was infused at a rate at least 10 times higher than was infused as ^{14}C oxalate in the micropuncture studies. In a third experimental series, clearances and free-flow micropuncture in PTX Sprague-Dawley rats were performed during calcium chloride and sodium citrate infusion, maneuvers designed to markedly change urinary calcium concentration. In Groups 1 and 2, ECVE and high oxalate infusion reduced fractional excretion of oxalate only in Sprague-Dawley rats, whereas Wistar rats did not respond to the experimental maneuvers with a significant change of FE_{ox} (Table 1).

Table 1. Effect of ECVE and Oxalate Infusion on $FE_{ox}\%$ in the PTX Rat

	Sprague-Dawley		Wistar	
	C	E	C	E
Group 1. Extracellular Volume Expansion (22.5 ml/45 min) n=6				
C_{ox}	2.81 ± .12	2.51 ± .27	2.40 ± .14	2.13 ± .26
C_{In}	2.57 ± .10	2.58 ± .26	2.24 ± .11	2.05 ± .24
FE_{ox}	1.11 ± .05	0.98 ± .05	1.07 ± .02	1.04 ± .03
Ca_U	5.50 ±1.5	2.47 ± .39	2.64 ± .37	2.55 ± .27
Group 2. Oxalate Infusion (1 μmol/min) n=6				
C_{ox}	3.06 ± .14	2.25 ± .18	2.38 ± .16	2.52 ± .11
C_{In}	2.79 ± .16	2.53 ± .29	2.26 ± .15	2.39 ± .11
FE_{ox}	1.10 ± .03	0.91 ± .04	1.06 ± .04	1.06 ± .04
Ca_U	6.43 ±1.5	1.83 ± .03	-- --	-- --

C and E refer to control and experimental periods; mean values ± SEM

In Group 3, five rats in which only clearances were performed, infusion of $CaCl_2$ (120 mg/dl @ 2.8 ml/hr) for one hour resulted in a $FE_{ox}\%$ of 110 ± 10. Infusion of sodium citrate (0.18 mmol/hr) for ninety minutes following cessation of calcium chloride infusion, markedly reduced $FE_{ox}\%$ to 79 ± 10 (Figure 1). In Group 4, five rats prepared for micropuncture, sodium citrate lowered $FE_{ox}\%$ from 100 ± 23 to 53 ± 13 (Figure 1). The fractional delivery of oxalate to the late proximal tubule was lowered by sodium citrate from 109 ± 8 to 86 ± 12%, indicating that sodium citrate induced tubular oxalate reabsorption mainly in the distal part of the nephron (Figure 2). A positive correlation was found between $FE_{ox}\%$ and urinary calcium concentration (Figure 1). We conclude from the results that the renal handling of oxalate can be affected by different states of calcium excretion.

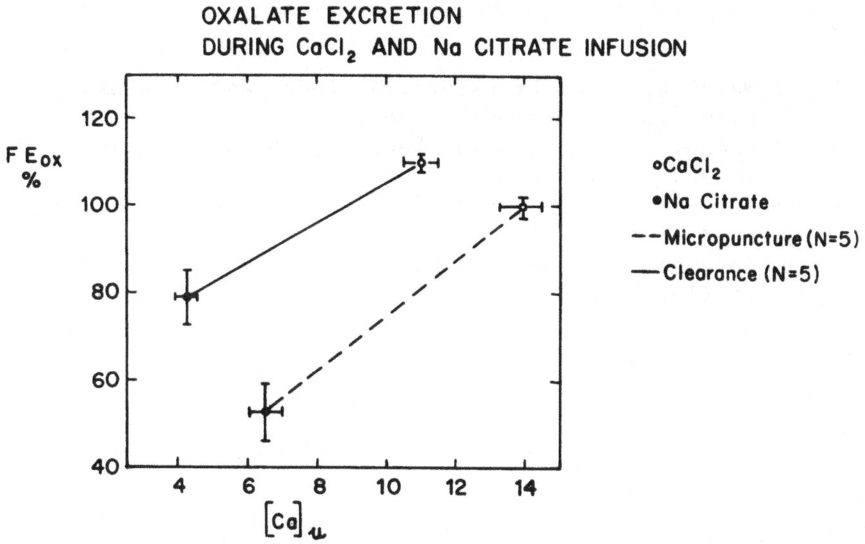

Figure 1. Effect of calcium chloride and sodium citrate infusion on fractional excretion of oxalate (FE_{ox}%) in PTX Sprague-Dawley rats. [Ca]μ is in mm/dl.

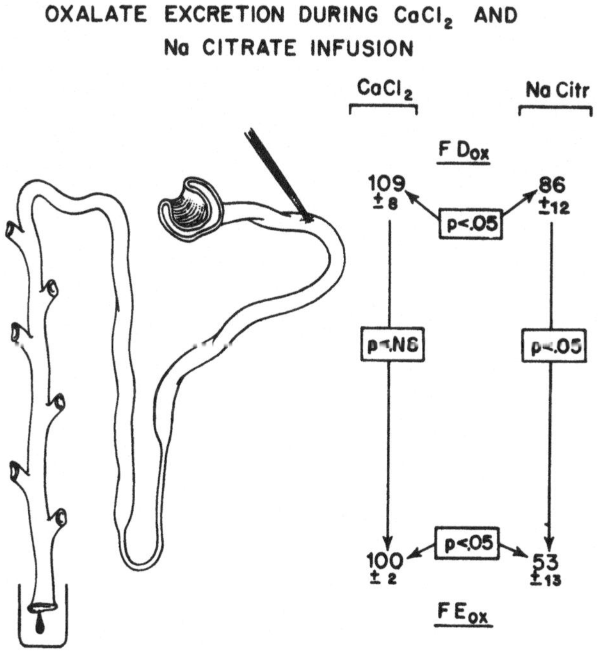

Figure 2. Effect of calcium chloride and sodium citrate infusion on oxalate delivery in the proximal tubule and final urine in PTX Sprague-Dawley rats.

REFERENCES

1. E. J. Weinman, S. J. Frankfurt, A. Ince, and S. Sansom, J. Clin. Invest. 61:801 (1978).
2. R. Hautmann, and H. Osswald, Naunyn-Schmiedebergs Arch. Pharmacol. 304:277 (1978).
3. R. Greger, F. Lang, H. Oberleithner, P. Deetjen, Pfluegers Arch. 374:243 (1978).
4. T. F. Knight, H. O. Senekjian, and E. J. Weinman, Kid. Int. 15:38 (1979).

EVALUATION OF A NEW OXALATE ASSAY

F. E. Cole, S. Snyder, D. J. Bennett, K. M. Gladden, E. D. Frohlich, and D. T. Erwin
Alton Ochsner Medical Foundation

New Orleans, Louisiana 70121

The literature contains sparse information concerning renal oxalate clearance. This situation is undoubtedly due to the lack of a widely accepted, accurate method for the determination of serum and plasma oxalate concentrations. We have developed a new radio-enzymatic isotope dilution assay (REIDA) that is specific, sensitive, and accurate[1,2]. This report describes its use in measuring urine and plasma oxalate concentrations in normal volunteer subjects and patients with renal calculi.

The subjects of the study were volunteer employees of the Ochsner Research facility who were normal subjects and patients from the Ochsner Stone Clinic. The patient population included 20 women and 41 men ranging in age from 13 to 74 years. The volunteer subjects included 7 males and 4 females who had no personal or family history of renal stone formation and ranged in age from 20 to 38 years.

No restrictions were imposed on the diet of the normal subjects. Twenty-four hour urines were collected and refrigerated without preservatives. The volume and pH were measured and recorded, and then the urines were titrated to pH <1. Aliquots of the titrated urine were then frozen at $-90^{o}C$ until analyzed. At the completion of the 24-hour period, a fasting blood sample was drawn into Vacutainer tubes containing EDTA and the plasma frozen at $-90^{o}C$ until analyzed.

The oxalate assay has been described in detail[1,2]. In brief, plasma ultrafiltrates and urines are titrated to pH 7.0, the oxalate precipitated with $CaCl_2$ in 75% ethanol, redissolved in diluted HCl, extracted with diethyl ether, and then dried. The dried extract is dissolved and analyzed in a citrate buffer by measuring the $^{14}CO_2$ evolved from ^{14}C oxalic acid in the presence of unlabelled oxalate standards or unknowns and the enzyme oxalate decarboxylase (EC 4.1.1.2.). A linear standard curve is obtained using an equation which quantitatively accounts for the effects of unlabelled oxalate on isotope dilution and the rate of the enzymatic reaction.

In addition to urine and plasma oxalate concentrations, the urine was also analyzed for sodium, potassium, chloride, ammonium, magnesium, sulfate, phosphate, calcium, citrate, uric acid, creatinine and acid mucopolysaccharide (AMPS) concentrations[3-7]. Plasma creatinine concentrations were determined thereby permitting calculation of creatinine clearances.

RESULTS AND DISCUSSION

We compared measurements of 24 hour urinary oxalate using REIDA with those of Bio-Science Laboratories (BSL) (Van Nuys, California) on paired samples from 56 renal stone-forming patients (Figure 1). The patient population reflected the stone-forming population in general, and while most of them were in the idiopathic stone-forming group, patients with urate stone disease, infected stone disease and renal tubular acidosis were intentionally included to check for conditions that might interfere with assay. The BSL procedure[8], which measures oxalate precipitated calcium by atomic absorption, yielded results that correlated ($r=0.40$, $p<0.01$) with those obtained using REIDA. However, a larger variation was associated with the BSL (BSL 26±33; REIDA 34±17 SD), rendering the means of the two procedures statistically indistinguishable. This large deviation was caused by a single oxalate value of one patient that was reported to be very high (233 mg/24 hr) by BSL but only slightly elevated (39.7 mg/24 hr) by REIDA. If we eliminated this patient from the comparison, as well as 6 others reported to have undetectable oxalate values by BSL, the correlation was improved considerably ($r=0.72$, $p<0.001$) with the mean for the BSL assay (25±7 SD) lower ($p<0.001$) than that obtained using REIDA (34±19 SD). The discrepancy in absolute values and means likely reflects the differences in precipitation techniques and specifically between the two procedures.

Large individual variation in the urinary oxalate excretion of normal volunteers on repetitive diets has been observed by others[9]. Our investigation of normal volunteers revealed a large individual variation in urinary oxalate excretion, as well as in plasma oxalate and renal oxalate clearance over a four month period (Table 1). This variability greatly exceeds the variation of the analytical method (<8%)[2]. These observations do not define whether the individual variations in oxalate concentrations result from differences in absorption, excretion or metabolism, or simply dietary differences.

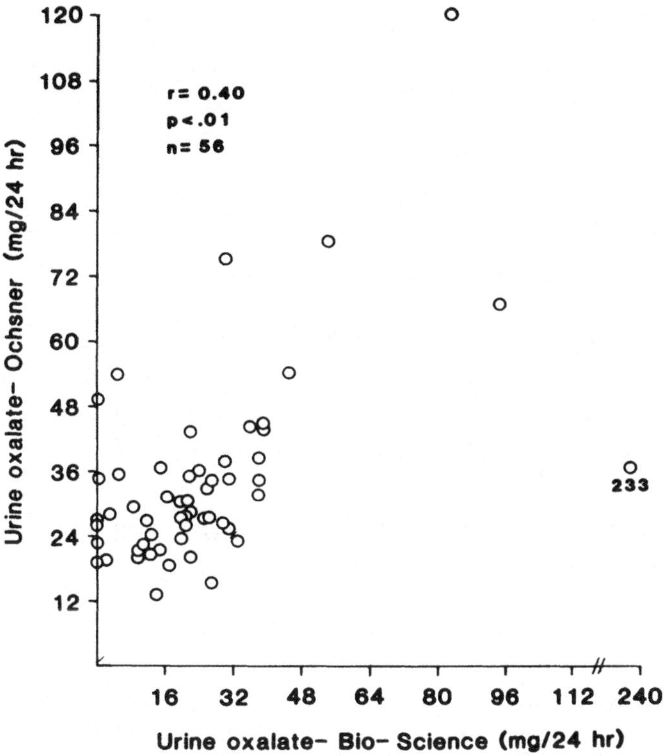

Figure 1. Comparison of Bio-Scienc Laboratory (oxalate-precipitated calcium by atomic absorpt n) and radioenzymatic isotope dilution assay for urine alate in stone forming patients.

We also observed previously recognized effects[10] of dietary calcium on urine and plasma oxalate concentrations as well as on other urinary measurements. This was demonstrated by analyzing samples from patients receiving high (~1200 mg Ca^{++}/day) and low (~400 mg Ca^{++}/day) dairy diets over three day periods, respectively (Figure 2). Dietary calcium impairs intestinal oxalate absorption[10] and lower plasma and urine oxalate concentrations were measured in patients receiving a high Ca^{++} intake. Elevated urinary Ca^{++} and urinary Ca^{++}/creatinine ratios most probably reflect increased intestinal absorption and/or renal excretion of the dietary Ca^{++} in these patients.

Table 1. REIDA Oxalate Measurements: The Variation of Individuals Compared to the Variation of the Population

Male Normals	X ± S.D.	(n)	CV	Female Normals	X ± S.D.	(n)	CV
URINARY OXALATE (mg/24 hr)							
Individual A	25 ± 3	5	12%	Individual A	22 ± 4	5	18%
Individual B	35 ± 9	5	26%	Individual B	22 ± 7	5	32%
Individual C	55 ± 31	5	56%				
Total Male Normal Population	39 ± 20	19	51%	Total Female Population	22 ± 4	11	18%
PLASMA OXALATE (μg/ml)							
Individual A	0.49±0.20	5	41%	Individual A	0.37±0.14	5	38%
Individual B	0.34±0.18	5	53%	Individual B	0.61±0.49	5	80%
Individual C	0.75±0.27	4	36%				
Total Male Normal Population	0.53±0.24	18	45%	Total Female Normal Population	0.49±0.34	11	69%
OXALATE CLEARANCE (ml/min)							
Individual A	41 ± 21	5	51%	Individual A	47 ± 16	5	35%
Individual B	73 ± 30	5	42%	Individual B	44 ± 34	5	77%
Individual C	41 ± 8	4	19%				
Total Male Normal Population	51 ± 24	18	47%	Total Female Normal Population	45 ± 24	11	53%

X ± S.D. = Mean ± Standard Deviation

C.V. = Coefficient of Variation

n = Total number of observations

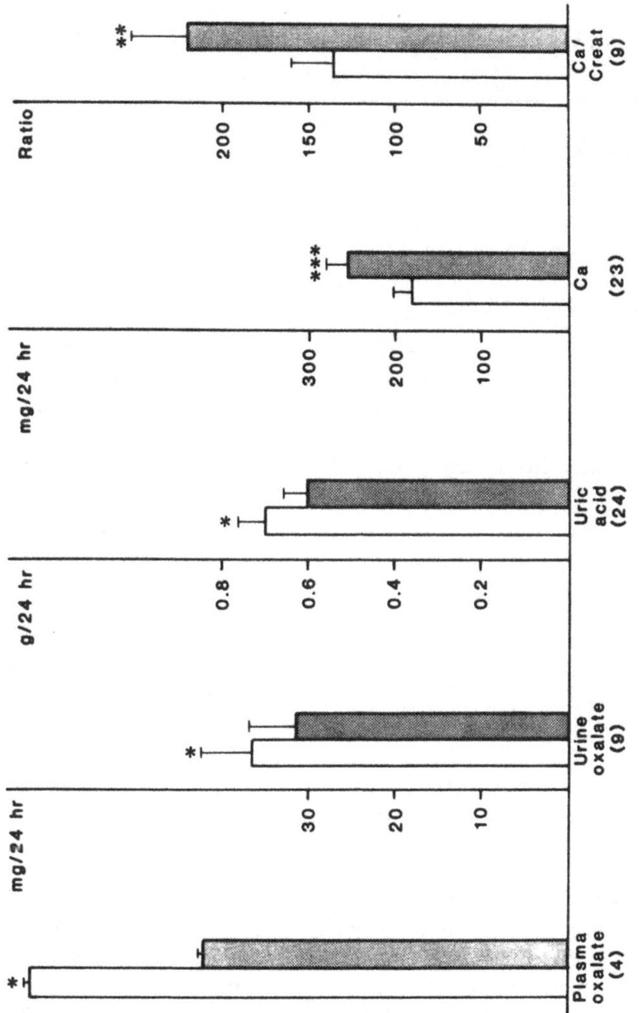

Figure 2. The effect of high (1200 mg Ca^{++}/day) and low (250 mg Ca^{++}/day) dairy diets (3 days) upon various plasma and urine measurements in calcium oxalate stone forming patients receiving no drug therapy. Open bar - low dairy; solid bar - high dairy. *$p < 0.05$; **$p < 0.01$; ***$p < 0.001$. Number in parentheses = n.

Table 2. Multiple Linear Regression Analysis of Various Urine and Plasma Measurements in Normal and Stone Forming Patients (No Drug Therapy, Low Dairy) Populations

	P Oxal	NH^4	Creat	Cit	Uric	Ca^{++}	AMPS	Mg^{++}	Oxal Clear	Cl^-
Normals n = 27										
U oxalate	.01	.05	.001					.05		
P oxalate									-.001	
NH_4^+			.01				.01			
Creatinine							.01	.05		
Uric acid							.001	-.001		.01
Calcium										.05
AMPS										.05
Patients, No Drugs, Low Dairy, n = 16										
U oxalate									.05	
P oxalate									-.05	
NH_4^+								-.05		
Creatinine					.001	.01	.05			
Uric acid						.01	.05			
Calcium										
AMPS								.05		

The various urinary measurements were analyzed statistically for correlations by multiple linear regression analysis (Table 2). In the normal population, urinary oxalate correlated directly with plasma oxalate, urinary NH_4^+, creatinine and magnesium. Plasma oxalate was inversely correlated with oxalate clearance. Uric acid was directly correlated with acid mucopolysaccharide and magnesium. In contrast, in the patient population (calcium oxalate stone formers on a low dairy diet and receiving no drug therapy), urinary oxalate correlated directly with oxalate clearance. Plasma oxalate was again inversely correlated with oxalate clearance. Absence of a significant correlation between urine and plasma oxalate in the patient group resulted from a greater variance in plasma oxalate values in the patient population as compared with the normal population ($p < 0.01$). Ca^{++} excretion also demonstrated greater variance in the patient population ($p < 0.01$).

CONCLUSION

We have evaluated REIDA in a varied clinical population. The results indicate that REIDA is a promising technique for elucidation of those factors which influence oxalate absorption, urinary excretion and metabolism.

REFERENCES

1. D. J. Bennett, F. E. Cole, E. D. Frohlich, and D. T. Erwin, J. Lab. Clin. Med. 91:822 (1978).
2. D. J. Bennett, F. E. Cole, E. D. Frohlich, and D. T. Erwin, Clin. Chem. 25:1810 (1979).
3. P. B. Hawk, B. L. Oser, and J. Summerson, in:"Practical Physiological Chemistry," McGraw-Hill, New York (1947).
4. D. J. Bennett, Am. J. Chem. Pathol. 61:616 (1974).
5. T. T. Neilson, Scand. J. Clin. Lab. Invest. 36:513 (1976).
6. F. Berglund, and B. Sorbo, Scand. J. Clin. Lab. Invest. 12:147 (1960).
7. P. Whiteman, Biochem. J. 131:351 (1973).
8. J. Fraser, and D. J. Campbell, Clin. Biochem. 5:99 (1972).
9. H. E. Archer, A. E. Dorman, E. F. Scorven, and R. W. E. Watts, Clin. Sci. 16:405 (1957).
10. R. W. Marshall, M. Cochran, and A. Hodgkinson, Clin. Sci. 43: 91 (1972).

INTESTINAL OXALATE ABSORPTION IN CALCIUM OXALATE STONE DISEASE

J. W. Dobbins, K. Cooper, R. Lang, L. H. Smith,
H. J. Binder, and A. E. Broadus
Department of Medicine, Yale University School of Medicine, New Haven, Connecticut, and Department of Medicine, Mayo Medical School, Rochester, Minnesota

Several laboratories have reported a slight but significant increase in urinary oxalate excretion in patients with calcium oxalate stone disease[1-4]. The mechanism responsible for this increased oxalate excretion remains largely unknown. Zarembski and Hodgkinson[5], and Robertson et al.[1] reported that patients with calcium oxalate stones had a greater increase in urinary oxalate excretion than did normal subjects when placed on an increased oxalate diet. However, Barilla et al, in a similar study, did not confirm this observation[6]. Hodgkinson also reported that the increased oxalate excretion in patients with calcium oxalate stones was abolished by fasting[7]. These studies, in the aggregate, suggest that increased oxalate absorption might account for the increased oxalate excretion in certain patients with calcium stone disease.

Approximately half of the patients with calcium oxalate stone disease are found to have hypercalciuria[8], but no clear relationship between hypercalciuria and hyperoxaluria has been established. Recent studies have identified several distinct subtypes of idiopathic hypercalciuria and, although the pathophysiological features differ in these various subtypes, an increase in intestinal calcium absorption is a feature shared by each[8]. An increase in intestinal calcium absorption is also principally responsible for the hypercalciuria and predisposition to renal stone formation in some patients with primary hyperparathyroidism[9].

Since the luminal concentration of calcium is known to affect oxalate bioavailability and absorption, we postulated that patients with increased absorption of calcium might also have increased absorption of oxalate. To test this hypothesis, we evaluated oxalate absorption in groups of patients with and without intestinal hyperabsorption of calcium. Because of 1) endogenous oxalate production and 2) the poor reproducibility of many chemical assays for oxalate, we chose to determine oxalate absorption by measuring the urinary excretion of ^{14}C oxalate after oral administration. Oxalate is an end product of metabolism in man which is excreted almost exclusively by the kidneys[10]. Therefore, urinary excretion of ^{14}C oxalate should provide an accurate representation of the amount absorbed.

Normal subjects and patients with various disorders of mineral metabolism (primary hyperparathyroidism, absorptive hypercalciuria, and idiopathic calcium oxalate nephrolithiasis) were included in the study. The patients were classified as having either increased or normal calcium absorption on the basis of their response to the oral calcium tolerance test[11]. With this test the calciuric response to 1000 mg of calcium serves as an index of intestinal calcium absorption.

Two consecutive 24 h urines were collected while on both a 400 mg and a 1000 mg calcium diet. Each diet contained, in addition to the calcium, 300 mg oxalate, 800 mg phosphorus, 1 g protein per kg body weight, and 69 to 109 mg sodium. Five μCi ^{14}C oxalate and 20 mg potassium oxalate in 100 ml of distilled deionized water were given with a standardized breakfast (eggs, toast, butter, orange juice, milk, coffee) on the first morning of each diet. The urinary excretion of ^{14}C oxalate was determined over the next 48 h.

Intestinal oxalate absorption was also determined with an oral oxalate tolerance test: Well hydrated patients ingested a liquid test meal containing 75 mg calcium (supplied as Calcitest ^{R}), 75 mg oxalate, and 5 μCi ^{14}C oxalate. Urine was collected for four 2 hour periods after the meal and total ^{14}C oxalate excretion determined.

The patients with increased calcium absorption displayed an abnormal calciuric response to the calcium tolerance test and had a greater than normal increase in 24 h urinary calcium excretion when the calcium intake was increased from 400 mg to 1000 mg daily. These same patients were found to have an increased absorption of ^{14}C oxalate as determined by 1) the oral oxalate tolerance test ($p < 0.001$) and 2) ^{14}C oxalate excretion when ^{14}C oxalate was administered with breakfast while on both the 400 mg calcium and 1000 mg calcium diet ($p < 0.05$ and $p < 0.01$ respectively).

The patients without increased calcium absorption were normocalciuric and had a mean response to the oral calcium tolerance test identical to that seen in the normal subjects. Their absorption of ^{14}C oxalate from the liquid test meal was also similar to that of the control subjects. The 24 h urinary oxalate excretion was greater in the patients with increased calcium absorption on both the 400 mg and 1000 mg calcium diet. A direct linear correlation was found between the intestinal absorption of calcium and the absorption of oxalate, as determined by the calcium and oxalate tolerance tests ($p < 0.01$).

These findings indicate that patients with increased absorption of calcium have increased absorption of oxalate. A highly significant linear correlation between the absorption of calcium and oxalate was found. The patients with increased oxalate absorption had increased 24 h urinary oxalate excretion. The increase was small, but significant, and similar to that previously reported[1-4]. Thus, patients with hypercalciuria secondary to increased intestinal calcium absorption, also appear to be at risk for calcium oxalate nephrolithiasis because of increased absorption of oxalate.

Robertson et al. analyzed risk factors in 65 patients with recurrent calcium stones, idiopathic hypercalciuria, and hyperoxaluria[12]. They concluded that hyperoxaluria was the greatest single risk factor for stone formation in these patients. Furthermore, Robertson et al. have presented evidence suggesting that small changes in urinary oxalate concentration have a greater impact on calcium oxalate supersaturation than similar changes in urinary calcium concentration[13]. Thus, it is possible that the small increase in urinary oxalate excretion seen in the patients with hypercalciuria secondary to increased calcium absorption may represent a risk as great or greater than the hypercalciuria. Certainly, concurrent abnormalities in calcium and oxalate excretion should be at least additive in terms of risk.

These studies suggest that therapy for patients with hypercalciuria secondary to increased absorption should be directed at reducing both calcium and oxalate excretion. Decreasing dietary calcium alone is probably not sufficient therapy because this will result in increased oxalate absorption. Both ^{14}C oxalate excretion and 24 h urinary oxalate excretion were greater in our patients on the 400 mg calcium diet compared to the 1000 mg diet. Zarembski and Hodgkinson have made similar observations utilizing a low calcium diet and EDTA to chelate dietary calcium[5]. The Leeds' group has long advocated a diet that is restricted in both calcium and oxalate in the treatment of recurrent calcium stone formers[5]. Indeed, the generally poor clinical results observed with restricted calcium diets alone in calcium oxalate stone formers may be because these diets increase oxalate absorption[14].

There are at least two plausible explanations for the observed correlation between calcium and oxalate absorption. First, calcium binds oxalate in an insoluble complex, limiting its bioavailability and absorption. An increase in Ca absorption would decrease the luminal concentration of Ca, thereby increasing the concentration of soluble oxalate for (passive) absorption. Second, a fundamental defect in absorption at the level of the intestinal cell may result in increased oxalate absorption. 1,25 dihydroxy vitamin D stimulates Ca and phosphate absorption in the intestine by altering the rate limiting transport of these ions in the brush border membrane of the mucosal cells. Since both oxalate and phosphate are divalent anions, it is possible that oxalate absorption is mediated by the phosphate transport system. Studies designed to examine these two possibilities are currently under way.

REFERENCES

1. W. G. Robertson, M. Peacock, and B. E. C. Nordin, Clin. Sci. 40:365 (1971).
2. R. W. Marshall, M. Cochran, W. G. Robertson, A. Hodgkinson, and B. E. C. Nordin, Clin. Sci. 43:433 (1972).
3. C. Y. C. Pak and K. Holt, Metabolism 25:665 (1976).
4. J. S. Elliot, J. Urol. 100:687 (1968).
5. P. M. Zarembski and A. Hodgkinson, Clin. Chim. Acta. 25:1 (1969).
6. D. E. Barilla, C. Notz, D. Kennedy, and C. Y. C. Pak, Am. J. Med. 64:579 (1978).
7. A. Hodgkinson, Clin. Sci. Mol. Med. 54:291 (1978).
8. A. E. Broadus and S. O. Thier, New Engl. J. Med. 300:839 (1979).
9. A. E. Broadus, R. L. Horst, R. Lang, E. T. Littledike, and H. Rasmussen, New Engl. J. Med. 302:421 (1980).
10. H. E. Williams and L. H. Smith, in:"The Metabolic Basis of Inherited Disease," 3rd edition, J. B. Stanbury, J. B. Wyngaarden, and D. S. Fredrickson, eds., McGraw-Hill, New York (1972).
11. A. E. Broadus, M. Dominquez, and F. C. Bartter, J. Clin. Endocrinol. Metab. 47:751 (1978).
12. W. G. Robertson, M. Peacock, P. J. Heyburn, D. H. Marshall, and P. B. Clark, Br. J. Urol. 50:449 (1978).
13. W. G. Robertson, M. Peacock, and B. E. C. Nordin, in:"Urolithiasis: Physical Aspects," B. Finlayson, L. L. Hench, and L. H. Smith, eds., National Academy of Sciences, Washington, D.C. (1972).
14. J. Lemann, in:"Nephrolithiasis; Contemporary Issues in Nephrology," F. L. Coe, B. M. Brenner, and J. H. Stein, eds., Churchill-Livingstone, Inc., New York (1980).

ACKNOWLEDGMENT

These studies were supported by USPHS Research Grants (AM 20510, AM 20605 and RR 125) from the National Institute of Arthritis, Metabolism and Digestive Diseases and from the National Institutes of Health, Division of Research Resources. Dr. Dobbins is the recipient of a Research Career Development Award (AM 00647) from the National Institute of Arthritis Metabolism and Digestive Diseases.

OXALATE LOADING TEST FOR THE DIAGNOSIS OF OXALATE HYPERABSORPTION

A. Hesse, A. Strenge, D. Bach, and W. Vahlensieck

Urinary Stone Research Department, Urological University Clinic, Bonn, West Germany

The initiation of a stone may be the result of excessive excretion of oxalic acid and/or insufficient dilution of the urine. The evidence for the importance of oxalic acid in calcium oxalate stone formation, however, is often contradictory. Our own studies on 24-h urines on the patient's own diet and on a standard diet have shown that hyperoxaluria is present in some patients and that the circadian rhythm of oxalate excretion in both studies follows a sinusoidal curve.

Ten to fifteen percent of the oxalic acid in urine is reported to be of exogenous origin. In situations of excessive loads, however, the fraction may be much higher. In these situations hyperabsorption of oxalic acid represents a risk factor for stone-formation.

MATERIALS AND METHODS

We attempted to define hyperabsorption of oxalic acid with an oxalate loading test. Healthy controls (n = 9) were studied on a calcium-and oxalate-restricted diet (see Table 1 of Strenge et al. page 790 of this volume). To this was added a load of 500 mg sodium oxalate. Urine samples were collected at specified times according to the protocol and oxalic acid and calcium measured in the urine. Calcium oxalate stone-formers (n = 10) were investigated under the same conditions.

RESULTS

The course of excretion of oxalic acid following the load of oxalate in healthy controls and stone-formers is shown in Figure 1.

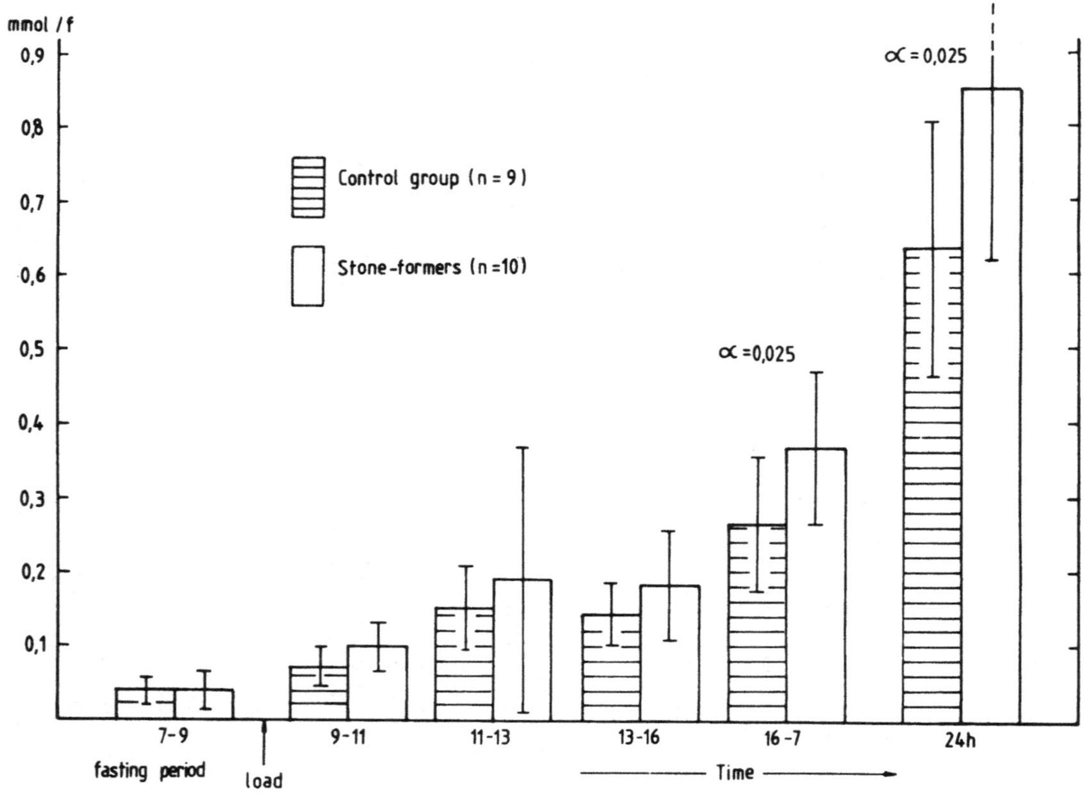

Figure 1. The urinary excretion of oxalate before and after the oral oxalate loading test in stone-formers (▯) and normal controls(▤).

Two hours after the oral load a significant increase in oxalate concentration was observed. In stone-formers the increase in concentration was more rapid and they show a clear decrease after 4 h. There was no significant difference in the urinary concentration of oxalic acid in the 24-h urines of the stone-formers and healthy controls. However, the 24-h excretion of oxalic acid was significantly elevated in the stone-formers. Crystalluria was not observed in any specimen of urine from either controls or stone-formers.

The normal range of oxalate excretion following the load of 500 mg sodium oxalate was 0.636 ± 0.170 mmol/24 h. In calcium oxalate stone-formers we interpreted all values > 0.800 mmol/24 h as showing hyperabsorption of oxalic acid. Based on this criterion, 5 out of 10 patients (50%) were hyperabsorbers of oxalate.

CONCLUSION

Hyperabsorption of oxalic acid is a possible risk factor for calcium oxalate stone-formation. An exact definition of hyperabsorption of oxalic acid based on oxalate-loading studies in normal controls requires a standard protocol with a fixed fluid intake. The reported results indicate that 50% of calcium oxalate stone-formers are hyperabsorbers of oxalic acid. However, the results have to be interpreted with reservation, since comparatively small numbers were studied.

EFFECT OF VITAMIN B_6 DEFICIENCY ON THE INTESTINAL ABSORPTION AND EXCRETION OF OXALATE IN RATS

S. Farooqui, A. Mahmood*, R. Nath, and S. K. Thind

Departments of Biochemistry and Gastroenterology*,
Postgraduate Institute of Medical Education and
Research, Chandigarh, India

INTRODUCTION

Northern India has a high incidence of stone disease and nearly 96% of these stones contain calcium oxalate[1]. Several reports have suggested that the primary cause of stone-formation is the hyper-absorption of oxalate[2] due to the marginal nutritional deficiency of vitamin B_6[3]. In this study the effect of B_6 deficiency on the intestinal absorption and the renal clearance of oxalate has been studied along with the mechanism of its transport.

MATERIALS AND METHODS

Male albino rats (BW 100g) were fed vitamin B_6 deficient diet[4], for 45 days and 15 days to achieve chronic and marginal deficiencies respectively. Acute vitamin B_6 deficiency was produced by administering deoxypyridoxine (10 mg/kg BW), i.p., for three days. Control rats were given 20 μg of pyridoxine-HCl/day. Vitamin B_6 deficiency was monitored by GPT stimulation index[5].

Oxalate Absorption Studies

Intestinal absorption of oxalate was studied by a tissue accumulation method[6], and an everted gut sac technique[7]. The incubating buffer contained Tris-HCl (4 mM), NaCl (130 mM) and KCl (6 mM) at pH 7.4. Incubation was carried out at 37°C for 45 minutes using different concentrations of sodium oxalate with a trace of ^{14}C-oxalic acid. Correction for extracellular space was made as described earlier[6]. Urine was collected over 10 h and analyzed for calcium and oxalate, by the standard methods used in this laboratory.

RESULTS AND DISCUSSION

Oxalate absorption at different stages of vitamin B_6 deficiency is shown in Table 1.

Table 1. Oxalate Transport from the Intestine in Different Stages of Vitamin B_6 Deficiency

Group+	Transport (μmol/h/g dry wt)	GPT Index	Increase %
Control	8.58±1.06	5.05±1.06	-
Acute deficiency	15.39±2.36*	24.90±1.00	79
Subclinical deficiency	20.65±5.54*	43.30±2.40	133
Chronic deficiency	22.65±2.20*	65.80±5.50	163

+8 animals in each group; *P <0.001 as compared to controls

With an increase of vitamin B_6 deficiency (as indicated by rise of GPT Index from 43 to 65) oxalate transport was enhanced from 80 to 163% compared with that in pair-fed controls (Table 1).

In order to study the mechanism of the observed enhancement of oxalate transport in vitamin B_6-deficient rats, oxalate absorption was studied at various concentrations of oxalate (0-6 mM). At concentrations between 0.1 - 0.8 mM oxalate uptake in chronic vitamin B_6 deficient rats exhibited a saturable type of transport mechanism (OTM). However, with further increase in the oxalate concentration in the incubation medium, the absorption rate increased linearly with the medium concentration (Figure 1).

The presence of biphasic transport processes involving a carrier-mediated and passive diffusion type of mechanism has been described earlier for various other nutrients[8]. In contrast to the biphasic type of mechanism in B_6 deficient animals the oxalate transport in control rats followed simple passive diffusion as reported by Binder[9]. To characterize further OTM observed in vitamin B_6 deficient rats, the effect of structural analogues of oxalate was studied. The double reciprocal plot for oxalate absorption in presence and absence of glycolate and glyoxylate is shown in Figure 2. Glycolate and glyoxylate competitively inhibited oxalate absorption as shown by an increase in the slope of the lines with no change in the intercept. The various kinetic parameters calculated from the data are given in Table 2.

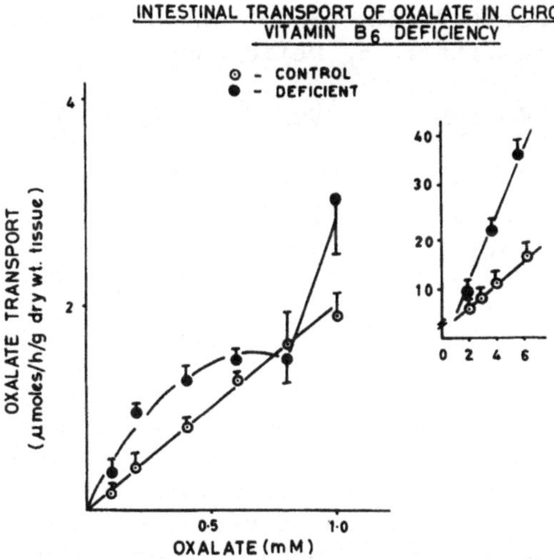

Figure 1. Oxalate transport studies in control (⊙) and chronic vitamin B_6 deficient rats (●). Oxalate concentrations (0.1 - 1.0 mM). The inset represents the oxalate transport between 1-6 mM concentrations. Each point is the mean of 6-8 determinations.

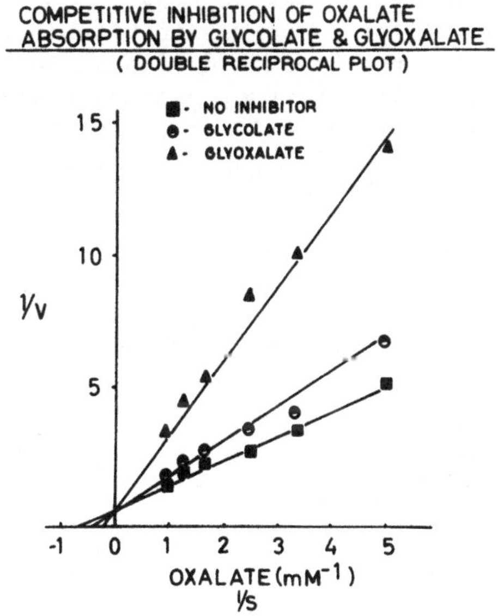

Figure 2. Double reciprocal plot for oxalate transport in chronic vitamin B_6 deficient rats. Oxalate uptake was studied at concentration (0.2-1.0 mM) in absence (■) and presence of 1.5 mM glycolate (●) or 1.0 mM glyoxylate (▲). Each point represents the mean of 6-8 determinations.

Table 2. Kinetic Parameters of Oxalate Transport in Vitamin B_6 Deficiency

Inhibitor	Km (mM)	Vmax	Ki (mM)
Control	1.25	1.48	-
Glycolate	1.75	1.48	3.08
Glyoxylate	3.93	1.48	0.59

Glyoxylate inhibited oxalate absorption to a greater extent than glycolate. No change was observed in the maximum velocity (Vmax = 1.48 μmol/h/g wet wt). Such observations indicate the presence of a transport ligand, which was induced in vitamin B_6 deficiency. The OTM was found to be independent of metabolic energy and thiol groups. Actinomycin D administration to the vitamin B_6 deficient rats impaired the oxalate transport process, suggesting the involvement of a protein component.

The present data on oxalate absorption suggests a facilitative transport process in vitamin B_6 deficiency. The development of this protein ligand in vitamin B_6 deficiency may be due to the differential degradation of proteolytic enzymes in vitamin B_6 deficiency which are responsible for the breakdown of oxalate binding proteins. Similar enhancement in the activity of ornithine amino transferase in B_6 deficiency has been reported earlier[10]. There was a marked increase in the excretion of calcium and oxalate in the chronic B_6 deficient group of animals (Table 3).

Table 3. Calcium and Oxalate Excretion in Chronic Vitamin B_6 Deficiency

Group*	Calcium (μmol/10 h)	Increase %	Oxalate (μmol/10 h)	Increase %
Control	21.0±4.0	-	8.0±1.0	-
Experimental	45.0±8.0	114	16.0±1.0	100
p value	<0.001		<0.001	

*Eight animals in each group.

These results are in agreement with earlier reports[11], which indicate marked hyperoxaluria as well as hypercalciuria in vitamin B_6 deficiency.

CONCLUSIONS

Vitamin B_6 deficiency induced a carrier-mediated oxalate transport system in the intestine of rats, which operates at low intraluminal oxalate concentrations[5]. The hyperoxaluria observed in the vitamin B_6 deficiency is a consequence of hyperabsorption of oxalate from the gut possibly due to the development of a new type of carrier-mediated facilitative type of transport system in the enterocytes of these animals. In contrast to this biphasic type of oxalate transport mechanism, the absorption of oxalate in control rats followed a simple passive type of diffusion. Kinetic studies indicated that glyoxylate was a better competitive inhibitor of oxalate transport than glycolate.

REFERENCES

1. S. K. Thind and R. Nath, Indian J. Med. Res. 57:1179 (1969).
2. A. Hodgkinson, Clin. Sci. Mol. Med. 54:29 (1978).
3. E. J. Will and O. L. M. Bijvoet, Metabolism 28:123 (1979).
4. T. J. Runyan and S. N. Gershoff, J. Biol. Chem. 240:1869 (1965).
5. M. J. Woodring and C. A. Storvick, Am. J. Clin. Nutr. 23:1385 (1970).
6. F. Alvardo and A. Mahmood, Biochem. 13:2828 (1974).
7. T. J. Wilson and C. Wiseman, J. Physiol. 123:116 (1954).
8. A. M. Hoyumpa, Jr., K. J. Breen, S. Schenker, and F. A. Wilson, J. Lab. Clin. Med. 86:803 (1975).
9. H. J. Binder, Gastroenterology 67:441 (1974).
10. N. Kutunuma, E. Kominami and S. Koninami, Biochem. Biophys. Res. Com. 45:70 (1971).
11. A. Hodgkinson, Clin. Sci. Mol. Med. 46:357 (1974).

EXCRETION OF OXALIC ACID FOLLOWING THE INGESTION OF VARIOUS AMOUNTS OF OXALIC ACID-RICH FOODS

A. Strenge, A. Hesse, D. Bach, and W. Vahlensieck

Urinary Stone Research Department, Urological University Clinic, Bonn, West Germany

A slight elevation of urinary oxalate is more important as a risk factor for stone-formation than a corresponding rise in the urinary Ca. Therefore, dietary restriction of oxalic acid-rich foods for calcium oxalate stone-formers is an important measure in the prevention of stone recurrences. There is often disagreement on those foods that have to be restricted or avoided by stone-formers.

To study the effect of food intake on urinary oxalate, we chose conditions of extreme dietary intake for our initial investigations thus simulating the biased eating habits which might occur at the time of the main seasonal supply of each foodstuff. Instructions regarding the restriction of those foods believed to elevate urinary oxalate are based on measurements of 24-h urines only. Thus the most critical period for crystallization after the consumption of oxalate-rich foods is not known. We therefore examined urine samples collected at 3-hourly intervals after the load.

METHOD

Only normal subjects participated in our investigations. Food and fluid intake as well as urinary sample collections were standardized (Table 1).

Investigations on the effect of extreme dietary oxalate loads were made with rhubarb, spinach, chocolate, tomatoes, and asparagus. The amount of food intake and the corresponding oxalic acid and calcium content of each load, as calculated from standard food composition tables are given in Table 2.

Table 1.

Dietary instructions and sample collections for different oxalate loads

Day 1	calcium and oxalate - restricted diet	
	19 00 - 09 00 hours of Day 2	fasting
	20 00 - 22 00 hours	1000 ml of mineral water (< 10 mg Ca / kg)
Day 2	07 00 hours	200 ml of mineral water
	07 00 - 09 00 hours	1. urine collection (fasting period)
	09 00 hours	breakfast (bread, coffee, marmelade, butter) + dietary oxalate load
	09 00 - 11 00 hours	2. urine collection
	11 00 hours	300 ml of mineral water
	11 00 - 13 00 hours	3. urine collection
	13 00 - 16 00 hours	4. urine collection
	16 00 - 19 00 hours	5. urine collection
	19 00 - 22 00 hours	6. urine collection
	22 00 - 07 00 hours	7. urine collection
Day 3	24 - h urine collection	

Table 2.

Oxalic acid and calcium content of different dietary loads

Food	Total intake g	Oxalic acid content — mmol	Calcium content —
Rhubarb	600	35,796	7,20
Spinach	600	38,064	13,92
Chocolate (60% cocoa)	170	7,060	6,90
Tomatoes	600	0,258	1,92
Asparagus	600	0,114	2,76

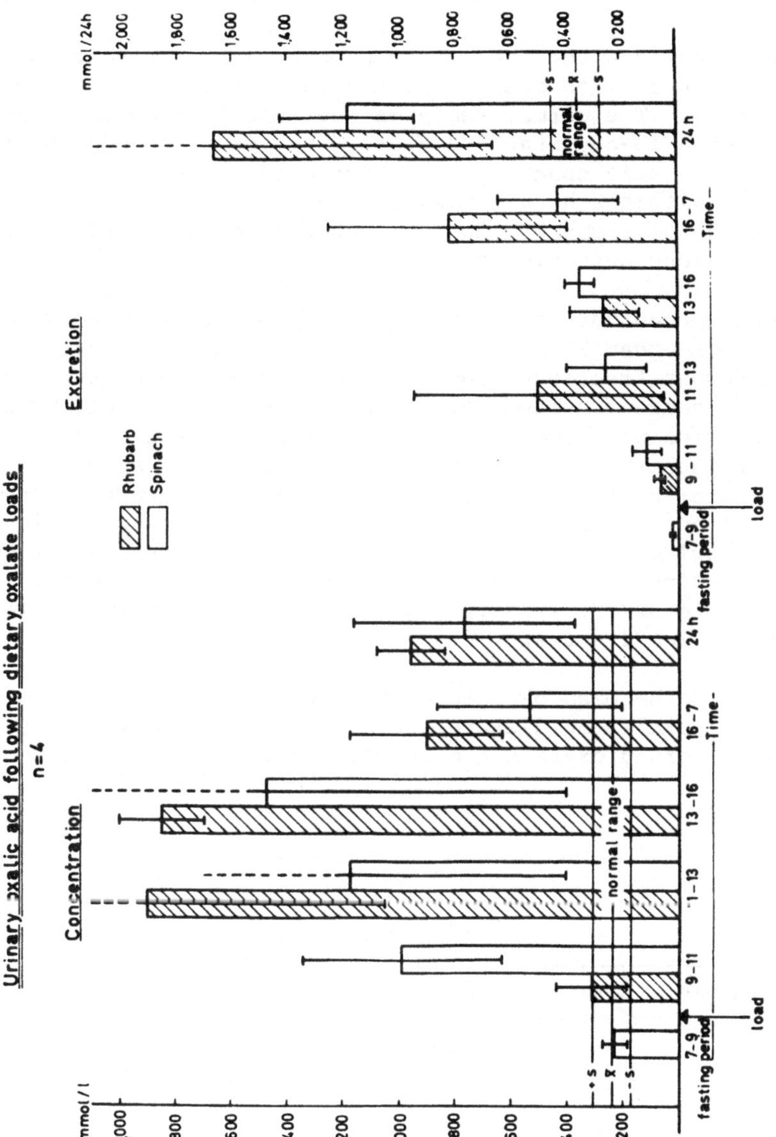

Figure 1. The concentration and excretion of oxalate following oral loads of rhubarb and spinach.

Following the load, urine was collected in 7 fractions and analyzed for oxalic acid, uric acid and other lithogenic and inhibitory substances. Oxalic acid was determined by gas chromatography.

RESULTS

Within 2 to 4 h after the intake of spinach and rhubarb urinary oxalic acid concentration reached values far exceeding the normal range (Figure 1). The normal range was defined from normal controls investigated on a 10-day standard diet. Whereas after consumption of spinach oxalic acid concentration increased to pathological concentrations within 2-h, a somewhat delayed course was observed after the intake of rhubarb. In the latter case, however, oxalic acid concentrations were higher.

The mean concentrations of the 24-h urine following rhubarb and spinach were more than 200% above the normal range. Collecting the urine in different fractions, however, shows that there were maxima in oxalic acid concentration that exceeded the normal range by 800%. The mean excretion was 350% above the upper normal range following the intake of rhubarb and 200% above this range after spinach intake. Although the oxalic acid content of spinach exceeded that of rhubarb (Table 2), the concentration as well as the excretion of oxalic acid was lower following a spinach load. This can be accounted for by the Ca content of spinach which is 2 times higher than in rhubarb. Relatively little oxalic acid is absorbed from the extremely high intake in these loading tests.

Subtracting the mean oxalate excretion after each load from the mean normal oxalic acid excretion gives us information about the additionally absorbed oxalate (Table 3). In the urine specimens with

Table 3.

Increment of oxalic acid excretion (mmol/24 h) after ingestion of rhubarb, spinach and chocolate

	oxalic acid content mmol	increase of oxalic acid above the mean normal range mmol	absorption %
rhubarb	35,796	1,301	3,64
spinach	38,064	0,819	2,16
chocolate	7,060	0,228	3,23

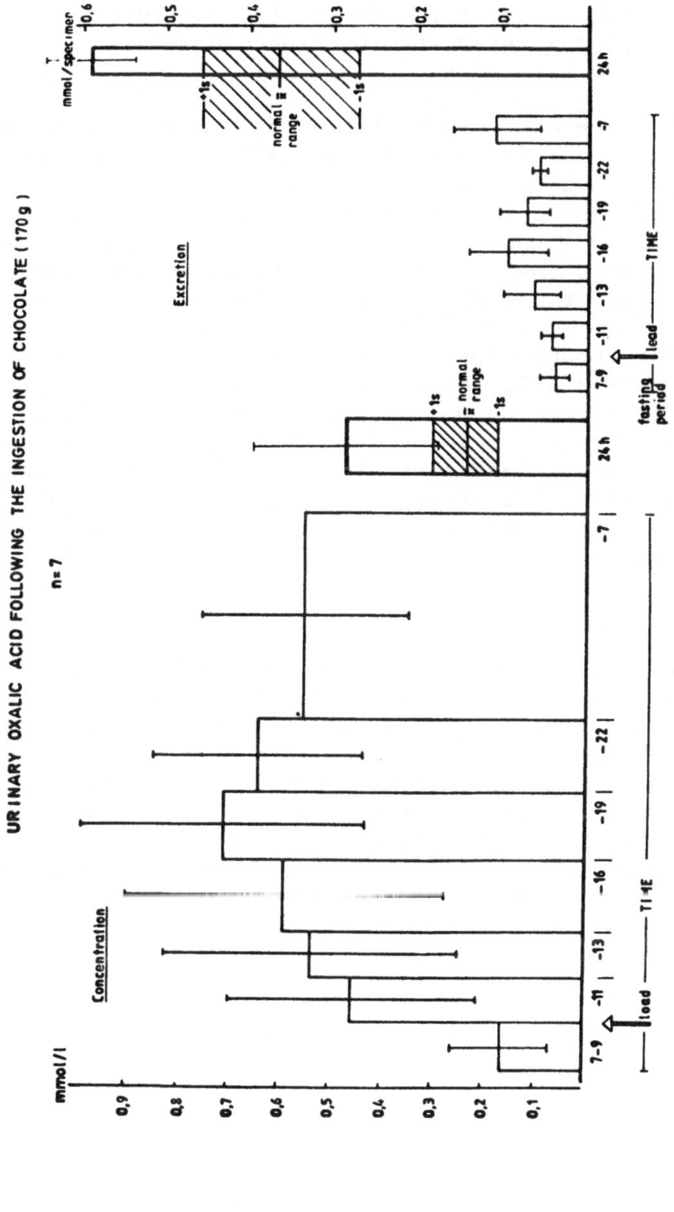

Figure 2. The concentration and excretion of oxalate following an oral load of chocolate.

extremely elevated oxalate concentration, crystalluria was observed. In parallel with oxalate concentration, it was found to be highest in the periods 11.00 - 13.00 h and 13.00 - 16.00 h. Initially weddellite crystals appeared and, with increasing concentration, these crystals grew in number and size. Aggregation was observed and whewellite crystals appeared. These crystals were regarded as an indication of hyperoxaluria and for stone-formers it should be interpreted as a risk situation.

The concentration and 24-h excretion of oxalate following the consumption of chocolate is shown in Figure 2. Two hours after the intake of chocolate, the urinary concentration of oxalic acid was increased about 50% above the upper normal range, reaching a maximum of 250% in the period 16.00 - 19.00 h. The total concentration in 24 h urine exceeded the normal range by 60% while the 24-h excretion was 25% above the upper normal range.

Following the consumption of asparagus there was no significant rise in urinary oxalic acid concentration other than what might resemble the reflection of a normal circadian rhythm. Values for the circadian rhythm of oxalic acid were taken from a study on normal subjects on a 10-day standard diet with a daily fluid intake of 1500 ml. The mean concentration after asparagus intake is within the normal range. Following the consumption of chocolate and asparagus no crystalluria was observed.

CONCLUSIONS

Asparagus represents no risk for stone-formation. Loads of rhubarb and spinach show peaks in concentration and crystalluria within 2 - 4 h after ingestion, thus representing a considerable risk situation for stone-formers. Chocolate must be restricted for stone-formers in the diet. Although no crystalluria could be observed, the concentration and excretion of oxalic acid increases within 10 h after intake to values above the normal range. From examination of Ca-oxalate crystalluria, the passage of aggregates and whewellite crystals are interpreted as a special risk situation.

RESPONSE OF GASTROINTESTINAL HORMONES AND INTESTINAL CALCIUM ABSORPTION DURING AN ORAL CARBOHYDRATE MEAL

D. Scholz[1], P. O. Schwille[1], and A. Sigel[2]

Mineral Metabolism and Hormone Research Laboratory[1],
Departments of Surgery and Urology[2],
University of Erlangen (FRG)

Little is known about changes of gastrointestinal (GI) hormones in patients with calcium lithiasis. In a preliminary study[1] we reported altered responses of GI hormones to a test meal in not rigidly classified calcium stone patients. It might be possible, that these observed changes modify the intestinal calcium absorption (CaA), which is one main cause for hypercalciuria in calcium stone formers. Therefore, we studied the influence of a synthetic test meal on the CaA and the secretion of gastrin, insulin, C-peptide, glucagon and glucose in healthy volunteers and patients with recurrent calcium lithiasis.

MATERIALS AND METHODS

The study was performed in male metabolically healthy volunteers and male patients with recurrent calcium lithiasis, classified into the different calciuria types[2] by a modified investigation program[3].

In protocol A 13 controls (- C), 8 patients with normocalciuria (= NC), 5 patients with renal hypercalciuria (= RHC) and 8 patients with absorptive hypercalciuria (= AHC) of comparable age and weight were investigated with their informed consent. After an overnight fast (12 - 15 hr) a balanced, carbohydrate rich synthetic meal[+] (2 g/kg body weight dissolved in 5 ml distilled water/kg body weight) was swallowed by the subjects.

In protocol B an identical dose of calcium as in A together with an amount of distilled water equal to the total mean volume of A was given to the participants of trial A (8 C, 5 NC, 5 RHC, 5 AHC). After 3 fasting baseline values, blood samples were collected at different time intervals over 180 min.

Gastrin-17, insulin, C-peptide and glucagon++ were determined by radioimmunoassay techniques established in this laboratory, glucose by the enzymatic method (Beckman Glucose Analyser). CaA was measured by a double isotope technique.

Statistics: Values indicate means ± 1 standard error (SEM). From the three preexperimental samples of each individual a mean baseline concentration was calculated for hormones and glucose, and experimentally induced changes were expressed as percent deviation from this baseline value (= 100 percent). The area under these values was integrated and results log-transformed. When individual values were normally distributed, the t-test was used to compare differences between controls and patients, otherwise the test of Mann and Whitney.

RESULTS

1. Baseline values (Table 1)

In protocol A gastrin values are higher in NC, RHC and AHC ($p < 0.01$ each), insulin values in NC and AHC ($p < 0.05$ each), and C-peptide in NC and AHC (not significant) in comparison with C. Glucose concentration is not different from C, whereas glucagon is lowered in NC ($p < 0.01$) and RHC ($p < 0.05$). Similar observations are found in protocol B, in which there is also a significantly higher glucose concentration in AHC ($p < 0.05$, Table 1).

2. CaA, responses of hormones and glucose (Figure 1, Table 2)

In protocol A the three hour values of CaA are elevated in NC ($p < 0.05$), RHC ($p < 0.05$) and AHC ($p < 0.001$), in the latter approximately twice the value of C. These differences of the CaA are reflected by the respective time curves (Figure 1). In AHC gastrin (60 - 120 min) and insulin (30 - 90 min) are significantly elevated above C and these findings correspond with the higher integrated outputs of the hormones. The slightly raised time curves and integrated outputs of gastrin and insulin in NC are not significantly different from C. C-peptide is elevated in NC (90 min) and AHC (90, 120 min), confirming an enhanced secretory activity of B-cells, but the integrated outputs, although elevated, are not significantly different from C. Glucose is higher in NC (10 min) and AHC (30 min) and the respective output is also greater in the latter ($p < 0.05$). The time curve and output of glucagon is low in NC, RHC and AHC in comparison with C (all differences not significant). A positive correlation between gastrin and CaA is found in C ($r = 0.54$, $p < 0.05$, $n = 13$).

+Vivasorb^R; Pfrimmer, Erlangen (FRG)
++Antibody 30 K, Dallas Diabetes Foundation, Dallas (USA)

Table 1. Baseline values of controls (C), patients with normocalciuric (NC), renal hypercalciuria (RHC) and absorptive hypercalciuria (AHC) before a synthetic test meal (=A) or distilled water with the respective calcium load of A (=B). Values are indicated as means ($\bar{x}$) ± 1 standard error (SEM); n = number of observations. [a]: $p<0.05$; [b]: $p<0.01$ vs C.

		Gastrin-17 pg-equiv/ml $\bar{x}$ ± SEM; n	Insulin uU/ml $\bar{x}$ ± SEM; n	C-Peptide ng/ml $\bar{x}$ ± SEM; n	Glucose mg/dl $\bar{x}$ ± SEM; n	Glucagon pg/ml $\bar{x}$ ± SEM; n
A	C	34 ± 1 ; 39	16 ± 1 ; 34	1.5 ± 0.2; 18	83 ± 1; 39	70 ± 6 ; 32
	NC	50 ± 5[b]; 22	19 ± 1[a]; 23	1.4 ± 0.1; 15	83 ± 2; 20	45 ± 6[b]; 23
	RHC	46 ± 4[b]; 13	17 ± 1 ; 13	1.5 ± 0.2; 12	86 ± 2; 11	48 ± 7[a]; 14
	AHC	49 ± 4[b]; 24	20 ± 1[a]; 24	1.9 ± 0.1; 13	82 ± 1; 24	62 ± 9 ; 24
	C	39 ± 2 ; 15	23 ± 1 ; 23		83 ± 1 ; 24	
	NC	52 ± 4[a]; 15	27 ± 2 ; 15		85 ± 3 ; 15	
	RHC	44 ± 6 ; 11	25 ± 1 ; 15		80 ± 3 ; 11	
	AHC	53 ± 2[b]; 11	31 ± 2[b]; 15		88 ± 1[a]; 14	

Table 2. Intestinal calcium absorption (Ca_A) and integrated responses of hormones and glucose during a synthetic test meal (= A) or distilled water with the respective calcium load of A (= B) in controls (C), patients with normocalciuria (NC), renal hypercalciuria (RHC) and absorptive hypercalciuria (AHC). For calculations see Methods section. Values are indicated as means ($\bar{x}$) ± 1 standard error (SEM); n = number of observations. [a]: $p<0.05$; [b]: $p<0.01$; [c]: $p<0.001$ vs C.

	Ca_A % of dose $\bar{x}$ ± SEM; n	Gastrin-17 $\bar{x}$ ± SEM; n	Insulin $\bar{x}$ ± SEM; n	C-peptide $\bar{x}$ ± SEM; n	Glucose $\bar{x}$ ± SEM; n	Glucagon $\bar{x}$ ± SEM; n
C	34±4 ; 13	4.22±0.04 ;13	4.77±0.07;13	4.66±0.09;7	4.11±0.03 ;13	4.26±0.05;11
NC	46±2[a]; 8	4.30±0.10 ; 8	4.91±0.09; 8	4.70±0.08;5	4.15±0.02 ; 8	4.19±0.06; 8
RHC	46±5[a]; 5	4.19±0.04 ; 5	4.88±0.05; 5	4.54±0.05;5	4.13±0.04 ; 5	4.11±0.09; 5
AHC	70±3[c]; 8	4.40±0.05[b]; 8	4.95±0.15; 8	4.76±0.04;5	4.20±0.03[a]; 8	4.20±0.03; 8
C	42±2 ; 8	4.01±0.03 ; 8	3.95±0.04; 8		3.96±0.01 ; 8	
NC	45±3 ; 5	3.95±0.04 ; 5	3.94±0.04; 5		3.99±0.03 ; 5	
RHC	51±3[a]; 5	3.99±0.09 ; 5	3.97±0.04; 5		3.98±0.03 ; 5	
AHC	57±2[b]; 5	4.02±0.04 ; 5	3.88±0.08; 5		3.96±0.02 ; 5	

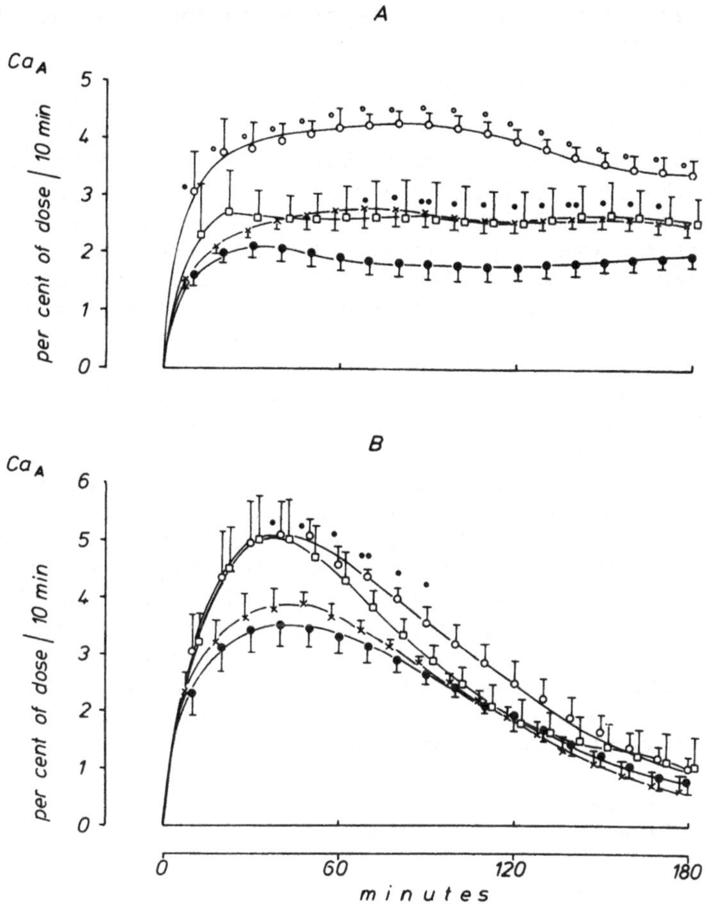

Figure 1. Intestinal calcium absorption (Ca_A) during a synthetic test meal (= A) or distilled water with the respective calcium load of A (= B) in controls (•), patients with normocalciuria (X), renal hypercalciuria (□) and absorptive hypercalciuria (O). ⊥ represents mean ± 1 standard deviation. •: p<0.05; ••: p<0.01; °: p<0.001 vs C.

In protocol B CaA is elevated in NC, RHC, and AHC, but because of the small number of participants in this trial, differences are only significant in RHC (p <0.05) and AHC (p <0.01). The percent deviation from baseline values of hormone and glucose responses is minimal in all groups, and the integrated outputs are not significantly different from C.

COMMENTS

An elevated CaA in comparison with C is found in NC, RHC, AHC during both the test meal and the supply of distilled water with the respective amount of calcium of the test meal. Therefore the alteration of the CaA in patients is largely independent of the acute load irrèspective of either nutrients administered or the associated water calcium supply alone. The a priori and chronically altered CaA thus may become only slightly modified by the nutrient load, as is the case with NC and AHC, in which groups the difference in the CaA between C and NC respectively. AHC is greater during the test meal than during the water plus calcium supply.

Glucose in diabetic man[4] and insulin[5] in the streptozotocin diabetic rat are reported to raise CaA. As in our study elevated values of glucose and insulin are found in NC and AHC in the fasting state and during the carbohydrate rich test meal, alterations in carbohydrate metabolism could well be considered responsible for the additional elevation of CaA in those patients. However, more detailed investigations are necessary to substantiate this hypothesis, especially as serum glucose is high in these patients, despite the facts all participants had roughly identical body weight and no symptoms of overt diabetes.

Besides glucose other insulinogenic factors, e.g. gastrin[6] deserve attention by investigators.

REFERENCES

1. P. O. Schwille, R. Thun, and N. M. Samberger, in:"Urolithiasis Research," H. Fleisch, W. G. Robertson, L. H. Smith, and W. Vahlensieck, ed. Plenum Press, New York (1976).
2. C. Y. C. Pak, M. Ohata, E. C. Lawrence, and W. Snyder, J. Clin. Invest. 54:387 (1974).
3. D. Scholz, P. O. Schwille, and A. Sigel, Urologe A 19:196 (1980).
4. J. Mirouze, and I. Monnier, J d'Urologie et de Nephrologie 12:921 (1975).
5. L. E. Schneider, L. M. Nowosielski, and H. P. Schedl, Endocrinology 100:67 (1977).
6. J. F. Rehfeld, and F. Stadil, J. Clin. Invest. 52:1415 (1973).

ACKNOWLEDGMENT

We are grateful to K. Schwille, M. L. Rasenack, I. Goldberg, and B. Schreiber for technical assistance.

HOW TO PREVENT THE HYPERRESORPTION OF DIETARY OXALATE AND THE OXALATE PEAKS IN URINE

P. Leskovar, R. Hartung, M. Hropot,
H. Schneider, H. G. Reichling, and H. Huber
Urologische Klinik und Poliklinik rechts der Isar
der Technischen Universität München
München, Germany

INTRODUCTION

Our detailed investigations concerning the kinetics of Ca-oxalate and Ca-phosphate crystal growth from metastable and unstable solutions showed clearly that differences in oxalate concentration as small as 0.05 - 0.15 mM resulted in a distinct shift of the size-distribution curve of formed crystals toward bigger crystals and crystal aggregates. In the case of Ca^{2+} ions, the comparable increase in the average size of formed crystals can be achieved by changes in the Ca^{2+} concentration as high as 1.0 - 3.0 mM, this corresponds to a factor of 15 - 20. The effect of minimal changes in the oxalate concentration is enhanced furthermore if the oxalate load is prolonged. In urine, the stoichiometrically unfavorable molar oxalate/calcium ratio of 1/20 - 1/30 could be responsible for the highly sensitive response of crystal growth to the minimal changes in the oxalate concentration.

These observations are in accordance with the observations of Robertson et al.[1] who, measuring the activity product of Ca-oxalate in an average urine during the continuous addition of Ca^{2+} or $C_2O_4^{2-}$ ions, found that the increasing oxalate concentration rapidly caused the Ca-oxalate product to exceed the formation product, with crystal precipitation; whereas, the analogous increase of the Ca^{2+} concentration resulted in flattening of the activity product curve with the consequence of a strongly delayed transgression of the formation product.

A further instructive experiment of Dr. Robertson and his co-workers[2] demonstrated clearly that an oral oxalate load led to a highly significant increase in number and size of urinary crystals, especially in the group of the stone-patients, whereas the corresponding oral calcium load failed to show a comparable rise in urinary crystals and their size. Also noticeable was the high intestinal absorption rate and the resulting high urinary oxalate concentration after oral administration of oxalate to a group of stone patients in comparison to a normal group.

The most striking difference between the recurrent stone-formers and healthy persons appears to be the intestinal absorption of the dietary oxalate. As it is known, the oxalate absorption is increased in patients with small intestine diseases or after ileal resection, a fact that can be explained in part by the binding of the dietary calcium to free fatty acids being incompletely resorbed (formation of "calcium soap") instead of binding to the dietary oxalate.

One can imagine that the endogenous oxalate, normally representing 80 - 90% of the total urinary oxalate, continuously provides a basic level of urinary oxalate (20 - 30 mg/day). The nutritional oxalate on the contrary represents a highly variable part of the total urinary oxalate. The increased urinary excretion of oxalate as measured in the 24 hour urine, amounting normally to 40 - 45 mg/24 h, seldom to 50 - 65 mg/24 h does not exhibit temporary peaks to much higher hourly rates than these values. In our laboratory calcium oxalate crystal growth in urine is especially enhanced after a prolonged (exogenous) oxalate load (1 - 3 hours). Therefore, it is possible that urinary oxalate could be reduced by binding exogenous oxalate in the gut, in analogy to urinary calcium reduction by its gastrointestinal binding to sodium cellulose phosphate (NCP) or to strong acid cationic exchangers.

MATERIALS AND METHODS

The following reagents were used: Strontium sulfate ($Sr\,Cl_2 \cdot 6H_2O$, Merck 7865 + $Na_2SO_4 \cdot 10H_2O$, Merck 6648, equimolar amounts), calcium sulfate ($CaCl_2 \cdot 2H_2O$, Merck 2382 + $Na_2SO_4 \cdot 10H_2O$, Merck 6648, equimolar amounts), di-sodium oxalate (Merck 6556), calcium chloride dihydrate (Merck 2382), strongly acidic cationic exchanger: a) Typ I, Merck 4765); b) Lewatit S1020, strongly basic anionic exchanger: a) Typ III (Merck 4767); b) Lewatit MP 5080, weakly basic anionic exchanger: Typ II (Merck 4766), Permutid T/Decalso (Merck 2939), Manganic (IV) oxide (pyrolysite, Merck 5957), Ferric (III) oxide (Merck 3924), aluminum oxide Typ T (Merck 1105), aluminum oxide (γ-alumina) (Merck 1095), aluminiumphosphate (basic, Merck 1098), magnesium oxide (Merck 5865), zinc oxide (Merck 8849), iron-powder (Merck 3800), manganese-powder (Merck 12237).

Determination of soluble oxalate was done by turbidimetry (after addition of the standard $CaCl_2$-solution) (semiquantitative method) or a double enzymatic method (semimicro, OxDC/FDH).

RESULTS AND DISCUSSION

Systematic investigations of a great number or coarse (powdered) scarcely soluble substances showed that in direct short-term in vitro experiments (30-120 min treatment) only strontium sulfate, calcium sulfate and to a certain degree the strong acidic cationic exchangers (in Ca-form) are able to bind a high-percent of the dissolved oxalate ion. In the long-term in vitro experiment (100 days) however several additional coarse, scarcely soluble substances like MnO_2, MgO, Fe_2O_3, ZnO, Fe- and Mn-powder and other inorganic materials were capable to bind a relatively high percent of the dissolved $C_2O_4^{2-}$ ion. In the short-term experiment, strontium sulfate and calcium sulfate proved to be the most effective compounds binding the oxalate almost completely. The ranking of oxalate binding the other reagents is as follows: strongly acidic cationic exchangers (Typ I, Merck 4765 and Lewatit 51020) in the Ca form, strongly basic anionic exchangers (Typ III, Merck 4767 and Lewatit MP 5080) in the Cl form, basic aluminum phosphate and finally weakly basic anionic exchangers (Typ II, Merck 4766). The binding of oxalate by the ionic exchangers was, in general, slow and incomplete, compared with Sr- and Ca- sulfate. The $C_2O_4^{2-}$ binding capacity of the strongly basic anionic exchangers didn't exceed 60%, that one of the weakly basic exchangers was less than 20%. Permutites showed low activity (e.g. the Permutit T, Decalso, Merck 2939).

In the long-term experiment (100 days), Sr- and Ca- sulfate bound the dissolved oxalate in both, physiological (< 50 mg/l) and pathological (< 100 mg/l) range, analogously to the short-term experiment, nearly completely (> 95%). A similarly high $C_2O_4^{2-}$ binding capacity showed (only in the long-term experiment) by MNO_2. A surprise effect was found for long-term binding of oxalate by some other coarse inorganic materials (Fe_2O_3, Al_2O_3, MgO, ZnO, Fe^- and Mn^- powder).

By the rapid, complete and selective binding of oxalate, the $SrSO_4$ and the $CaSO_4$ fulfil the expectations; the Sr-sulfate could be advantageous because of the very low solubility. In the 100 ml water, only 11.4 mg $SrSO_4$ are soluble. (In the case of $CaSO_4$, 202 mg can be dissolved in 100 ml water).

Pak[3] proposed a calcium therapy in stone patients who don't respond to calcium load by a hyperresorption. The administered soluble calcium salt should bind the nutritional oxalate in the gut and prevent its absorption. Pak sees in the oxalate resorption a greater risk than in the accompanying calcium absorption.

The introduction of the relatively insoluble calcium sulfate would doubtless reduce the inevitable calcium absorption. Even this reduced calcium absorption could be omitted by the replacement of

$CaSO_4$ with highly insoluble $SrSO_4$. The toxicity of the "cold" isotope of strontium is not higher than that of calcium (Rauen: Biochemisches Taschenbuch I and II; Braun/Dönhardt: Vergiftungs-register). The "bad reputation" of strontium seems to originate from its radioactive nuclide ^{90}Sr (^{89}Sr). Normal strontium, present in the commercially available strontium chemicals, is a mixture of the non-radioactive isotopes 88 (82.56%), 86 (9.86%), 87 (7.02%) and 84 (0.56%).

The proposal to add strontium to fluoridated drinking water to increase its protective activity against dental caries, an idea based on the observation that school children in Wisconsin (USA) drinking water with 5 - 6 mg/l strontium had significantly reduced caries frequency, is an additional indication of strontium's relative lack of toxicity. The mechanism of oxalate binding by the reagents tested in this report is not known; it could be the result of the formation of a highly insoluble calcium oxalate salt from the relatively more soluble $CaSO_4$ salt or the direct result of the alkaline earth cation being in excess with oxalate. Fixation of dietary oxalate in the gut might be favored by the large active surface on the strontium and calcium sulfate, and the crystallization of SrC_2O_4 on CaC_2O_4 may be accelerated by the presence of $SrSO_4$ or $CaSO_4$ solid phase.

CONCLUSION

From our systematic screening of coarse, insoluble organic materials that would bind the dissolved oxalate it can be concluded that Sr- and Ca-sulfate fulfil in the best way our expectations: they bind rapidly and completely the dissolved oxalate, are not toxic and are selective. They could reduce the exogenous oxalate in some analogy to the reduction of dietary calcium by sodium cellulose phosphate or strong cationic exchangers. The exogenous oxalate is in our opinion critical for the short term oxalate peaks in urine; their prevention could reduce, from the crystal-kinetic point of view, the risk of stone formation.

REFERENCES

1. W. G. Robertson, M. Peacock, and B. E. C. Nordin, in: "Urolithiasis: Physical Aspects," B. Finlayson, L. L. Hench, L. H. Smith, eds., National Academy of Sciences, Washington, D. C. (1972).
2. W. G. Robertson, M. Peacock, and B. E. C. Nordin, Lancet 2:21 (1969).
3. C. Y. C. Pak, in:"Urolithiasis Research," H. Fleisch, W. G. Robertson, L. H. Smith, and W. Vahlensieck, ed., Plenum Press, New York-London (1976).
4. B. Carlquist and A. Nelson, Acta. Radiol. 54:305 (1960).
5. A. Catsch, Int. J. Rad. Biol. 4:75 (1961).

6. A. Catsch, Atomkernenergie 7/2:65 (1960).

ACKNOWLEDGMENT

The authors would like to thank Mrs. D. Scherm, Mr. K.-L. Schade, Mrs. H. Richter and Mr. M. Gottinger (München) for their kind technical assistance.

ISOLATION OF THE OXALATE BINDING PROTEIN

Bernardo Pinto and José L. Paternain

Laboratorio de Exploraciones Metabolicas

Barcelona, Catalunya, Spain

Intestinal hyperabsorption of oxalate occurs secondary to some intestinal disorders[1] but can also be associated with mild hyperoxaluria in the absence of intestinal disease[2]. Intestinal transport of oxalate appears to be a diffusive mechanism[3] dependent on the oxalic acid concentration gradient. This transport appears to be affected by the presence of an oxalate binding protein[4] whose physiological significance has not been established. The following paper describes the partial purification of this protein from rabbit small intestine.

EXPERIMENTAL PROCEDURE

Partial Purification

Oxalate binding protein from a crude intestinal extract was purified by precipitation with ammonium sulfate and sephadex chromatography.

Rabbit small intestine stored at 20C was washed with 0.9 percent sodium chloride and suspended at 4C in the double volume of 10 mM sodium phosphate buffer (pH 7.5). The intestine was cut in small pieces and homogenized in a blender for 30 seconds, four times. The homogenate was centrifuged at 4C and 6,000 r.p.m. for 10 minutes in a Sorvall SM-24 rotor. Supernatant was recentrifuged for 30 minutes at 20,000 r.p.m. under the same conditions. The second supernatant at 4C was brought to a 50% concentration with an ammonium sulfate supersaturated solution. The resulting precipitate was pelleted by centrifugation at 10,000 r.p.m. for 10 minutes under the conditions described above. The 50% ammonium sulfate supernatant was concentrated 70 percent with the same ammonium sulfate supersaturated solution. The suspension was recentrifuged as described above and the pellet dissolved in the minimum volume of 10 mM sodium phosphate buffer (pH 7.5).

The total volume of the 70% ammonium sulfate precipitate was layered on the top of a 90 x 5 cm size sephadex G - 200 column, equilibrated with 10 mM sodium phosphate buffer (pH 7.5). Elution with the same buffer was carried out by collecting 4 ml fractions at room temperature. The elution profile was monitored at 280 nm.

Oxalate binding activity was identified with the corresponding 280 nm absorbing peak by incubating 150 mg of protein from the ammonium sulfate step with 25 x 10^6 cpm. ^{14}C-oxalic acid in the same volume of 10 mM phosphate buffer (pH 7.5) as that of the ammonium sulfate precipitate layered on the sephadex G - 200 column. This mixture was incubated for 24 hr at 4C and then layered on the top of the same sephadex G - 200 column. Equilibration and elution was performed in the same manner.

The oxalate binding peak was concentrated at room temperature by ultradialysis in collodion bags. This procedure yielded a 12 fold purification and a 27% recovery (Table 1).

Oxalate Binding Assay

In a final volume of 1 ml the incubation mixtures contained: 10 μmoles of phosphate buffer (pH 7.5), 25 nmoles of oxalic acid, 2 x 10^6 cpm of ^{14}C-oxalic acid (U) (specific activity 75 mCi/mmole from Amersham Radiochemical Centre, England) and increasing amounts of the sample to be tested. The correct amount of sample added to incubation mixture has to show linear kinetics. The incubation mixtures were incubated at 4C for 24 hr. Free and bound oxalate portions were separated on 22 by 1.6 cm sephadex G-25 columns. The columns were equilibrated and eluted with 10 mM phosphate buffer (pH 7.5) by collecting 1 ml fractions. Radioactivity in the fractions was determined in a mixture of 0.2 per cent P.P.O. (2,5-diphenyl-oxazole) and 0.002 per cent P.O.P.O.P. (1,4 bis(2-5-phenyl-oxazolyl)benzene) in dioxane. The vials were counted for 10 minutes in a scintillation counter (Nuclear Chicago, type Isocap-300).

COMMENT

The oxalate binder from small intestine has been partially purified with the procedure described herein. Further purification is needed before definitive physicochemical properties can be established. If the physicochemical properties can not be established, the physiological significance may remain obscure. It can be speculated that this protein mediates the diffusion of oxalate across the gut.

Table 1. Purification Procedure

Sample	Volume ml	Protein mg/ml	Specific activity oxalate bound pmoles/mg protein	Total activity pmoles	Purification fold	Yield %
Crude extract	460	22.7	8.8	91,889	--	100
Ammonium sulfate 50 - 70%	55	33.6	44.8	82,790	5.09	90
Sephadex G-200	260	0.91	108.0	25,552	12.27	27.8

REFERENCES

1. L. H. Smith, A. F. Hofmann, J. T. McCall, and P. J. Thomas, Clin. Res. 18:541 (1970).
2. B. Pinto, G. Crespí, F. Solé-Balcells, and P. Barceló, Kid. Int. 5:285 (1974).
3. H. J. Binder, Gastroenterology 67:441 (1974).
4. B. Pinto and J. L. Paternain, Invest. Urol. 15:502 (1978).

VII. METABOLISM

THE PATHOPHYSIOLOGICAL BASIS OF HYPERCALCIURIA IN PRIMARY HYPERPARATHYROIDISM

Arthur E. Broadus, Ronald L. Horst, Robert Lang,
E. Travis Littledike, and Howard Rasmussen
Department of Internal Medicine, Yale University,
New Haven, Connecticut and the National Animal
Disease Center, Ames, Iowa

INTRODUCTION

When initially described in the mid-1920's, primary hyperparathyroidism (1°HPT) was regarded as a rare and severe disorder of bone. Shortly thereafter, Albright and colleagues recognized a different clinical presentation of 1°HPT in patients with renal stones who lacked evidence of overt bone disease[1]. It subsequently became clear that renal stones are a far more frequent complication of 1°HPT than overt osteitis, being the presenting complaint in approximately 50% of patients[2]. Further, it was recognized that patients presenting with stones rarely display evidence of clinical bone involvement and that patients presenting with clinical bone disease only rarely gave a history of renal stones (nephrocalcinosis was variably observed in a minority of patients with both presentations). Thus, early investigators were impressed by reasonably distinctive "bone" and "stone" presentations of the disorder and offered several hypotheses in attempt to explain their observations. These included Albright's "dietary calcium" hypothesis[1]. Dent's "dual hormone" hypothesis[3], and the general proposal that clinical bone involvement developed as a function of the duration of the disease. Although Albright's general tenets concerning external calcium balance were later supported by the observation of negative balance in patients with overt bone disease and zero or even positive balance in patients with stone disease[4]. All three hypotheses were subsequently either disproven or could not be supported by the accumulated evidence[2]. Thus, the clinical "spectrum" of the disorder remained enigmatic well through the 1960's.

Most recent reports of large series of patients with 1°HPT have emphasized that the growth rate of the parathyroid lesion may be an important variable influencing the presentation of the disease and have suggested that patients with overt bone disease have an inherently aggressive basic disease process, whereas the process may be relatively indolent in patients with stone disease[5,6,7]. Indeed, patients with parathyroid carcinoma typically present with the general features of the "bone" presentation. Although this "growth rate" proposal has obvious and implicit merit in explaining the severe disease process typifying patients with 1°HPT and clinical bone disease, this proposal sheds little light in the pathogenesis of stones in 1°HPT, unless relative indolence and chronicity have something to do with stone formation.

In 1975, Peacock reported data on fractional intestinal calcium absorption in 111 patients with 1°HPT[8]. Because of the difficulties involved in defining clinically significant bone involvement, the patients were classified as those with stone disease (57% of patients) and those with "other" presentations of the disease. He noted that patients with 1°HPT and stones invariably displayed an increase in intestinal calcium absorption, whereas the majority of patients with "other" presentations had normal intestinal calcium absorption[8]. Although these findings were incorrectly attributed to putative intestinal effects of parathyroid hormone, the results suggested that the status of intestinal calcium absorption was another important variable which might influence the presentation and pathogenesis of complications in 1°HPT.

The present series represents an attempt to confirm and extend the implications of this brief historical review.

METHODS

Eighty unselected patients with 1°HPT were studied. There were 54 women and 26 men, and the average age was 50 years. Thirty-one (39%) patients had a history of one or more renal stone events. Twelve patients with "subtle" primary HPT, presenting with mild, intermittent hypercalcemia, were also studied. These patients have been described in detail previously[9]; 9 of the 12 (75%) had a history of one or more stone events. Informed consent was obtained from all patients.

All patients were studied with an oral calcium tolerance test employing 1000 mg of elemental calcium[2]. Data from the fasting control period included fasting serum calcium, phosphorus, iPTH, 25-OHD, and $1,25\text{-}(OH)_2D$, and fasting calcium excretion, TmP/GFR, and nephrogenous cyclic AMP (NcAMP). The calciuric response (increase in calcium excretion from the control period to the experimental collection period, expressed as Δ mg calcium/100 ml glomerular filtrate, GF) served as an index of intestinal calcium absorption, the calcemic response as an index of calcium "tolerance", and the induced decrease in NcAMP from the control period to the experimental collection period as an index of parathyroid suppressibility[2,9,10]. All patients were studied after 7-10 days on a restricted (approximately 400 mg) calcium intake.

Fifty-five of the 80 unselected patients with 1°HPT and all 12 patients with "subtle" 1°HPT were studied on a metabolic ward with a minimum of two 24-hour urine collections each on both a 400 mg and a 1000 mg calcium diet[9,10]. The diets were otherwise identical.

The analytical techniques have been previously described[9,10]. Pertinent normal ranges include serum calcium 9.0-10.6 mg/dl, serum phosphorus approximately 3.0-4.5 mg/dl, serum iPTH $<$ 100 µleq/ml, plasma 25-OHD $>$ 15 ng/ml, plasma 1,25 OH_2D $<$ 65 pg/ml, fasting calcium excretion $<$ 0.18 mg calcium/100 ml GF, TmP/GFR $>$ 2.5 mg/dl, and NcAMP $<$ 2.5 nmol/100 ml GF[9,10]. The normal calciuric response to the calcium tolerance test is $< \Delta 0.20$ mg calcium/100 ml GF[9,10]. Hypercalciuria was defined as a calcium excretion rate $>$ 300 mg/day or $>$ 4 mg/kg/day on the 1000 mg calcium diet.

Statistical analysis was performed with the paired and unpaired t-test.

RESULTS AND COMMENTS

There was a strong positive correlation ($r=0.73$, $p < .001$) between the plasma concentration of 1,25-OH_2D and the calciuric response to the calcium tolerance test (Figure 1). There were also strong positive correlations between circulating 1,25 $(OH)_2D$ and calcium excretion on the 1000 mg calcium intake ($r=0.67$, $p < .001$, Figure 2) and the increase in calcium excretion on the 1000 mg intake relative to the 400 mg calcium intake ($r=0.64$, $p < .001$, data not shown). In the 55 patients studied in detail, the calciuric response to the tolerance test was strongly correlated with the rate of calcium excretion on the 1000 mg calcium diet ($r=0.70$, $p < .001$, data not shown). There was a weaker but significant correlation ($r=0.52$, $p < .01$) between fasting calcium excretion and 24-hour calcium excretion on the 1000 mg diet. Fasting calcium excretion did not correlate with either circulating 1,25-$(OH)_2D$ or the fasting serum calcium. This series of correlations suggests that the intestine serves as the principal source of urinary calcium in patients with 1°HPT.

There was considerable heterogeneity in the patient group with respect to the status of intestinal calcium absorption (Figure 1) and the presence and/or degree of hypercalciuria (Figure 2). Although the data clearly represent a continuum, patients with stone disease were noted to cluster in the upper reaches of both figures, denoting concurrent abnormalities in the circulating level of 1,25-$(OH)_2D$ and calcium absorption and excretion. In order to further examine pathophysiological correlates, the patients were subdivided into "absorptive" and "nonabsorptive" subpopulations on the basis of whether they displayed an abnormal calciuric response to the calcium tolerance test.

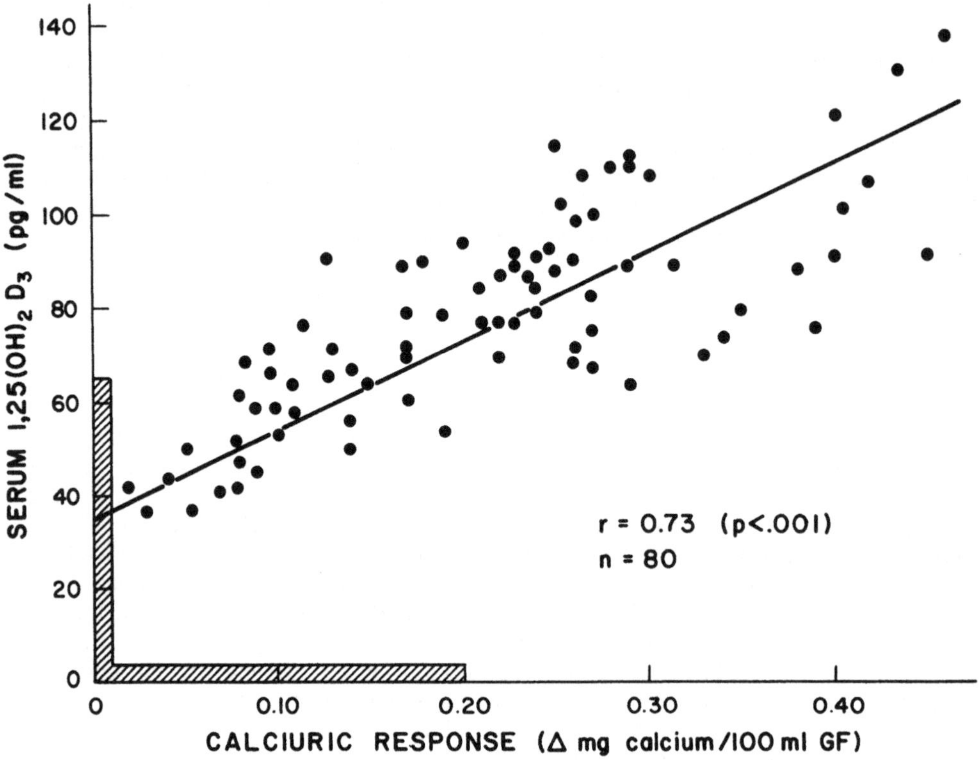

Figure 1. Correlation between plasma 1,25-$(OH)_2D$ and the calciuric response to the oral calcium tolerance test in 80 patients with 1°HPT.

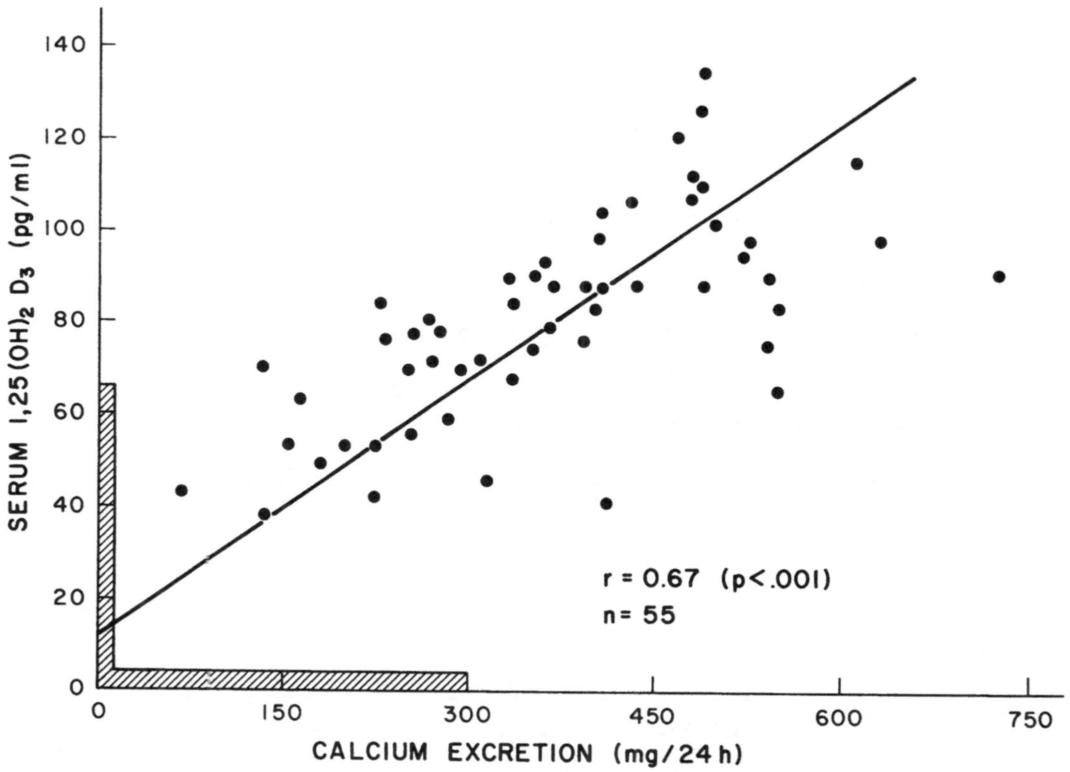

Figure 2. Correlation between plasma $1,25(OH)_2D$ and calcium excretion determined on a 1000 mg calcium diet in 55 patients with 1^oHPT.

Table 1. Subpopulations of Patients with Primary Hyperparathyroidism*

Category of Patients	No. of Patients	Calciuric Response (mg Ca/100 ml GF)	Plasma 1,25-(OH)$_2$D (pg/ml)	Calcium Excretion ‡ Fasting (mg/100 ml GF)	Calcium Excretion ‡ 400 mg Diet (mg/24 hr)	Calcium Excretion ‡ 1000 mg Diet (mg/24 hr)	No. of Patients With Stones
Absorptive	45	0.29	89	0.19	314	449	26/45 (58%)
Nonabsorptive	35	0.11	59	0.16	203	260	5/35 (14%)
P value		<.001	<.001	NS	<.001	<.001	<.001

*All data are shown as mean values.

‡Fasting calcium excretion was measured in all patients. Twenty-four hour data on both calcium intakes were obtained in 33 absorptive and 22 nonabsorptive patients.

Table 2. Features of Absorptive and Nonabsorptive Subpopulations*

Category of Patients	Plasma 25-OHD (ng/ml)	Serum Calcium (mg/dl)	Serum Phosphorus (mg/dl)	TmP/GFR (mg/dl)	GFR (ml/min)	Serum iPTH (µl-eq/ml)	NcAMP (nmol/100 ml GF)	Age (yr)	Sex (M/F)
Absorptive	19	11.0	2.6	2.3	97	118	4.06	48	14/31
Nonabsorptive	20	11.3	2.7	2.3	100	117	3.95	52	12/23

* All data are shown as mean values.

As shown in Table 1, the 45 patients in the absorptive subpopulation displayed a striking mean elevation in the plasma concentration of 1,25-$(OH)_2D$ and marked hypercalciuria, whereas the 35 patients in the nonabsorptive subpopulation had normal or high-normal plasma 1,25-$(OH)_2D$ levels and were predominantly normocalciuric. Fasting calcium excretion was slightly but not significantly higher in the absorptive than in the nonabsorptive patients. The influence of calcium intake and the status of intestinal calcium absorption on the patterns of calcium excretion in the two subpopulations was most apparent when viewed in the sequence fasting calcium excretion→ calcium excretion on the 400 mg diet→calcium excretion on the 1000 mg diet (Table 1).

The circulating concentration of 1,25-$(OH)_2D$ varied over a 4-fold range and was the key pathophysiological feature which distinguished the absorptive and nonabsorptive subpopulations (Figures 1 and 2). Table 2 summarizes the variables which might be expected to relate to the 1,25-$(OH)_2D$ production rate in the patients. The two subpopulations were noted to be descriptively and biochemically virtually identical, so that none of the factors currently regarded as regulating 1,25-$(OH)_2D$ synthesis could be invoked to explain the observed differences in 1,25-$(OH)_2D$ levels. Similarly, none of these variables correlated with circulating 1,25-$(OH)_2D$ when the patient population was considered as a whole[10],

In the entire group of 80 patients, the oral dose of calcium produced a 20% suppression in NcAMP (from 3.99 to 3.19 nmol/100 ml GF), resulting in values for NcAMP which were within the normal range in 35% of patients during the experimental collection period. The absorptive patients displayed a significantly ($p < .001$) greater calcemic response or calcium "intolerance" than did the nonabsorptive patients, which was associated with a significantly greater suppression in NcAMP (-0.94 versus - 0.55 nmol/100 ml GF, respectively, $p < .01$). Similarly, increasing the daily calcium intake from low-normal (400 mg) to high-normal (1000 mg) was associated with a significant ($p < .001$) reduction in 24-hour total cAMP excretion, resulting in values which were within the normal range in 30% of patients on the 1000 mg calcium diet. Again, the diet induced suppression in total cAMP excretion was significantly greater ($p < .02$) in the absorptive than in the nonabsorptive patients (data not shown).

Twenty-six of the 45 patients (58%) in the absorptive subpopulation had a history of renal stones, whereas only 5 of the 35 patients (14%) in the nonabsorptive subpopulation had a history of stones.

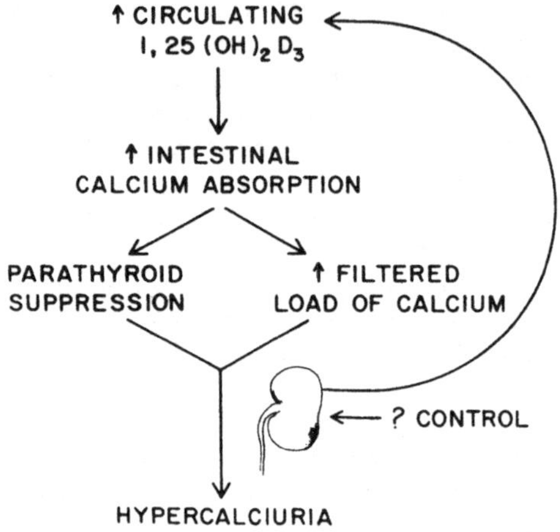

Figure 3. Schematic representation of the pathophysiological sequence leading to hypercalciuria in absorptive patients with 1°HPT.

Figure 3 is a schematic representation of the pathophysiological sequence which leads to hypercalciuria in patients with the absorptive pattern. The increased circulating $1,25-(OH)_2D$ is associated with intestinal hyperabsorption of calcium and an accentuated calcemic response, leading to both a significant post-prandial increase in the filtered load of calcium and a significant postprandial suppression in parathyroid function, with an attendant reduction in the effects of the hormone on calcium reabsorption in the distal nephron. The net result is an enhanced spillage of the absorbed calcium into the urine, hypercalciuria, and predisposition to stone formation. This pathophysiological pattern of calcium absorption and excretion is remarkably similar to the pattern observed in patients with absorptive hypercalciuria, albeit at a clearly higher level of parathyroid function. Although there is an apparent "resorptive" component in the hypercalciuria in certain patients with 1°HPT, and an occasional patient is encountered in whom this component appears to be predominant (based on marked hypercalciuria on a restricted calcium diet, increased fasting calcium excretion, a low-normal calciuric response, and normal circulating 1,25-$(OH)_2D$, the aggregate data suggests that the sequence depicted in Figure 3 is primarily responsible for hypercalciuria in the vast majority of patients with 1^oHPT.

Patients with "subtle" 1^oHPT represent a forme fruste of the typical patient in the absorptive subpopulation and are an extreme example of the disproportionality between the level of the fasting serum calcium and the rate of calcium excretion in 1^oHPT. Although this category of patient has spawned a literature which is justly regarded as controversial[2,9], an appreciation of the pathophysiological sequence of events depicted in Figure 3 provides both an understanding of the principal abnormalities in this subtle variant of 1^oHPT and a sound approach to the diagnosis of these patients. In these patients, the calcium tolerance test serves as a rather classical endocrine suppression test, and the combination of 1) induced-hypercalcemia (mean 11.4 mg/dl from a mean baseline value of 10.2 mg/dl) and 2) abnormal suppressibility of NcAMP diagnosis a relatively simple matter (Figure 4). Circulating levels of 1,25-$(OH)_2D$ are typically markedly elevated in patients with subtle 1° HPT (to a mean value of 90 pg/ml in the patients illustrated in Figure 4). Our rule-of-thumb is to seriously consider this diagnosis in any hypercalciuric patient with a mean total serum calcium equal to or greater than 10.0 mg/dl on 3 determinations performed fasting and with scrupulous sampling and analytical technique. Eighty percent of patients with "subtle" 1^oHPT harbor a single, small (< 1 gm) parathyroid adenoma[2].

Reasoning that the increases in circulating 1,25-$(OH)_2D$ constitute an important component of the disease process, 10 patients in the absorptive subpopulation were placed on oral phosphorus therapy (1250-1500 mg elemental phosphorus daily as the neutral salt) for 12 or more months. Phosphorus therapy produced a reduction in plasma levels of 1,25-$(OH)_2D$ (from 79 to 53 pg/ml), the calciuric response to the tolerance test (from 0.30 to 0.21 Δ mg calcium/100 ml GF), and hypercalciuria (from 442 to 272 mg/day on the 1000 mg diet) and was not associated with a discernible rebound increase in parathyroid function. The long-term implications of this therapeutic approach remain unknown, and the data from this series will be reported in detail in a subsequent publication.

The principal thrust of the present series was a consideration of the pathophysiological basis of hypercalciuria in patients with 1^oHPT, together with the clinical, diagnostic, and therapeutic implications that the data convey. There is no intent to imply a direct causal relationship between hypercalciuria and stone formation in 1^oHPT. Other risk factors, such as a tendency to

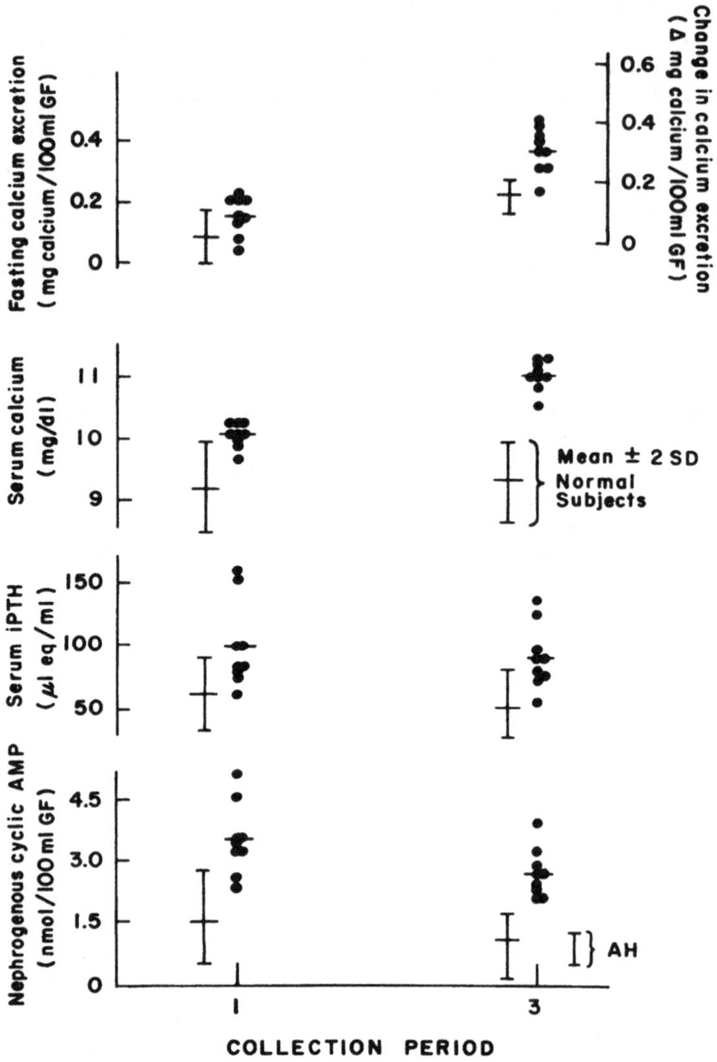

Figure 4. Results of the oral calcium tolerance test in 12 patients with subtle 1°HPT. In the top panel, fasting calcium excretion is represented by the ordinate on the left, and the calciuric response, expressed as the change (Δmg/100 ml GF) from fasting values, is represented by the ordinate on the right. The normal ranges are depicted by cross-hatched bars adjoining the ordinates, and the responses (mean ± 2SD) of 18 normal subjects to the test are shown by vertical bars in the experimental period. Also shown for comparison in the bottom panel is the range of results for NcAMP from 4 patients with absorptive hypercalciuria (AH) who developed mild hypercalcemia (mean 10.8 mg/dl, range 10.6-11.0 mg/dl) during test.

hyperabsorb dietary oxalate, as reported by Dobbins and colleagues[11] elsewhere in this volume, may also be of importance. Nevertheless, hypercalciuria clearly confers a significant statistical risk for stone formation in patients with 1°HPT (Table 1). Our inability to explain the wide range of observed values for plasma 1,25-$(OH)_2D$ suggests that knowledge concerning the regulation of 1-hydroxylase activity is imperfect and/or that there is a degree of polymorphism in the basic disease process of hyperparathyroidism.

The major conceptual limitation in previous attempts to understand the clinical spectrum of primary HPT was the assumption that all pathophysiological aspects of the disease should be explainable solely on the basis of the tissue effects of circulating parathyroid hormone and/or the degree of attendant hypercalcemia. Simply stated, the principal conclusion of the present series is that 1°HPT is a bihormonal disease process and that the effects of the "secondary" hormone, 1,25-$(OH)_2D$, appeared to define in large part the presentation and complications in certain patients with the disorder. There is a clear irony in this conclusion with respect to both Albright's "dietary" proposal[1], and Dent's "bihormonal" hypothesis[3], as well as a recognition of the soundness of Albright's basic concepts. Whether or not our data and subclassification of patients are germaine to the development of osteopenia and/or osteitis in patients with 1°HPT remains to be explored.

REFERENCES

1. F. Albright and E. C. Reifenstein, in:"The Parathyroid Glands and Metabolic Bone Disease," Williams and Wilkins, Baltimore (1948).
2. A. E. Broadus, in:"Nephrolithiasis (Contemporary Issues in Nephrology:Vol. 5)," F. L. Coe, B. M. Brenner, and J. H. Stein, eds., Churchill-Livingstone Inc., New York, (1980).
3. C. E. Dent, Br. Med. J. 2:1495 (1962).
4. J. A. Parsons, in:"The Biochemistry and Physiology of Bone: Vol. 4," G. H. Bourne, ed., Academic Press, New York (1977).
5. H. M. Lloyd, Medicine 47:53 (1968).
6. D. C. Purnell, L. H. Smith, D. A. Scholz, L. R. Elveback, and C. D. Arnaud, Am. J. Med. 50:670 (1971).
7. L. E. Mallette, J. Bilezidian, D. A. Heath, and G. D. Aurback, Medicine 53:127 (1974).
8. M. Peacock, in:"Calcium Regulating Hormones: Proceedings of the Fifth Parathyroid Conference," R. V. Talmage, M. Owen, and J. A. Parsons, eds., Excerpta Medica, Amsterdam (1975).
9. A. E. Broadus, R. L. Horst, E. T. Littledike, J. E. Mahaffey, and H. Rasmussen, Clin. Endocrinol. 12:225 (1980).
10. A. E. Broadus, R. L. Horst, R. Lang, E. T. Littledike, and H. Rasmussen, N. Eng. J. Med. 302:421 (1980).

11. J. W. Dobbins, K. Cooper, R. Lang, L. H. Smith, H. J. Binder, and A. E. Broadus, in:"Proceedings Fourth International Urolithiasis Research Symposium," L. H. Smith, W. G. Robertson, and B. Finlayson, eds., Plenum Press, New York (in press).

ACKNOWLEDGMENT

This work was supported in part by grants RR 125 and AM 20570 from the National Institutes of Health.

PLASMA $1,25(OH)_2D$ IN IDIOPATHIC AND HYPERPARATHYROID STONE-FORMERS

M. Peacock, P. J. Heyburn, M. Barnet,
G. A. Taylor, W. B. Brown, and A. E. J. Davies
M.R.C. Mineral Metabolism Unit
The General Infirmary
Leeds LS1 3EX, U.K.

INTRODUCTION

The differentiation of stone formation associated with primary hyperparathyroidism from that due to idiopathic stone disease is easily made when the degree of hyperparathyroidism is severe. In such patients the plasma calcium and parathyroid hormone (PTH) concentration are both persistently high. Furthermore at parathyroidectomy the histology is unequivocal since the weight of abnormal gland tissue is well above the weight of the normal total parathyroid tissue.

In milder forms of primary hyperparathyroid disease, however, the plasma biochemistry and the gland weight at parathyroidectomy are more equivocal. The diagnostic difficulty is accentuated by the fact that hyperparathyroid stone formers have several biochemical features in common with those of idiopathic stone formers. Calcium absorption is increased and tubular reabsorption of phosphate decreased in a proportion of both types of stone formers[1]. These similarities and the difficulty of accurately measuring plasma PTH by radioimmunoassay make the diagnosis of mild hyperparathyroidism with stone disease from idiopathic stone disease a difficult problem.

The observation that plasma $1,25(OH)_2$ vitamin D ($1,25(OH)_2D$) is abnormal in both primary hyperparathyroid patients and idiopathic stone-formers[2] gave some hope that the plasma concentration of this hormone might help to differentiate between the two diseases. We have therefore compared the plasma $1,25(OH)_2D$ concentration in idiopathic stone-formers and hyperparathyroid patients during dietary changes in calcium and phosphate.

PATIENTS AND METHODS

Twenty-three patients were selected for study. In 13 ("hyperparathyroid"), the majority of whom had active urinary stone disease, the ionized calcium (Ca^{++}) and the PTH concentrations were persistently outside the two standard deviation range of 48 normal control subjects. In 10 with active stone disease ("idiopathic"), these biochemical variables were within the normal range. Any subject who showed an abnormality in any one of these variables was excluded from the study. Glomerular filtrate rate was calculated from creatinine clearances performed during the period of study and the mean value taken and corrected for 1.73 m^2 of body surface area. Any patient with impairment of renal function was excluded from the study.

The patients were studied on a metabolic ward on 4 dietary regimens - 3 days on a low calcium diet, 3 days on a high calcium diet, 3 days on a high phosphorus diet and 3 days on a low phosphorus diet.

INVESTIGATIONS

Fasting plasma and urine were taken at the beginning of the study and at the end of each 3 day period. Twenty-four hour urines were collected continuously throughout.

Plasma $1,25(OH)_2D$ and PTH were measured as previously described [3,4]. Plasma total calcium, ionized calcium, phosphate, creatinine and 24-hour urine calcium, phosphate and creatinine were measured by standard methods.

RESULTS

Figure 1 shows the basal values of plasma $1,25(OH)_2D$ and the values obtained at the end of each of the 4 dietary regimens. There was no significant difference in plasma $1,25(OH)_2D$ between the "hyperparathyroid" and the "idiopathic" patients on a normal diet. Both groups had elevated concentrations many of which were above the upper limit of the normal range.

On a low calcium diet there was no significant change from the basal levels in the plasma $1,25(OH)_2D$ concentrations in the two groups. On a high calcium diet the mean concentrations fell significantly in both groups but there was no difference between the groups.

A high phosphorus intake also reduced the plasma $1,25(OH)_2D$ concentrations from basal levels although not to the same extent as a high calcium diet. When the patients were placed on a low phosphorus intake there was a rise in plasma 1,25(OH)$_2$D concentration which was more obvious in the "hyperparathyroid" than the "idiopathic" group but the concentrations did not reach those seen on the basal or low calcium intake.

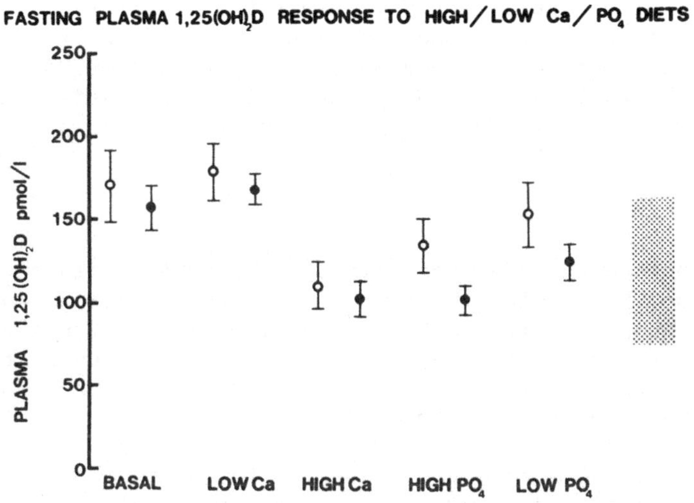

Figure 1. The mean (±2SE) plasma 1,25(OH)$_2$D concentrations in a group of "hyperparathyroid" patients (o) and a group of "idiopathic" stone formers (•) on basal, low calcium, high calcium, high phosphorus and low phosphorus diets.

Plasma Ca^{++}, and PTH did not change significantly during the study. Plasma phosphate was significantly lower in the "hyperparathyroid" group but did not change significantly during the study although there was a tendency for it to rise in both groups on the high calcium, high and low phosphorus diets.

Radiocalcium absorption was equally high in both groups basally and did not change significantly during the study. The 24-hour urine calcium was higher throughout in the "hyperparathyroid" group but the change on the four dietary regimens was similar in both groups.

DISCUSSION

The diagnosis of patients with mild primary hyperparathyroidism and calcium stone disease from patients with idiopathic calcium stone disease is a difficult biochemical problem. The major biochemical criteria for distinguishing these diseases remains a high plasma Ca^{++} and PTH concentration. The development of reliable methods for measuring ionized calcium have helped but the unreliability of radio-immunoassay methods for measuring PTH continue to cause confusion. Biochemical criteria in addition to plasma Ca^{++} and PTH therefore must also be used.

In our present studies on plasma $1,25(OH)_2D$ concentrations in stone patients with high plasma Ca^{++} and PTH concentrations i.e. definite hyperparathyroidism and normal plasma Ca^{++} and PTH concentrations i.e. idiopathic, the plasma $1,25(OH)_2D$ was equally high in both groups. Dietary calcium and phosphorus changes affected the plasma $1,25(OH)_2D$ equally in both groups and was not helpful in distinguishing between the two groups.

SUMMARY

1. Patients with suspected primary hyperparathyroidism, the majority of whom had a history of urinary stone formation, and patients with suspected idiopathic stone disease were studied on a low calcium diet, a high calcium diet, a high phosphorus diet and a low phosphorus diet. All patients with an impairment of glomerular filtration rate were excluded from the study.

2. The patients formed two groups on the basis of fasting plasma ionized calcium and parathyroid hormone concentrations - a "hyperparathyroid" group with both values above the normal range and an idiopathic group with both values within the normal range. Any patient who had an abnormality on either one of these variables was excluded from the study.

3. Plasma $1,25(OH)_2D$ concentration was equally high in both groups and did not rise from the basal values on a low calcium diet. On a high calcium diet plasma $1,25(OH)_2D$ concentration fell equally in both groups but the mean values remained in the normal range. A high phosphorus and a low phosphorus diet increased the plasma $1,25(OH)_2D$ concentration in both groups, particularly in the hyperparathyroid group, but there was no significant difference in the response in the two groups.

4. Plasma $1,25(OH)_2D$ concentration does not help to distinguish between stone forming patients with primary hyperparathyroidism from those with idiopathic stone disease.

REFERENCES

1. M. Peacock, W. G. Robertson, and R. W. Marshall, in:"Endocrinology," L. J. DeGroot, G. F. Cahill, Jr., L. Martini, D. H. Nelson, W. D. Odell, J. T. Potts, Jr., E. Steinberger, and A. I. Winegrad, eds., Grune and Stratton, New York (1979).

2. M. R. Haussler, D. J. Baylink, M. R. Hughes, P. F. Brumbaugh, J. E. Wergedal, F. N. Shen, R. L. Nielsen, S. J. Counts, K. M. Bursac, and J. A. McCann, Clin. Endocrinol. 5:151S (1976).
3. M. Peacock, G. A. Taylor, and W. Brown, Clin. Chim. Acta. 101: 93 (1980).
4. M. Peacock, in:"Calcium, Phosphate and Magnesium Metabolism," B. E. C. Nordin, ed., Churchill Livingstone, Edinburgh/ London (1976).

ORTHOPHOSPHATE THERAPY DECREASES URINARY CALCIUM EXCRETION AND SERUM 1,25-DIHYDROXY VITAMIN D CONCENTRATIONS IN IDIOPATHIC HYPERCALCIURIA

C. J. Van Den Berg, R. Kumar, D. M. Wilson,
H. Heath, and L. H. Smith
Mayo Clinic

Rochester, MN 55901

The term "idiopathic hypercalciuria" is used to describe the single metabolic abnormality detected by routine laboratory investigation in approximately one-half of the patients who present with idiopathic calcium urolithiasis[1]. At least two advances have helped our understanding of this disorder; first, is the realization that idiopathic hypercalciuria is not one single entity and more likely, encompasses multiple disorders with separate etiologies. Currently, at least two processes have been identified and idiopathic hypercalciuria is classified as either absorptive or renal hypercalciuria depending on whether increased urinary excretion of calcium is the direct result of intestinal hyperabsorption of calcium, i.e. absorptive hypercalciuria, or impaired renal tubular reabsorption of calcium, i.e. renal hypercalciuria[2]. A second advance is the finding of increased plasma 1,25-dihydroxy vitamin D levels in some patients with idiopathic hypercalciuria[3]. The metabolite, 1,25-hydroxy vitamin D, stimulates the intestinal absorption of calcium. Indeed, intestinal hyperabsorption of calcium is present in patients with both absorptive and renal hypercalciuria. Presumably, this increase in plasma 1,25-dihydroxy vitamin D reflects increased synthesis of this hormone by the renal enzyme 25-hydroxy vitamin D-1-α hydroxylase. Experimentally, the activity of this enzyme is increased as a consequence of both increased parathyroid hormone activity[4] and with dietary phosphate deprivation[5]. Phosphate deprivation increases plasma 1,25-dihydroxy vitamin D levels in the absence of parathyroid glands, suggesting a parathyroid hormone-independent effect of phosphate metabolism on 1,25-dihydroxy vitamin D synthesis. Studies of patients with idiopathic hypercalciuria suggest that those patients with renal hypercalciuria have secondary hyperparathyroidism which, in turn, could increase 1,25-dihydroxy vitamin D synthesis and increase intestinal absorption of calcium[6]. In absorptive hypercalciuria, serum immunoreactive parathyroid hormone levels are normal or low and altered phosphate metabolism has been proposed as a primary stimulus for increased synthesis of 1,25-hydroxy vitamin D.

Our group has used oral phosphorus supplements in the treatment of idiopathic calcium renal lithiasis for many years and this treatment consistently reduces urinary excretion of calcium. This prompted us to examine the relationship between oral phosphorus-associated decreases in urinary excretion of calcium and changes in vitamin D metabolism in patients with calcium urolithiasis and idiopathic hypercalciuria.

Eleven patients (10 men and 1 woman) with idiopathic renal lithiasis and hypercalciuria were studied as in-patients on a metabolic ward. An extensive etiologic urolithiasis evaluation failed to reveal any metabolic abnormality other than hypercalciuria. With one exception, these patients had so-called absorptive hypercalciuria as defined by a fasting urine calcium-to-creatinine ratio <0.11. No patient had an absolute increase in the serum level of immunoreactive parathyroid hormone. A professional dietician estimated their habitual dietary intake including calcium, phosphorus and vitamin D which was maintained during the in-patient study. Two consecutive 24 h urine collections and a fasting blood sample were obtained on two separate occasions before and during treatment. After the first study and for at least 14 days prior to and including the second study period, all patients took 2 g of oral phosphorus (Neutraphos[1]) daily in four divided doses.

Serum and urine calcium were measured by atomic absorptive spectroscopy. Immunoreactive parathyroid hormone was measured by the method of Arnaud using the anti-serum GP1M. Serum 1,25-dihydroxy vitamin D was measured using a rachitic chick duodenal cytosol assay. All data were analyzed by the paired two-tailed t-test.

RESULTS

Significant ($p < 0.001$) changes in the urinary excretion of calcium and phosphorus and serum 1,25-dihydroxy vitamin D levels occurred during oral phosphorus therapy. The urinary excretion of calcium decreased in every patient with a mean Δ of -123 mg per 24 h, the urinary excretion of phosphorus increased in every patient with a mean Δ of +1,039 mg per 24 h and the serum levels of $1,25(OH)_2D$ decreased in 10 of 11 patients with a mean Δ of -22 pg/ml. Pretreatment serum 1,25-dihydroxy vitamin D levels were initially high in some patients and were elevated as a group when compared with levels in age-matched controls whether assessed as the arithmetic mean (57 vs 33 pg/ml), the logarithmically normalized mean (42 vs 27

[1]Neutraphos, Willen Drug Company, Baltimore, MD 21202.

pg/ml) or the median value (45 vs 24 pg/ml). During phosphorus therapy, serum levels of 1,25-dihydroxy vitamin D decreased to values not significantly different from those of the normal controls. Levels of serum calcium and phosphorus were initially within the normal range and were not changed by treatment. Serum immunoreactive parathyroid hormone levels were all initially within the normal range and increased minimally within the normal range during treatment (mean Δ was 2 ± 1 μlEq/ml, $P < 0.025$).

We conclude serum 1,25-dihydroxy vitamin D levels are increased in some patients with idiopathic hypercalciuria and that the effect of oral phosphorus in decreasing the urinary excretion of calcium may involve the reduced synthesis of 1,25-dihydroxy vitamin D independent of altered parathyroid function.

REFERENCES

1. G. A. Rose and A. R. Harrison, Br. J. Urol. 46:261 (1974).
2. C. Y. C. Pak, M. Ohata, E. C. Lawrence, and W. Snyder, J. Clin. Invest. 54:387 (1974).
3. F. H. Shen, D. J. Baylink, R. L. Nielsen, D. J. Sherrard, J. L. Ivey, and M. R. Haussler, J. Lab. Clin. Med. 90:955 (1977).
4. D. R. Fraser and E. Kodicek, Nature (London) New Biol. 241:163 (1973).
5. R. W. Gray, D. R. Wilz, A. E. Caldas, and J. Lemann, Jr., J. Clin. Endocrinol. Metab. 45:299 (1977).
6. F. L. Coe, J. M. Canterbury, J. J. Firpo, and E. Reiss, J. Clin. Invest. 52:134 (1973).

ACKNOWLEDGMENT

This work was supported by grants AM 20605 and RR 585 from the National Institutes of Health.

CYCLIC NUCLEOTIDES AND RELATED VARIABLES IN UROLITHIASIS

P. O. Schwille, D. Scholz, W. Engelhardt, K. Schwille,
B. Schreiber, I. Goldberg, and A. Sigel
Mineral Metabolism and Hormone Research Laboratory,
Departments of Surgery and Urology, University of
Erlangen, Erlangen, West Germany

Although there is good knowledge of cyclic AMP (cAMP) in urine and plasma of various disorders of calcium metabolism[1] and calciurias in urolithiasis[2] only little is known about cyclic GMP (cGMP), the amounts contributed by the kidney (= nephrogenous moiety), the relationship among nucleotides in established lithiasis subgroups and the associated concentrations of serum parathyroid hormone (PTH) in venous peripheral blood.

SUBJECTS AND METHODS

Patients with metabolically active calcium stones were classified as normocalciuria (N-C), absorptive hypercalciuria (A-HC), renal leak hypercalciuria (R-HC), bone resorptive hypercalciuria (pHPT) based on previously described criteria[3]. They were complemented by patients forming either idiopathic uric acid stones only (UA-I) or uric acid and calcium stones (UA-II). Investigations were conducted in an outpatient manner with participants on their free home diet. Additional studies included a 2 h morning (9-11 a.m.) creatinine clearance period, fasting serum/plasma from the antebrachial vein, a 3 h postprandial urine period and in some instances 24 h urine collections. Renal functions in all groups was normal, except five pHPT patients (serum creatinine > 1.33 mg/dl or creatinine clearance < 39 ml/min).

Analyses: cAMP was measured by protein binding and cGMP by radioimmunoassay techniques (Amersham test kit). Serum PTH[4]: the routine non-carboxyl-terminal (= mid-portion) assay employs bovine (b) -PTH(1-85) as standard and tracer, the sheep anti-porcine PTH antibody S-478 (University Medical School, Hannover, FRG; final dilution 1:6000), whose antigenic recognition sites are confined to amino acid residues 1-52 (no detection of human (h)-PTH (53-84); <10% crossreactivity with h-PTH(1-34), Brewer sequence). The homologous amino-terminal assay utilized h-PTH(1-34) Brewer (standard, tracer) and the corresponding antibody (European PTH Study Group; final dilution 1:125000). Although the recovery of dilution factors in pHPT serum is perfect in this system, in the present individual samples B (= fractional tracer binding to antibody) was higher B_o (= fractional tracer binding in the absence of unlabelled PTH) necessitating to express results in arbitrary units (= (1/B) x 100). In a third amino- and carboxyl-terminal assay the antibody 211/41 (Wellcome; Beckenham; final dilution 1:150000) was used, which recognizes intact h-PTH and circulating PTH fragments (P. O. Schwille et al.: manuscript in preparation). Sensitivity was 20, 4, 15 pg respectively for the systems (same order). All other serum/urine constituents were measured by conventional methods.

Calculations and statistics: excretion of nucleotides was normalized for creatinine clearance. The nephrogenous part (NcAMP, NcGMP) was calculated as shown previously[5]; positive values mean net production, negative net reabsorption of nucleotides. Results are given as median and range (non-parametric distribution). Significance of differences between controls and stone groups was tested using the U-test.

RESULTS

As is shown in the table PTH is elevated above control in the mid-portion assay (A-HC, R-HC, UA-II, pHPT), but is in the range of controls or insignificantly lower, except pHPT, in the amino-terminal assay. PTH also appears lower than normal, except pHPT in the intact hormone system (see medians), where we decided not to test significance or differences owing to the many undetectably low results.

Serum calcium varies in a close range, except in the hypercalcemic pHPT patients. Conversely, serum phosphate and phosphate threshold are low in every stoneforming group. Fasting urinary cAMP (normalized for creatinine clearance) and NcAMP (normalized for creatinine) are elevated in pHPT only, but decreased in N-C subjects. If only non-pHPT stone formers are considered, there is a weak (not significant), but direct correlation between NcAMP ($r = 0.10$, $n = 151$) and phosphate threshold. In pHPT the latter variable and fasting urinary cAMP are linked by an inverse correlation ($r = -0.61$, $n = 18$, $p < 0.01$). Mean NcAMP as based on daily urine is lowest in the N-C group, but significance of differences is not achieved owing to the small number of controls in this protocol.

A pattern similar to urinary cAMP was found for urinary cGMP excretion (nadir in N-C, UA-II), whereas the NcGMP moiety in non-pHPT stones is unaltered, but elevated in pHPT. Total renal production

Table 1. Radioimmunoassayable PTH(s) (A), response parameters to parathyroid gland activity (B), and other parameters of cyclic nucleotides in controls and urolithiasis patients. For abbreviations see "Subjects and Methods" section. Median and range (beneath).

	Controls n = 34+	A - HC n = 15+	R - HC n = 23+	N - C n = 60+	UA - I n = 13+	UA - II n = 12	pHPT n = 19+
	(+: if not otherwise indicated in brackets)						
A. Parathyroid Hormones in Peripheral Serum (I = N-assay; II = non-C-assay; III = N + C-assay)							
Human PTH (I-34);	1.97 (15)	2.0 (8)	1.99 (10)	1.92 (15)	1.96 (9)	---	2.05[a] (10)
Arbitrary units	1.83-2.09	1.89-2.13	1.85-2.13	1.78-2.0	1.80-2.04		1.90-2.77
Bovine PTH (I-84); II	335	427[a]	451[b]	409	362	416[a]	1185[c]
pg-equiv/ml	<200-576	246-1017	<200-1300	<200-1281	<200-993	203-853	270-8744
Bovine PTH(I-84); III	201	281	256	150	150	150	1624[c]
pg-equiv/ml	<150-630	<150-555	<150-866	<150-820	<150-547	<150-345	555-7238
B. Accepted Response Parameters to Parathyroid Gland Activity (I: calculated from 2 h fasting urine; II: from 24 h urine)							
Serum calcium;	9.86	9.86	9.90	9.82	9.82	9.93	12.75[c]
mg/dl	8.72-10.58	9.09-10.84	9.14-10.36	8.95-10.46	8.94-10.35	9.45-10.39	10.16-16.65
Serum phosphate;	3.76	3.05[c]	3.23[c]	3.18[c]	2.84[c]	3.29[a]	2.40[c]
mg/dl	2.54-5.03	2.47-4.26	2.50-4.91	1.89-4.54	2.05-4.22	2.46-3.99	1.49-4.67
Phosphate threshold;	4.07	3.23[c]	3.13[c]	3.18[c]	2.90[c]	3.17[c]	1.89[c]
mg/dl I	2.40-5.30	2.40-4.40	2.05-4.90	2.0-4.55	1.80-4.20	2.10-4.10	0.80-2.80
Urinary cyclic AMP;	3.92	3.36	3.30	2.95[b]	3.04	3.95	6.32[c]
nM/100 ml creatinine	0.78-9.14	1.88-5.22	1.80-6.80	1.08-7.36	1.44-4.63	0.55-5.49	2.85-16.58
clearance I							
Nephrogenous cyclic	2.2	1.6	1.8	1.2[b]	1.5	2.1	4.3[c]
AMP; uM/g creatinine I	-0.6-6.3	-0.3-3.3	0.4-4.8	-0.7-4.3	-0.003-2.8	-1.2-3.5	0.6-9.3
Nephrogenous cyclic	2.14 (5)	1.28 (13)	1.07 (21)	0.94 (48)	0.98 (11)	1.36 (11)	3.18 (15)
AMP; μM/g creatinine II	-2.16-3.96	-0.28-2.12	-0.10-7.93	1.51-3.72	0.03-2.92	-0.25-3.01	0.41-6.82

(Table 1 is continued on next page)

Table 1 continued.

	Controls n = 34+	A - HC n = 15+	R - HC n = 23+	N - C n = 60+	UA - I n = 13+	UA - II n = 12	pHPT n = 19+
C. Other Parameters of Cyclic Nucleotides (I: calculated from 2 h fasting urine; II: calculated from 24 h urine)							
Plasma cyclic AMP;	17.8	17.1	16.1	16.9	17.2	16.5	20.9[a]
pM/ml	9.0-27.2	11.8-20.4	11.1-23.4	11.8-32.5	12.9-25.4	15.6-23.7	13.1-38.8
Plasma cyclic GMP;	5.3	4.6	5.3	4.9	5.5	4.9	5.4
pM/ml	1.7-8.7	2.9-10.1	3.6-8.0	3.7-11.4	4.0-8.5	3.5-7.3	3.7-11.1
Urinary cyclic GMP;	0.37	0.28	0.40	0.29[c]	0.32	0.29[a]	0.43
nM/100 ml creatinine clearance I	0.07-1.06	0.12-0.70	0.12-0.56	0.08-0.63	0.14-0.69	0.09-0.48	0.17-1.09
Nephrogenous cyclic	-0.15	-0.20	-0.15	-0.21	-0.12	-0.10	0.08[c]
GM:; μm/g creatinine II	-0.84-0.36	-0.57-0.17	-0.46-0.8	-0.77-0.08	-0.59-0.06	-0.52(-)-0.03	0.02-0.76
Nephrogenous cyclic	2.12	1.37	1.46	1.05[b]	1.23	2.06	4.69[c]
AMP + GMP; μM/g creatinine I	-0.82-6.48	-0.45-3.49	0.14-4.82	-1.03-4.30	-0.10-2.69	-0.73-3.42	1.77-9.31

[a]: $p < 0.05$; [b]: $p < 0.01$; [c]: $p < 0.001$

rate of nucleotides (NaAMP + NcGMP) in N-C stones is less than half the rate of controls, and is more than doubled in pHPT.

Plasma nucleotide (cAMP, cGMP) levels in controls and non-pHPT subjects are in the range of values documented as normal in the literature[2], but in pHPT are either elevated (cAMP) or normal (cGMP).

COMMENTS

NcAMP is considered a powerful discriminatory help in evaluating parathyroid gland activity at the renal tubular level[2]. In the present pHPT subjects, our aides for decision making in diagnosing parathyroid hyperfunction were serum calcium, PTH and NcAMP. But in contrast to biochemical signs of secondary hyperparathyroidism, as observed in R-HC[6,7], we cannot confirm such a condition when decision making is based primarily on fasting calcium/creatinine ratio and the former criteria. In addition, none of the non-pHPT stone-forming groups appears afflicted by parathyroid overactivity, although they have in common with pHPT a definitely lower than normal serum phosphate and lower phosphate threshold, and a slightly elevated non-bioactive PTH of the mid-portion variety. Therefore, unless more sensitive homologous assays for h-PTH in peripheral circulation become available and prove the opposite, we conclude as follows: 1) in non-pHPT stone diseases radioimmunoassayable PTH is not a reliable indicator of parathyroid gland bioactivity at the renal tubular site, since it may be elevated, normal or even low depending on the recognition sites of the antibody in use, and on the circulating PTH molecular species; 2) low bioactivity regulation of parathyroids at the tubules of so-called idiopathic (non-pHPT) stone formers is highly likely when expressing it is terms of NcAMP; 3) enhanced phosphaturia in the latter populations, best expressed in terms of phosphate threshold, should be caused beyond the step of PTH-mediated tubulo-cellular cAMP generation and subsequent diminution of phosphate reabsorption; 4) the combination of low serum phosphate, low parathyroid activity and hyperphosphaturia may help to focus research work on phosphate metabolism and factors regulating parathyroid glands apart from serum free calcium ions; 5) that renal tubular guanylate cyclase appears sensitive to PTH excess such as in pHPT situations, whereas NcGMP is high.

REFERENCES

1. W. A. Peck and S. Klahr, Adv. Cycl. Nucl. Res. 11:89 (1979).
2. A. E. Broadus, Adv. Cycl. Nucl. Res. 8:509 (1977).
3. D. Scholz, P. O. Schwille, and A. Sigel, Urologe A 19:196 (1980).
4. P. O. Schwille, in:"Diagnostik in der Gastroenterologie," W. Domschke, H. Koch, eds., Thieme, Stuttgart (1979).
5. P. O. Schwille, C. Bornhof, R. Thun, D. Scholz, R. Botticher, W. Schellerer and A. Sigel, Klin. Wschr. 56:601 (1978).

6. C. Y. C. Pak, M. Ohata, E. C. Lawrence, and W. Snyder, J. Clin. Invest. 54:387 (1974).
7. F. L. Coe, J. M. Canterbury, J. J. Firppo, and E. Reiss, J. Clin. Invest. 52:134 (1973).

DISTURBED TERMINAL MINERALIZATION OF BONE IN IDIOPATHIC HYPERCALCIURIA

H. H. Malluche, W. Tschope, W. Meyer,
E. Ritz, and S. G. Massry
Division of Nephrology and Department of Medicine,
University of Southern California School of Medicine,
Los Angeles, California, 90033

Hypercalciuric renal stone-formers are commonly divided into 3 different groups: Resorptive hypercalciuria, hyperabsorptive and renal hypercalciuria[1-4]. Patients with hyperabsorptive hypercalciuria have normal or low serum parathyroid hormone activities and normal to low urinary excretion of cAMP. In renal hypercalciuria elevated serum PTH levels and increased renal excretion of cAMP has been reported[4-6]. Bordier et al.[6] published elevated immunoreactive parathyroid hormone levels and increased numbers of osteoclasts in bone biopsies obtained from patients with renal hypercalciuria. No information is available on bone histology in patients with hypercalciuria of the hyperabsorptive type. The present study evaluates quantitatively bone sections in 15 patients with hyperabsorptive hypercalciuria and recurrent stone-formation.

There were 12 men and 3 women with ages ranging between 26-52 years, mean age 41.9 years. The number of stones passed by the patients and or visualized by x-ray ranged from 2 to 50. All patients had normal renal function as documented by normal creatinine clearance, none of them had renal tubular acidosis as evidenced by a normal response to an ammonium chloride test. Primary or secondary hyperparathyroidism was excluded by the findings of normal or low levels of parathyroid hormone and fasting serum ionized calcium and normal urinary excretion of cAMP. Selection criteria of patients for the study included one or more of the following: Urinary excretion of calcium more than 15 mEq/24 hrs. Urinary calcium to creatinine ratio >0.2 and decrease of urinary calcium to creatinine ratio of >40 % after oral administration of cellulose phosphate. Thus our patients fulfilled the criteria of hyperabsorptive hypercalciuria. The studies were carried out under outpatient conditions without dietary restrictions. None of the patients received medications, in particular thiazides, before the study.

Two 24 h urine collections were obtained, first under basal conditions and subsequently under oral administration of 10 g cellulose phosphate with meals 3 times a day. After completion of each of the two urine collections, blood samples were drawn in the fasting state at 8:00 a.m. without venous compression. Subsequently, the patients received, after an interval of no more than 1 to 2 weeks, oral tetracycline hydrochloride 1 g/day for 2 days, the drug was stopped for 12 days and subsequently given again at the same dose for another period of 4 days. Three days later, bone biopsies were obtained from the left iliac crest. Bone biopsy specimens were processed undecalcified and quantitatively evaluated for micromorphometric structural parameters of bone and parameters of bone formation and resorption. In addition, the fraction of osteoid seams, taking up tetracycline in a double label pattern and the distance between two tetracycline bands was determined.

The control group for serum and urine chemistry consisted of 360 men randomly selected from a telephone directory with aid of computer generated random numbers. Basal values of these individuals were obtained under the same conditions as the patients studies. The control data for bone histology were obtained from 22 healthy subjects who died from traffic accidents or other violent deaths. There were 10 women and 12 men with ages ranging from 24 to 65 years.

Table 1. Serum biochemical results in patients with absorptive hypercalciuria and renal stone-formation as compared to controls. In parenthesis values after cellulose phosphate administration. Results are given as mean value ± SE for patients and mean value ± SD for controls.

		Patients		Controls	
Ca	(mEq/l)	4.7±0.04	(4.55)	4.7±0.1	(SD)
Ca^{++}	(mEq/l)	2.2±0.02	(0.05)	2.2±0.1	
P	(mg/100ml)	2.8±0.12	(2.9)	3.1±0.4	
PTH	(pmol/l)	11±2.25		30±25	

Total and ionized serum calcium levels, serum phosphate and serum parathyroid hormone concentrations in the patients studied are given in Table 1. All serum biochemical results were in the normal range in the patients studied. The differences between patients and controls were not significant. Urine biochemical results are shown in Table 2. The patients had normal urinary excretion of cAMP and the values did not differ from controls although urinary calcium was much higher in the patients. Upon short-term administration of cellulose phosphate urinary cAMP rose by 40% while the urinary excretion of calcium fell by 60%. Both changes were significant. The correlation between the fall in calcium concentration and the rise in cAMP excretion was highly significant ($r = -0.7$; $p < 0.01$).

Table 2. Urine Biochemical Results in Patients with Absorptive Hypercalciuria and Renal Stone-Formation as Compared to Controls

		Patients		Controls
cAMP:Cr	(μmol/mol)	267±24	(362)	273±81
UV_{Ca}/24 h	(mEq)	22.3 ±1.4	(9.0)	11.2 ±6.0
Ca:Cr	(mg/mg)	0.27±0.02	(0.10)	0.13±0.09

Micromorphometric parameters of bone structure and of bone resorption were not significantly different between hypercalciuric patients and normals. However, there was a significant increase in the mean value of volumetric density of osteoid (Table 3) in the stone-forming patients and in 9 of the 15 patients osteoid volume was greater than the mean ± 2 SD of the control values. The fraction of the trabecular surface covered by osteoid in the patients was also significantly higher than in the control subjects. On the other hand, the surface fraction of osteoblasts was significantly lower in patients than in control subjects. Accordingly the fraction of inactive osteoid was significantly increased. Under polarized light the accumulating osteoid seams exhibited typical lamellar texture without evidence of woven osteoid. In all of the patients a decrease in the fraction of mineralizing osteoid seams was observed (Fm_{ini} Table 3) i.e. seams taking up tetracycline in a double-label pattern were rare. The linear rate of apposition, calculated from the distance between 2 tetracycline bands was diminished in 12/15 patients. The fraction of mineralizing osteoid seams i.e. appositional sites with a tetracycline double label correlated with the relative osteoblastic activity i.e. fractional osteoid-osteoblast interface.

The increase in volume fraction and surface fraction of trabecular bone consisting of non-mineralized osteoid due to an increase in the fraction of inactive osteoid points to a delay or cessation of secondary mineralization of osteoid seams and would imply a prolongation of the life-span of osteoid seams. A similar increase of inactive osteoid secondary to a slow down of terminal mineralization has been found in elderly individuals but advanced age cannot explain our results. The shown correlation between relative osteo-

Table 3. Quantitative static and dynamic histologic parameters of bone which were found to be significantly altered in hypercalciuric renal stone-formers of the hyperabsorptive type as compared to normal controls.

	Patients	Controls
V_{vos} (mm^3/cm^3)	5.1 ±0.8	1.3 ±0.3*
OB (%)	1.5 ±0.3	2.2 ±0.2*
OS (%)	17.2 ±2.2	7.7 ±1.3*
F_{ios} (%)	91.1 ±1.2	72 ±2.1*
F_{min} (%)	36.7 ±3.4	±>70*
M_{trab} (μ/day)	0.54±0.03	0.65±0.02*

* = Statistically significantly different from controls (p <0.01).

blastic activity and fraction of mineralizing osteoid seams indicate that induction of mineralization of the major portion of the osteoid seams covered by osteoblasts is not disturbed.

Rasmussen and Bordier[7] suggested that osteoblastic activity is stimulated by high serum phosphate. Patients with hyperabsorptive hypercalciuria may have low blood levels of inorganic phosphate[8,9] which was not observed in the present study. However, our data do not contradict the hypothesis that low serum phosphate levels reduce the rate of matrix synthesis and maturation but the coefficient of correlation between serum phosphate and inactive osteoid did not reach the level of statistical significance. Consequently, it remains undetermined whether low serum phosphate plays a role in the disturbance of matrix synthesis and maturation.

Theoretically, a deficiency of vitamin D or its metabolites may be responsible for part or all of the observed results. However, this possibility seems remote. Although we did not measure levels of vitamin D metabolites in our patients, available data indicate that patients with hyperabsorptive hypercalciuria have either normal or elevated levels of $1,25\text{-}(OH)_2D_3$. Information on blood levels of $24,25\text{-}(OH)_2D_3$ in such patients is not available and relative or absolute deficiency of this metabolite may be important in view of the recent data of the requirement of $24,25\text{-}(OH)_2D_3$ for bone metabolism[10,11].

Our data are consistent with normal net bone mineral resorption. This conclusion is based on the reduction of hypercalciuria during the administration of cellulose phosphate, normal or low levels of immunoreactive PTH, normal urinary excretion of cAMP and the normal number and surface density of osteoclasts. It is, therefore, plausible to suggest that osteoclastic activity is not increased in patients with hyperabsorptive hypercalciuria.

In summary, bone abnormalities in patients with hyperabsorptive hypercalciuria consist of (a) an increase in volume and surface density of osteoid due to increase in fraction of inactive osteoid which fails to incorporate tetracycline and (b) a low rate of mineral apposition.

In conclusion, disturbed secondary mineralization is observed in hyperabsorptive hypercalciuria. It remains to be clarified whether abnormal bone histology is the cause or consequence of the electrolyte abnormality in hyperabsorptive hypercalciuria. It also remains undetermined whether the patient group studied is representative of all patients with absorptive hypercalciuria. However, the present findings show that bone may not be merely an innocent bystander in this disease.

REFERENCES

1. P. Adams, T. M. Chalmers, L. F. Hill, and B. Truscott, Br. Med. J. 4:582 (1970).
2. M. Keynes, Lancet 1:1077 (1971).
3. A. Hodgkinson and L. N. Pyrah, Br. J. Surg. 46:10 (1958).
4. C. Y. C. Pak, M. Ohata, E. C. Lawrence, and W. Snyder, J. Clin. Invest. 54:387 (1974).
5. B. E. C. Nordin, M. Peacock, and R. Wilkinson, in:"Clinics in Endocrinology and Metabolism," J. MacIntyre, ed., Saunders, Philadelphia, (1972).
6. P. Bordier, A. Ryckewan, J. Gjuens, and H. Rasmussen, Am. J. Med. 63:398 (1977).
7. H. Rasmussen and P. Bordier, in:"The Physiologican and Cellular Basis of Metabolic Bone Disease," Williams and Wilkins, Baltimore, (1974).
8. F. Albright, P. Henneman, P. H. Benedict, and A. P. Forbes, Proc. R. Soc. Med. 46:1077 (1953).
9. F. H. Shen, D. J. Baylink, R. L. Nielson, D. J. Sherrard, J. L. Ivey, and M. R. Haussler, J. Lab. Clin. Med. 90:955 (1977).
10. H. H. Malluche, H. Henry, W. Meyer-Sabellek, D. Sherman, S. G. Massry, and A. W. Norman, in:"Vitamin D-Basic Research and its Clinical Application, A. W. Norman, K. Schaefer, D. V. Herrath, H. G. Grigoleit, J. W. Coburn, H. F. DeLuca, E. B. Mawer, and T. Suda, eds., Walter de Gruyter, Berlin/New York, (1979).
11. A. Ornoy, D. Goodwin, D. Noff, and S. Edelstein, Nature 276:517, 1978.

DIETARY CALCIUM RESTRICTION MAY BE GOOD FOR PATIENTS' STONES - BUT NOT FOR THEIR BONES

C. Velentzas, D. G. Oreopoulos, S. Meema, H. E. Meema,
T. Nutsuga, E. Alison, A. Katirtzoglou and P. Crassweller
Departments of Medicine, Radiology, Dietetics and
Urology, The Toronto Western Hospital and University of
Toronto, Toronto, Canada

The conservative management of patients with renal stone disease consists of an increased fluid intake and a low calcium diet[1,2]. The former was originally proposed by Hippocrates[3] and is now accepted as the cornerstone of the treatment of renal stone disease. However, the importance of restricting dietary calcium in the prevention of kidney stones is controversial. A decrease in calcium intake may theoretically increase oxalate absorption from the gut[4,5,6], and may also affect the bones of the patients. This may be of particular importance in view of recent observations that the bone mineral content of untreated patients with renal stone disease is lower than that of normal controls[7,8,9].

This paper contains the results of a prospective study on sequential measurements of bone mineral content in renal stone patients advised to maintain a low calcium diet either alone or in combination with various drugs.

MATERIAL AND METHODS

All patients attended the Renal Stone Clinic of the Toronto Western Hospital. To avoid age-dependent bone changes, only men between 20 and 50 years of age were included in the study. Hyperparathyroidism was excluded by a normal serum calcium on repeated examination, normal iPTH and normal urine and plasma cAMP.

Thirty-six patients were included in this study. Ten had uric acid stones and 26 had calcium stones. The latter group was divided into 2 groups: (a) 11 who had idiopathic hypercalciuria (24 h urine calcium in excess of 300 mg on ordinary diet) and (b) 15 who had normal urine calcium and no other metabolic abnormalities. Table 1 shows some additional information on these patients as well as the follow-up period which ranged from 11 to 144 months with an average of 35.6 months.

Bone mineral mass (M) was measured at a standard site in the proximal radial shaft using a radiological photodensitometric method [10,11,12]. This measurement is expressed as mineral thickness in mg/cm^2 through the full thickness of bone taken through a diameter of the radius along a one cm longitudinal scan-path. At the same site, the average combined cortical thickness (C) was measured from another radiograph perpendicular to the one used for bone mineral mass measurement. From these two values it is possible to calculate mineral density (D) of the cortical bone (in mg/cm^3) using the equation $D=M/C$. Since $M=D \times C$, it is apparent that a decrease of M could either be due to a decrease in D (due to intracortical porosity and/or undermineralization) or in C (due to endosteal resorption), or both.

All patients were advised to increase their fluid intake and to decrease their calcium intake (to about 550 mg/day) mainly by avoiding dairy products (milk, cheese, yogurt, ice cream etc.). Table 2 shows the mean daily calcium intake of the patients (estimated from dietary records by a dietician).

Table 2. Calcium Intake During the Time of Presentation at the Stone Clinic (Initial) and that Practised as a Result of the Recommended Low Ca Diet

	Initial Ca intake (mg/24 h)	Practiced Ca intake (mg/24 h)
Kidney stone patients with idiopathic hypercalciuria	62.6 (10)*	563.6 (7)
Normal urine calcium	685.2 (12)	538.4 (8)
Uric acid stones	935 (9)	611.8 (10)

* Numbers in parenthesis indicate the number of patients on whom dietary data were available.

Of the 11 patients with idiopathic hypercalciuria, 6 received hydrochlorothiazide either alone (4) or in combination with

Table 1. Initial Values of Bone Mineral and Cortical Thickness Measurements in the Proximal Radius in Three Groups of Renal Stone Patients (mean ± S.D.)

	Normal (x+S.D.)*	Calcium Stones (with Hypercalciuria)	Calcium Stones (without Hypercalciuria)	Uric Acid Stones	Significance of Difference Between Meals
Group		I	II	III	
No. of patients		11	15	10	
Age (years)		38.7± 5.5	40.4± 6.3	37.1±9.1	
Follow-up (months)		46.0±38.6	27.9±12.7	35.8±8.6	
Bone mineral mass (mg/cm^2)	804±104	697 ±115.6	795 ±145.7	894±133.0	I and III: $p < 0.01$
Combined cortical thickness (cm)	0.71±0.07	0.63 ±0.056	0.70 ±0.073	0.76±0.071	I and III: $p < 0.01$; I and II: $p < 0.01$
Bone mineral density (mg/cm^3)	1131±0.102	1107 104.5	1126 ±116.4	1174±86.9	n.s.

* In normal males, age 20-30 (13)

allopurinol (2). Two who could not tolerate hydrochlorothiazide were switched to either magnesium or phosphate supplements. An additional patient was prescribed magnesium supplements initially and having failed on this, was given phosphate supplements. Finally, 2 patients received no treatment. Of the 15 normocalciuric calcium stone-formers, 8 were treated with hydrochlorothiazide either alone (3) or in combination with allopurinol (5). Two were treated with allopurinol and 2 with phosphates. Three patients received no drugs. Finally, of the 10 patients with uric acid stones, 7 were treated with allopurinol either alone (1) or in combination with $NaHCO_3$ (6) and the remaining 3 were treated with $NaHCO_3$ alone.

RESULTS

Table 1 contains the initial bone mineral measurements in the 3 groups[13]. The uric acid stone-formers generally had thicker and denser bones than the calcium stone-formers, although the differences were not statistically significant; the significantly higher bone mineral mass in the uric acid stone group ($p < 0.01$) was mainly due to increased cortical thickness. The hypercalciuric group had the thinnest cortices which differed significantly from both those of the uric acid group and those of the normocalciuric group. The mean value of bone mineral mass in the hypercalciuric group was 1 S.D. below the normal mean, whereas the mean of the uric acid group was approximately 1 S.D. above the normal mean. The normocalciuric patients were in an intermediate position.

Results of the follow-up examinations are given in Table 3. The loss of bone mineral mass and density was highly significant ($p < 0.01$) for the uric acid group and of borderline significance ($p < 0.05$) for the hypercalciuric group. The normocalciuric patients showed similar trends, but the rate of change was not statistically significant.

The loss of bone in the uric acid stone formers was uniform, all patients exhibiting a tendency to lose bone. In the hypercalciuric group there was less uniformity in that 3/11 patients slightly increased their bone mass. The fall was least consistent in normocalciuric patients, 5/15 showing an apparent increase of bone mass.

It is likely that many of the apparent increases in bone mineral mass merely reflect methodological variation since the S.D. of the error has been estimated to be approximately 38.5 mg/cm^2 [12] and most of the increases are within this range. This is further supported by the fact that the increasing values are mainly found among those patients with relatively short follow-up periods, compared with the decreasing values in patients who were followed-up for longer.

Table 3. Mean Rates of Changes per Year of Bone Mineral Measurements in the Proximal Radius in Three Groups of Renal Stone Patients

	Calcium Stones With Hypercalciuria	Calcium Stones Without Hypercalciuria	Uric Acid Stones	
Group	I	II	III	I+II
No. of patients	11	15	10	26
Bone mineral mass (mg/cm^2)	-17.10*	-12.64	-33.95**	-14.87*
Combined cortical thickness (cm)	- 0.0019	+ 0.0047	+ 0.0036	- 0.0006
Bone mineral density (mg/cm^3)	-26.64*	-17.64	-48.94**	-20.56

* Significantly different from 0: * at 5% level ($p < 0.05$); ** at 1% level ($p < 0.01$)

DISCUSSION

A decrease in the bone mineral content of patients with kidney stones was first reported by Alhava et al.[7]. Although they did not analyze subgroups of their patients separately, the mean bone mineral content of the radius of their total patient population was significantly lower than that of the controls. Harrison et al.[8] reported a decrease in partial body calcium content (measured by neutron activation analysis) in a group of patients with calcium stones. Lawoyin et al.[9] observed that whereas patients with absorptive hypercalciuria had a bone mineral mass within the normal range, those with resorptive or renal hypercalciuria had significantly lower values than normal controls. Interestingly there was a positive correlation between the fractional decrease of bone mineral mass from normal and the duration of the disease but only in those suffering from renal hypercalciuria. These authors postulated that the bone loss in patients with renal hypercalciuria was due to secondary hyperparathyroidism, especially when hypercalciuria was not compensated by an increased calcium intake.

Our report is the first to correlate calcium intake with bone loss in kidney stone patients. Although we did not separate our patients with idiopathic hypercalciuria into renal and absorptive types, the fact that all of them had a normal urine cAMP suggests that they are hyperabsorbers. In addition, our study included not only hypercalciuric patients but also patients with normal urine calcium and patients with uric acid stones. The latter group can be considered as a "control" group since they had a normal calcium intake and normal bone measurements at the beginning of the investigation.

Restriction of milk and dairy products is a common advice given to patients with kidney stones[1,2]. Although the main purpose is to restrict calcium intake, there is no evidence that reduced intake of dairy products prevents stones[14,15]. Moreover, milk also contains phosphorus and lactose[16,17]. An increased phosphorus intake will result in an increase of urine phosphorus which may be undesirable when urine pH is elevated e.g. in renal tubular acidosis or urinary infection[17], and lactose is a potent lithogenic agent[16,18]. Restriction of calcium intake may result in a decrease of urine calcium especially in patients with absorptive hypercalciuria without an effect on bone mineral content[19]. Whether calcium restriction is beneficial in patients with calcium stones in general has not yet been established[14,15].

Whereas Lawoyin et al.[9] have shown that calcium restriction may be detrimental to the bones of patients with renal hypercalciuria, they did not study the bones of stone patients in general. Our finding that a significant decrease in bone mineral mass occurs not only in patients with idiopathic hypercalciuria, but also in those with uric acid stones suggests that it is the dietary calcium deficiency rather than induced hyperparathyroidism which is responsible for the bone loss.

The role of an inadequate calcium intake in the etiology of osteoporosis is still controversial. Although decreasing calcium intake may cause an increase in the percentage of dietary calcium absorbed[20,21], a prolonged low calcium intake may lead to negative calcium balance and osteoporosis. Thus, dietary calcium deficiency has been shown to produce osteoporosis in animals[22,23], and Nordin[24] has shown that patients with primary osteoporosis have a significantly lower calcium intake (17.9 ± 1.3 mg/kg/day) than controls (19.7 ± 1.3 mg/kg/day) of similar age and sex. The same investigators observed that calcium intake of over 1 g per day was rarely associated with osteoporosis. Bogdonoff et al.[25] studied calcium balance in 7 ambulatory male patients aged 66 and over. They observed that all patients on a low calcium intake were in negative balance, at intermediate calcium intakes the patients were in balance, while at high calcium intakes the patients were in varying degrees of positive balance. They concluded that in elderly men, approximately 850 mg of calcium per day should be adequate to maintain calcium equilibrium. The National Research Council of the United States has recommended a minimum daily calcium intake of 800 mg for adults[26]. Prolonged calcium intake of less than 500-600 mg per day would result in a negative calcium balance[24]. The mean calcium intake in our patients, after they had been advised to restrict their intake of dairy product, was near these levels (i.e.

500-600 mg/day). It is also of interest to note that at the time of initial observations there was a correlation between the dietary calcium and the initial bone mineral mass, the highest values for both being found in uric acid stone patients and the lowest in the hypercalciuric group.

Among the various drugs used in stone disease, only phosphate has been shown to produce secondary hyperparathyroidism resulting in bone loss[27]. However, only 4 of our patients were receiving phosphates. Hydrochlorothiazide, by decreasing urine calcium, may produce a positive calcium balance whereas allopurinol has not been incriminated in calcium metabolism before.

Although our findings should not be surprising in view of the previously mentioned experience, the deleterious effect of the prolonged calcium restriction in patients with kidney stones has not been appreciated before and this dietary treatment is widely practiced among patients suffering from kidney stones. Our data indicate that unless there is a special indication, a low calcium diet should be prescribed with caution and preferably with periodic assessment of the patients' bone status.

REFERENCES

1. J. E. A. Wickham, in:"Urinary Calculus Disease," Churchill Livingstone, New York (1979).
2. L. N. Pyrah, in:"Renal Calculus," Springer-Verlag, New York (1979).
3. E. R. Yendt, Can. Med. Assoc. J. 102:497 (1970).
4. B. E. C. Nordin, A. Hodgkinson, M. Peacock, and W. G. Robertson, in:"Xth Congress International de Therapeutique," Dcin, Paris (1971).
5. P. M. Zarembski and A. Hodgkinson, Clin. Chem. Acta. 25:1 (1969).
6. R. W. Marchall, M. Cochran, and A. Hodgkinson, Clin. Sci. 43:91 (1972).
7. E. M. Alhava, M. Juuti, and P. Karjalainen, Scand. J. Urol. Nephrol. 10:154 (1976).
8. J. E. Harrison, Personal Communication.
9. S. Lawoyin, S. Sismilich, R. Browne, and C. Y. C. Pak, Meta. 28:1250 (1979).
10. H. E. Meema, C. K. Harris, and R. E. Porrett, Radiology 82:986 (1964).
11. H. E. Meema and S. Meema, in:"Proceedings of Conference. Progress in Methods of Bone Mineral Measurement," D. G. Whedon and J. R. Cameron, eds., HEW, Bethesda, MD (1970).
12. H. E. Meema, S. Rabinovich, D. G. Oreopoulos, G. J. Lloyd, and S. Meema, in:"Proceedings of Bone Measurement Conference," J. R. Cameron, ed., U. S. Atomic Energy Commission Conf. 700515, Chicago (1970).

13. H. E. Meema and S. Meema, Invest. Radiol. 7:88 (1972).
14. W. C. Thomas, Jr., Urol. Clin. N. Amer. 1:261 (1974).
15. W. C. Thomas, Jr., Kid. Int. 13:390 (1978).
16. C. W. Vermeulen, D. L. Proctor, and L. Seibutis, J. Lab. Clin. Med. 57:883 (1961).
17. I. Oliver, A. Weinberger, S. Ber-Meir, O. Sperling, J. Jakor, and A. de Vries, Urol. International 29:414 (1974).
18. B. Finlayson, Urol. Clin. N. Amer. 1:181 (1974).
19. C. Y. C. Pak, D. Barilla, H. Bone, and C. Northcutt, in:"New Concepts in Endocrinology and Metabolism," L. Rose and R. Levine, eds., Grune and Stratton, New York (1976).
20. B. E. C. Nordin and D. A. Smith, in:"Diagnostic Procedures in Disorders of Calcium Metabolism," J. A. Churchill, London (1965).
21. B. E. C. Nordin, in:"Calcium Phosphate and Magnesium Metabolism" Churchill Livingston, New York (1976).
22. M. C. Carttar, F. C. McLean, and M. R. Urist, Am. J. Pathol. 26:307 (1950).
23. B. E. C. Nordin, Clin. Orthopaed. 17:235 (1960).
24. B. E. C. Nordin, Lancet 1:1011 (1961).
25. M. D. Bogdanoff, N. W. Schock, M. G. Nicholas, J. Gerontol. 8:272 (1953).
26. Recommended daily allowances, Food and Nutritional Board. Nat. Acad. Sci. Nat. Res. Council Washington, D.C. publication 2216 (1974).
27. J. Jowsey, E. Reiss, and J. M. Canterbury, Acta. Ortheop. 801 (1974).

ACKNOWLEDGMENTS

This work was supported by the Canadian Medical Research Council Grants No.: MA-3889 and MA-6123.

THE PATHWAYS OF OXALATE BIOSYNTHESIS

Keith E. Richardson and Michael P. Farinelli

Department of Physiological Chemistry
The Ohio State University
Columbus, Ohio

Urinary oxalate in man originates from the absorption of dietary oxalate (3-11%) and endogenous synthesis from several precursors[1]. Ascorbic acid has been reported to provide from 10 to 40% of the total urinary oxalate while glycine provides another 40 %[2]. Glycolate, glyoxylate, tryptophan, tyrosine, phenylalanine, and serine and possibly citrate, xylitol, hydroxyproline, ethanolamine, and glucose also contribute to oxalate biosynthesis. The pathways of oxalate biosynthesis are summarized in Figure 1.

Three compounds, ascorbate, glyoxylate and glycolate, are immediate precursors of oxalate. In solution, ascorbic acid undergoes rapid decomposition producing oxalate from carbon atoms 1 and 2[3]. The urine from rats injected with L-[$1-^{14}C$] ascorbic acid contained only labeled oxalate and ascorbic acid. Attempts to trap metabolic intermediates such as glycolate and glyoxylate employing isotope dilution techniques were unsuccessful, suggesting that the formation of oxalate occurs directly from ascorbic acid and is probably nonenzymic in nature[4].

Glycolate may be converted directly to oxalate by glycolic acid dehydrogenase (GAD), an enzyme restricted to the liver in both the rat and man[5]. This enzyme, which has a Km for glycolate of 6.3 x 10^{-5} M, is present in the liver at sufficient concentration to potentially account for all of the oxalate synthesis which occurs in man and is inhibited by DL-phenyllactate and glyoxylate. The low Michaelis constant indicates that this enzyme would be effective with low levels of glycolate. If glyoxylate is an intermediate in this reaction, it remains tightly bound to the GAD and is not present as a free metabolite. Indirect evidence is available demonstrating the

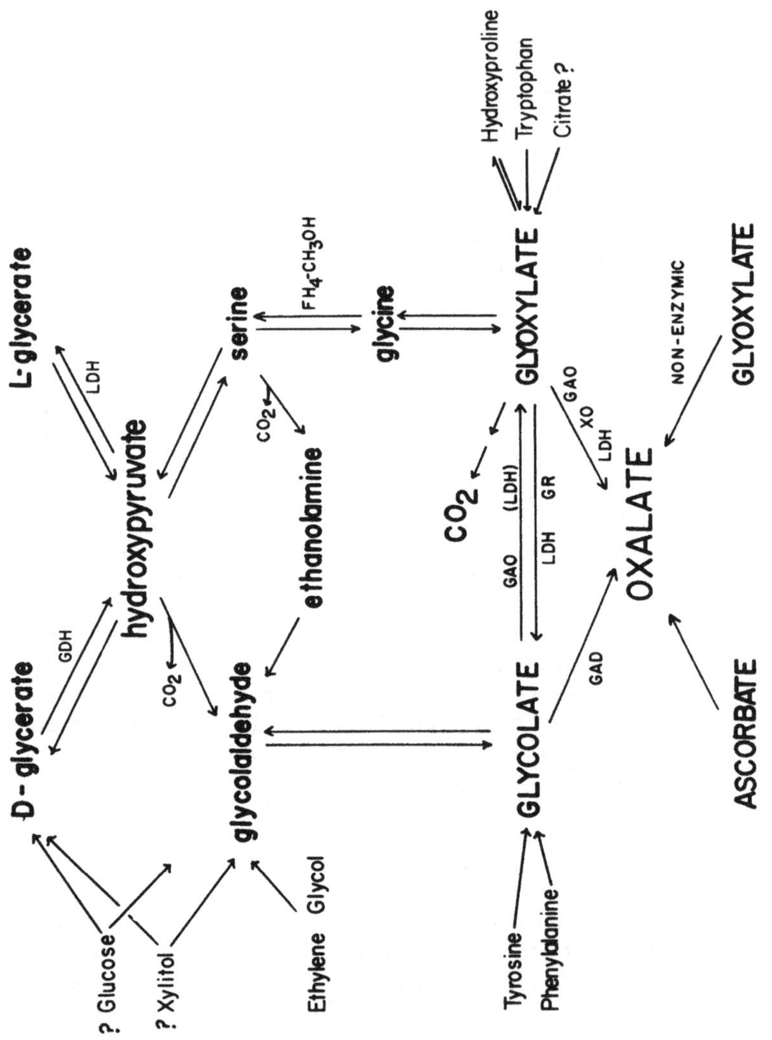

Figure 1. Pathways of Oxalate Biosynthesis

in vivo activity of GAD in the rat. In male rats fed with a vitamin B_6 deficient diet, the conversion of glycolate, ethylene glycol and ethanolamine to oxalate increased 18, 10, and 14-fold respectively, while the conversion of glyoxylate and glycine only increased 1.2 and 1.4 fold respectively[6]. These results are inconsistent with the catabolism of glycolate, ethylene glycol, and ethanolamine to oxalate via glyoxylate, but are consistent with their oxidation to oxalate via glycolate. Further, in isolated perfused rat liver, [1-^{14}C]glycolate and [U-^{14}]ethylene glycol were oxidized to [^{14}C]oxalate more efficiently than [U-^{14}C]glyoxylate[7]. The addition of hydroxypyruvate to the isolated perfused rat liver metabolizing [U-^{14}C]glyoxylate completely inhibited the formation of [^{14}C]oxalate, but total oxalate synthesis was increased[8]. On the other hand, hydroxypyruvate stimulated the conversion of [1-^{14}C]-glycolate to [^{14}C]oxalate. These results, which are inconsistent with the metabolism of glycolate to oxalate via glyoxylate but consistent with the direct oxidation of glycolate to oxalate, confirm the activity of GAD in the rat *in vivo* as well as its contribution to endogenous oxalate synthesis.

When glycolate is included in the diet of the rat, essentially 100% dietary absorption occurs and 3% of the glycolate consumed is recovered in the urine as oxalate within 24 hours[9]. Among the established oxalate precursors, ethylene glycol, tyrosine and phenylalanine are metabolized to oxalate via glycolate[4]. However, glycolate may also be converted to oxalate by a two step oxidation via glyoxylate catalyzed by glycolic acid oxidase (GAO)[10].

Glyoxylate is generally considered to be the major immediate precursor of oxalate. Glycine, hydroxyproline, tryptophan and probably citrate are metabolized to oxalate via glyoxylate. Serine is metabolized to oxalate via either glyoxylate or glycolate. Three enzymes, xanthine oxidase (XO), GAO, and lactate dehydrogenase (LDH) catalyze the oxidation of glyoxylate to oxalate. Since inhibitors of XO such as allopurinol do not significantly alter oxalate excretion, the contribution of this enzyme to oxalate synthesis *in vivo* is considered to be minor[11].

Glycolic acid oxidase is an FMN requiring enzyme found in liver with a Km for glycolate of 3.3×10^{-4} M and for glyoxylate of 3.54×10^{-3} M[12]. The enzyme has a broad specificity towards α-hydroxyacids and a pH optimum between 8.2 and 8.8 depending on the substrate employed. It has been suggested, because of the ubiquitous nature of LDH and its higher concentration in liver, heart, and kidney compared to GAO, that GAO does not contribute significantly to endogenous oxalate biosynthesis[13]. However, considerable evidence suggests that the major enzyme contributing to oxalate synthesis from glyoxylate is GAO, at least where high substrate levels are involved. First, the increased rate of oxaluria in male rats correlates with an increased level of liver glycolic acid oxidase[14].

No increase in liver LDH was observed. Second, partial hepatectomy had a marked effect on the toxicity of ethylene glycol and glyoxylate[15]. Since GAO is essentially limited to the liver in man as well as the rat while LDH is ubiquitous, one would only expect a marked effect from partial hepatectomy if GAO were the major contributing enzyme. Third, DL-phenyllactate at a 1:1 ratio with glyoxylate inhibits the oxidation of glyoxylate to oxalate by both human and rat liver GAO, but has no effect on the oxidation of glyoxylate to oxalate by human and rat liver LDH[16]. The addition of DL-phenyllactate to the perfusate of isolated perfused rat liver oxidizing either [^{14}C]ethylene glycol, [^{14}C]glycolate or [^{14}C]glyoxylate completely inhibits the formation of [^{14}C]oxalate, indicating that in rat liver oxalate synthesis from glyoxylate is catalyzed by GAO exclusively. The formation of oxalate from glycolate and glyoxylate was also inhibited by DL-phenyllactate in hepatocytes[17], and the intact rat[18], but less effectively. The role of GAO is supported by *in vivo* studies in which the excretion of [^{14}C]oxalate in the urine of normal male rats fed [^{14}C]ethylene glycol was reduced by 50% or more when DL-phenyllactate was administered. Finally, the concentration of GAO in the liver is sufficient to account for the total oxalate synthesis observed in man and the rat.

Primary hyperoxaluria is a relatively rare inborn metabolic error that is inherited in the autosomal recessive mode and is characterized by an abnormally high excretion of oxalate in the urine. The excretion in the urine of glycolate and glyoxylate is increased in primary hyperoxaluria type I, but remains normal or slightly reduced in primary hyperoxaluria type II, which is characterized by increased excretion in the urine of L-glycerate. The clinical course of both type I and type II is characterized by calcium oxalate nephrolithiasis and nephrocalcinosis ofter associated with early death as a result of renal failure. The specific defect in type I involves an increase in the glyoxylate pool resulting from a deficiency of 2-oxoglutarate:glyoxylate carboligase in the cytosol. The glyoxylate which accumulates is reduced to glycolate and inhibits GAD both of which cause glycolate to accumulate. The increase in glyoxylate also increases the rate at which it is oxidized to oxalate by GAO. Thus, the deficiency of the 2-oxoglutarate:glyoxylate carboligase enzyme results in an increase in the excretion of oxalate, glycolate and glyoxylate.

Primary hyperoxaluria type II results from a deficiency of D-glycerate dehydrogenase resulting in an increased excretion in the urine of L-glycerate and oxalate, but not glycolate and glyoxylate. Williams and Smith[19] have suggested that in the absence of D-glycerate dehydrogenase, hydroxypyruvate accumulates and is reduced by LDH to L-glycerate. This reduction causes an increase in the NAD:NADH ratio which stimulates the oxidation of glyoxylate to oxalate by LDH. Results from our laboratory, however, indicate that hydroxypyruvate is a precursor of oxalate and inhibits the oxidation of glyoxylate to oxalate[8]. Glycolate also inhibits the oxidation of glyoxylate to oxalate, presumably because of its greater affinity for GAO. This suggests that the increased oxaluria is caused by the conversion of the accumulated hydroxypyruvate to glycolate which is then oxidized to oxalate by GAD. Since the normal pathways of glycolate and glyoxylate metabolism are not altered, there is no accumulation and subsequent increased excretion of these compounds in the urine. This mechanism suggests that GAD is the enzyme responsible for oxalate accumulation in primary hyperoxaluria type II and that GAO is the active enzyme in type I.

Studies with isolated perfused rat liver demonstrate that oxalate synthesis in the liver does not involve LDH, but depends upon GAO and GAD[15]. This might have been anticipated, since the major role of LDH in the liver is the oxidation of lactate to pyruvate for utilization in gluconeogenesis. This oxidation would utilize NAD, limiting the availability of this coenzyme for the oxidation of glyoxylate to oxalate by LDH. Thus, although when NAD is provided to a liver homogenate glyoxylate is oxidized to oxalate by LDH, in the *in vivo* situation, the ratio of NAD:NADH determined by the oxidation of lactate to pyruvate prevents the oxidation of glyoxylate to oxalate by LDH. However, in other tissues where gluconeogenesis is not significant, the role of LDH would be in the reduction of pyruvate to lactate producing NAD which could be used for the oxidation of glyoxylate to oxalate. Further, the reduction of glyoxylate to glycolate could provide an additional source of NAD at the expense of the glyoxylate concentration. If the above hypothesis is correct, the removal of GAO and GAD by hepatectomy would reduce the contribution of liver to total oxalate synthesis, but would not curtail the formation of oxalate in those tissues favoring glycolysis over gluconeogenesis.

The effect of total hepatectomy on the metabolism of glyoxylate and glycolate in the rat is summarized in Tables 1 and 2. The liver appears to be the major site for the decarboxylation of glyoxylate and glycolate, which presumably occurs via 2-oxyglutarate:glyoxylate carboligase, since hepatectomy reduced CO_2 production by 67% and 85% from glyoxylate and glycolate, respectively. However, contrary to the situation in primary hyperoxaluria type I where the deficiency of the carboligase enzyme significantly increases oxalate excretion, removal of the enzyme by hepatectomy decreased the oxalate in the urine from glyoxylate by 50% and from glycolate by 89%. Total oxalate synthesis was reduced by 15% from glyoxylate and 83% from glycolate but the former does not appear to be significant. The results confirm that the liver plays a significant role in oxalate biosynthesis. That this contribution involved GAO and GAD is indicated by the comparisons of the oxalate to glycolate ratios.

Table 1. The Effect of Total Hepatectomy on the Metabolism of Glyoxylate in the Rat

	Oxalate (μmoles/kg) Average (Range)	Glyoxylate (μmoles/kg) Average (Range)	Glycolate (μmoles/kg) Average (Range)	CO_2 (μmoles/kg) Average (Range)
BLOOD				
Hepatectomized	3.5 (3.0- 4.0)	1.8 (1.7- 1.8)	47.2 (38.1- 56.2)	
Control	27.2 (26.6-27.8)	10.0 (8.3-11.7)	18.3 (17.2- 19.4)	
VISCERA				
Hepatectomized	203.4 (180.0-226.8)	11.8 (9.0-14.5)	57.6 (49.1- 66.0)	
Control	168.8 (130.6-207.0)	6.1 (4.4- 7.8)	9.4 (8.8- 10.0)	
URINE				
Hepatectomized	61.0 (36.5- 85.5)	10.2 (9.0-11.3)	90.7 (64.3-117.0)	
Control	120.0 (98.0-142.0)	12.3 (9.0-15.6)	17.5 (13.5- 21.5)	
TOTAL				
Hepatectomized	267.9 (219.5-316.5)	23.8 (19.7-27.6)	195.5 (152.2-239.2)	44.3 (37.5- 51.0)
Control	316.0 (255.6-376.8)	32.0 (25.1-31.7)	45.2 (39.5- 50.9)	135.0 (121.5-148.5)

The animals were placed in metabolism cages after the injection of radio-labeled precursors and urine and CO_2 were collected. At the end of 6 hours the animals were sacrificed and their blood and viscera removed. All values are the averages of 2 or more animals.

Table 2. The Effect of Total Hepatectomy on the Metabolism of Glycolate in the Rat

	Oxalate (μmoles/kg)	Glyoxylate (μmoles/kg)	Glycolate (μmoles/kg)	CO_2 (μmoles/kg)
	Average (Range)	Average (Range)	Average (Range)	Average (Range)
BLOOD				
Hepatectomized	1.8 (0.9- 2.3)	0.8 (0.2- 1.3)	150.4 (105.6-176.5)	
Control	4.5 (2.4- 8.0)	10.7 (2.9-24.1)	73.7 (10.6-108.8)	
VISCERA				
Hepatectomized	3.6 (3.3- 3.9)	2.5 (2.0- 3.0)	59.1 (49.0- 69.1)	
Control	5.1 (3.1- 7.0)	16.7 (15.4-17.8)	11.6 (8.7- 14.5)	
URINE				
Hepatectomized	6.0 (2.1- 9.0)	3.9 (1.7- 5.0)	116.3 (35.9-276.5)	
Control	53.5 (15.2- 72.2)	13.8 (10.8-15.3)	258.4 (206.1-334.4)	
TOTAL				
Hepatectomized	11.4 (6.3- 21.5)	7.2 (3.9- 9.3)	325.8 (190.5-522.1)	33.0 (30.1- 36.6)
Control	63.1 (20.7-107.9)	41.2 (29.1-57.2)	343.8 (225.4-457.7)	215.1 (152.0-301.3)

The animals were placed in metabolism cages after the injection of radio-labeled precursors and urine and CO_2 were collected. At the end of 6 hours the animals were sacrificed and their blood and viscera removed. All values are the averages of 2 or more animals.

The oxidation of glyoxylate to oxalate by LDH is dependent upon the NAD level and if no other source of the oxidized coenzyme is available, it can be obtained by the reduction of glyoxylate to glycolate. Thus, where LDH is catalyzing the oxidation of glyoxylate to oxalate and recovering the NAD by reducing glyoxylate to glycolate, the synthesis of glycolate would be increased and the ratio of oxalate/glycolate produced would be 1. If GAO were involved no requirement for glycolate formation would be present and in addition any glycolate produced could either be reoxidized to glyoxylate by liver GAO or to oxalate by liver GAD. In the control rat the ratio of oxalate/glycolate was 7.9 while in the hepatectomized rat the ratio was 1.5 which, along with the significant increase in glycolate synthesis and excretion in the hepatectomized rat (Table 1) indicates that LDH is the major enzyme for oxalate synthesis in the hepatectomized rat, but that GAO is the significant enzyme in the normal or control rat.

When the oxidation of glyoxylate is transferred to other organs or tissues due to hepatectomy, more oxalate, glyoxylate and glycolate are found in these tissues (Table 1). This suggests that oxalosis may result when oxalate synthesis from glyoxylate catalyzed by LDH occurs within the various tissues or organs. The results further suggest that when present at low concentrations glycolate and glyoxylate are primarily metabolized in the liver by GAO and GAD. At higher concentration where the GAO and GAD may be saturated or under conditions where the liver enzymes are not functioning effectively, the LDH catalyzed oxidation of glyoxylate to oxalate in other tissues would be enhanced. Since the specific inhibition of GAO and GAD in the liver would apparently only shift the site of oxalate synthesis to the LDH catalyzed oxidation in other tissues, the effectiveness of such inhibitors in treating or controlling primary hyperoxaluria seems questionable. However, since elimination of GAO and GAD activity by hepatectomy did appear to reduce oxalate excretion, inhibition of these enzymes may lower urinary oxalate levels sufficiently to effectively reduce oxalate stone formation.

REFERENCES

1. H. E. Williams, and L. H. Smith, Jr., in:"The Metabolic Basis of Inherited Disease," J. B. Stanbury, J. B. Wyngaarden, and D. S. Fredrickson, eds., McGraw Hill, New York (1978).
2. J. C. Crawhall, E. F. Scowen, and R. W. E. Watts, Lancet 2:806 (1959).
3. E. M. Baker, J. C. Saari, and B. M. Tolbert, Am. J. Clin. Nutr. 19:371 (1966).
4. R. L. Gambardella, and K. E. Richardson, Biochim. Biophys. Acta. 499:156 (1977).
5. D. W. Fry, and K. E. Richardson, Biochim. Biophys. Acta. 567:482 (1979).

6. T. J. Runyan, and S. N. Gershoff, J. Biol. Chem. 240:1889 (1965).
7. L. L. Liao, and K. E. Richardson, Arch. Biochem. Biophys. 153:438 (1972).
8. L. L. Liao, and K. E. Richardson, Biochim. Biophys. Acta. 538:76 (1978).
9. K. S. Harris, and K. E. Richardson, Invest. Urol. (1980) (in press).
10. K. E. Richardson, and N. E. Tolbert, J. Biol. Chem. 236:1280 (1961).
11. D. A. Gibbs, and R. W. E. Watts, Clin. Sci. 31:285 (1966).
12. D. W. Fry, and K. E. Richardson, Biochim. Biophys. Acta. 568:135 (1979).
13. D. A. Gibbs, and R. W. E. Watts, Clin. Sci. 44:227 (1973).
14. K. E. Richardson, Endocrinology 74:128 (1964).
15. K. E. Richardson, Toxicol. Appl. Pharmacol. 24:530 (1973).
16. L. L. Liao, and K. E. Richardson, Arch. Biochem. Biophys. 154:68 (1973).
17. A. M. Rofe, and J. B. Edwards, Biochem. Med. 20:323 (1978).
18. R. L. Gambardella, and K. E. Richardson, Biochim. Biophys. Acta. 544:315 (1978).
19. H. E. Williams, and L. H. Smith, Jr., Science 171:390 (1971).

ACKNOWLEDGMENT

This work was supported by the USPH, NIH Grant AM-12960.

ALTERATIONS IN KIDNEY ENZYMES OF OXALATE METABOLISM IN PATIENTS WITH UROLITHIASIS

S. K. Thind, R. Nath, G. Verma, M. S. Rao* and
B. C. Bapna*
Departments of Biochemistry and Urology*, Postgraduate
Institute of Medical Education and Research,
Chandigarh, India

McCarrison[1] described northern India as a "stone-belt", in which the stones are of a mixture of calcium oxalate and calcium phosphate [2]. Many etiological factors have been implicated in the formation of idiopathic renal calculi. Recent work on experimental urolithiasis in rats has shown that enzymes of oxalate metabolism are altered in stone formers[3]. In the present study the role of enzymes involved in urolithiasis in humans has been ascertained by measuring the activities of alkaline phosphatase (AP), lactate dehydrogenase (LDH), glycolate oxidase and glyoxylase I, from biopsy specimens of kidneys collected during operation.

MATERIALS AND METHODS

Twenty-four adult male patients (45-65 years) admitted to the Urology Ward for the removal of kidney stone, were selected for this study. Twelve control subjects of the same age group, undergoing operation for other causes, but having normal kidneys, served as controls. Fragments (10-20 mg) of biopsy tissue were collected from different sections of the kidney, during the course of surgical exploration. The tissues were immediately chilled in ice and homogenized in normal physiological saline (1:10). The homogenate was centrifuged at 15,000 rpm for 10 min in the cold. The supernatant was used to assay the kidney enzymes. Glyoxalase I was assayed by the method of Racker[4], glycolate oxidase by the method of Dixon and Kornberg[5], alkaline phosphatase by the method of Bessy et al.[6], LDH by that of Wroblewski and Gregory[7] and protein by Folin's method [8]. The enzyme units are expressed as milliunits (one milliunit = Δ O.D./min/mg protein x 10^{-3}).

RESULTS

The enzyme activities of control subjects and patients of urolithiasis are given in Table 1. A significant decrease (40%) in alkaline phosphatase and increase (100%) in lactate dehydrogenase were noted in the kidneys of stone-formers compared with the controls. The other two enzymes i.e. glycolate oxidase and glyoxylase I showed decreases of 18% and 40% respectively, which, however, were not statistically significant.

Table 1. Activities of the Human Kidney Enzymes in Oxalate Urolithiasis (Milli - International Units[+] ± S.E.M.)

Group	Glyoxylase I	Glycolate Oxidase	Alkaline Phosphatase	Lactate Dehydrogenase
Control (12)	53.25±11.04	3.40±0.74	70.67±7.93	113.33±17.33
Stone-formers (24)	34.68± 4.35	2.82±0.72	45.50±5.62*	203.92±16.97**

+, Milli-International Unit = O.D./min/mg protein x 10^{-3}.
Figures in brackets indicate the number of subjects.
*, $P < 0.05$; **, $P < 0.01$ as compared to controls.

The frequency distribution patterns of the enzymes are shown in Figure 1 (a, b, c, d).

DISCUSSION

Glyoxylate is the main precursor of oxalate in man and mammals. In normal subjects, 40% of urinary oxalate is derived from glycine via glyoxylate. Regulation of oxalate synthesis in mammalian system involves the enzymes, glycolate oxidase and lactate dehydrogenase besides glyoxylase. Both the enzymes i.e. glycolate oxidase and lactate dehydrogenase, oxidize glycolate to oxalate via glyoxylate. Formation of glyoxylate by LDH is inhibited by oxalate[9] providing a feed-back regulation of the formation of oxalate, however, LDH favors formation of glycolate. Inhibition of glyoxylase, and/or, increase in LDH in kidneys of stone-formers will promote the accumulation of glycolate. Direct oxidation of glycolate to oxalate by glycolate dehydrogenase has also been reported in rat and human liver[10]. Increase in AP in kidneys of stone-formers will lead to the lowering of the Pi pool, thereby making calcium more available for calcium oxalate formation. Thus, this study shows that lactate

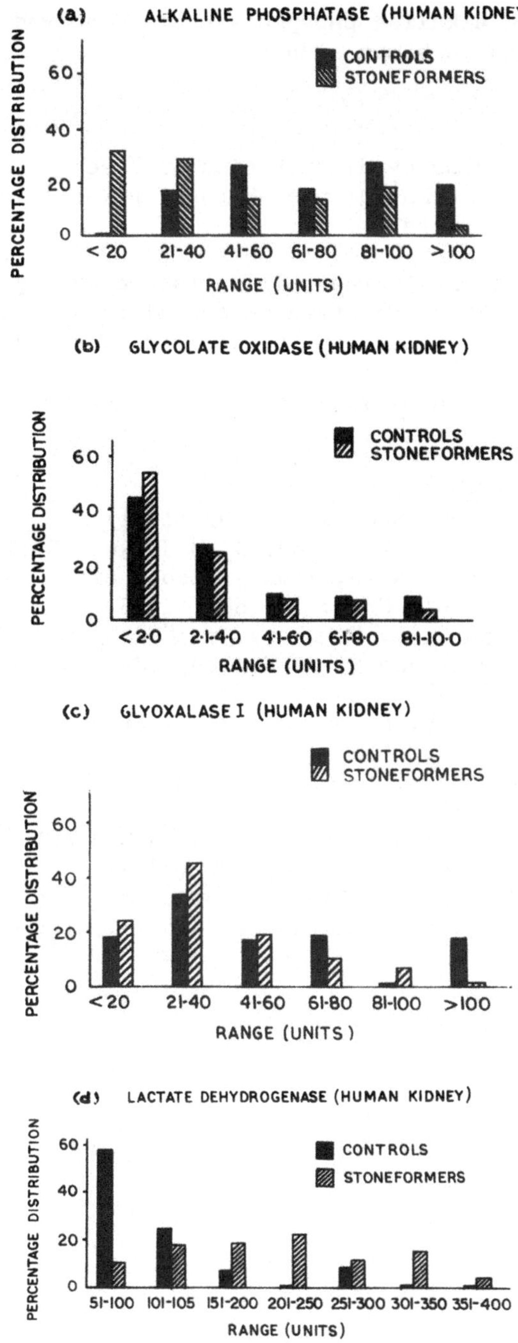

Figure 1. Frequency distributions of (a) alkaline phosphatase; (b) glycolate oxidase; (c) glyoxylase I; (d) lactate dehydrogenase in human kidney of stone patients.

dehydrogenase and alkaline phosphatase are involved in the process of stone-formation in human kidney.

CONCLUSIONS

1. A high frequency distribution has been noted in the lower range activities of alkaline phosphatase, glyoxylase and glycolate oxidase in stone-formers.

2. A significant increase in lactate dehydrogenase and a decrease in alkaline phosphatase in the kidneys of stone-formers indicates their involvement in the process of stone-formation.

3. Glyoxylase and glycolate oxidase remained unaltered.

REFERENCES

1. R. McCarrison, Br. Med. J. 1:1009 (1931).
2. S. K. Thind and R. Nath, Ind. J. Med. Res. 57:1790 (1979).
3. S. K. Thind and R. Nath, Ind. J. Expt. Biol. 16:66 (1978).
4. E. Racker, J. Biol. Chem. 190:685 (1955).
5. G. H. Dixon and H. L. Kornberg, in:"Methods in Enzymology," S. P. Colowick and N. O. Kaplan, eds., Academic Press Inc., New York (1966).
6. O. A. Bessey, O. H. Lowry, and M. J. Brock, J. Biol. Chem. 164:321 (1946).
7. F. Wroblewski and K. F. Gregory, Ann. N. Y. Acad. Sci. 94:912 (1961).
8. I. D. P. Wooton, in:"Microanalysis in Medical Biochemistry," J. & A. Churchill Ltd., London (1964).
9. C. Lluis and J. Bozal, Biophys. Biochem. Acta. 480:333 (1977).
10. D. W. Fry and K. E. Richardson, Biophys. Biochem. Acta. 567: 482 (1979).

ACKNOWLEDGMENT

This work was supported by the Indian Council of Medical Research (India).

THERAPEUTIC ROLE OF VITAMIN B_6 ON OXALATE METABOLISM IN UROLITHIASIS AND ITS EFFECT ON HYPEROXALURIA INDUCED IN RATS BY ETHYLENE GLYCOL

S. K. Thind, R. Nath, S. Farooqui and M. S. R. Murthy

Departments of Biochemistry and Experimental Medicine*
Postgraduate Institute of Medical Education and
Research, Chandigarh, India

Marginal deficiency of vitamin B_6 has been shown to promote hyperoxaluria in man[1]. Even though large doses of pyridoxine may reduce the hyperoxaluria[1], the dose of pyridoxine to be administered has not been well defined. Hyperoxaluria in animals can be induced by ethylene glycol or sodium glycolate[2]. The present study has been undertaken to find out the effect of large doses of pyridoxine on ethylene glycol-induced hyperoxaluria in rats and also in hyperoxaluric stone-forming patients.

MATERIALS AND METHODS

Thirty-six male Wistar rats (200 g) fed stock diet ad libitum were grouped as follows: Group I - 8 rats on stock diet only served as controls, Group II - 8 rats received 10 mg pyridoxine - HCl/100 g BW/day, Group III - 10 rats administered 0.1% ethylene glycol in their drinking water, and Group IV - 10 rats given 0.1% ethylene glycol in their water and 10 mg pyridoxine HCl/100 g BW/day. During the treatment period (6 weeks) 24 h urine samples were individually collected every week from Group III and IV rats. After the sixth week, all the rats were sacrificed and blood, liver and kidneys, were removed for biochemical analysis. Urines were analyzed for creatinine, calcium and phosphorus, by standard methods[3] and oxalate by the method of Hodgkinson and Williams[4]. Glutamate oxaloacetate transminase (GOT) in RBC, liver and kidneys and glutamate pyruvate transminase (GPT) in livers and kidneys were assayed[5].

Recurrent stone-forming patients with established hyperoxaluria were given 10 mg pyridoxine HCl/day for a period of 180 days. Urine and blood samples were collected at intervals of 0, 15, 30, 90 and 180 days. Urine samples were analyzed as mentioned above and GPT and GOT were assayed in erythrocytes[5]. Stimulation in the activity of the transaminases after addition of pyridoxal-5'-phosphate was calculated.

RESULTS AND DISCUSSION

Urinary oxalate, calcium and phosphorus values, in ethylene glycol-treated rats, with and without pyridoxine supplementation are given in Table 1. All the parameters within groups III and IV increased significantly by the sixth week compared with the basal values, but there were no significant differences between these two groups, indicating that pyridoxine supplementation alone does not give protection against ethylene glycol-induced hyperoxaluria. This is probably due to the excessively high doses of pyridoxine fed to these rats. Pyridoxine administration with magnesium oxide has been shown to decrease urinary oxalate levels in ethylene glycol treated rats[6]. The proposed role of pyridoxine in reducing hyperoxaluria by converting glyoxylate to glycine has been refuted on the basis that glycolate dehydrogenase converts glycolate (from the metabolism of ethylene glycol), to oxalate without forming free glyoxylate[7].

Table 1. Urinary Oxalate, Calcium, and Phosphorus in Ethylene Glycol Treated Rats With or Without Pyridoxine Supplementation (Groups III & IV) (Values are mg/dg creatinine (mean ± S.E.M.)

	Oxalate		Calcium		Phosphorus	
Week	Group III	Group IV	Group III	Group IV	Group III	Group IV
0	30± 6.3	25± 6.3	22± 5.9	13±4.5	70± 9.2	110±18.1
2	128±23.6	139±48	18± 2.9	15±3.9	96± 7.9	113±20.3
4	59±16.2	72±10.7	9± 1.3	25±7.8	48±23.2	64±18.9
6	267±36	217±48	242±74	90±24	177±49	357±91

The effect of pyridoxine supplementation to ethylene glycol-treated rats on the transaminase activities is shown in Table 2. GPT and GOT levels showed a significant decline in all the tissues, suggesting that pyridoxine may provide only partial protection in maintaining the transaminase activities. High doses of pyridoxine alone (group II) also caused a significant decrease in the activity of transaminases in all tissues except the erythrocyte GOT. Pyridoxine given in large amounts is known to produce changes similar to its own deficiency, probably due to the inhibition of pyridoxine-5'-phosphate oxidase, while erythrocytes have an additional system for the inactivation of excess of pyridoxine to 4-pyridoxic acid[8].

Eighty percent of stone-forming patients in this study with hyperoxaluria and hypercalciuria for up to 30 days showed a reduction

Table 2. GPT and GOT Activities in the Tissues of Rats Fed Pyridoxine or Ethylene Glycol With or Without Pyridoxine (Units/mg Protein x 10^{-2}; Mean ± S.E.M.)

Group	Glut. Oxaloacetate Transaminase R.B.C.	Liver	Kidney	Glut. Pyruvate Transaminase Liver	Kidney
I. Normal	1.16±0.10	15.30±2.30	9.89±0.40	1.89±0.20	0.69±0.08
II. Pyridoxine (10 mg/100 g BW/day)	2.22±0.25**●●	7.67±1.00***	7.52±0.30*	1.23±0.20*	0.44±0.02**
III. Ethylene glycol (0.1%)	0.19±0.04***●●	5.01±0.50***●●●	8.14±0.50*●●	0.76±0.10*	0.17±0.03***●
IV. Ethylene glycol + pyridoxine	0.30±0.03***++●	9.44±0.70***+++	5.44±0.30**++	0.84±0.10**	0.26±0.02***+

*P < 0.05, ** P < 0.01, *** P < 0.001 as compared with normal group.

●P < 0.05, ●● P < 0.01, ●●● P < 0.001 as compared with pyridoxine group.

+P < 0.05, ++ P < 0.01, +++ P < 0.001 as compared with ethylene glycol group.

in their urinary oxalate levels by 90 days on pyridoxine therapy (10 mg/day) (Table 3). Administration of this vitamin, also improved the pyridoxine status of the patients, as evidenced by their erythrocyte transaminase activities.

Table 3. Effect of Pyridoxine Supplementation on Urinary Oxalate and Erythrocyte Transaminase Activity in Kidney Stone Patients

Supplementation Period (days)	Urinary Oxalate (mg/24 h)	Percentage Activation by added Pyridoxal-5'-Phosphate	
		EGOT	EGPT
0	65.8± 8.5*	32	47
15	55.0±11.3	24	28
30	57.7± 9.9	25	28
90	38.2± 7.2**	23	16
180	22.2± 5.3**	6	11

*Mean ± SEM; ** P < 0.01 as compared to 0 day.

If the body retention of pyridoxine by humans and rats is considered, the dose administered to rats in this study (10 mg/100 g BW/day) resembles the high doses usually administered to patients (1.5 - 2.5 g/day). The toxic effects of pyridoxine in rats should be considered before employing high doses of this vitamin to humans as a pharmacological measure.

CONCLUSIONS

Pyridoxine supplementation (10 mg/70 kg BW/day) to hyperoxaluric kidney stone patients, reduced their urinary oxalate excretion after 90 days therapy. High doses of pyridoxine (10 mg/100 g BW/day) to ethylene glycol treated rats led to decrease in transaminase levels in tissues, thus indicating that caution should be exercised when giving pharmacological doses of this vitamin to humans.

REFERENCES

1. S. N. Gershoff, Vitamins and Hormones 22:581 (1964).
2. F. H. C. Chow, D. W. Hamar, and R. H. Udall, Invest. Urol. 12:50 (1974).
3. I. D. P. Wootton, in:"Microanalysis in Medical Biochemistry," A. Churchill, London (1960).
4. A. Hodgkinson and A. Williams, Clin. Chim. Acta. 36:127 (1972).
5. H. Kishi and K. Folkares, J. Nutr. Sci. Vitaminol. 22:225 (1976).

6. S. N. Gershoff and S. B. Andrus, Proc. Soc. Exptl. Biol. Med. 109:99 (1962).
7. D. W. Fry and K. E. Richardson, Biochim. Biophys. Acta. 567:482 (1979).
8. M. Stanulovic, V. Jeremic, V. Leskovac, and S. Chaykin, Enzyme 21:357 (1976).

ACKNOWLEDGMENT

This work was supported by the Indian Council of Medical Research (India).

DECOMPOSITION OF EXOGENOUS ^{14}C-OXALATE (^{14}C-OX) TO ^{14}C-CARBON DIOXIDE ($^{14}CO_2$) IN VITRO AND IN ANIMALS

V. Hagmaier[1], D. Hornig[2], C. Bannwart[1], K. Schmidt[3], F. Weber[2], H. Graf[1], and G. Rutishauser[1]
[1]Division of Urology, Department of Surgery, University of Basel, Basel, Switzerland; [2]Department Vitamin Nutrition Research, Hoffmann-La Roche, Basel, Switzerland; [3]Department of Surgery, University of Tübingen, Tübingen, Germany

SUMMARY

The question concerning bacterial decomposition of oxalate by intestinal microorganisms is unresolved. Varying amounts of oxalate were incubated with human feces. The formed CO_2 was determined by liquid scintillation counting. Oxalate was found to be metabolized by bacteria from the human feces. However, the deterioration was very small (0.15%). In a second experiment rats and guinea pigs received ^{14}C-Ox by gastric intubation. The exhalation of $^{14}CO_2$ was measured. In guinea pigs the major pathway of metabolism of exogenous Ox was found to be respiratory exhalation (72%). In contrary, the rat excreted only 5% as CO_2. Therefore, balance studies with Ox in guinea pigs are only valuable when following the CO_2 exhalation.

INTRODUCTION

The mechanism of oxalate stone formation is, despite intensive research and improvement of analytical determination of oxalate[1] not yet elaborated. The available information on daily intake of oxalate with food[2], on absorption[3] and distribution[4] is often contradictory. Also, the question on a bacterial decomposition of oxalate by intestinal microorganisms is unresolved. However, this is not only of physiological importance, but also has a practical impact in balance studies.

METHODS

In Vitro

Varying amounts of oxalate (50, 150, 500 mg oxalate containing 50 μCi ^{14}C-oxalate sodium) were incubated (37°C, pH 7.4, 8h) with human feces in 100 ml broth-solution (Iso-Sensitest CM 473) under anaerobic conditions. The formed $^{14}CO_2$ was precipitated as Ba $^{14}CO_3$ and the radioactivity was determined by liquid scintillation counting.

In Vivo

Two male rats each (Wistar, 250 g) and two male guinea pigs each (Himalayan spotted, 350 g) were placed separately in a metabolic cage and received ^{14}C-oxalate sodium (spec. activity 22.3 μCi/mmol) in 1 ml isotonic NaCl by gastric intubation. The animals were fed ad libitum normal diets (Nafag 850, Nafag 845, Nafag AG, Gossau) and had free access to water.

The metabolic cage was deviced in a manner to allow collection of urine, feces and continuous sampling of CO_2 (hourly until 8h, then in a pool up to 24h) which was absorbed in ethanolamine. By counting an aliquot of this solution by liquid scintillation counting using Instagel, the radioactivity was determined.

RESULTS AND DISCUSSION

In Vitro-Experiments

The data from this investigation are summarized in Table 1. The bacterial degradation of oxalate to $^{14}CO_2$ was found to be very small (0.15%, 0.13% and 0.22% depending on the amount of incubated oxalate, respectively). Microorganisms have been detected in the stomach of various animals which can degrade oxalate in appreciable amounts[5,6]. Barber[7] incubated human feces with oxalate and demonstrated after a 3 day incubation period approximately 80% of the oxalate to be degraded. However, following incubation for only one day no detectable oxalate decomposition was observed. Most of the oxalate is metabolized in vivo within 6h (see below). The time for passage of oxalate in the intestine of man and animal normally does not exceed 24h[4]. Therefore, only an investigation of the oxalate degradation during these 24h seems to be of physiological importance.

In contrary to the study of Barber[7] in our study employing labelled oxalate we could demonstrate a small bacterial decomposition of oxalate within the first 8h.

Table 1.

Oxalate(mg) metabolized by bacteria

50	0.08 mg(0.15%*)
150	0.20 mg(0.13%*)
500	1.10 mg(0.22%)

* $p < 0.001$

In Vivo-Experiments

Figure 1 shows the time course of $^{14}CO_2$ exhalation in guinea pigs and rats following a single oral dose of ^{14}C-oxalate. It is seen that in the guinea pig the respiratory exhalation of $^{14}CO_2$ is a major pathway of oxalate (70-75%) of the dose excreted as $^{14}CO_2$ in 24h, whereas in the rat $^{14}CO_2$ exhalation was only minute (5.4% of the dose in 24h). Peak exhalation of $^{14}CO_2$ occurred between 3 and 4h after dosage in the guinea pig. The exhalation curve in rats showed two peaks at 1h and 5h following administration of the label, respectively.

In the literature no reports could be found on the respiratory catabolism of orally administered oxalate to CO_2. The data on the fate of metabolism of oxalate following parenteral application are contradictory. In the rat CO_2 excretions between 1 and 8% of the dose are reported[8]. In man following intravenous application of ^{14}C-oxalate no respiratory $^{14}CO_2$ could be detected[9]. In the present study we could demonstrate in the guinea pig the main route of metabolism of exogenous ^{14}C-oxalate to be the respiratory exhalation as $^{14}CO_2$.

In conclusion, evidence is presented for the existence of a species specific difference in oxalate metabolism in guinea pigs and rats following oral application. Whether the metabolism of oxalate to CO_2 may be due to in vivo metabolism after absorption from the intestine or whether it might be microbial destruction in the gut is unclear and awaits further investigation.

Balance studies with oxalate in guinea pigs are only valuable when following the CO_2 excretion. In contrary in the rat in such studies CO_2 excretion can be neglected.

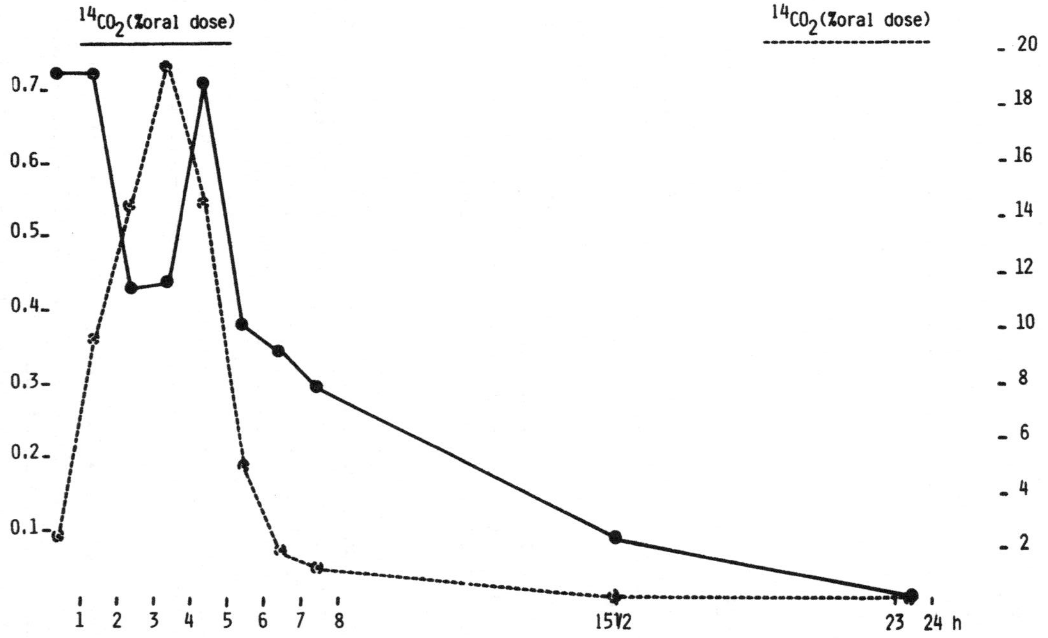

Figure 1. Time course of $^{14}CO_2$ exhalation in guinea pig (---) and rat (———) following single oral dose of ^{14}C-Ox.

REFERENCES

1. K. Schmidt, V. Hagmaier, G. Bruchelt, and G. Rutishauser, Urol. Res. (in press).
2. P. M. Zarembski, and A. Hodgkinson, Br. J. Nutr. 16:627 (1962).
3. C. Bannwart, V. Hagmaier, G. Rutishauser, H. Seiler, Eur. Urol. 5:276 (1979).
4. V. Hagmaier, C. Bannwart, W. Remagen, and G. Rutishauser, Eur. Urol. 6:172 (1980).
5. M. P. Morris, and J. Garcia-Riviera, J. Dairy Sci. 38:1169 (1955).
6. T. S. Chandra, and Y. J. Shethna, J. Microbiol. and Serol. 41: 101 (1975).
7. H. H. Barber, and F. J. Gallimore, Biochem. J. 34:144 (1940).
8. G. Brubacher, M. Just, H. Bodur, and K. Bernhard, Physiol. Chem. 304:173 (1956).
9. T. D. Elder, and J. B. Wyngaarden, J. Clin. Invest. 39:1337 (1960).

ENHANCEMENT OF URINARY CITRATE IN OXALATE STONE FORMERS BY THE INTAKE OF ALKALINE SALTS

M. Butz and H.-J. Dulce

Department of Urology and Department of Clinical Chemistry, Klinikum Steglitz, Free University of Berlin, Berlin, West Germany

ABSTRACT

Oxalate stone formers have a decreased concentration and excretion of urinary citrate. By oral ingestion of K-Na-citrate (Uralyt-U^R) a 100% increase of citrate and a 40% decrease of calcium is achieved. Urinary oxalate, uric acid, magnesium and phosphate remain unaltered under therapy. Two additive effects improving the solubility of calcium oxalate are obtained by the intake of alkaline citrate. Thus it is suggested to extend prophylactic Uralyt-U^R therapy to oxalate stone formers.

INTRODUCTION

Only in the minority of oxalate stone formers either hyperoxaluria or hypercalciuria are found. Nevertheless urine is frequently oversaturated with these compounds in healthy as well as in stone forming persons. Despite this oversaturation formation of crystals is prevented to a great extent by various inhibitors excreted in urine such as magnesium, pyrophosphates and citrate. Recently, investigation into the role of citrate in calcium stone formation has increased. Citrate can form a soluble complex with calcium ions, thus the solubility of calcium oxalate can be maintained even if the thermodynamic solubility product is exceeded.

Kissin and Locks[1] were the first to observe reduced excretion of citrate in calcium stone formers. In recent years this finding has been confirmed by several investigators[2-4]. In 1931 Oestberg[5] showed that ingestion of alkali increases the citrate content of urine in man. On the basis of these observations we consider it a worthy goal to concentrate efforts on the potential therapeutic benefit of increasing citrate excretion in oxalate stone disease.

MATERIALS AND METHODS

In a control group of 20 healthy males and females 24 hr urinary citrate excretion was determined. Sixty single and recurrent oxalate stone formers ingested K-Na-citrate (Uralyt-U^R) for consecutive eight days. The dose was calculated according to body weight aiming at a minimum urinary pH of 6.8 (mean dose: 3.7 gm b.i.d. and 5 gm h.s.). Before and on the seventh day of therapy 24 hr urine samples were collected without preservatives, after measurement of pH, it was adjusted to 1.5 by adding concentrated HCl. Oxalate[6], citrate, uric acid were measured enzymatically and calcium, phosphate and magnesium by atomic-spectro-photometry.

RESULTS

In the control group the median citrate concentration was 3.37 mmol/l in males and 3.4 mmol/l in females respectively. In male oxalate stone formers a significantly reduced citrate concentration of 2.28 mmol/l and 1.68 mmol/l in females was observed (Table 1). During therapy with alkaline citrate the median value of citrate concentration was found to be 4.0 mmol/l, which signifies a 100% increase compared to the control value. Citrate excretion increased from 3.54 mmol/24 hr to 7.22 mmol/24 hr. In contrast calcium concentration decreased from 2.94 mmol/l to 1.64 mmol/l and excretion from 4.48 mmol/l to 2.71 mmol/l. This reduced rate amounts to 40% of control values. No significant change during therapy was detected for oxalate, uric acid, phosphate and magnesium (Figure 1).

Table 1. Urinary Citrate

(24 hr sample, mmol/l)

Group	Male	Female
Healthy n = 20	3.37$^+$	3.4
Stone n = 60	2.28	1.68

$^+$Values represent medians

DISCUSSION

Renal clearance of citrate is regulated by acid-base metabolism (Figure 2). It has been experimentally proven that serum bicarbonate is the essential factor influencing renal citrate excretion[7,8].

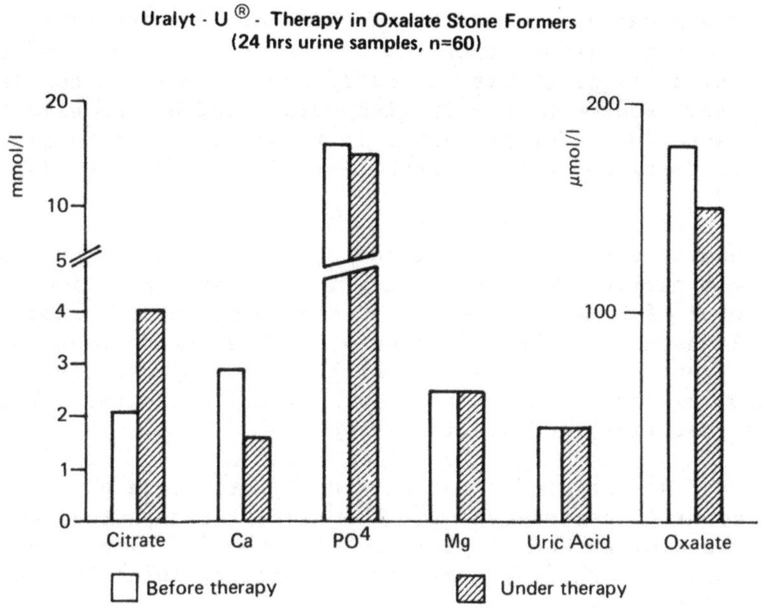

Figure 1

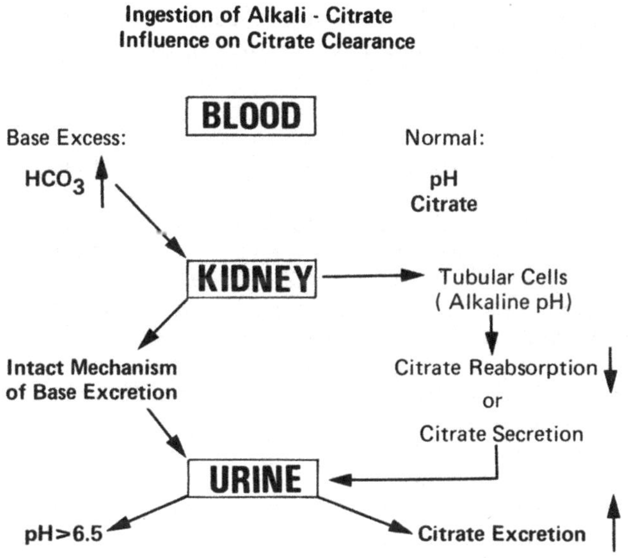

Figure 2

A base excess can be induced by any kind of alkaline salt. In the case of alkaline citrate there is no specific influence of the citrate anion itself on citrate excretion since it is completely metabolized. Furthermore, alkaline urinary pH has no effect on citrate excretion. For instance, in renal tubular acidosis urinary citrate is decreased due to metabolic acidosis despite high alkaline urinary pH.

A reduction in urinary calcium excretion has not been shown to result from citrate therapy. There is experimental evidence that the turnover of bone calcium is reduced in metabolic alkalosis[9]. The simultaneous increase of urinary citrate and decrease of calcium excretion represent conditions, which should improve the solubility of calcium oxalate. The increase of urinary pH to the alkaline range requires justification and discussion:

1. For stable binding of calcium by citrate a pH value at the neutral point is necessary. 2. The risk of phosphate stone formation can be disregarded if patients with the following conditions are excluded from therapy: a) chronic urinary infection, b) presence of a stone.

Phosphate deposition around uric acid stones has been observed only in the case of excessive urinary alkalinization[10]. Alkaline citrate therapy has been applied to patients with uric acid stones without serious side effects for almost two decades. Based upon this experience the indication for alkalinizing therapy can be extended to oxalate stone disease without difficulties. In order to prove the efficacy of this therapy a long term study in stone formers with a high recurrence rate is being performed[11].

REFERENCES

1. B. Kissin, and M. O. Locks, Proc. Soc. Exp. Biol. Med. 46:216 (1941).
2. J. S. Elliot, and B. E. Ribeiro, Invest. Urol. 10:102 (1972).
3. P. O. Schwille, D. Scholz, M. Paulus, W. Engelhardt, and A. Sigel, Invest. Urol. 16:457 (1979).
4. S. G. Welshman, and M. G. McGeown, Br. J. Urol. 48:7 (1976).
5. O. Oestberg, Scand. Arch. Physiol. 62:81 (1931).
6. G. Kohlbecker, and M. Butz, (in press).
7. M. A. Crawford, M. D. Milne, and B. H. Scribner, J. Physiol. 149:413 (1959).
8. D. P. Simpson, Am. J. Physiol. 204:875 (1964).
9. U. S. Barzel, and J. Jowsey, Clin. Sci. 36:517 (1969).
10. P. H. Petritsch, Urol. 10:536 (1977).
11. M. Butz, (in preparation).

MAGNESIUM METABOLISM IN RENAL STONE FORMERS

G. Johansson, U. Backman, B. G. Danielson,
B. Fellström, S. Ljunghall, and B. Wikström
Department of Internal Medicine, University Hospital

S-750 14 Uppsala, Sweden

INTRODUCTION

A possible role for magnesium in the formation of calcium stones was suggested by the investigations of Hammarsten[1], who reported a beneficial effect of magnesium on the solubility of calcium oxalate in vitro. Furthermore, experimentally-induced magnesium depletion in the rat is known to cause calcification in the proximal tubular cells in the kidneys[2].

The present study was undertaken to determine whether or not magnesium deficiency, or a reduced urinary magnesium excretion, was a common feature of recurrent renal calcium stone formers. Since urinary magnesium output is age- and sex-dependent[3], the stone patients were compared with an age- and sex-matched control group.

SUBJECTS

Ambulant patients with renal stone disease were investigated in our out-patient, kidney-stone clinic. Seventy consecutive cases, 52 males and 18 females with mean ages of 45 and 39 years, respectively, were studied. All patients had a diet of their own choice and followed their normal daily activity.

Three patients had prior to admission passed more than 100 stones each, while the remainder had altogether formed about 500 stones during a total of 640 years, i.e. a stone-episode rate of 0.8 stones/year.

Apparently healthy subjects recruited from a general health survey, members of the medical staff and medical students formed a control group. For comparison of the serum and urinary electrolytes, the groups were matched for age and sex. No control subject presented with a history of renal stone disease or had any regular medication.

METHODS

Measurements were made on serum magnesium, intracellular magnesium concentration in muscle specimens, retention of an intravenously administered magnesium load, urinary magnesium excretion and fractional gastrointestinal magnesium absorption with the radionuclide ^{28}Mg[3].

RESULTS AND DISCUSSION

Table 1 summarizes magnesium and calcium data in the renal stone formers and the control group. All values for serum magnesium fell within the normal range. Compared with the controls, stone formers had values within the same range for both the intracellular magnesium content and the magnesium retention of an intravenously given magnesium load. Thus, whichever method was used for assessing the magnesium balance, stone formers did not differ from the control group and it seems unlikely that magnesium deficiency in man is of common, pathogenic importance as regards renal stone formation.

Table 1. Magnesium and Calcium Data in Renal Stone Formers and Controls. When comparing serum and urinary values the groups were matched for sex and age. Mean ± S.D. Figures within brackets denotes numbers of subject studies.

	Stone formers		Controls	
Serum Mg (mmol/l)	0.83 ± 0.06	(70)	0.83 ± 0.05	(70)
Muscle Mg (mmol/100 g FES)[a]	3.8 ± 0.7	(57)	3.7 ± 0.5	(35)
Mg retention (%)	21 ± 13	(60)	20 ± 11	(34)
Urinary Mg (mmol/24 h)				
Males	5.1 ± 1.4[b]	(70)	4.5 ± 1.1	(70)
Females	3.7 ± 1.2	(70)	4.3 ± 1.5	(70)
Urinary Ca (mmol/24 h)	7.2 ± 2.6[c]	(70)	5.2 ± 2.2	(70)
Urinary Mg/Ca	0.7 ± 0.2[c]	(70)	1.1 ± 0.7	(70)
Intestinal Mg absorption (%)	41 ± 6	(26)	42 ± 7	(16)

a) FES = fat free solid weight
b) $p < 0.05$ compared with controls
c) $p < 0.001$ compared with controls

The values for urinary magnesium were normally distributed with a mean of 4.7 ± 1.5 (S.D.) mmol/24 h. Male stone formers had a higher output than age-matched male controls. For all ages, male stone formers had a higher output than female stone-forming patients. The urinary calcium excretion was greater in stone formers than in controls and there was a positive correlation between the magnesium and calcium excretion both in stone formers and controls. The possible role of magnesium in inhibiting calcium crystallization seems to depend on the concentration of magnesium in relation to calcium rather than on the absolute amounts of the two ions in the urine. Therefore, it seemed appropriate to calculate the urinary magnesium/calcium ratio in stone formers, when evaluating these patient's stone-forming propensity. The ratio was found to be low in the stone formers when compared with the controls (Table 1), which is in agreement with results from previous studies[4,5].

The fractional gastrointestinal absorption of magnesium in the stone formers was similar to that found in the controls[6]. The range of 28 to 54% and a mean absorption of the radionuclide of 41 ± 6% agreed closely with values in normal subjects obtained earlier from conventional balance studies[7,8]. As most stone formers have an increased absorption of calcium[9], these results support the view that magnesium and calcium, at least in part, have different mechanisms for intestinal absorption.

In conclusion, magnesium deficiency seems to be uncommon in renal calcium stone formers. The urinary excretion of magnesium in stone patients did not differ from an age- and sex-matched control group, but male stone formers had a higher excretion than female stone-forming patients. However, a low urinary excretion of magnesium in relation to calcium may be of importance for the increased stone-forming propensity.

REFERENCES

1. G. Hammarsten, C. R. Lab. Carlsberg 17:1 (1929).
2. G. E. Bunce and G. A. King, Exp. Mol. Pathol. 28:322 (1978).
3. B. G. Danielson, G. Johansson, and S. Ljunghall, Scand. J. Urol. Nephrol. Suppl. 51:49 (1979).
4. S. Ljunghall and A. U. Waern, Scand. J. Urol. Nephrol. Suppl. 41:55 (1977).
5. H. G. Tiselius, L. E. Almgård, L. Larsson, and B. Sörbo, Eur. Urol. 4:241 (1978).
6. B. G. Danielson, G. Johansson, B. Jung, S. Ljunghall, and H. Lundqvist, Mineral Electrolyte Metab. 2:116 (1979).
7. L. A. Graham, J. J. Caesar, and A. S. V. Burgen, Metabolism 9:646 (1960).
8. P. G. Brannan, P. Vergne-Marini, C. Y. C. Pak, A. R. Hull, and J. S. Fordtran, J. Clin. Invest. 57:1412 (1976).
9. S. Ljunghall, U. Backman, B. G. Danielson, G. Johansson, B. Jung, R. Källsen, L. Wibell, and O. Wålinder, Scand. J. Urol. Nephrol. Suppl. 41:77 (1977).

URATE METABOLISM AND URINARY ACIDIFICATION

B. Fellström, U. Backman, B. G. Danielson,
G. Johansson, S. Ljunghall, and B. Wikström
Department of Internal Medicine
University Hospital
S-750 14 Uppsala, Sweden

Hyperuricemia[1] as well as hyperuricosuria[2], have been claimed to be common features among calcium stone formers. The frequency of hyperuricemia or hyperuricosuria was the same among our stone formers and controls but hyperuricemic or hyperuricosuric stone patients had a more severe stone disease in terms of stone operations[3]. Patients with renal acidification defects had also been operated more often than patients with a normal acidification capacity[4].

Since uric acid is an organic acid with a $pK_a = 5.7$, it could be expected that the urinary excretion of uric acid would be related to the urinary pH. The purpose of this study was to investigate if there is a connection between disturbances in urate metabolism and renal acidification capacity.

SUBJECTS AND METHODS

Serum and urinary urate were determined in 284 calcium stone formers (200 males and 84 females) that were ambulatory on an ambient diet. Hyperuricemia was defined arbitrarily as a serum urate > 300 μmol/l in females and > 400 μmol/l in males. Hyperuricosuria was defined as a urinary urate > 4.5 mmol/24h in males and > 4.0 mmol/24h in females. Hyperuricemic stone patients were compared to normouricemic patients matched for age and sex. Hyperuricosuric patients were compared to normouricosuric patients matched in the same way.

Altogether 215 of these patients (145 males and 70 females) had been investigated with respect to their renal acidification capacity.

Urate in serum and urine was measured with an enzymatic (uricase) method[5]. Renal acidification capacity was studied with a short time ammonium chloride load[6]. Urinary pH as well as titratable acid (TA) and ammonium ion excretion were measured during the ammonium chloride load and related to the systemic acid base status. Frequencies were compared using a chi-square method.

RESULTS

Hyperuricemia was found in 19 patients (16 males and 3 females). Renal acidification defects were diagnosed in 7/15 hyperuricemic patients, 5 with a proximal and 2 with a distal tubular acidification defect. The expected frequency of acidification defects in our stone patients is 20% ($X^2_{df=1} = 5.3$; $p < 0.05$). Among the normouricemic stone formers 3/17 patients had a renal acidification defect.

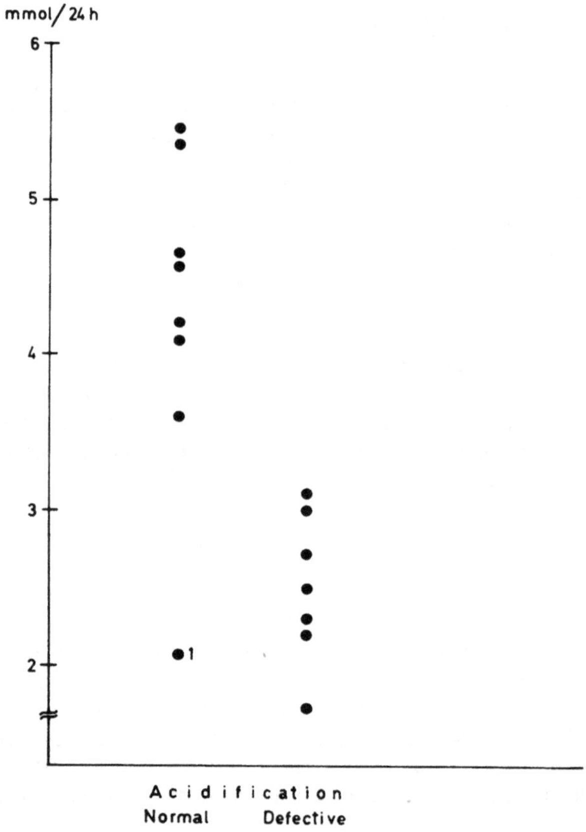

Figure 1. Urinary urate excretion/24 hours in hyperuricemic stone formers with a normal or deficient acidification of the urine. One patient with normal acidification (1) had a slight azotemia with GFR = 48 ml/min.

With one exception, all hyperuricemic stone formers with a normal renal acidification had a higher urate excretion than hyperuricemics with a renal acidification defect. The one exception was a hyperuricemic patient with a slight azotemia (GFR = 48 ml/min) (Figure 1).

When classified according to renal acidification capacity male stone formers with a proximal acidification defect were found to have a higher serum urate than both males with a normal acidification of the urine ($p < 0.05$) and males with a distal tubular acidification defect ($p < 0.05$) (Table 1). The same pattern was found among female stone formers but the differences were not statistically significant.

Table 1. Serum Urate (mol/l), Urinary Urate (mmol/24h) and Renal Clearance of Urate (ml/min) in Calcium Stone Formers Classified According to Renal Acidification Capacity

	Males			Females		
	Acidification			Acidification		
	Normal	Defective		Normal	Defective	
		Prox	Dist		Prox	Dist
n	107	29	9	34	22	14
Serum urate	294±66*	342±68*	270±50	225±53	240±45	225±45
Urinary urate	3.3±1.0	3.2±0.8	3.7±1.5	2.9±1.0	2.7±0.6	3.0±0.9
Urate clearance	8.0±3.0	7.1±2.4†	10.3±3.2	9.7±3.9	8.2±2.6	9.5±3.2

* $p< 0.05$
† $p< 0.02$

Hyperuricosuria was found in 22 patients (19 males and 3 females). The frequency of renal acidification defects in hyperuricosuria and in normouricosuria was 25% which did not differ from the expected frequency in the over all stone forming population. The typical response to an ammonium chloride load in hyperuricosuric stone patients was an "acid" curve, i.e. 11/14 hyperuricosuric patients had a urinary pH and an ammonium excretion in the low normal range and 12/14 had an excretion of titratable acid in the high normal range (comparison at Base Excess = 0).

Urinary excretion and renal clearance of urate related to renal acidification capacity are summarized in Table 1.

DISCUSSION

Since uric acid is an organic acid with $pK_a = 5.7$ it could be expected that alkalinization of the urine would cause an increased dissociation of uric acid and thereby a decreased back diffusion and subsequently an enhanced excretion. This could not be verified in man, neither through alkalinization with sodium bicarbonate or acetazolamide[7]. Gutman and Yü[8] could, however, show that gouty patients with uric acid urolithiasis had a more acid urine and a low ammonium excretion.

In the present study renal acidification defects were more common in hyperuricemia than in normouricemia. There was also a remarkable discrimination according to urate excretion between hyperuricemic patients with a normal or defective renal acidification capacity. This would suggest that the reason for hyperuricemia may be an underexcretion of urate if the renal acidification capacity is inadequate. Whether this is due to a defective secretion or an enhanced reabsorption remains to be investigated.

Hyperuricosuric patients on the other hand revealed a remarkably acid curve in response to ammonium chloride load, with 11/14 patients having a urinary pH and an excretion of ammonium ions in the low normal range. Whether this is due to a shift in glutamine metabolism in favor of urate instead of ammonium remains to be investigated. The role of the diet as a common cause for hyperuricosuria and an acid urine also remains to be explored.

When the patients were classified according to their renal acidification capacity a comparison of serum and urinary urate between the classes only revealed very meager differences.

It is concluded that there was a connection between hyperuricemia and proximal acidification defects, possibly caused by an underexcretion of urate. Hyperuricosuria on the other hand was associated with a more acid urine in combination with a low excretion of ammonium ions and a high excretion of titratable acid compared to a healthy reference group.

REFERENCES

1. M. J. V. Smith, L. D. Hunt, J. S. Cling, and W. H. Boyce, J. Urol. 101:637 (1969).
2. F. L. Coe, and A. G. Kavalach, NEJM 291:1344 (1974).
3. B. Fellström, U. Backman, B. G. Danielson, G. Johansson, S. Ljunghall, and B. Wikström, Scand. J. Urol. Nephrol. Suppl. 54 (1980) (in press).
4. U. Backman, B. G. Danielson, G. Johansson, S. Ljunghall, and B. Wikström, Nephron 25:96 (1980).

5. N. Kagemaya, Clin. Chim. Acta. 31:421 (1971).
6. U. Backman, B. G. Danielson, and M. A. Sohtell, Scand. J. Urol. Nephrol. Suppl. 35:33 (1976).
7. T. H. Steele, M. A. Manuel, and G. Boner, Nephron 14:48 (1975).
8. A. B. Gutman, and T.-F. Yü, J. Clin. Invest. 44:1474 (1965).

URATE METABOLISM IN CALCIUM STONE DISEASE

B. Fellström, U. Backman, B. G. Danielson, G. Johansson,
S. Ljunghall, and B. Wikström
Department of Internal Medicine
University Hospital
S-750 14 Uppsala, Sweden

INTRODUCTION

Urate metabolism has been extensively investigated in calcium stone disease. Some investigators have reported that hyperuricemia was a common feature among stone formers[1]; whereas this could not be reproduced by others[2]. Increasing attention has been focused on the amount of urate in urine in calcium stone formers. Hyperuricosuria has been reported[3] to be more frequent among stone formers than healthy controls and suggested to reflect overconsumption of dietary purines as animal protein[4,5]. Two mechanisms have been proposed to explain the connection between urinary urate and calcium oxalate stone formation. One is the possibility of epitaxial growth of calcium oxalate on uric acid or sodium urate crystals[6]. The other is that urate should act as an anti-inhibitor through complex binding of naturally occurring acid mucopolysaccarides in the urine[7]. The purpose of the present study was to evaluate to what extent disturbances in urate metabolism were present among our stone formers and characterize their clinical picture.

SUBJECTS AND METHODS

The 24 hour urinary excretion and the serum concentration of urate were measured in 284 recurrent stone formers (200 males and 84 females) and compared to 89 healthy controls (54 males and 35 females). Patients and controls were investigated while ambulatory and on a free diet.

Hyperuricemia was defined arbitrarily (> 300 μmol/l in females and > 400 μmol/l in males) and so was hyperuricosuria (> 4.0 mmol/24h in females and > 4.5 mmol/24h in males). Patients with hyperuricemia or hyperuricosuria were compared to normouricemic or normouricosuric patients respectively, matched for age and sex.

Urate in serum and urine was measured with an enzymatic (uricase) method. Lithium carbonate was used as a preservative for the urine collections.

The evaluation of the clinical history was based on stone episode rates and frequency of stone operations. The student's t-test was used to compare laboratory values and the chi-square test for comparison of frequencies.

RESULTS

Serum urate was lower in male stone formers than male controls and lower in female stone formers than in female controls (Table 1). In females serum urate increased with age ($p < 0.05$). The 24 h urinary excretion of urate was lower in male stone formers than in male controls, whereas in females there was no difference. In all but male stone formers there was an inverse relation between urinary urate and age. The overall decrease was 0.2 mmol x $(24h)^{-1}$ x (10 years of age)$^{-1}$. Females excreted 0.4 mmol less urate than males per 24 hours.

Table 1. Serum and Urinary Urate in Stone Formers and Controls (Mean 1 SD)

	Males		Females	
	Stone formers (n=200)	Controls (n=54)	Stone formers (n=84)	Controls (n=35)
Serum urate (µmol/l)	307±74***	347±56	233±73*	262±48
Urinary urate (mmol/24h)	3.2±1.0*	3.5±1.1	2.9±0.9	2.9±0.9

* p< 0.05
*** p< 0.001

The frequency of hyperuricemia in stone patients, as defined above, was 19/284 (16 males and 3 females) which was not different from the controls and the frequency of hyperuricosuria was 22/284 (19 males and 3 females), which did not differ from the controls either.

The number of stone episodes per 100 patient years (pt yrs) was not higher in hyperuricemic stone formers compared to normouricemics. Neither did hyperuricosuric patients have a higher stone episode rate than normouricosurics. On the other hand, hyperuricemic patients had been operated 12.5 times/100 pt yrs compared to 2.7 operations/100 pt yrs in normouricosemic stone formers ($p < 0.001$). Hyperuricosurics had been operated 7.4 times/100 pt yrs compared to 3.6 operations/100 pt yrs in normouricosuric patients ($p < 0.005$) (Table 2).

Table 2. Clinical Characteristics

	Hyper-uricemia	Normo-uricemia	Hyper-uricosuria	Normo-uricosuria
No. patients	19	19	22	22
Patient years	184	148	217	194
No. stone episodes	161	150	159	290
No. operations	23	4	16	7
No. patient operated	8	4	10	4
No. operations/ 100 patient years	12.5***	2.7	7.4**	3.6

** $p < 0.005$
*** $p < 0.001$

DISCUSSION

Urate production is dependent upon both endogenous and exogenous factors. The dietary content of purines seems to have an impact on the urate turnover[4,5] and varies with the amount of animal protein in the diet, which in turn is related to socio-economic factors[5]. Furthermore, when studying urate in serum and urine, sex and age variations must be considered and adequately matched controls used for comparison. Variations in the extrarenal[0] elimination of urate may play a role for the total variation of urate in serum and urine. These factors may explain the diverging results by various investigators of urate in urolithiasis[1-3].

In the present study it could not be confirmed that calcium stone formers have a higher frequency of hyperuricosuria than healthy controls. Even though our limits for hyperuricosuria were at the 67% tolerance limit of the control population only 10% of the male stone formers were hyperuricosuric.

Hyperuricemia or hyperuricosuria seem, however, to be associated to a more severe clinical picture. Patients with either of these urate disturbances had gone through more stone operations than matched patients with normouricemia or normouricosuria respectively. This observation has also been made by Coe[9] regarding hyperuricosuric stone formers. The explanation to this observation remains to be uncovered.

REFERENCES

1. M. J. V. Smith, L. D. Hunt, J. S. Cling, and W. H. Boyce, J. Urol. 101:637 (1969).
2. A. Hodgkinson, Br. J. Urol. 48:1 (1976).
3. F. L. Coe and A. G. Kavalach, New Engl. J. Med. 291:1344 (1974).
4. F. L. Coe, E. Moran, and A. G. Kavalach, J. Chron. Dis. 29:793 (1976).
5. W. G. Robertson, P. J. Heyburn, M. Peacock, F. A. Hanes, and R. Swaminathan, Clin. Sci. 57:285 (1979).
6. F. L. Coe, R. L. Lawton, R. B. Goldstein, and V. Tembe, Proc. Soc. Exp. Biol. Med. 149:926 (1975).
7. W. G. Robertson, in:"Urolithiasis Research," H. Fleisch, W. G. Robertson, L. H. Smith, and W. Vahlensieck, eds., Plenum Press (1976).
8. L. B. Sorensen and D. J. Levinson, Nephron 14:2 (1975).
9. F. L. Coe, Ann. Int. Med. 87:404 (1977).

VIII. STONE MORPHOLOGY AND STRUCTURE

INVESTIGATION WITH POLARIZING MICROSCOPY FOR THE CLASSIFICATION OF URINARY STONES FROM HUMANS AND DOGS

W. Hicking[1], A. Hesse[1], M. Gebhardt[2], and W. Vahlensieck[1]

[1]Harnsteinforschungsstelle der Urologischen Universitats-Klinik, Bonn, Venusberg; [2]Mineralogisch-Petrologisches Institut der Universitat Bonn, Poppelsdorfer Schlob, Bonn

OBJECTS

Routine examination of urinary calculi without disturbing the crystal structure is performed by x-ray diffraction analysis and IR-spectroscopy. For a better understanding about the conditions leading to the formation of various kinds of stones the aggregation of the individual crystals must be studied with a polarizing microscope.

We examined urinary stones from humans and dogs to show similarities as well as differences in the stone forming conditions. With this study of urinary calculi which had formed naturally, we wanted to demonstrate the relevance of animal experiments for a better understanding of the formation of urinary stones in humans.

METHODS

In the present study the composition of 235 urinary calculi from dogs were investigated.

For separate analytical investigations the calculi - selected at random - were divided in half. One half was crushed by a mortar and taken for a quantitative x-ray diffraction analysis. The other half was prepared for polarizing microscopy in thin sections in order to examine crystal phases in the different zones of growth. For the preparation of thin sections the stone was imbedded into ARALDIT (Fa. Ciba-Geigy) after which thin sections of about 40 µm can be made with a saw-microtome (Fa. Leitz, Wetzlar).

Table 1. Results of X-ray Diffraction Analysis of Calculi From Human and Dog

Calculi Substance	Dog Stones %; n = 235	Human Stones %; n = 4000
Whewellite ($CaC_2O_4 \cdot 1\ H_2O$)	0.4	12.8
Weddellite ($CaC_2O_4 \cdot 2\ H_2O$)	-	3.3
Uric acid	0.4	4.2
Uric acid dihydrate	-	0.4
NH_4-/Na-/urates	5.1	0.6
Apatite ($Ca_3(PO_4)_2$)	0.4	3.6
Struvite ($MgNH_4PO_4 \cdot 6\ H_2O$)	36.2	1.6
Brushite ($CaHPO_4 \cdot 2\ H_2O$)	0.4	0.6
Whitlockit	-	0.08
Cystine	39.6	0.9
Whe + Wed	1.3	25.6
Uric acid + u a dihydrate	-	4.5
Apa + Stru	10.2	8.0
Phosphate-mixed-stones	0.9	1.8
Oxalate-phosphate-mixed stones	2.1	24.2
Oxalate + NH_4-/Na-/urates	0.4	0.9
Other mixed stones	0.9	7.1
Cystine + x	1.7	0.05

RESULTS

Table 1 represents the results of x-ray diffraction analysis of urinary calculi from dogs in comparison to human stones. Except for uric acid dihydrate all other stone components, which occur in humans, could also be found in our investigations so far. However, differences were seen in the distribution between humans and dogs.

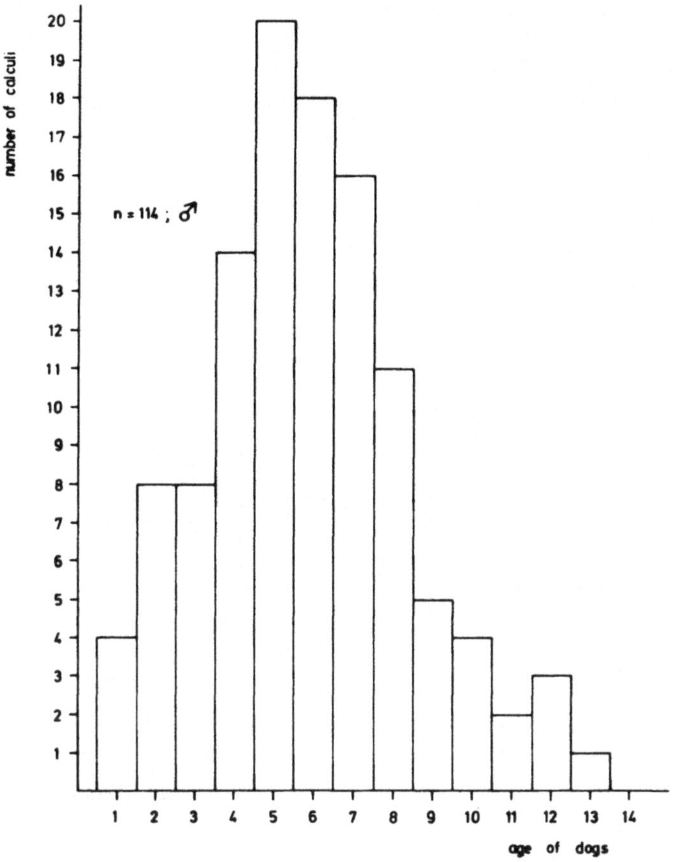

Figure 1a. Distribution of urinary calculi in dog. Investigations with polarizing microscopy for the classification of urinary stones from humans and dogs.

It is striking that more than 77% of the animal stones are composed of one mineral only, while this is found in only 28% of the human stones. The age distribution of the dogs suffering from urolithiasis and the number of stones having been examined so far are shown in Figures 1 a and b. The maximum is found at the age of 5.

In humans the two Ca-oxalate hydrates and the phosphate-oxalate mixed stones represent the most frequent types (66%).

In dogs, however, mostly struvite stones (36.2%) and cystine stones (39.6%) are found. Interestingly cystine stones are found in male dogs only, and here predominantly in Dachs-hunds.

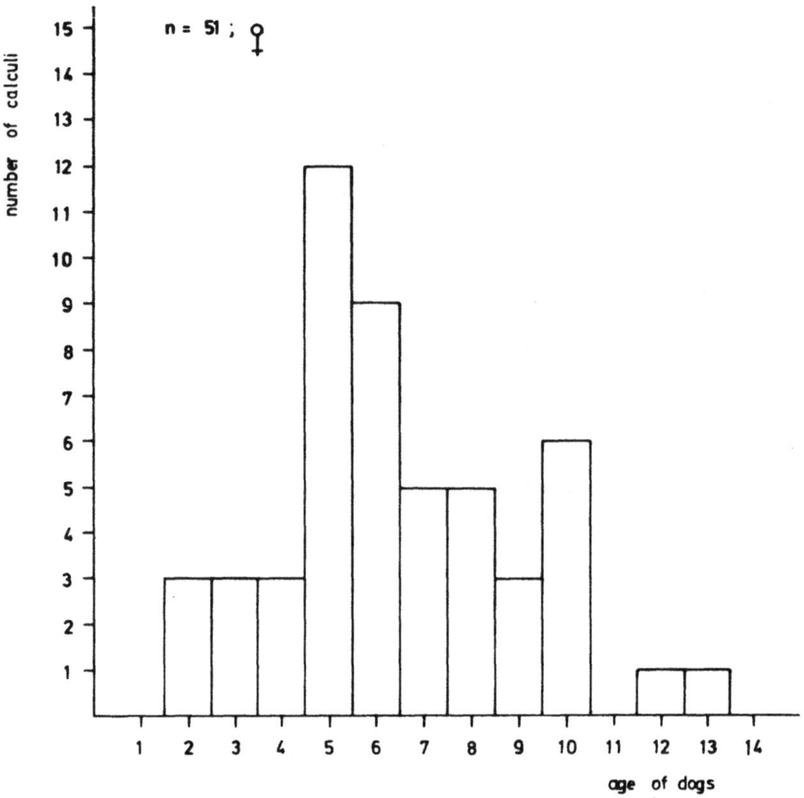

Figure 1b. Distribution of urinary calculi in dog. Investigations with polarizing microscopy for the classification of urinary stones from humans and dogs.

The age distribution of dogs suffering from cystine stones show a maximum between the age of 4 and 7 years (Fig. 2). This also can be applied to struvite stones (Fig. 3). However, the ratio of male to female is in the latter type of stones changed in disfavour of the females (♂/♀ = 0.55:1).

The stones, listed in Table 1, which are composed of uric acid and urate respectively, we found in Dalmatian dogs and Dachs-hunds. While all other mammals excrete allantoin, Dalmation dogs instead excrete uric acid as do humans and primates.

The elevated excretions of cystine in dogs is caused by a metabolic abnormality, which is found in human urolithiasis in only 1-2%. The frequent occurrence of these stones in dogs might be connected with the breeding conditions. The presumption, however, gives no explanation as to the predominant existence in male animals. By examining thin sections with a polarizing microscope no differences between cystine stones of dogs and humans can be seen. Their crystals are often monocentric and show a radiate structure and are enlarged occasionally in dogs.

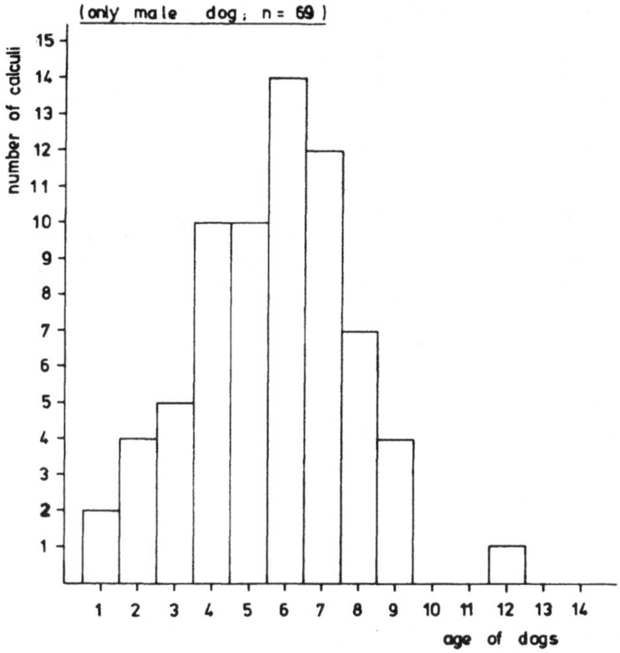

Figure 2. Distribution of cystine stones in dogs (only male dogs). Investigations with polarizing microscopy for the classification of urinary stones from humans and dogs.

Struvite stones, which are caused by infections only, are found in dogs in 36.2%. With the polarizing microscopic analysis no difference to human stones can be observed.

Struvite stones in dogs, which are usually composed of one mineral only, often contain very large and well developed single crystals besides fine crystalline struvite material. Idiopathic metabolic abnormalities leading to Ca-oxalate stone formation in humans are found very rarely in dogs. Optical investigations of Ca-oxalate stones with polarized light show no differences from human stones. As often found in human stones, the oxalate stones of dogs were polycentrically built. While in humans only 10.6% of the males and 3.5% of the females suffer from vesicle calculi, in dogs stones are most commonly removed from the bladder or urethra.

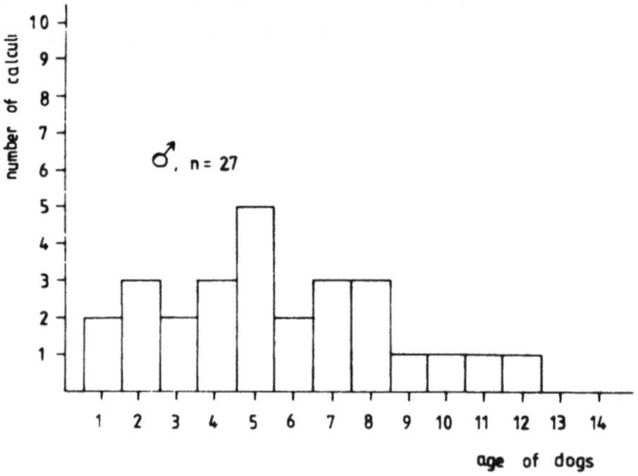

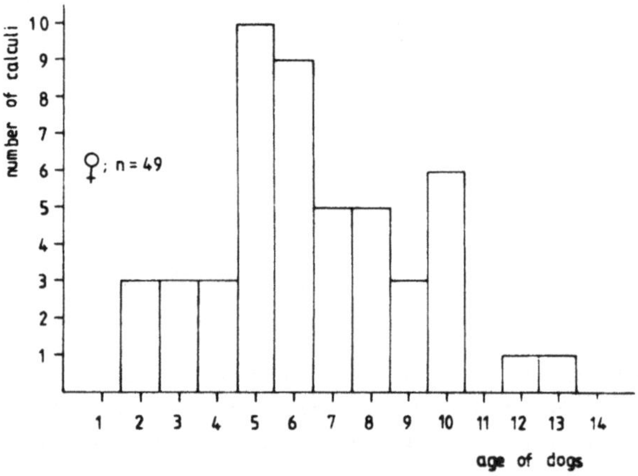

Figure 3. Distribution of struvite stones in dogs. Investigations with polarizing microscopy for the classification of urinary stones from humans and dogs.

Investigations of thin sections of urinary stones from humans and dogs do not suggest any typical differences in the crystalline structure. In dogs urinary calculi are largely monocentric and composed of one mineral only. They often show a very well developed crystal habit inferring slow growth. In human stones, however, frequently different nucleation centers are found. Whenever an infection is involved, these stones grow rapidly in the kidney and smaller crystals are developing.

STATISTICAL RESULTS OF THE ANALYSIS OF MORE THAN 7,500 URINARY CALCULI

M. A. H. Gebhardt and H.-P. Bastian

Mineralogisch-Petrologisches Institut and Museum,

5300 Bonn, West Germany

Over 7,500 analyses of urinary calculi were made with various x-ray diffraction techniques[1-4]. For very small specimens the "Gandolfi" chamber was used. A little bit larger stones were examinated with the Debye-Scherrer-method. Normally diffractometer methods with monochromators were used. The results were grouped in intervals of 5% in weight, if only a trace of a phase could be found, it was set to 0%. Over 7,500 stone analyses were processed statistically into tables of the following: 1) frequency of occurrence, 2) average stone, 3) average quantity, and 4) stone types. The following source descriptions for each stone were also recorded: 1) sex, 2) localization in kidney, ureter or bladder, 3) profession of the stone former, 4) age group of the stone former, and 5) housing region of the stone former. Some results are shown in the following tables without comment.

DEFINITIONS

Frequency of occurrence - the percentage of stones in which the special crystal phase (type) could be detected, regardless of whether present as a main component or as a trace component.

Average quantity = the average amount of the special crystal phase in such stones in which the phase was detected. This value shows whether the phase is in general the main or minor component.

Average stone = the sum of average amounts of all phases related to all stones. It is the expected result of an analysis of a mixture of all stones, if they were equal large.

Table 2. Crystal Type Composition (%) of an Average Stone by Location in Urinary Tract

Type	Abbreviation	Female Kidney	Female Ureter	Female Bladder	Male Kidney	Male Ureter	Male Bladder
Whewellite	WHE	31.90	47.25	20.22	39.73	51.39	20.03
Weddellite	WED	17.28	18.58	11.27	25.98	21.86	8.70
Apatite	APA	26.25	15.86	26.41	13.42	8.86	15.09
Struvite	STR	14.61	4.67	19.89	6.60	1.10	15.75
Uric Acid	UA	3.98	8.37	14.03	8.47	11.35	31.27
Uric Acid Dihydrate	UAD	1.17	2.36	2.00	2.04	3.80	4.65
Ammonium Acid Urate	AMU	0.69	0.42	1.11	0.44	0.20	0.30
Socium Acid Urate	NAU	0.21	0.24	0.03	0.16	0.13	0.30
Brushite	BRU	1.29	1.02	3.27	1.31	0.78	3.52
Octa Calcium Phosphate	OCP	0.10	0.07	-	0.07	0.03	0.12
Whitlockite	WHI	0.63	0.48	0.16	0.46	0.17	0.16
Newberyite	NEW	0.26	-	-	-	-	-
Bobierrite	BOB	-	-	-	-	-	-
L-Cystine	CYS	1.64	0.67	1.62	1.32	0.32	0.12

Table 1. Frequency of Stones with "N" Components (%)

N	Total	Kidney Female	Kidney Male	Ureter Female	Ureter Male	Bladder Female	Bladder Male
1	23.33	18.10	16.87	28.54	27.22	22.70	26.44
2	50.70	53.22	53.80	50.31	48.80	62.70	57.07
3	23.57	26.49	27.56	20.15	22.85	14.05	15.18
4	2.23	1.94	1.65	0.85	1.06	0.54	1.31
5	0.18	0.24	0.11	0.15	0.07	-	-

Table 3. Synopsis by Single Crystal Type

Type	Frequency of Occurrence (%)[a] Female	Male	Total	Average Quantity (%) Female	Male	Total	Composition (%) of Average Stone Female	Male	Total
WHE	62.33	70.08	67.02	62.48	64.58	63.75	38.94	45.26	42.73
WED	43.14	49.55	47.00	41.69	44.22	43.31	17.98	21.91	20.35
APA	50.44	36.72	41.72	39.96	28.62	33.75	20.16	10.51	14.08
STR	15.55	6.21	9.86	61.45	65.28	63.70	9.56	4.06	6.26
UA	14.16	22.11	19.36	50.48	55.34	53.77	7.15	12.23	10.41
UAD	5.43	9.33	7.88	35.03	36.15	35.91	1.90	3.37	2.83
AMU	3.85	3.83	3.84	16.63	9.38	11.85	0.64	0.36	0.46
NAU	3.60	3.87	3.74	8.47	8.09	8.19	0.30	0.31	0.31
BRU	2.31	1.86	2.03	65.08	61.36	63.14	1.50	1.14	1.28
WHI	1.43	0.81	1.14	32.95	29.38	29.94	0.47	0.24	0.34
OPC	0.66	0.51	0.55	15.28	13.20	14.07	0.10	0.07	0.08
NEW	0.37	-	0.26	28.50	-	21.25	0.10	-	0.05
BOB	0.04	-	0.01	10.00	-	10.00	-	-	-
CYS	1.21	0.55	0.84	97.42	97.22	97.58	1.18	0.53	0.82

REFERENCES

1. M. Gebhardt and H. P. Bastian, Fortschr. Urol. u. Nephrol. 9:296 (1977).
2. M. A. H. Gebhardt, H. P. Bastian, and W. Vahlensieck, Fortschr. Urol. u. Nephrol. 14:315 (1979).
3. K.-F. Seifert and M. Gebhardt, Fortschr. Urol. u. Nephrol. 14:275 (1979).
4. M. Gebhardt, in:"Epidemiologie Allgemeine Kausal - und Formalgenese Diagnostik, Urolithiasis I," Springer-Verlag, Berlin, Heidelberg, New York (1979).

"MILK OF CALCIUM": MORPHOLOGY, STRUCTURE AND MINERALOGICAL COMPOSITION

R. Diaz Gonzalez, H. Carvajal, O. Leiva,
P. Paniagua, and V. Borobia
Urology Service, C.S. "1ºde Octubre"

Madrid, Spain

The term "milk of calcium" has been borrowed from a somewhat similar condition encountered in the gallbladder. In most cases the condition is asymptomatic and is found only accidentally. In the plain film taken with the patient supine, the appearance suggests an ordinary round or oval solid calculus. However, with the patient upright or sitting, the calcific material gravitates to the bottom of the cyst resulting in the characteristic "half-moon" contour (Figure 1). It was first described by Fresnais[1] in 1937. Since then a number of cases (around 30) have been described in the world literature. Most of them showed the milk of calcium either in a calyceal diverticulum or in a pyelogenic cyst[2,3], but in several cases it was in hydronephrotic kidneys[1,4,5]. "Milk of calcium" is made of fine sand-like concretions[4,5,6] of calcium carbonate[2,3], hydroxyapatite[4], calcium oxalate[7] or magnesium ammonium phosphate[5].

MATERIAL AND METHODS

The structure, morphology and mineralogical composition of three cases of "milk of calcium," are presented. Two of these were located in pyelogenic cysts and in one caliectasis due to an obstructive lithiasis of calyceal neck. Surgical operation was the source in all cases for examination of fresh material followed by suction of cyst and calyceal contents. The aspirates were a yellowish suspension containing a large amount of macroscopic grains. Some of these grains had an approximate diameter of one millimeter. The following techniques were utilized for all of three cases: 1) X-ray diffraction (Debye-Scherrer method), 2) Infrared rays absorption spectroscopy (KBr discs 0.5%), 3) Thin sheet (30 μ), prepared prior inbedded in araldite, 4) Scanning with electronic microscope Philips SEM 500, 5) EDAX (energy dispersive analysis of x-ray).

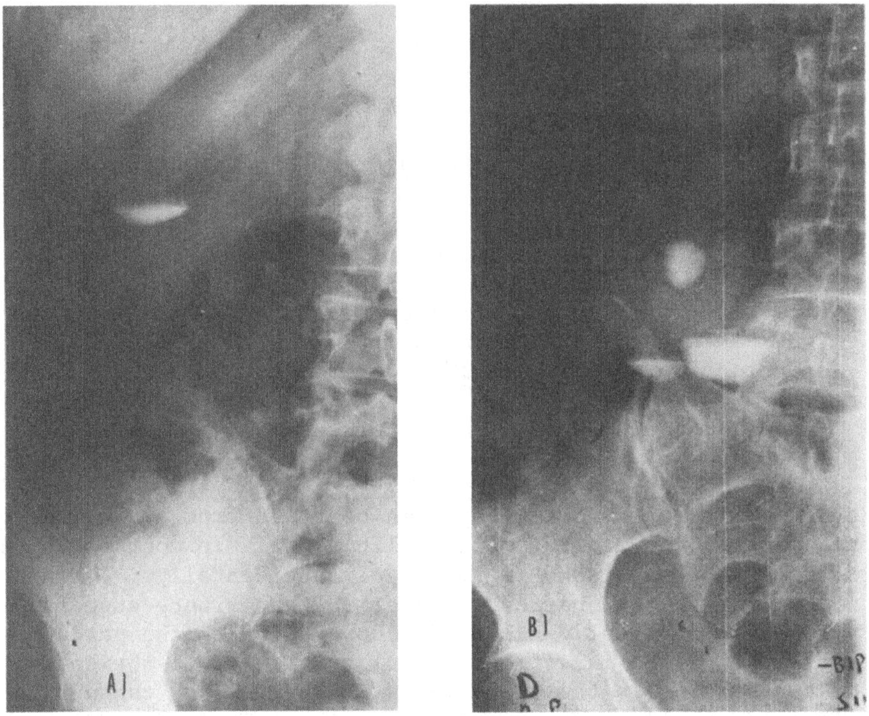

Figure 1. "Milk of calcium". A and B, upright film. Calcium material has "layered out" resulting in typical "half-moon" shape.

RESULTS

Granulated samples from the three cases were found by x-ray diffraction to be carbonate apatite. This was verified with infrared absorption spectroscopy which also showed the traces of calcium oxalate monohydrate (whewellite), in the grains of the "milk of calcium" from the ectatic calyx. Thin sheet observation on granulated concretions with the aid of optic microscope with polarized light using magnifications of 50 X and 100 X, shows that the grains are constructed with a nucleus and a series of concentric layers in the manner of an onion, giving rise to optical anisotroy (Figure 2). When the nucleus is observed with higher magnification (400 x), we found that it was formed, in two of the cases, by microspherulites, which structure remains that of the complete concretion, agglomerated by means of a non-crystalline material. In the third case the nucleus was made of microcrystals also agglomerated by an amorphous substance. The structural morphology observed in thin sheet was revealed in greater detail with a scanning electron microscope which showed microspherulites and microcrystals of the nuclei surrounded with concentric laminations (Figure 3, 4, and 5). Examining the nuclei with EDAX these nuclei indicated the presence of carbonate apatite and calcium oxalate.

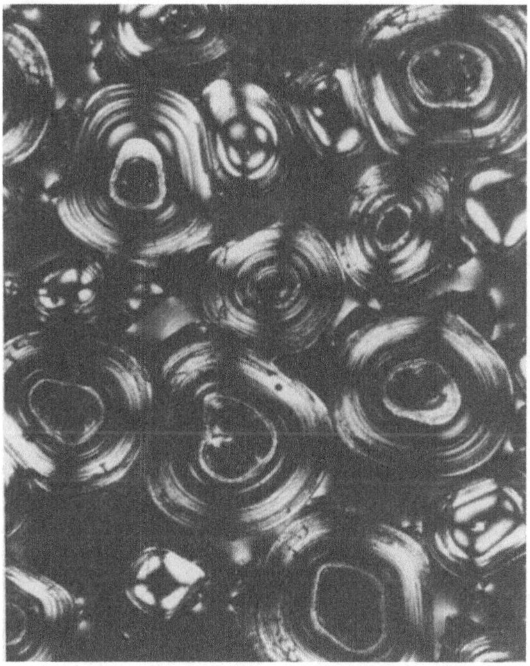

Figure 2. Thin sheet: Observation of granulated concretions with the optic microscope with polarized light (100 X). Nucleus with a series of concentrical layers superimposed, that possess optical anisotropy.

CONCLUSIONS

"Milk of calcium" material in our 3 cases was formed by a suspension of granulated concretions, some of them reaching an approximate diameter of one millimeter. Their structural morphology is a nucleated formation with peripheral concentrical layers, like onion skin. X-ray diffraction, infrared absorption spectroscopy, and EDAX show that the mineral composition of the granulated concretions is carbonate apatite in the three cases and some calcium oxalate monohydrate (whewellite) detected in one case was located in the nucleus of the concretions.

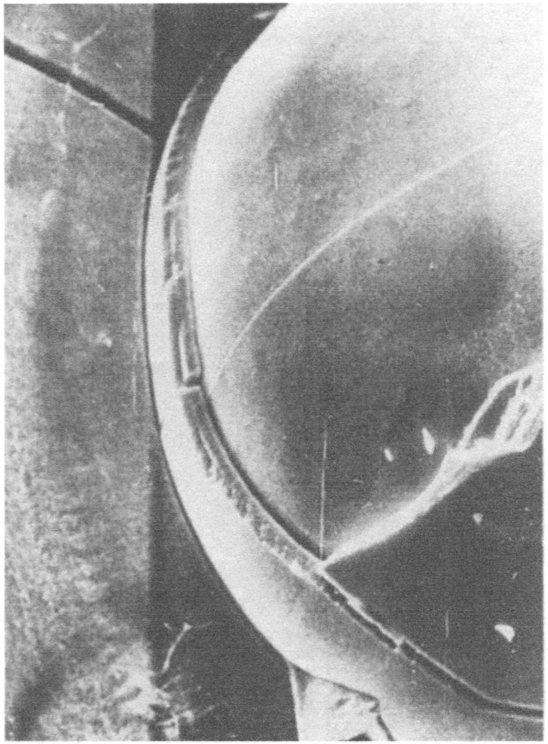

Figure 3. Scanning electron microscopy. Granular concretion with their peripheral concentrical laminations (150 X).

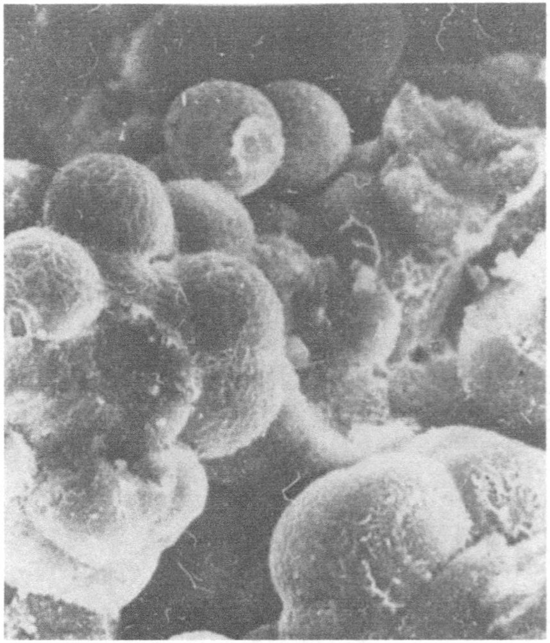

Figure 4. Scanning electrom microscopy. Microspherulites of the nuclei from pyelogenic cyst cases (5000 X).

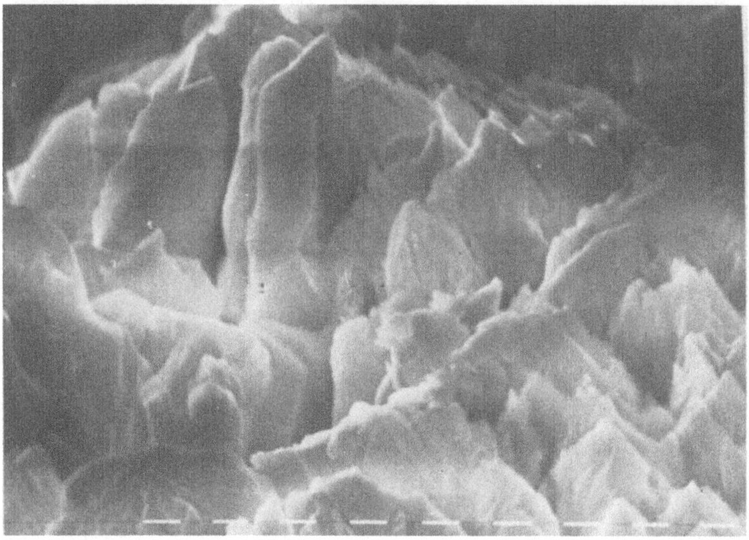

Figure 5. Scanning electron microscopy. Crystals of the nuclei from the caliectasis case (5000 X).

REFERENCES

1. J. Fresnais, Bul. de la Soc. Franc. D'Urologie :231 (1937).
2. B. Benendo and A. Litwak, Br. J. Radiol. 37:70 (1964).
3. M. A. Rosenberg, Am. J. Roentgenol. 101:714 (1967).
4. E. Somacarrera and J. Alonso, in:"Problemas Actuales de Urologia," L. Cifuentes Delatte, C. Alferez, E. Garcia de la Pena, and R. Vela Navarrete, ed., Salvat, Barcelona (1977).
5. Z. M. Mohamed, F. Cano, E. Blanco, and L. Resel, Actas de la Asociacion Esp. de Urol. :73 (1977).
6. L. Iozzi, M. Blocklyn, and F. Rosenberg, J. Urol. 93:556 (1965).
7. G. Piazza, Minerva Urologica 27:158 (1975).

OOLITIC STRUCTURE OF MILK OF CALCIUM SAND

AND MILK OF CALCIUM STONES

L. Cifuentes Delatte and J. A. Medina

Urolithiasis Laboratory, Fundación, Jiménez Díaz.
Department of Geochemistry, Universidad Atónoma,
Madrid, Spain

Renal milk of calcium was believed to be an x-ray opaque fluid[1,2,3] by their horizontal levels in some hydronephrosis, but was recognized as being mainly composed of a fine sand[4] of ovoid or irregularly spheroidal shaped granules about 1/2 to 1 mm in diameter.

Further studies on the structure of these granules point out their striking similarity to the oolites that can be found in sedimentary rocks. Furthermore, some small renal stones are found to be clusters of milk of calcium granules embedded in a continuous multilayered calcium phosphate material.

Intact and fractured granules and stones were examined with a scanning electron microscope, Philips SEM 500, and their composition was investigated with EDAX.

The individual granules of renal milk of calcium are spheroidal or elongated ellipsoidal structures with a central core and many concentrically superimposed thin layers. They were composed of apatitic calcium phosphate but the central part contained, in one of our cases, calcium oxalate. The concentrical layers were always composed by calcium phosphate. (Figure 1).

The similarity between renal milk of calcium granules and oolites of sedimentary rocks is astonishing. Guillén Cavero, in Spain[5] found oolitic elements in some kidneys, but not so typical as these that are discussed here. Oolites are described as small spherical or oblate elliptical accretionary bodies, 0.25 to 2.00 mm in diameter most commonly 0.5 to 1.00 mm[6]. An oolite is composed of an organic or mineral nucleus surrounded by at least two concentric layers that are of calcite or aragonite in the sedimentary rocks.

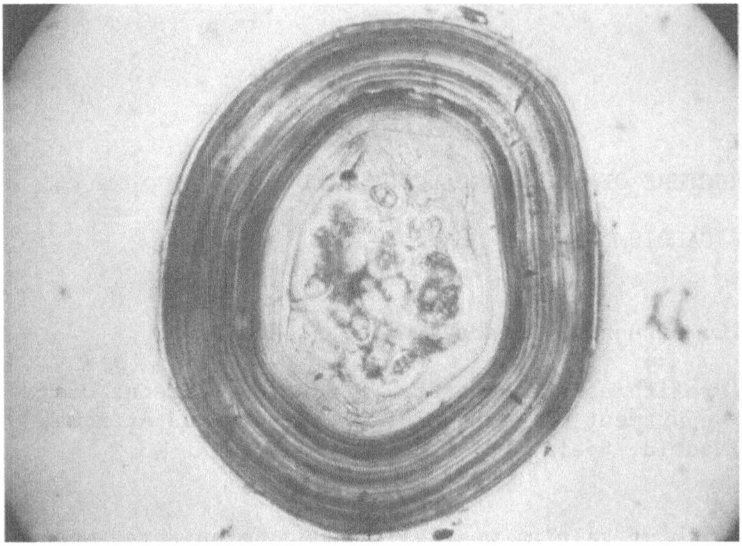

Figure 1. Milk of calcium granule with multilayered envelope.

The nuclei of oolites, can be very different, organic bodies of all sorts, broken oolites, rock fragments, quartz crystals, and structurless carbonate grains. Accretion in a turbulent medium causes thin concentric layers to develop around the nucleus. This is known as oolitization. Oolites show a coating of concentric layers but they are also not coated grains. In the envelope one can find a superposition of extremely thin individual layers, corresponding to successive phases of accretion separated by phases of interruption of the oolitization process[7]. Under crossed nicols, the oolites, like the renal milk of calcium granules, give a hazy black cross limited to the envelope.

Such a description is also applied to the elementary granules of the urinary milk of calcium sand. They show very different kinds of nuclei, sometimes with still smaller calcium phosphate granules or with calcium oxalate crystals. Around the core the oolitization process develops concentric, seemingly amorphous, thin layers. Pictures of oolites and renal granules of milk of calcium are similar each to another (Figures 2 and 3).

In our routine examination of thin sections of urinary calculi we found a small number of them essentially composed by a clustering of milk of calcium granules, cemented together and surrounded by a common envelope, building a small composite milk of calcium or

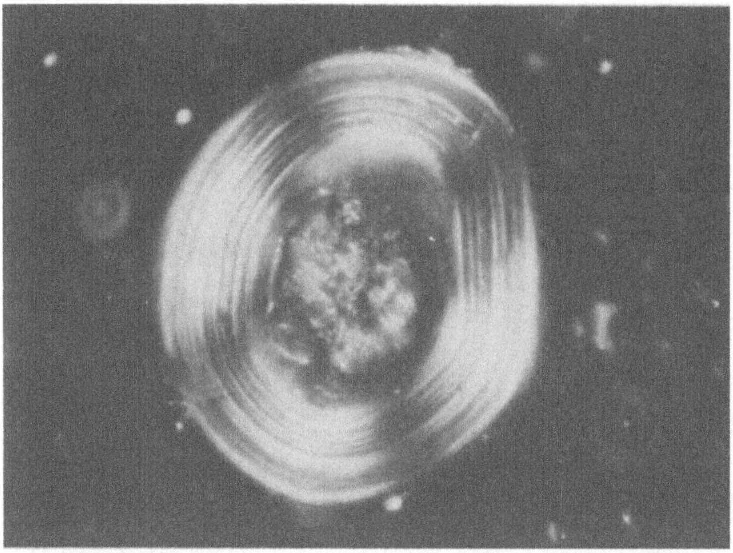

Figure 2. Milk of calcium granules give a black cross under the polarizing microscope like oolites.

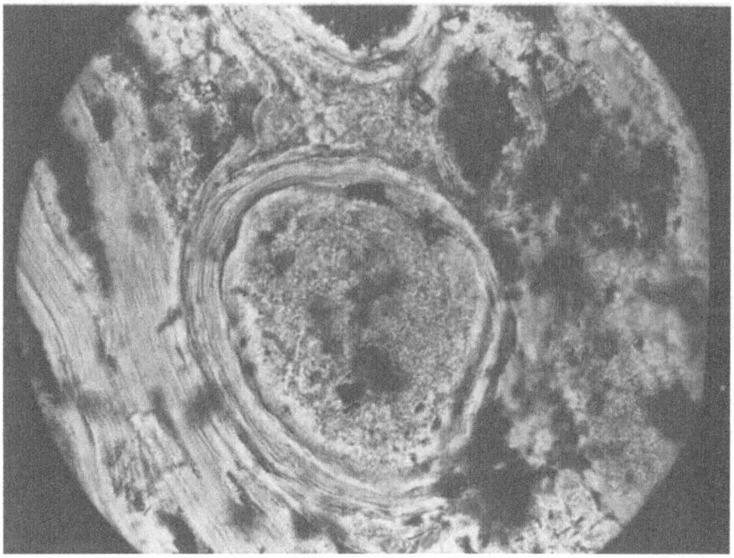

Figure 3. Oolitic granule in a kidney stone.

oolitic renal stone. This calculous structure can be easily suspected by the granular aspect of its surface (Figure 4).

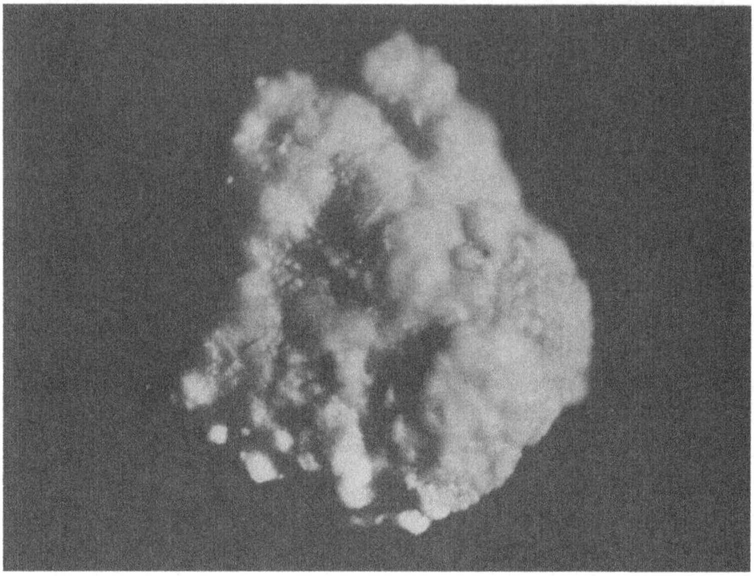

Figure 4. External surface of a milk of calcium stone (granular appearance).

In the sedimentary rocks several theories had been proposed to explain the formation of oolites but many agree in that they seem to be the product of direct precipitation of dissolved materials on nuclei in a "free rolling" environment. Oolites are believed to originate as precipitation products in a shallow turbulent environment. It is interesting to note that milk of calcium is usually found in the cavities of hydronephrosis where minute solid bodies can roll in every direction thanks to the motions of the body. Oolitic calculi were grown in our cases in the small cavities of sponge kidneys.

The similarity of oolitic structures occurring in such different environments as pathological human kidneys and sedimentary rocks is worthy of note.

REFERENCES

1. R. Garrett and J. Holland, J. Urol. 109:927 (1973).
2. R. M. Pomerantz, L. P. Kirschner, and H. L. Twigg, J. Urol. 103:18 (1970).

3. W. H. Walker, R. E. Pearson, and N. R. Johnson, J. Urol. 84:517 (1960).
4. E. Somacarrera and J. Alonso, in:"Problemas Actuales de Urología," L. Cifuentes Delatte, C. Alferez, E. García de la Peña, and R. Vela Navarrete, ed., Salvat, Barcelona (1977).
5. G. Cavero, Arch. Esp. Urol. 25:135 (1972).
6. F. J. Pettijohn, in:"Sedimentary Rocks," Harper-Row, New York (1975).
7. A. V. Carrozzi, in:"Microscopic Sedimentary Petrology," J. Wiley & Sons, New York-London (1960).

SILICA IN URINARY CALCULI

J. A. Medina, J. R. Sanchidrian, and L. Cifuentes Delatte

Department of Geochemistry, Universidad Autónoma,
Urolithiasis Laboratory , Fundación Jiménez Díaz,
Madrid, Spain

Silica appears in urinary calculi in two forms, opaline and quartz-like silica. The first one, as opaline silica, is an arrangement of small microscopical spheres whose packing shows a not so regularly ordered array as can be found in opals, formed of silica spherulites. There is also a silica deposition on organic fibers present in the calculi. There are until now only eleven observations of these kinds of silica calculi since the first description by Hammarsten et al (1953) in a man who was taking silicates because of a gastric ulcer[1]. The eleventh observation was published in Spain by Medina et al in 1978[2] (Figures 1-2). We have another unpublished one.

The second form of silica is surely the more frequent, although not yet too well known. Zinsser et al stated in 1961[3] somewhat surprisingly, that up to 6% calcium silicate was found in some of these stones by x-ray diffraction, neutron activation and emission spectrography.

We have studied with a Scanning Electron Microscope Philips SEM 500 ten renal calculi all containing struvite and apatite and some of them also ammonium urate. In 4 of these stones we found several broken concoid quartz-like crystals giving an EDAX (Energy dispersive analysis of x-ray) spectrum of silicon that was absent in the other types of crystals in the same stones. This finding was confirmed with other methods like Line Scan Ratemeter and Element Mapping. No other component but Si was detected on the focused point analyzed by EDAX in the crystals so we do not think that they are composed of Ca, Mg, Al silicates but of silicon dioxide or some combination between silicon and ammonium

(Figures 3, 4, 5, 6). We have found also this type of silica crystals in a renal stone mainly composed of uric acid.

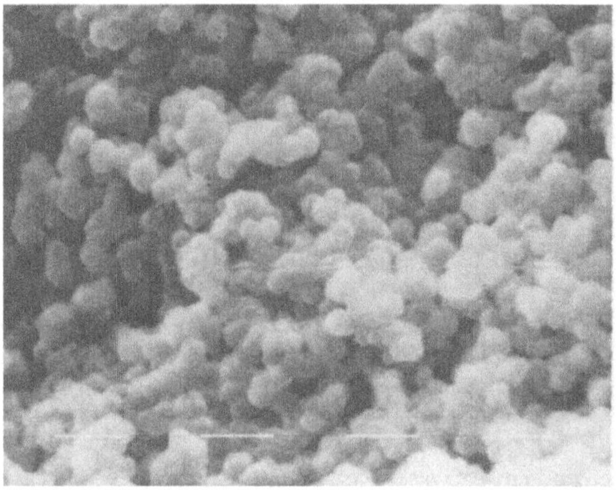

Figure 1. Spherulites of silica in a stone.

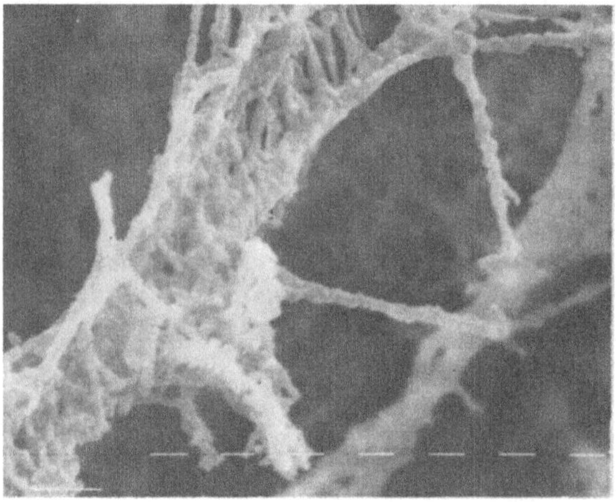

Figure 2. Deposition of silica on organic fibers.

The occurrence of such silica crystals is common in certain areas of the calculi. We have performed determinations of Si. content in 17 struvite stones by atomic absorption spectrometry. Our figures can be seen in Table 1. For silicum the highest concentration was 2166 p.p.m. (0.216%) and for SiO_2 4633 p.p.m. (0.463%).

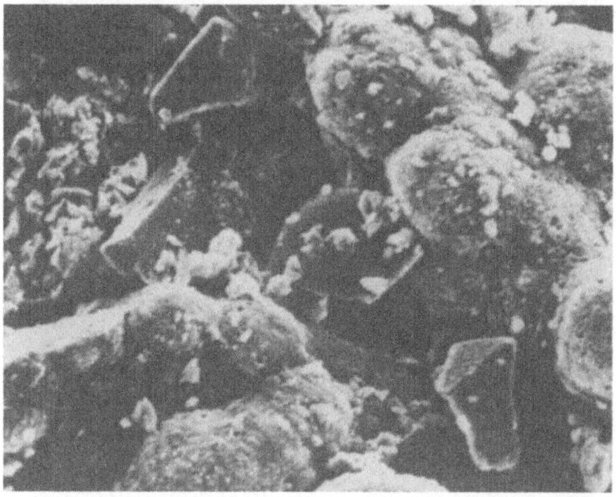

Figure 3. Broken crystals of silica in a struvite stone.

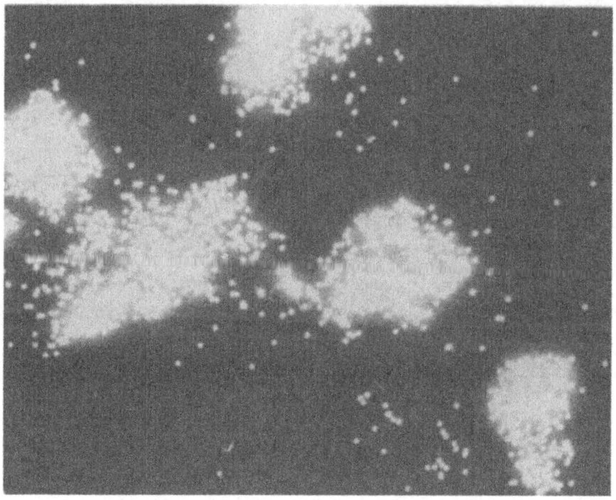

Figure 4. Si element mapping of the same field.

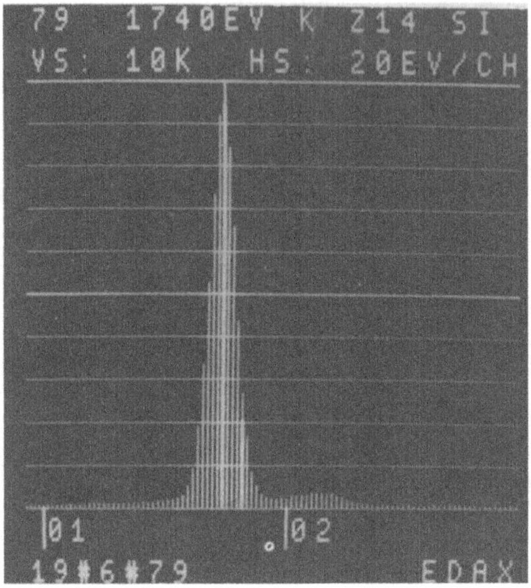

Figure 5. EDAX spectrum (Si) of a silica crystal.

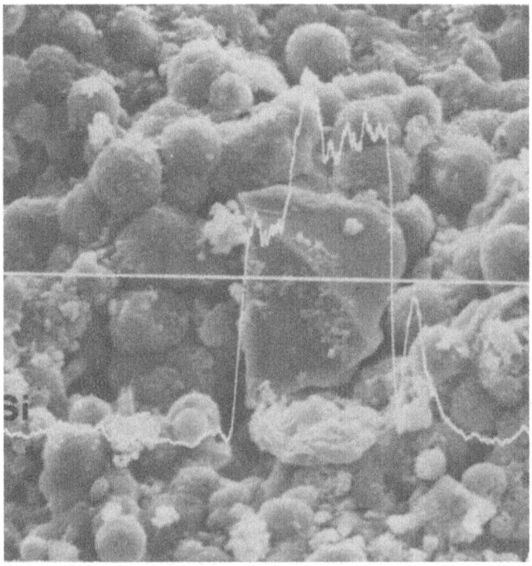

Figure 6. Line scan ratemeter of a silica crystal with apatite spherulites all around.

Table 1.

SILICIUM CONTENT

NUMBER OF THE STONE	SILICIUM (P.P.M.)	SILICA SiO_2
363	169	361
525	123	263
1131	33	70
1139	50	107
2462	159	340
2529	322	689
2532	< 15	< 30
2537	< 15	< 30
2540	101	216
2547 A	< 15	< 30
2618	< 15	< 30
2767	823	1760
2797	1785	3818
2819	38	81
3020	2166	4633
3080	35	53
3130	< 15	< 30

SILICIUM CONTENT OF 17 STONES, ANALYZED BY ATOMIC ABSORPTION SPECTROMETRY, CALCULUS - 3020 HAD THE GREATEST CONCENTRATION OF SILICA (0.46% = 4633 P.P.M.).

REFERENCES

1. G. Hammarsten, I. Helldorff, W. Magnusson, and T. Rilton, Svenska Lak. Tidn. 50:1242 (1953).
2. J. A. Medina, J. Rodriguez, M. Santos, and L. Cifuentes Delatte, Rev. Clin. Esp. 151:411 (1978).
3. H. H. Zinsser, H. Seneca, T. Light, G. Mayer, F. Karp, G. McGeoy, and H. Tarrasoli, N. York J. Med. 58:3001 (1968).

NEWBERYTE IN OLD RENAL AND BLADDER CALCULI

M. Miñón Cifuentes and M. Santos

Department of Urology and Laboratory of Urolithiasis,
Fundación Jiménez Díaz, Universidad Autónoma,
Madrid, Spain

Newberyte or magnesium hydrogen orthophosphate trihydrate $Mg.HPO_4.3H_2O$, is a natural mineral. It was first identified as a new species of Skipton Caves, Victoria, Australia, where it is present as large crystals in bat guano. Other well-known deposits also associated with guano are found in Mejillones, Chile, Ascension Island and the Tunnel du Comeran in Reunion[1].

MATERIAL AND METHODS

A study is made of a total of 542 human urinary calculi (298 renal calculi and 244 bladder calculi) which belonged to the collection which Dr. P. Cifuentes Diaz had compiled between 1913 and 1950. The study was carried out on thin sections observed under the conventional phase and polarising microscopes. Complementary analyses were also performed on selected samples in pressed KBr discs by infrared spectroscopy[1] using a Perkin-Elmer spectrophotometer, model 457. For scanning microscopy studies, a Jeal JSM-SOH instrument was available.

RESULTS

From these 542 old urinary calculi 126 were septic calculi developed in alkaline infected urine by bacteria which form the enzyme urease which splits urea, and 78 were calculi with secondary infection. In both groups there was struvite (Figure 1) which was the major component in most of the cases.

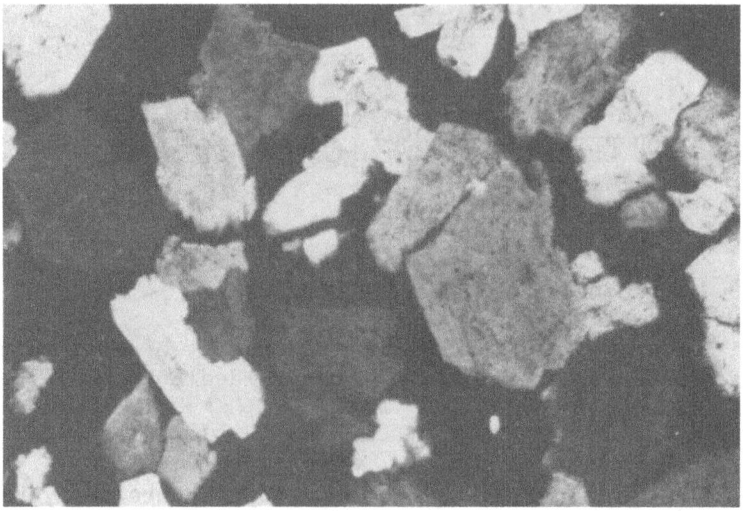

Figure 1. Laminae crystals of magnesium ammonium phosphate (struvite).

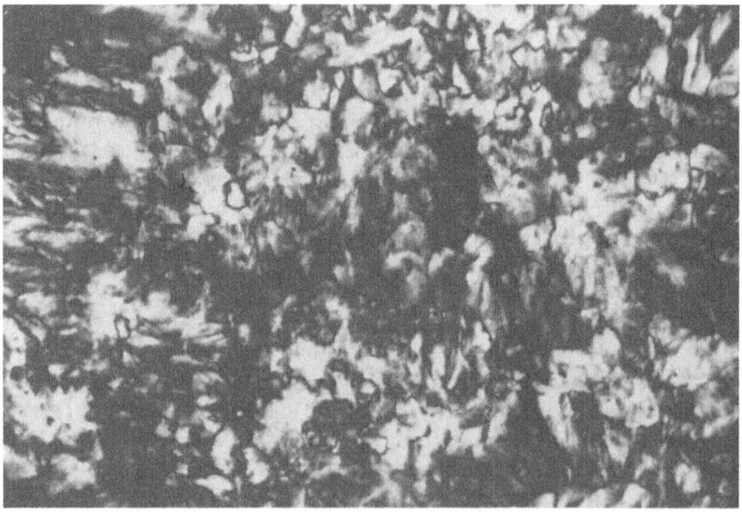

Figure 2. Small irregular crystals of magnesium hydrogen orthophosphate (Newberyte).

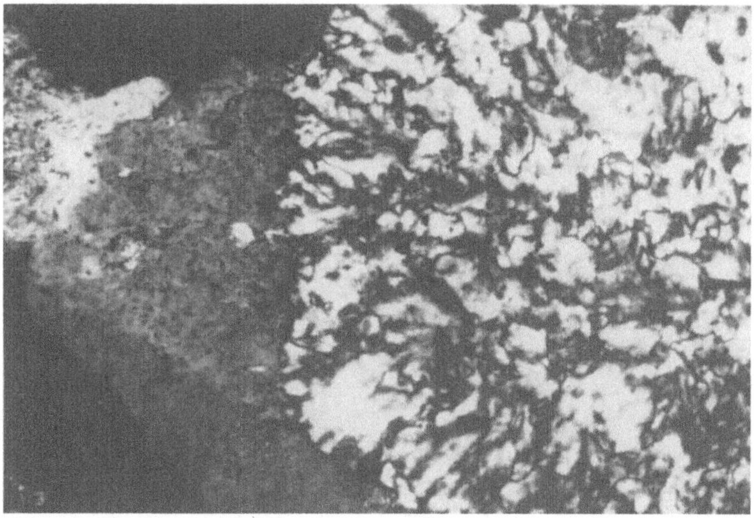

Figure 3. Newberyte associated with struvite in the peripheral portion of calculi.

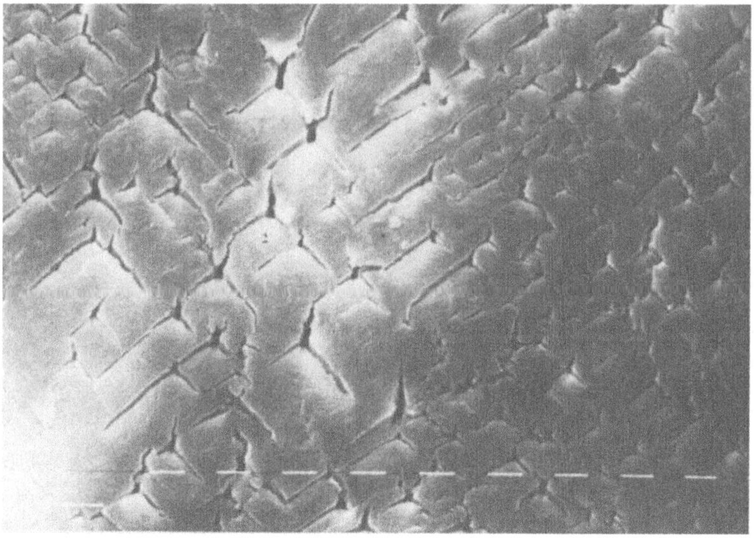

Figure 4. Small crystals observed with the scanning microscope that in our opinion can be newberyte.

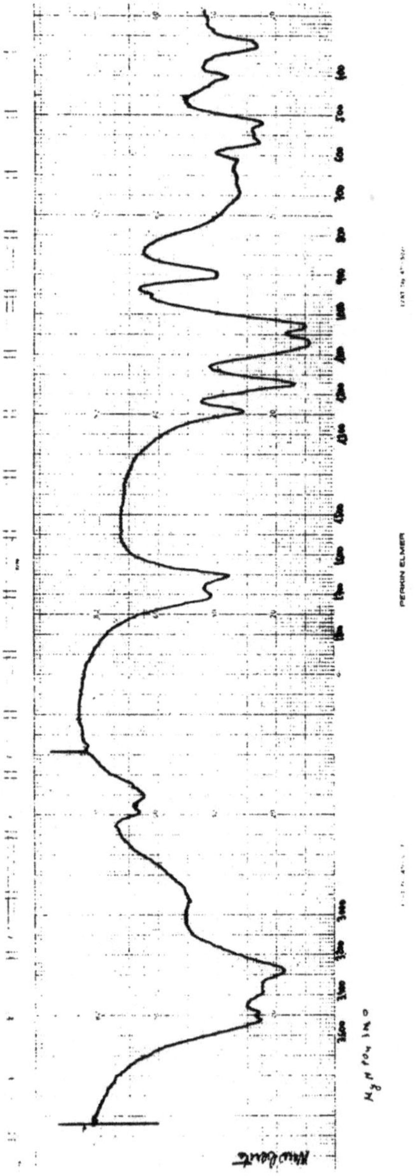

Figure 5. The infrared spectra of newberyte.

Newberyte was found in 53 out of 244 bladder stones (21.7%) and 28 out of 298 renal stones (9.4%). This is 81 cases out of 542 stones (14.9% of the total). When observed under the polarising microscope, newberyte showed small irregular orthorhombic crystals (Figure 2) resembling a shattered struvite crystal similar to a "design in mosaic." It is frequently associated with struvite and is mainly found in the peripheral portion of calculi because of loss of water and ammonia by struvite in contact with the air[3] (Figure 3). When these old calculi are observed under the scanning microscope, we found small crystals that in our opinion can be newberyte (Figure 4) because of their mosaic disposition. The infrared spectra of newberyte shows the main bands at 3.350, 3.280, 1.650, 1.170, 1.030, 570, 400 and 330 cm^{-1} (Figure 5).

DISCUSSION

Several investigators[4-8] have reported the occurrence of newberyte, ($Mg\ HPO_4\ 3H_2O$) in the human urinary calculi and we have found this one exclusively in old samples of stones studied in this laboratory[9].

Newberyte was first reported by Parsons[10] in 1956 in renal calculi as magnesium dibasic phosphate by x-ray diffraction method.

In 1962 Murphy and Pyrah[11] using x-ray diffraction and the immersion method, found newberyte in 0'04% of calculi studies. In the examination of 10,000 calculi with x-ray diffraction and optical crystallography, Herring[12] found newberyte only in one calculi.

In 1968 Bokkones et al[13] studied 70 bladder stones from India and Indonesia. Some calculi of this collection were obtained from the Museum of the Miraj Medical Center, Maharashtra, India and from patients operated in Indonesia during 1926-1927. Using x-ray diffraction they found newberyte in 8% of calculi. In 1968 Lonsdale and Sutor[14] found newberyte in 17% of the stones studied. In 1955 Torigoe[15] found an undefined component in urinary calculi and later in 1962 Hsu[16] found nine cases (1·7%) of possible newberyte. In our opinion, the findings of the latter two investigators were trimagnesium phosphate and not newberyte.

Trimagnesium phosphate in renal calculi, which is very different from the shape of newberyte, has been described by Cifuentes Delatte et al[17] in 1977 as very fine needles, which sometimes form bundles and other times are in a radial disposition when observed under the polarising microscope (Figure 6). Micrographies of these last authors showed that the trimagnesium orthophosphate ($Mg_3\ PO_4 - 5H_2O$) are the same mineral erroneously described by Torigoe[15] and Hsu[16] as "newberyte."

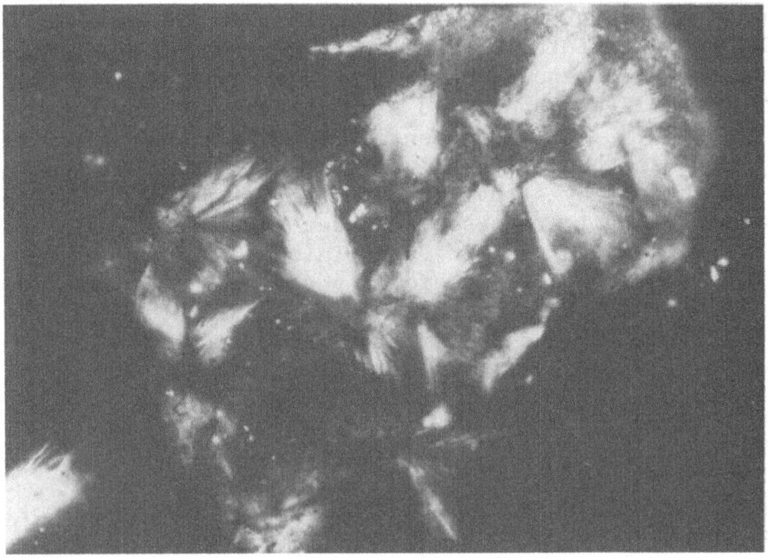

Figure 6. Needle-like crystals of trimagnesium phosphate.

REFERENCES

1. J. Sutor, Cryst. 23:418 (1967).
2. L. Cifuentes Delatte, A. Hidalgo, J. Bellanato, and M. Santos, in:"Urinary Calculi. Recent Advances in Aetiology, Stone Structure and Treatment," Karger, Basel (1973).
3. J. Sutor, Nature 218:295 (1968).
4. R. Morris, and M. Beeler, An. J. Clin. Path. 48:413 (1967).
5. J. Parsons, Henry Ford Hospital Med. Bull. 12:187 (1964).
6. E. Prien, J. Urol. 61:821 (1949).
7. J. Sutor, and S. Scheidt, Brit. J. Urol. 10:22 (1968).
8. J. Sutor, and S. Wooley, Brit. J. Urol. 41:397 (1969)
9. J. RGZ. Miñon Cifuentes, Ardh. Esp. Urol. 29:537 (1976).
10. J. Parsons, J. Urol. 76:228 (1956).
11. B. Murphy, and L. Pyrah, Brit. J. Urol. 34:129 (1962).
12. L. Herring, J. Urol. 88:545 (1962).
13. T. Rokkones, and D. Andersen, Act. Med. Scand. 183:431 (1968).
14. K. Lonsdale, and J. Sutor, Science 154:1353 (1966).
15. S. Torigoe, Jap. J. Urol. 46:190 (1955).
16. Te-Chin-Hsu, J.F.M.A. 61:937 (1962).
17. L. Cifuentes Delatte, P. Carmona, J. Bellanato, M. Santos, and A. Hidalgo, in:"Pathogenese and Klinik der Harnsteine," (1977).

ACKNOWLEDGMENT

We wish to thank Professor L. Cifuentes Delatte for his advice and great help in the preparation of this paper.

FORMS OF AMMONIUM URATE PRESENTATION IN URINARY CALCULI OF NON-INFECTIOUS AND INFECTIOUS ORIGIN

E. García de la Peña and L. Cifuentes Delatte

Department of Urology, Laboratorio de Urolithiasis,

Fundación Jiménez Díaz, Madrid, Spain

Until now infrequent reference has been made to ammonium urate and its presence in urinary calculi. Important elements such as the crystallization pattern of ammonium urate, whether or not more than one is possible and under what conditions each pattern is produced have not been specified. It is accepted that ammonium urate was often found in Europe in urinary calculi until the beginning of this century[1-3]. Now it is found only rarely at least in industrialized countries[4-19], but it is still one of the main components of urinary calculi in some oriental countries[15,17,18,20,22]. This drop in the frequency rate in Europe is due to a higher standard of living; therefore, the incidence of ammonium urate in urinary calculi seems to be directly related to socio-economic factors[23].

MATERIALS AND METHODS

The material consisted of 1,100 consecutive urinary calculi from our collection from 1,100 patients. The method used was the study of thin layers of calculi using a petrographic polarized light microscope "NIKON" model SFPO-KT, with - EFM Microflex photographic equipment. Confirmation of the presence of ammonium urate was done by infrared spectroscopy.

RESULTS

Based on the study of the composition and structure of 1,100 urinary calculi in our collection, we have found two crystallographic patterns of ammonium urate that are of different origins. Even though they are the same substance they present distinct, clearly differentiated patterns. On the one hand there is an ammonium urate found in calculi that originate in acid, sterile urines. On the other hand there is an ammonium urate found in calculi of infectious origin, because of the presence of ureolytic germs in the urine which releases ammonia when the urea contained in the urine breaks down under the action of a bacterial urease.

Pattern A.

The ammonium urate found in calculi of non-septic-origin, that is, calculi produced in acid, sterile urines, is composed of slender needles with a radial layout which stem from a common center and take on a spherulitic shape (Figure 1). These grouped spherulites make up a large part of the calculus. Under the polarizing microscope with crossed Nicol prisms it presents a characteristic golden yellow color. This kind of ammonium urate tends to be largely found in the central nucleus and is often associated with calcium monohydrate oxalate (Figure 2) which may be found in the most superficial layers of the calculus.

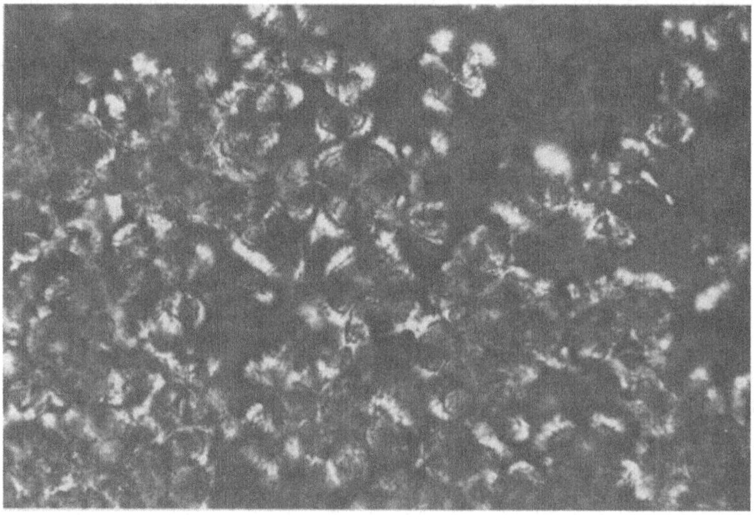

Figure 1. "Aseptic" ammonic urate pattern A.

Pattern B.

It is composed of small, slender needles with no apparent order and with no tendency toward spherulitic formation, scattered among crystals of ammonium magnesium phosphate and apatitic calcium phosphate. (Figures 3, 4, 5, 6).

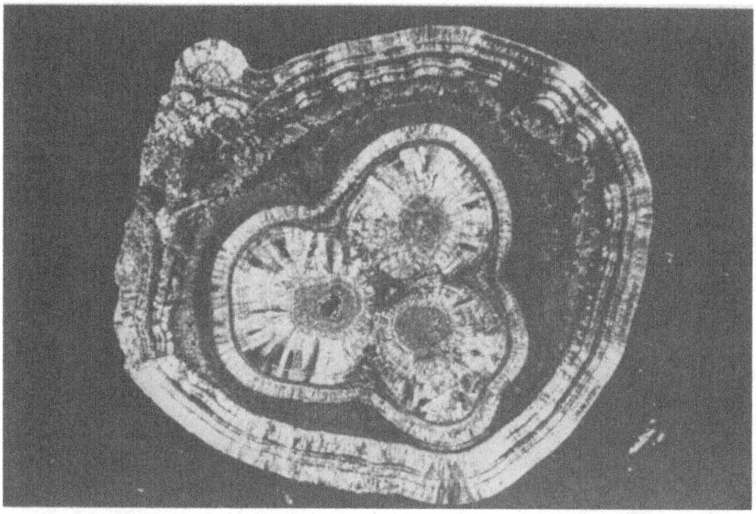

Figure 2. "Aseptic" ammonic urate pattern A in the nucleus and calcium monohydrate oxalate.

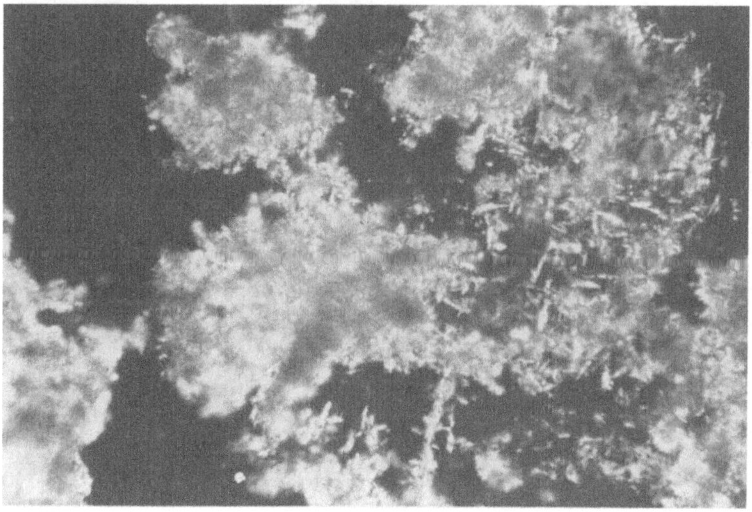

Figure 3. "Septic" ammonic urate Pattern B.

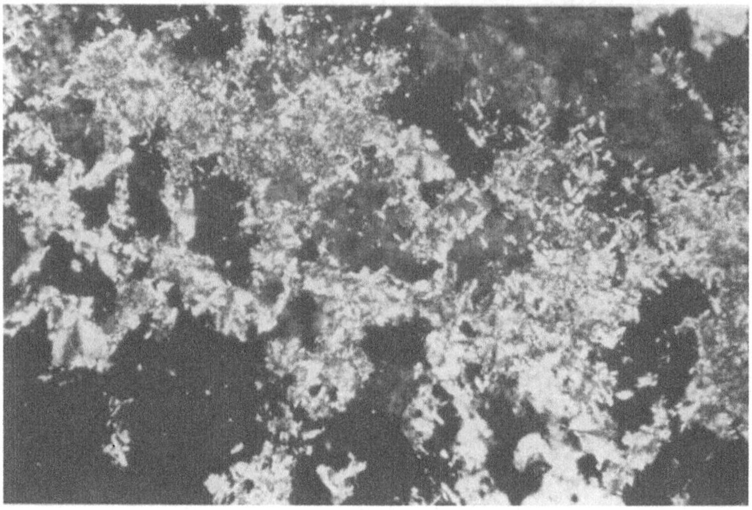

Figure 4. "Septic" ammonic urate pattern B.

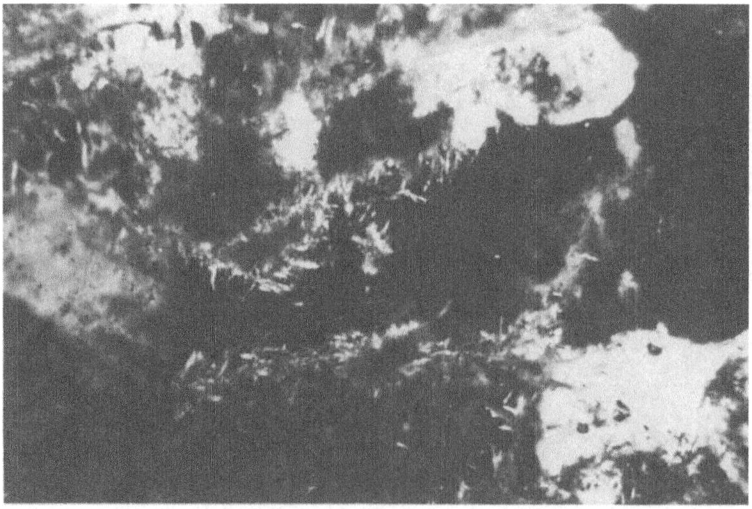

Figure 5. "Septic" ammonic urate Pattern B and ammonic magnesium phosphate.

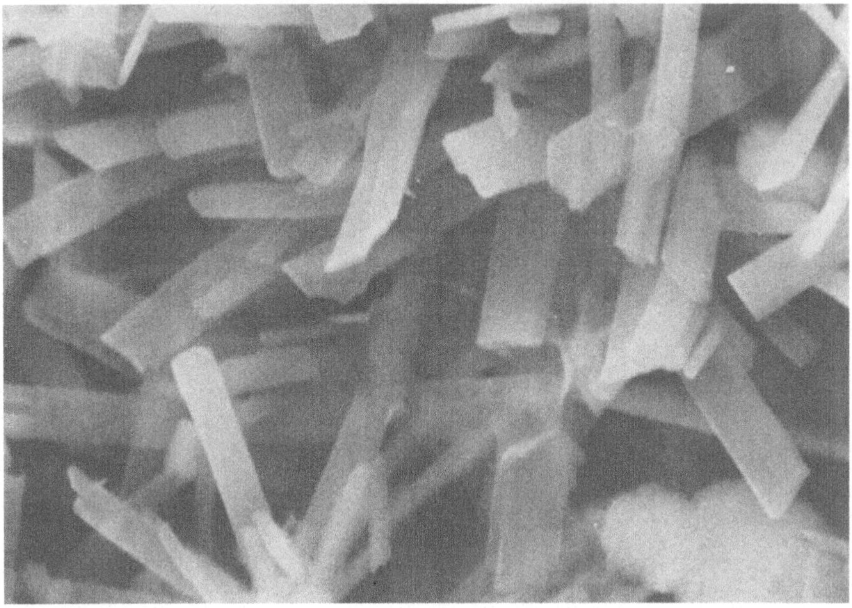

Figure 6. "Septic" ammonium urate Pattern B, scanning.

The ammonium urate we call "aseptic" (Pattern A) (Figures 1, 2, 7, 8) was found in 123 calculi (11.2%). The ammonium urate found in calculi of infectious origin with alkaline urines showed the crystallographic pattern B and was systematically associated with magnesium ammonium phosphate. It was found in 112 of the 1,100 calculi (10.2%).

Therefore, according to our experience, ammonium urate was found in 235 of 1,100 calculi (21.4%). Ammonium urate was as common in calculi of aseptic origin in association with calcium oxalate monohydrate or uric acid (123 = 11.2%) as in calculi of infectious origin appearing in alkaline urines and associated with ammonium magnesium phosphate (112 = 10.2%).

What we called "aseptic" ammonium urate, (pattern A), was located in the nuclei in 50% of the calculi containing ammonium urate. In the other 50% it was found on the surface or in the intermediate layers, associated with calcium oxalate monohydrate or with uric acid. The ammonium urate present in infectious stones, (pattern B), showed no preference of location. However, it was always found along with ammonium magnesium phosphate and the crystals seemed to be arranged at random among the struvite crystals. Both patterns of ammonium urate showed the same infrared spectra.

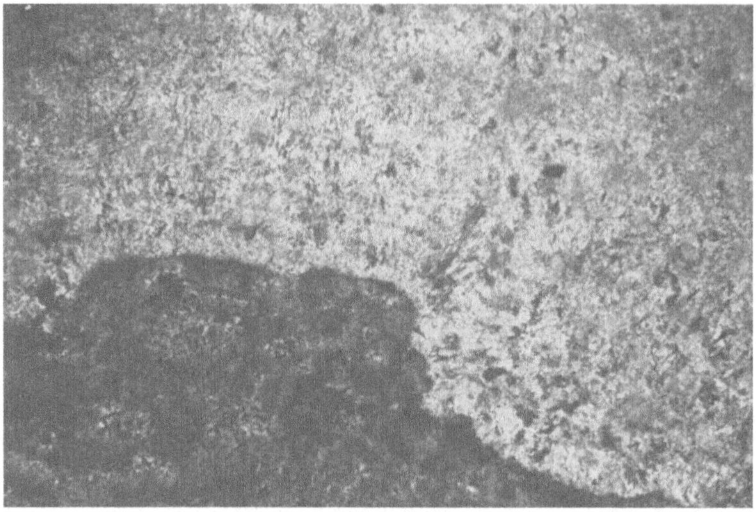

Figure 7. "Aseptic" ammonic urate: Pattern A and calcium monohydrate oxalate.

DISCUSSION

Although we have not been able to demonstrate that these two kinds of ammonium urate are two different substances, there is no doubt that each one has features with respect to its location in the layers of the calculi, the crystals with which it is associated and its genesis. These special features individualize both patterns. We think that this has not been previously pointed out, at least with enough emphasis.

In "aseptic" ammonium urate stones the cation proceeds from the ammonium obtained by the renal tubes, mainly from glutamine, as one of the mechanisms for maintaining the acid-base equilibrium of the organism. In the "septic" ammonium urate stones the ammonium comes from the ammonia produced when the urea contained in urine is broken down by ureolytic germs.

The ammonium urate found in endemic bladder calculi in children in Southeast Asia coincides with the one we call "aseptic ammonium urate." Its genesis is related to factors of deficiency, malnutrition, and the standard of living. Especially, phosphate depletion with reduction of the urinary phosphate buffer increases ammonia secretion by the kidney. On the other hand, the "septic" ammonium urate stones that are associated with calcium phosphate and

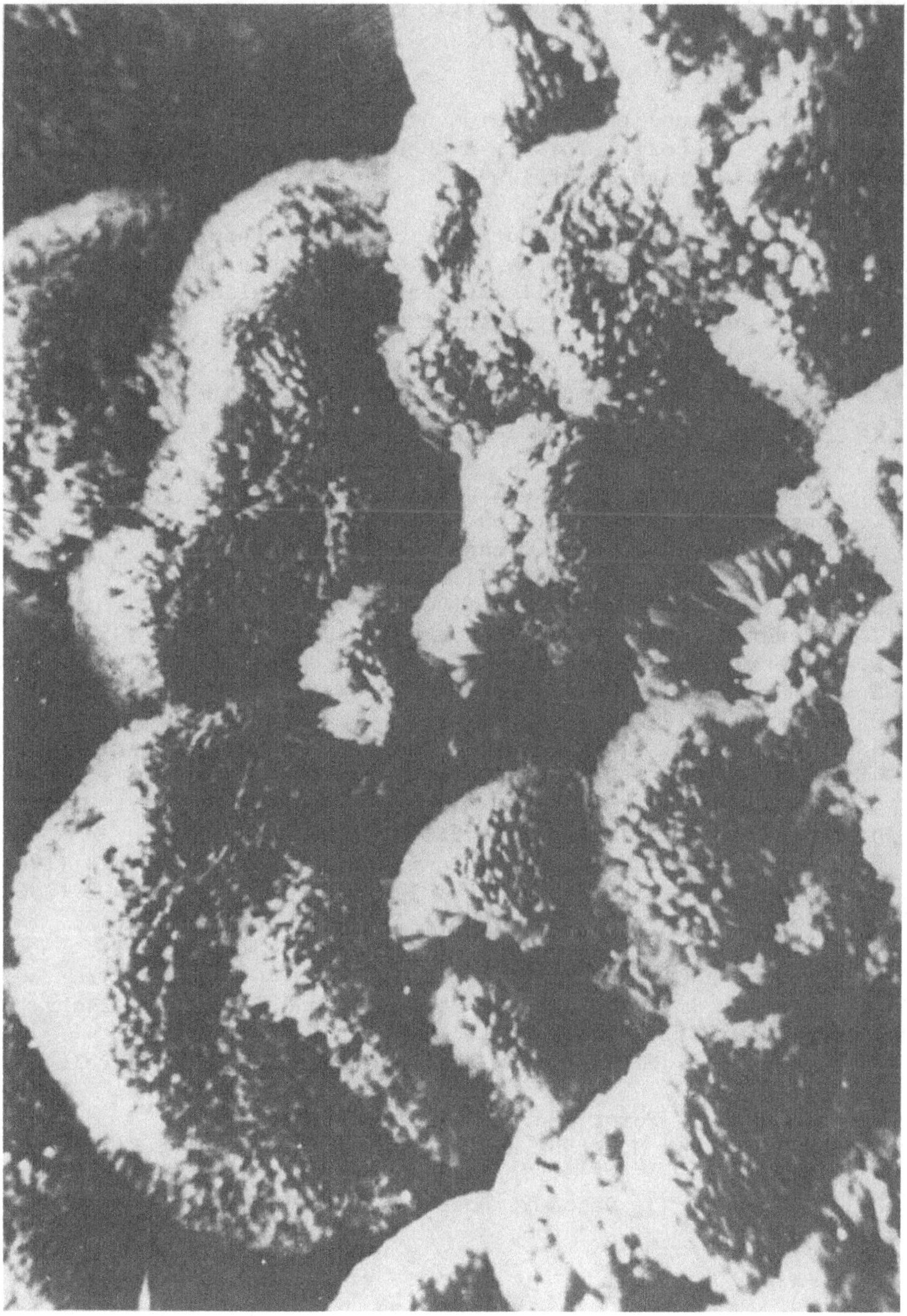

Figure 8. "Aseptic" ammonic urate. Pattern A scanning.

magnesium-ammonium phosphate, have nothing to do with eating habits. Rather, they are related to all those causes which make a person susceptible to the appearance of repeated urinary infections, especially those produced by ureolitic germs.

CONCLUSIONS

1. We have found that ammonium urate appears in 21.4% of studied urinary calculi. This is a much higher percentage than that given for other western countries[4-19].

2. We have found that in urinary calculi without a ureolitic infection, the ammonium urate is arranged in a spherulitic structural pattern (A); whereas in calculi with infected alkaline urine crystals are disordered according to structural pattern B.

REFERENCES

1. K. Lonsdale and P. Mason, Ancient and Modern Sciences, 152:511 (1966).
2. K. Lonsdale, J. Sutor, and S. Wooley, Br. J. Urol. 40:33 (1968).
3. K. Lonsdale, Science 195:1199 (1968).
4. A. T. Jensen, Acta. Chir. Scand. 84:207 (1941).
5. E. L. Prien and C. Frondel, J. Urol. 57:949 (1947).
6. E. L. Prien, J. Urol. 61:821 (1949).
7. C. Lagergren, Acta. Radiol. Stockholm. Suppl. 133:1 (1956).
8. L. C. Herring, J. Urol. 88:545 (1962).
9. B. T. Murphy and L. N. Pyrah, Br. J. Urol. 34:129 (1962).
10. E. L. Prien, J. Urol. 89:917 (1963).
11. M. F. Beeler, D. A. Veith, R. H. Morris, and G. R. Biskind, Am. J. Clin. Path. 41:553 (1964).
12. J. Parsons, Henry Ford Hosp. Med. Bull. 12:187 (1964).
13. D. Lenaghan, Med. J. Austral. 2:64 (1965).
14. R. H. Morris, and M. F. Beeler, Am. J. Clin. Path. 48:413 (1967).
15. K. Lonsdale, J. Sutor, and S. Wooley, Br. J. Urol. 40:402 (1968).
16. D. J. Sutor and S. E. Wooley, Br. J. Urol. 42:302 (1970).
17. D. J. Sutor and S. E. Wooley, Br. J. Urol. 43:268 (1971).
18. D. J. Sutor and S. E. Wooley, Br. J. Urol. 44:287 (1972).
19. A. Hesse, J. J. Schneider, S. Schnoder, and R. Wegner, Zschr. Urol. 69:1 (1976).
20. S. N. Gershoff, E. L. Prien, and A. Chandrapanund, J. Urol. 90:285 (1963).
21. Te-Chin Hsu, J. Form. Med. A. 61:937 (1962).
22. S. Shahjehan and M. Ataur Rahman, Am. J. Clin. Nutr. 24:32 (1971).
23. D. A. Andersen, J. Oslo Cy. Hosp. 16:101 (1966).

PROSTATIC CALCULI

M. Spector, C. E. Magura, and J. C. Lilga

Medical University of South Carolina

Charleston, South Carolina

INTRODUCTION

Few previous studies of urinary tract concretions have focused on prostatic calculi. While less clinically significant than renal lithiasis, prostatic stones can, under certain circumstances, produce severe urinary tract problems. In addition, insights into the mechanism of formation of prostatic concretions can provide a better understanding of aspects of renal calculus disease.

Prostatic concretions include corpora amylacea and corpora calculi as well as prostatic calculi. Corpora amylacea are uncalcified, rounded laminated bodies from 0.2 to 1 mm in diameter. As a result of early morphological observations, it was proposed that corpora are formed from desquamated acinar cells and prostatic concretions[1]. It has been noted that, with aging, corpora amylacea can undergo calcification to become corpora calculi[2]. Larger, more clinically significant calcified concretions, prostatic stones, may be either endogenous, derived from prostatic secretions, or exogenous, derived primarily from urinary constituents[2-4]. The etiology of corpora amylacea and corpora calculi, and their relationship to endogenous prostatic calculi, remain somewhat in question. The objective of the present study was to delineate the ultrastructure of these prostatic concretions as a means of determining their pathogenesis and interrelationship.

MATERIALS AND METHODS

Prostatic specimens were obtained from 31 individuals. Tissue samples were taken from all lobes of 16 prostates; 13 from autopsy and 3 following radial prostatectomy or radical cystectomy. Six other prostates were sampled by transurethral resection of the prostate (TURP); four of these yielded numerous prostatic calculi. Free prostatic calculi were also obtained from 9 additional individuals. Histological specimens were fixed in neutral buffered formalin and embedded in paraffin using conventional techniques. Corpora and prostatic calculi were plastic-embedded in preparation for microradiography. Other free calculi were powdered for x-ray diffraction studies. Selected tissue specimens, corpora calculi, and prostatic stone fragments were also fixed in glutaraldehyde and processed for scanning and transmission electron microscopy (SEM and TEM).

RESULTS

X-ray diffraction analysis of the free prostatic calculi identified the sole crystalline constituent of all but one of the stones as hydroxyapatite. In one stone, brushite predominated. Microradiography revealed the variation in the degree of calcification in alternate concentric lamellae of the concretions. Individual layers were found by SEM (Figure 1) to be composed of small spherical aggregates (0.5 to 5μ in diam.) of minute, ill-defined hydroxyapatite crystallites. In the one brushite stone, blade-like brushite crystals arranged in regular arrays radiated from an area of the stone consisting of randomly oriented brushite crystals and hydroxyapatite deposits. TEM revealed that the laminated structure of the prostatic calculi was due to variations in the number and arrangement of crystallites in alternate rings. Selected area electron diffraction confirmed the identity of the small crystallites as hydroxyapatite. However, in one stone, a discrete layer of whitlockite was found interposed between hydroxyapatite lamellae. Small rounded membranous-appearing features reminiscent of cell debris were found in the prostatic stones by TEM (Figure 2).

Histological studies revealed the typical, concentric, lamellar appearance of corpora amylacea in various stages of maturation. All were alcian blue and PAS positive. SEM revealed amorphous appendages, similar to colloidal substances seen in light microscopy, adhering to the outer surface of the corpora (Figure 3). TEM demonstrated that the corpora amylacea were composed of an amorphous substance and contained constituents reminiscent of cell debris. The concentric lamellar appearance was found to be the result of a variation in density of the organic matrix. TEM also revealed nuclei and debris from desquamated cells adherent to the surface of the corpora (Figure 4). A few corpora amylacea were calcified, staining positively with alizarin red, and were therefore designated as corpora calculi. SEM revealed that the calcified deposits often consisted of small spherical aggregates (~0.5 μm diam.) of crystallites. Individual crystallites of the corpora calculi were small, with ill defined borders, and could not be clearly delineated by TEM. The

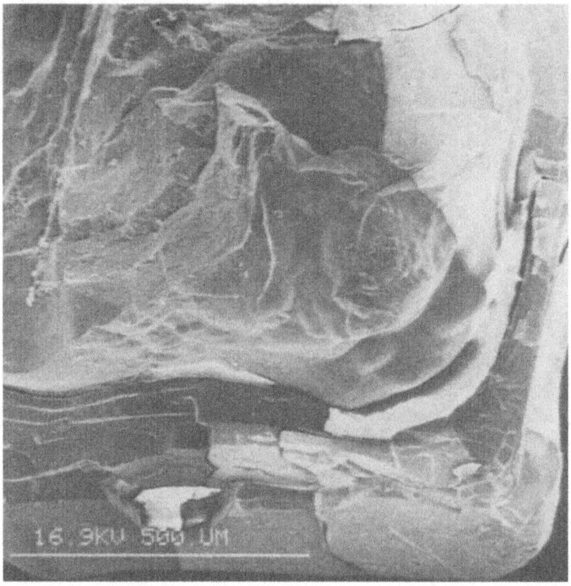

Figure 1. SEM of a cleaved prostatic calculus.

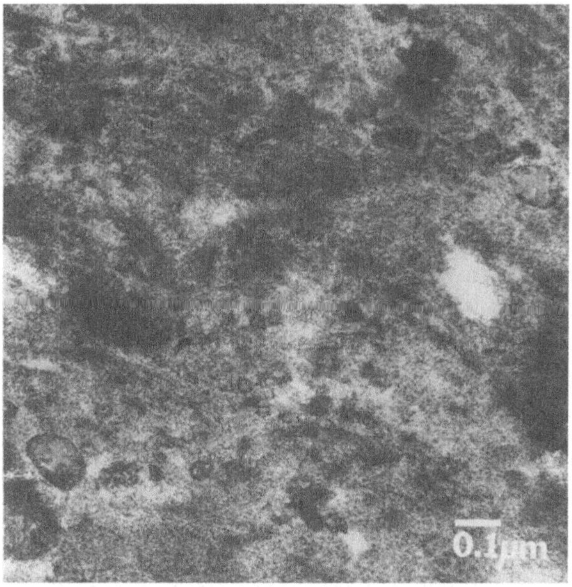

Figure 2. TEM of a prostatic calculus revealing rounded membranous bodies reminiscent of cell debris.

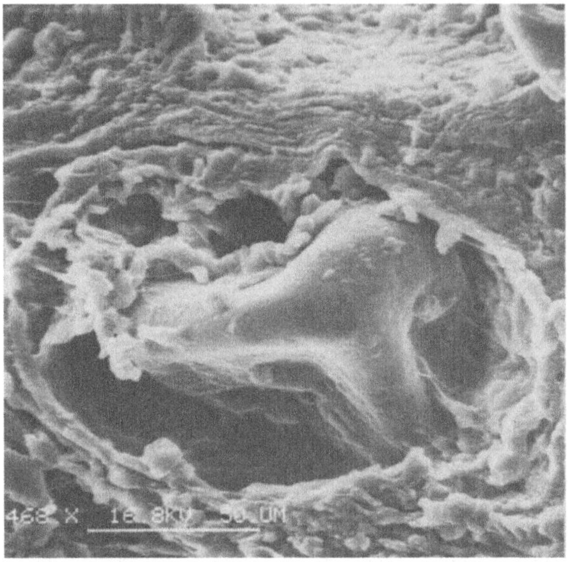

Figure 3. SEM of a corpus amylaceum in an acinus with cellular and amorphous appendages.

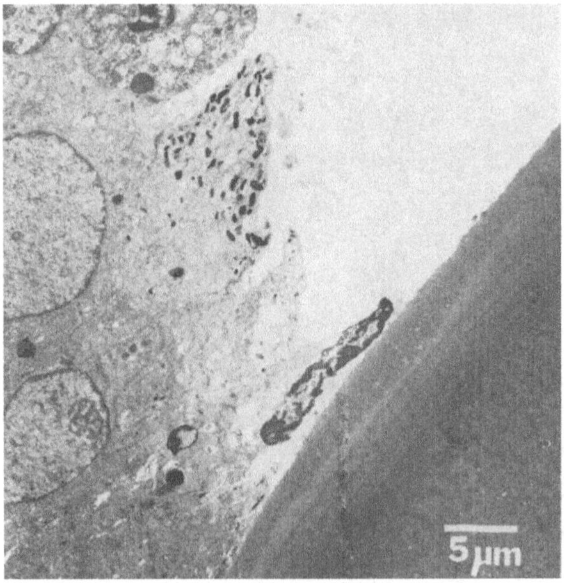

Figure 4. TEM of a corpus amylaceum and adjacent prostatic epithelium. Degenerated nudeus on surface of corpus.

crystallites were identified as hydroxyapatite by selected area electron diffraction. However, diffraction patterns of whitlockite were also obtained. Initial calcified deposits in the corpora amylacea appeared as small islands of crystallites. These crystallite aggregates appeared in increasing numbers as individual rings of the corpora became more calcified.

DISCUSSION

Similarities in the structure and composition of corpora and prostatic calculi were revealed by SEM and TEM. Each concretion displayed a variation in the degree of mineralization of concentric lamellae. Both types of calculi consisted of minute, ill-defined crystallites of hydroxyapatite which often appeared in small spherical aggregates. In addition, features reminiscent of cellular debris were seen in prostatic calculi as well as in corpora calculi. These results indicate that prostatic calculi may be corpora which have undergone further growth and mineralization. This would suggest that corpora amylacea, considered to be the result of normal aging processes, can be the precursors of pathologic concretions.

The brushite calculi identified in the present study were obtained from a patient after a TURP. Examination of prostatic chips from a second TURP revealed brushite encrustation of an extensive hydroxyapatite deposit exposed to the acidic urinary flow after the first TURP. The brushite stones appeared to be spawned from this brushite encrustation of the prostatic bed.

It is interesting to note that the small spherical aggregates of hydroxyapatite crystallites revealed in the calcified prostatic concretions by SEM are similar to deposits found in renal stones and other pathologic tissues[5,6]. This might suggest similar morphogenic mechanisms of mineral precipitation. While prostatic concretions may be of minimal clinical significance, further investigation into their pathogenesis may lead to a better understanding of other calcifying phenomena, including urinary calculus disease.

REFERENCES

1. R. A. Moore, Arch. Path. 22:24 (1936).
2. M. J. V. Smith, Mono. Surg. Sci. 3:209 (1966).
3. A. J. Leader and D. M. Queen, J. Urol. 80:142 (1958).
4. D. J. Sutor and S. E. Wooley, Br. J. Urol. 46:533 (1974).
5. M. Spector and L. H. Jameson, in:"Scanning Electron Microscopy/ 1976," O. Johari, ed., IIT Research Inst. Press, Chicago (1976).
6. M. Spector, N. M. Garden, and S. N. Rous, Br. J. Urol. 50:12 (1978).

ACKNOWLEDGMENTS

The technical assistance of J. T. Eldridge is gratefully acknowledged. Dr. Spector was supported by NIH-NIDR Research Career Development Award DE00067.

IX. ANALYTICAL METHODS

ISOTACHOPHORETIC DETERMINATION OF OXALATE IN UNPROCESSED URINE

W. Tschöpe and E. Ritz

Medizinische Universitat-Klinik, Sektion Nephrologie,
Bergheimer Straße 58,
D-6900 Heidelberg, Federal Republic of Germany

INTRODUCTION

Measurement of urinary oxalate is important in the elucidation of the mechanisms of renal stone formation. Methods recently described for measuring oxalate depend mainly on colorimetry or enzymatic destruction utilizing the specific enzyme oxalate decarboxylase (E.C. 4.1.1.2). All of the colorimetric methods[1,2,3] and most of the decarboxylase methods[4,5,6] require treatment of urine prior to measurement. This introduces the possibility of incomplete recovery and conversion of other substances into oxalate[7]. The pre-treatment procedures described involve precipitation with calcium[1], pre-treatment with anion-exchange columns[2], or precipitation of calcium oxalate with ^{14}C-oxalate[4].

No simple and specific method exists which allows urinary oxalate to be measured without pre-treatment of urine. Using isotachophoresis, Beckers and Everaerts[8] were able to measure a variety of carboxylic acids including oxalate in aqueous solutions. In the present study, the principle of isotachophoresis was applied to the measurement of oxalate in urine samples.

PATIENTS AND METHODS

Principle of Isotachophoresis

Isotachophoresis involves the separation of ionic species in an electrical field. "Iso"-"tacho" denotes equal velocity. In the isotachophoretic system, all ionic substances travel at the same velocity but are separated into different "zones". A solution, containing two or more different ionic species, is injected into a capillary tube. The sample is interposed between a "leading electrolyte solution" and a "terminating electrolyte solution". The leading electrolyte, the sample ions, and the terminating electrolyte all migrate towards the anode. As they do so, the sample ions separate according to their net mobilities until, at equilibrium, two or more distinct sample ion zones are present. The only ions to migrate in discrete zones are those with mobilities between that of the leading electrolyte, which has the highest mobility (in our system this is chloride, see below), and the terminating electrolyte, which has the lowest mobility (in our system this is acetate, see below). The zones containing the ions under study can be detected either by UV-absorption, or by a specific thermal signal. When a constant current is applied to the system, the migration velocity of the ions determined by the mobility of the respective ions and the electric field strength (Kohlrausch's law). Since ionic species differ in their mobilities and since the velocity of migration is constant, the local electrical field strength and the development of Joule's heat must both increase. This can be detected as a thermal signal, which is specific for each substance and can be used for identification of the ionic species under study (Figure 1). Furthermore, two separate zones containing different ions with different UV-absorbances can be clearly distinguished by a UV-positive or UV-negative signal. This may be quantitated using the equation of Kohlrausch. According to this equation, the concentration of the ions under study is directly proportional to the concentration of the leading electrolyte. Consequently, at equilibrium, the ionic concentration in each zone must be constant. The amount of a given ion in each zone is thus directly proportional to the length of the zone. The principle of isotachophoretic separation and quantitation of oxalic acid using the operational system given below, is illustrated in Figure 1.

Experimental

The isotachophoretic separations and determinations were performed in an LKB 2127 Tachophor (LKB Company, Bromma, Sweden) equipped with the 23 cm Teflon capillary. UV-absorption was measured at 254 nm. Reliable identification of oxalate by the thermal signal was possible, when the amount of injected oxalate exceeded 2 nmol. Oxalate decarboxylase (E.C. 4.1.1.2) was purchased from Sigma Corporation, Munich, No. 0-3500.

The leading electrolyte solution consisted of HCl (Suprapur) (5×10^{-3} M), NaCl (1×10^{-3} M) and 0.4% HPMC. No adjustment of pH was carried out. The terminating electrolyte consisted of acetic acid ($5\text{-}20 \times 10^{-3}$ M).

The samples were injected using a 10 µl Hamilton microsyringe equipped with either a planinum needle and tungsten plunger (model AA 701 SN) or with a steel canula and steel plunger (model 700).

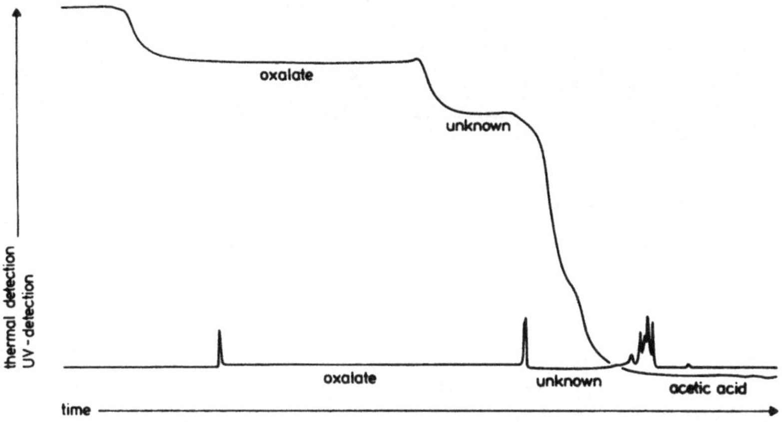

Figure 1. Principle of detection and quantitation in isotachophoresis, using the operational system as given above for the separation and quantitation of oxalic acid in rhubarb juice. Upper curve: traces of the thermal signal: the leading electrolyte Cl^- has the highest mobility and the lowest development of Joule's heat, chloride does not give UV-absorption. The second zone (oxalate) is recorded with a significant different specific thermal step height. The third zone (unknown, but probably phosphate) is well separated from the preceeding oxalate and the following impurities and acetic acid (terminating electrolyte).

The quantity of oxalate was determined by measuring the zone length with a graticule or ruler. Calculation of the oxalate content was performed using the combined zone lengths of both the UV-absorbing and non-UV-absorbing zone of oxalate (see below), which were present in each sample examined.

Urines

Urines were collected under outpatient conditions on a free diet from 17 healthy children, 27 healthy adults and 18 adult idiopathic renal stone-formers. Urines were collected in plastic bottles kept at 4°C during the collection period. Concentrated ZnCl2 (final concentration 10 mmol/l) was then added and urinary oxalate measured within 12 h after collection of the urines.

RESULTS AND DISCUSSION

Development of the Method

With the electrolyte system described above, oxalate has a high isotachophoretic mobility and appears in the first zone when the

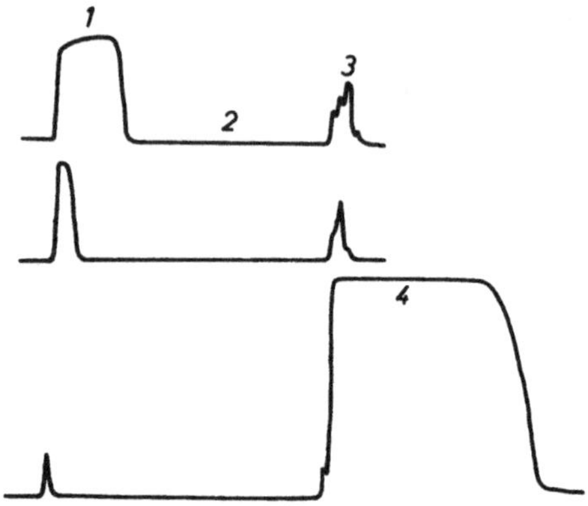

Figure 2. UV-positive and -negative zones of oxalate. 1 = UV-absorbing zone of the assumed ferrioxalate complex, 2 = non-UV-absorbing zone of oxalate, 3 = impurities, 4 = UV-absorbing complex of Fe and EDTA. Injection of 10 nmol of oxalate in aqueous solution with Hamilton microsyringe, model 700, which had been in use for three weeks (a). Addition of $ZnCl_2$ (10 mmol/l) reduces the UV-absorbing zone of the ferrioxalate complex (b). Addition of EDTA (10 mmol/l) results in further reduction of the UV-absorbing zone in aqueous solutions (c). In most of the urines examined EDTA or EGTA does not significantly influence the UV-absorbing zone of the Fe-containing oxalate complex.

thermal signal and the UV-signal is recorded. In aqueous solutions as well as in urine samples (Figures 2 and 3) oxalate is recorded as a UV-positive zone, which is followed by a non-UV-absorbing zone. Both zones increase in length as one increases the concentration of oxalate in the sample. When model 700 Hamilton microsyringes (steel needle, steel plunger) were used, considerable problems were encountered, as the relative contribution of the UV-absorbing zone increased up to 30%, after model 700 syringes had been used repeatedly. It was observed, that the UV-absorbing zone could be greatly increased by adding ferric ions in the form of ferric chloride (Figure 3). Following the treatment of aqueous oxalate solutions with oxalate decarboxylase both zones disappeared completely after 30 minutes. As all steel surfaces in contact with air are covered by a layer of ferri-oxide, it was assumed from these observations, that this first UV-absorbing zone of oxalate is a ferri-oxalate complex with high stability[9]. In aqueous solutions, but not in urines, addition of EGTA or EDTA abolished completely the UV-positive zone of the assumed ferri-oxalate complex (Figure 3). The problem of a vary-

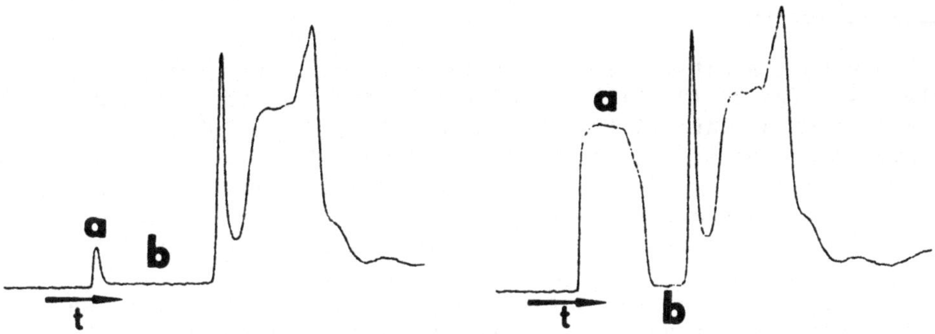

Figure 3. The effect of addition of iron ions. Isotachopherogram of the initial zones of a 24 h urine sample with and without the addition of $FeCl_3$ (5×10^{-4} mmol/l). The initial UV-absorbing zone of oxalate is significantly increased. Injection of 5 µl urine, calculated oxalate concentration of the sample 350 µmol/l, injection with Hamilton microsyringe, model AA 701 SN. Operational systems as above.

ing contribution of the UV-positive zone to the total oxalate zone was solved by two modifications: firstly, only thoroughly siliconized glassward was used, and secondly, injections were performed with platinum canulae and tungsten plungers instead of iron containing syringes. In native urine samples, the recovery of added oxalate was only 85%. While the addition of EDTA, magnesium, or citrate were ineffective, rates of recovery could be markedly improved by the addition of $ZnCl_2$. Using $ZnCl_2$ as additive to urines, 102% of added oxalate (range 90-111%) was recovered. In the presence of $ZnCl_2$, the recovery of exogenous oxalate was still complete in the presence of high concentrations of calcium. The physico-chemical explanation for the effect of zinc may be a relative high solubility product for Zn oxalate[10] and possibly the formation of relatively stable complexes[9]. Repeat measurements of oxalate in urine samples yielded a coefficient of variation of 3.2%, showing good reproducibility. The reproducibility was even better, however, in aqueous solutions (1.2%).

Detection of oxalate was specific without interference from other carboxylic or dicarboxylic acids. Specifically, parabanic acid and oxaluric acid did not interfere with the oxalate signal. Oxaluric acid was not attacked by oxalate decarboxylase. However, heating urines for only 15 min., to which 1 mmol/l oxaluric acid had been added, resulted in a significant increase in the apparent content of oxalate.

Clinical Studies

In normal adults, the 24 h oxalate excretion was 436 ± 176 µmoles/24 h (range 190-815); idiopathic stone-formers excreted slightly more oxalate (471 ± 195 µmoles/24 h, range 207-871). Urinary excretion of oxalate in children was significantly lower than in adults (292 ± 162 µmoles/24 h, range 87-650). The difference was reversed after normalization with urinary creatinine (children: 66 ± 21 µmol/mmol, adults: 33 ± 11 µmol/mmol urinary creatinine).

For all subjects, including children, the correlation between urinary excretion of oxalate and age, weight, body surface or urinary creatinine was calculated. The best correlation was found between urinary oxalate and urinary creatinine (Figure 4).

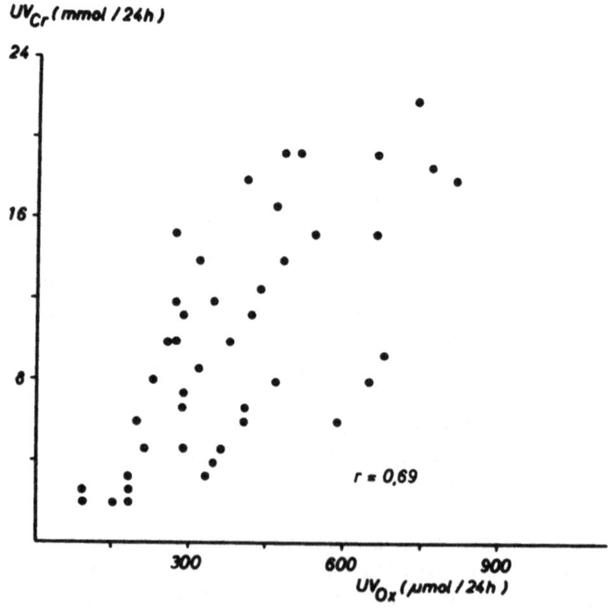

Figure 4. Correlation between the urinary excretion of oxalate and creatinine (17 healthy children, age 3-14, 27 healthy adults, age 17-48 years). ($r = 0.69$, $p < 0.01$, $n = 44$).

CONCLUSIONS

The present study provides clear evidence that isotachophoretic separation of unprocessed urine permits satisfactory measurements of urinary oxalate with good recovery and reproducibility. The method is also suitable for measuring other substances which are relevant to renal stone-formation. Co-determination in one single run of oxaluric acid, citrate, glycolate and urate is possible (data not given). The method may also be useful to observe and follow oxalate complex formation *in vitro*.

REFERENCES

1. A. Hodgkinson and A. Williams, Clin. Chim. Acta. 36:127 (1972).
2. F. M. G. Olthuis, A. M. G. Markslag, J. T. K. Elhorst, P. G. L. C. Krugers-Dagneaux, Clin. Chim. Acta. 75:123 (1977).
3. H. Baadenhuijsen and A. P. Jansen, Clin. Chim. Acta. 62:315 (1975).
4. D. J. Bennett, F. E. Cole, E. D. Frohlich, and D. T. Erwin, J. Lab. Clin. Med. 91:822 (1978).
5. P. C. Hallson and G. A. Rose, Clin. Chim. Acta. 55:29 (1974).
6. J. Costello, M. Hatch, and E. Bourke, J. Lab. Clin. Med. 87:903 (1976).
7. A. Hodgkinson and P. M. Zarembski, Analyst 86:16 (1961).
8. F. M. Everaerts, J. L. Beckers, and Th. P. E. M. Verheggen, J. Chromat. Library Vol. 6 (1976).
9. L. G. Sillen and A. E. Martell, in:"Stability Constants of Metal-Ion Constants," Alden and Mowbray Ltd., Alden Press, Oxford (1971).
10. K. V. Krishnamurty and G. M. Harris, Chem. Rev. 61:213 (1961).

ANALYTICAL ISOTACHOPHORESIS: AN IMPROVED METHOD FOR QUANTITATIVE DETERMINATION OF URINARY OXALATE

K. Schmidt, V. Hagmaier, G. Bruchelt, and G. Rutishauser

Department of Surgery, University of Tuebingen, Germany F.R., and Division of Urology, Department of Surgery, University of Basle, Switzerland

Calcium oxalate stones are the most common type of renal calculi, accounting for about 70% of all stones. Whereas calcium metabolism and excretion have been investigated extensively in patients with recurrent nephrolithiasis, relatively little attention has been paid to oxalate[1]. Determination of urinary oxalate has been considered of some value in the elucidation of the role of oxalate in controlling stone formation in patients with recurrent nephrolithiasis.

For quantitative determination of urinary oxalate concentrations a great number of different procedures have been described in the literature. However, a rapid and sufficiently simple technique for routine determinations is lacking. Volumetric and colorimetric procedures are of limited specificity[2,3], methods involving enzyme reactions have the disadvantage that the enzymes are difficult to isolate and catalytic activity is inhibited by various urinary constituents[4]. Gas liquid chromatographic and isotope dilution techniques are time consuming and need sophisticated processing of the biological material.

Analytical isotachophoresis has recently been successfully applied to the analysis of organic acids extracted from human urine. In this paper separation and quantitative determination of oxalate in urine is demonstrated using this simple, rapid, and sensitive technique.

MATERIALS AND METHODS

Urine was obtained from ten young, healthy, male volunteers that was collected during 24 h and kept frozen until analyzed.

The volunteers were on a free diet but were instructed to avoid excess intake of food containing large amounts of oxalic acid. Isotachophoretic runs were performed in a Tachophor 2127 apparatus (LKB, Sweden) equipped with an 800 mm PTFE capillary of 0.5 mm internal diameter. The leading electrolyte was 0.01 M hydrochloric acid titrated to pH 3.68 with 0.01 M beta-alanine. 0.3% Methylcellulose (methocell MC 4000 cP) was added to increase viscosity and thus to reduce electroendosmosis. The terminating electrolyte was 0.01 M n-hexanoic acid. The initial current was 175 μA, and the analyzing current 75 μA. The temperature was kept constant at 15°C. For injection of aliquots of the urine samples (10 μl injection volume) high-quality syringes with a PTFE-tipped piston were used to avoid iron-oxalate complex formation. For quantification of separated ions the width of the UV peaks (254 nm) corresponding to the zone length in the capillary was used. Identification and calibration were performed by use of oxalate and ^{14}C oxalate as internal standards as well as the thermosignal. All chemicals and reagents were of highest commercially available purity, water was twice distilled in an all-quanrtz apparatus. Buffers were prepared fresh weekly.

Different pretreatment schemes were employed prior to the isotachophoretic analyses: a) acidification alone, b) acidification and addition of EDTA, c) acidification and superposition of a spacer electrolyte gradient, and d) acidification, adjustment of pH to 5.3, precipitation of calcium oxalate and dissolution of the precipitate.

RESULTS

Highest precision and accuracy was obtained after precipitation of the oxalate anion.

A typical result of an isotachophoretic separation of dissolved precipitate is given in Figure 1. The thermal step height representing the temperature of the corresponding zone produced by Joule's heat in the capillary was used for identification. The temperature is related to the electrical field strength in each zone and is therefore a measure of the mobility of the ions in the zone. In our electrolyte system the step height of oxalate amounts to 8% of the total thermosignal obtained with chloride-caproate. The UV recordings exhibit the characteristic absorbance of the oxalate anion. Various internal standards were added to the urine samples for calibration purposes. A standard calibration curve is drawn showing linearity in the range from 20 mg/l to 100 mg/l of oxalate added to the urine (Figure 2). This curve parallels the one obtained with pure oxalate when dissolved in water. The concentration of the intrinsic urinary oxalate is measured on the negative abscissa. From the measurements a 24 h urinary oxalate excretion of 29 ± 12 mg

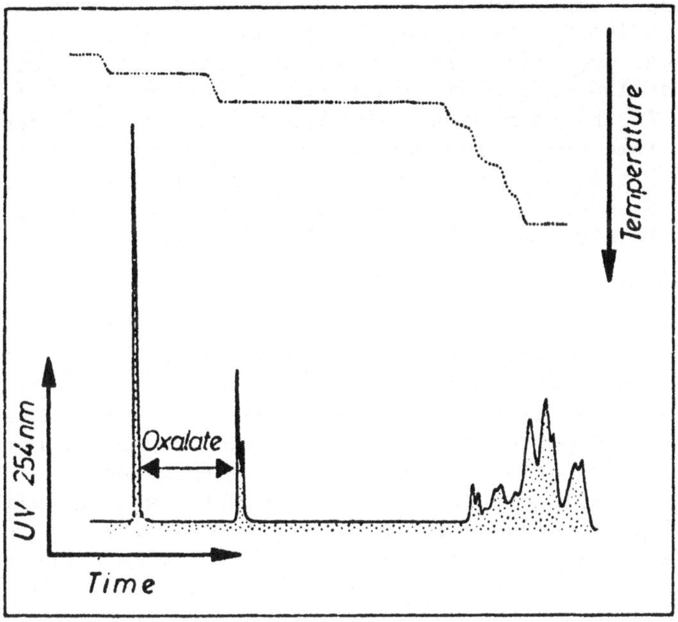

Figure 1. Isotachophoretic separation of the urinary Ca^{++} precipitate dissolved in hydrochloric acid.

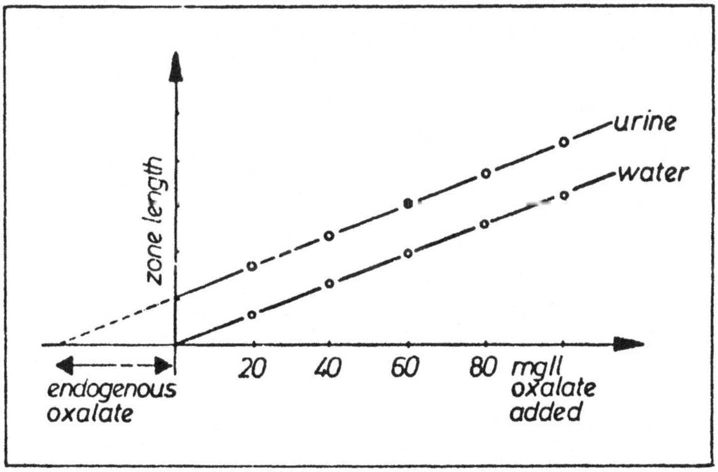

Figure 2. Standard calibration curves of oxalate dissolved in water or urine.

can be derived (n=30) which is in the range of the enzymatic methods. With an injection volume of 10 µl minimum measurable oxalate concentration was approximately 20 nmol/ml. Up to an oxalate concentration of 150 mg/l equilibrium can be obtained with the 800 mm capillary. In the case of a very high urinary oxalate concentration injection volume can be reduced. The recovery rates after precipitation of the oxalate with calcium ions are comparable to those reported by Baadenhuijsen[5]. Our recovery studies confirm the hyperbolic precipitation curve found by this author.

DISCUSSION

In isotachophoresis the sample ions are separated according to their net mobility (net mobility = ionic mobility x degree of dissociation). The technique described here for determination of urinary oxalate provides several advantages over other methods. The coefficient of variation of the isotachophoretic analysis is less than 3%. The simple pretreatment of the urine samples allows the rapid handling of a large number of samples routinely. The use of internal standards avoids errors due to varying recovery rates. The method is sufficiently sensitive since the detection limit (20 nmol/ml) is far below the normal urinary concentration of oxalate.

REFERENCES

1. A. Hodgkinson, Academic Press, London (1977).
2. A. V. Harcourt, J. Chem. Soc. 20:460 (1867).
3. S. Burrows, Analyst 97:958 (1972).
4. C. F. Knowles and A. Hodgkinson, Analyst 97:474 (1972).
5. H. Baadenhuijsen and A. P. Jansen, Clin. Chim. Acta. 62:315 (1975).

THE EFFECT OF STORAGE ON SERUM OXALATE VALUES

M. Maguire, N. Fituri, B. Keogh, and J. Costello

The Irish Stone Foundation and Department of Medicine and Nephrology, Trinity College, Meath Hospital, Dublin, Ireland

INTRODUCTION

Controversy still exists regarding the true concentration of oxalate in mammalian blood. Indirect radioisotope methods[1-4] have given values of 11.0 - 16.5 μg per 100 ml plasma while chemical-enzymic techniques[5-9] have obtained oxalate levels of around 120 μg. More recently, however, Akcay and Rose[10] have produced evidence to explain this discrepancy. In the presence of inhibitors of glyoxylate oxidation to oxalate they demonstrated considerably lower levels by their enzymic procedure. Using a modification of the method of Hatch et al.[8] we have observed similar serum oxalate levels to Akcay and Rose[10] but in the absence of these inhibitors.

MATERIALS AND METHODS

Serum and plasma oxalate were determined as previously described[8] but with the following modifications.

1. Serum or plasma is ultrafiltered at its normal pH (7.4) and not at 10.6.

2. Post-precipitation with ethanol/calcium sulphate the precipitate is lyophilized instead of being dried in an oven at 105°C.

3. The lyophilized precipitate is extracted for 30 minutes at 37°C and not as previously at 75°C.

4. The pH of the phosphate buffer (0.5M pH 7.0), for the formate determination, is changed to 7.5.

The first three modifications were introduced to reduce further the possibility of conversion of any precursors to oxalate during the assay procedure. The citrate extract was analyzed in triplicate and oxalate recoveries carried out on each extract. The sensitivity of the assay is 0.2 µg.

Serum oxalate was determined in a number of healthy non-fasting individuals. Plasma oxalate was also analyzed after the blood had been collected with and without the inhibitors, allopurinol, DL-β-phenyllactic acid and boric acid as described by Akcay and Rose[10]. Serum ascorbate of three sera was increased by 5.7 mg per 100 ml and the sera then stored at -20°C for periods of 2 days to 5 months before being analyzed. The sera were also stored without additions. Serum ultrafiltrate was similarly treated. Plasma with added glyoxylate 23 µg per 100 ml was stored for a period of ten days and compared with its control. The ability of whole blood to convert added glyoxylate to oxalate and the inhibition of this oxidation by the inhibitor mixture was studied.

RESULTS

There was no significant difference between the oxalate concentration in serum and that in the corresponding plasma - Table 1. While there are individual differences in plasma oxalate with and without the inhibitors there is no definite trend and the mean value of both is almost identical. When glyoxylate, 7.5 mg/100 ml, was added to whole blood and the plasma separated immediately there was a dramatic increase in oxalate concentration - Table 2. The presence of the three inhibitors decreased but did not prevent this conversion. When glyoxylate, 50 µg/100 ml, was added to whole blood which had been preincubated for 5 minutes with the inhibitors and the plasma then rapidly removed at 4°C there was a very significant increase in oxalate concentration - Table 2. Storage of plasma for ten days at -20°C with added glyoxylate, 23 µg/100 ml showed a 52% increase in oxalate concentration, 62% of this increase could be attributible to oxidation of the glyoxylate.

When serum was stored at -20°C very significant increases were observed - Table 3. If the ascorbate concentration of the serum is increased by 5.7 mg per 100 ml over 100% increase in oxalate is found within 48 hours and progressively increases with storage time. Serum ultrafiltrate was found to be even more unstable showing dramatic increases in oxalate even without added ascorbate.

DISCUSSION

Recently Akcay and Rose[10] reported that plasma oxalate of 70 µg per 100 ml was reduced to 20.3 µg when the blood was collected in the presence of inhibitors, allopurinol, boric acid and DL-β-phenyllactic acid. They speculated that these inhibitors when added immediately

Table 1. Oxalate Concentration of Healthy Volunteers (μg/100 ml)

Serum		Plasma	Without Inhibitors	With Inhibitors
A.W.	24.6			
G.G.	22.4			
H.G.	31.2	J.C.	38.8	20.5
J.F.	32.4	N.F.	26.5	8.4
C.M.	42.8	N.R.	25.7	42.1
P.G.	27.7	J.J.	39.1	24.6
E.R.	25.9	G.G.	24.0	34.1
H.A.	32.1	N.A.	17.0	37.0
N.E.	35.9	J.R.	18.6	25.9
Mean	30.6		27.1	27.5
S.D.	±6.3		±8.8	±11.4

Table 2. Effect of Glyoxylate on Plasma Oxalate

	Glyoxylate Added per 100 ml	Oxalate (μg per 100 ml)
Whole blood	Nil	35.6
Whole blood	7.5 mg	2104.3
Whole blood and inhibitors	7.5 mg	495.5
Whole blood	Nil	12.1
Whole blood	50 μg	37.3
*Whole blood and inhibitors	50 μg	29.5

*This blood was pre-incubated with inhibitor mixture before glyoxylate addition.

to whole blood prevented the enzymic oxidation of glyoxylate to oxalate. While we find plasma and serum levels of 27 μg per 100 ml we were unable to detect any significant difference in the presence of these inhibitors. It is noteworthy that these workers[10] found no change in two out of seven samples with the inhibitors. We confirm their findings of very large increases in plasma oxalate when 7.5 mg of glyoxylate was added to whole blood. However, we have demonstrated the inability of their inhibitor mixture[10] to prevent oxidation of low concentrations, 50 g, of glyoxylate to oxalate. We feel it reasonable to conclude that glyoxylate is not the major contributory factor to the higher oxalate concentrations reported by chemical-enzymic techniques[5-9].

Table 3. Effect of Storage on Oxalate Concentration

Time	Subject	% Increase in Oxalate	
		Serum	Serum + Ascorbate (5.7 mg%)
2 days	Pool	Nil	110
1 week	J.C.	32	
2 week	J.C.	109	
16 week	J.F.	794	
20 week	N.A.	148	2253
20 week	N.F.	453	2447
20 week	A.K.	753	3210
		Ultrafiltrate	Ultrafiltrate + Ascorbate (5.7 mg%)
4 days	B.M.	455	1765

No studies have been reported on the effect of storage on serum and plasma oxalate concentration. We observed large increases in serum oxalate when stored at -20°C for more than 48 h. The presence of added ascorbate greatly increases this conversion of precursors to oxalate as does glyoxylate. Due to the very rapid oxidation of glyoxylate to oxalate in whole blood, it appears very unlikely that there is any significant amount of glyoxylate remaining in plasma. It appears possible that ascorbate may be one of the main precursors causing the increase in serum oxalate on storage. These results emphasize the importance of sample handling and storage prior to analysis. The oxalate levels of the lyophilized precipitate and its citrate extract are stable for at least 3 months when stored at -20° C.

The above results go some way to explain the discrepancy between serum oxalate levels found by chemical-enzymic methods and those obtained by isotope techniques. However, further studies are necessary to explain the lower values of 11-16.5 µg per 100 ml reported using in vivo techniques.

REFERENCES

1. H. E. Williams, G. A. Johnson, and L. H. Smith, Clin. Sci. 41:213 (1971).
2. A. Hodgkinson and R. Wilkinson, Clin. Sci. Mol. Med. 46:61 (1974).
3. A. R. Constable, A. M. Joekes, J. P. Kasidas, P. O'Regan, and G. A. Rose, Clin. Sci. Mol. Med. 56:299 (1979).

4. R. Hautmann and H. Osswald, Invest. Urol. 16:395 (1979).
5. C. F. Knowles and A. Hodgkinson, Analyst 97:474 (1972).
6. V. V. S. Eswara Dutt and H. A. Mottola, Biochem. Med. 9:148 (1974).
7. P. G. L. C. Krugers Dagneaux, J. T. Klein Elhorst, and F. M. F. G. Olthuis, Clin. Chim. Acta 71:319 (1976).
8. M. Hatch, E. Bourke, and J. Costello, Clin. Chem. 23:76 (1977).
9. D. J. Bennett, F. E. Cole, E. D. Frohlich, and D. T. Erwin, Clin. Chem. 25:1810 (1979).
10. T. Akcay and G. A. Rose, Clin. Chim. Acta. 101:305 (1980).

ACKNOWLEDGMENTS

We wish to thank the Irish Stone Foundation and the Medical Research Council of Ireland for generous financial support. We are grateful to our normal volunteers and to Nurse Grant for taking many blood samples.

DIRECT MEASUREMENT OF IONIZED CALCIUM

(STANDARDIZATION, NORMAL VALUES AND CLINICAL RESULTS)

B. M. Ulshöfer and A. Peemöller

Urologische Universitätsklinik und Poliklinik
Robert-Koch-Straße 8, D-355o Marburg a.d.
Lahn, Germany (FRG)

INTRODUCTION

Ionized calcium (Ca^{++}) is the biologically active fraction of total serum calcium (Ca_t), thus it is of special clinical interest. In the diagnosis of primary hyperparathyroidism (pHPT) none of the previously reported methods[1-5] for measuring $(Ca)^{++}$ have become clinically useful because of cost. The development of a $(Ca)^{++}$-selective membrane[6] provided a simpler and more specific measurement of $(Ca)^{++}$. The Orion SS-20 (R) made this technique available for clinical purposes. In order to evaluate this procedure we determined the factors that influence ionization[7-10] and studied the usefulness[11-14] of the procedure in the diagnosis of pHPT.

STANDARDIZATION

Heparin (= Liquemin (R)) and CO_2 concentration are known factors that influence ionization of calcium. The suggested concentration of heparin (7-10 U/ml sample) caused no significant decrease of ionization (Figure 1). Increasing pCO_2 increased pH and decreased Ca^{++}, so after one month of deepfrozen storage correction for pH must be done (Figure 2). Measurements within 24 hours (Figure 3) have shown no change. We found no significant difference between heparinized blood and anaerobically drawn serum (Vacutainer(R)) (Figure 4). Neither venous stasis (Figure 5) nor the gas diffusible tubes of the SS-20 (Figure 6) affected the results.

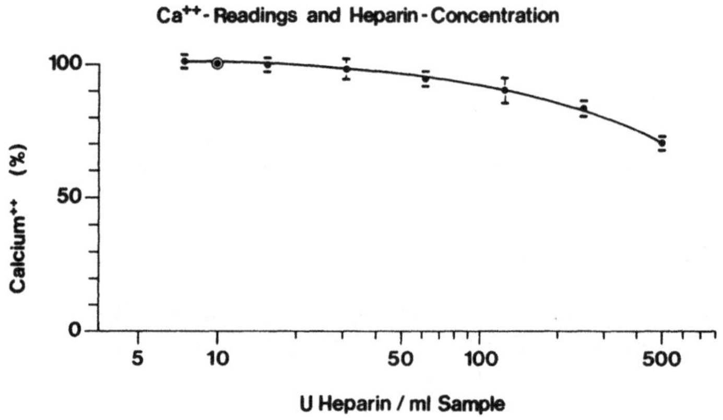

Figure 1.

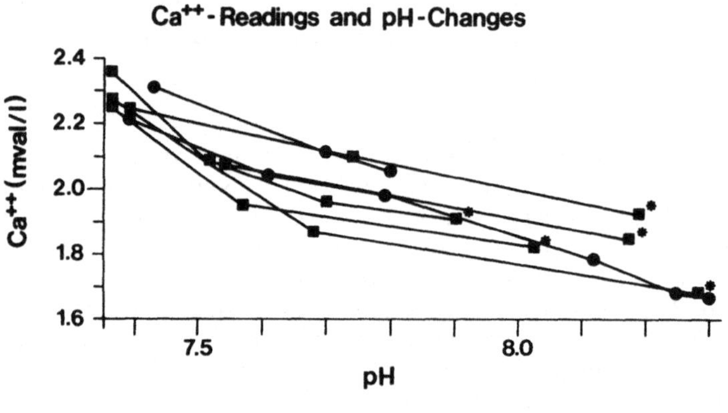

Figure 2.

Ca^{++}-Reading and Sample Storage n=9

Temperature (°C)	Hours	Ca^{++} (%) $\bar{x}\pm SD$	pH $\bar{x}\pm SD$	pCO_2 $\bar{x}\pm SD$	pO_2 $\bar{x}\pm SD$
+20	<3	100.0 8.0	7.366 0.025	50.1 5.0	82 17
+20	8	100.5 1.1	7.378 0.029	49.5 4.6	89 17
+ 4	8	100.4 2.0	7.375 0.028	49.2 4.6	92 15
+ 4	24	99.1 1.6	7.386 0.038	49.2 5.0	144 44

Figure 3.

n=13	Whole Blood	Serum
Ca^{++} (mval/l) $\bar{x}\pm SD$	2.05 0.10	2.05 0.10
pH $\bar{x}\pm SD$	7.290 0.032	7.358 0.026
pCO_2 $\bar{x}\pm SD$	50.4 6.0	48.5 5.9

Figure 4. Comparison of blood and serum.

Venous Stasis ($p\frac{RR_{syst}+RR_{diast}}{2}$) and Ca^{++} n=5

	Before	1/2 Min.	1 Min.	2 Min.	1 Min. after release
Ca^{++} (%) $\bar{x} \pm SD$	100.0	99.9 1.7	100.5 2.2	101.2 2.2	100.5 3.5
pH $\bar{x} \pm SD$	7.291 0.029	7.291 0.031	7.288 0.036	7.278 0.019	7.271 0.008
pCO_2 $\bar{x} \pm SD$	52.4 5.2	51.1 2.2	52.1 2.5	54.2 4.7	53.6 7.1
pO_2 $\bar{x} \pm SD$	38 15	38 7	34 7	28 6	39 10

Figure 5. The effect of venous stasis.

Blood-Gases and Ca^{++} Before and After Passing the Tube-System n=5

	pH	pCO_2	pO_2
before	7.292 ±0.023	53.0 ±7.2	26 ±4
after	7.336 ±0.010	32,2 ±2.3	38 ±6

Figure 6.

CLINICAL RESULTS

There were no differences in various groups of age, sex or urological diseases except hypo- and hyperparathyroidism. Compared with albumin-corrected and Ca_t, Ca^{++} discriminated much better between normals and pHPT-patients as shown in Figures 7 and 8. The effect of successful adenectomy is illustrated in Figure 9, which shows the greater variation of Ca_t and inorganic phosphate compared to Ca^{++}, pre- as well as postoperative. Intraoperative measurements (Figure 10) revealed a slight temporary fall of Ca^{++} 5-15 minutes after removal of the adenoma, while the definite fall started 2-5 hours later. This phenomenon, also published by Moore[15], is yet unexplained.

CRITICAL COMMENT

Threads of fibrin, not visible in the syringe, may obstruct the capillary flow-through system. For "trouble-free" use careful maintenance by experienced personnel is necessary. Protein deposits on the membrane shorten useful life of the electrode. The costs (reagents, electrodes, service, time) limit the general use.

CONCLUSIONS

Normal value of Ca^{++} ± 2SD): 2.35 ± 0.18 resp. 1 99 ± 0.27[§]

Standard procedure: Serum by Vacutainer(R) without additional evacuation; whole blood containing 7-10 U Liquemin(R)/ml sample. All samples handled anaerobically. Analysis within 8 hours (20°C) resp. 24 hours (+4°C). Stored deepfrozen for more than 1 month correction for raising pH is necessary.

Clinical results: Compared with total and albumin corrected serum calcium much better discrimination between normal and pHPT patients especially in borderline- and/or "normocalcemic" pHPT. No additional information in case of distinct hypercalcemia.

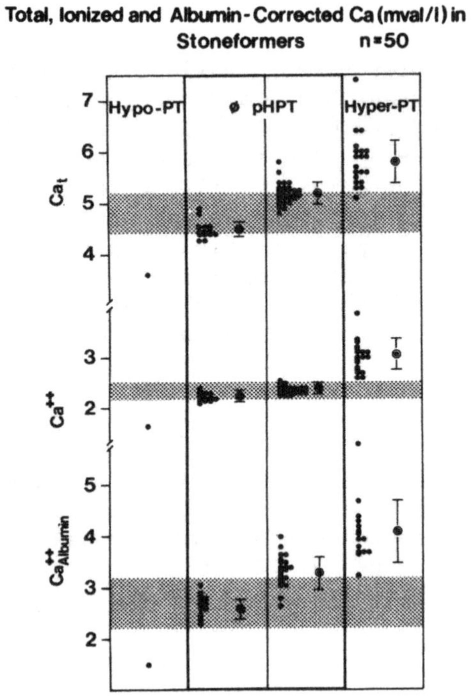

Figure 7

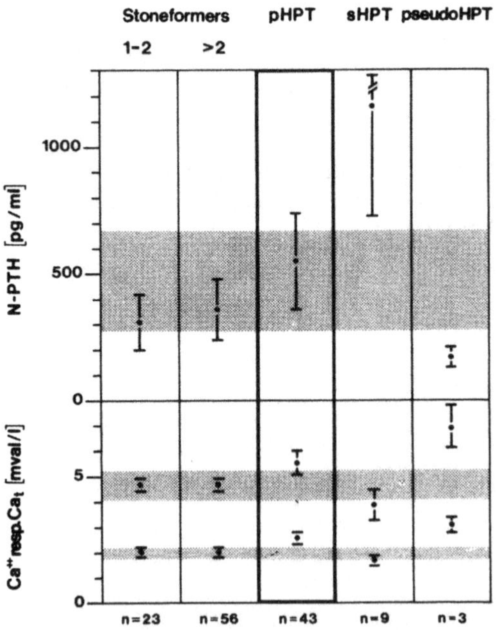

Figure 8

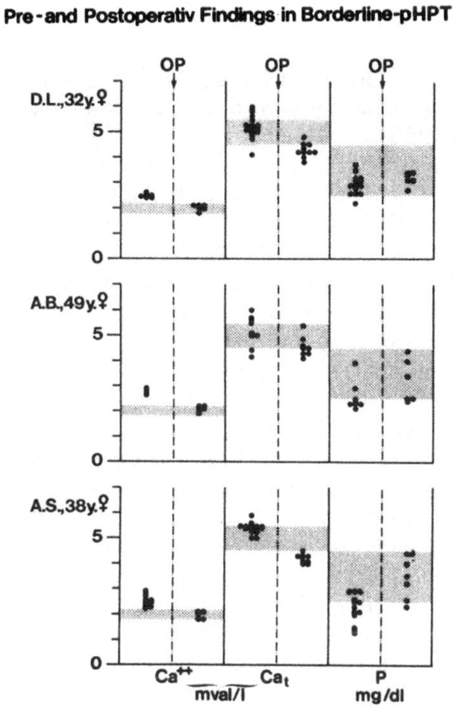

Figure 9.

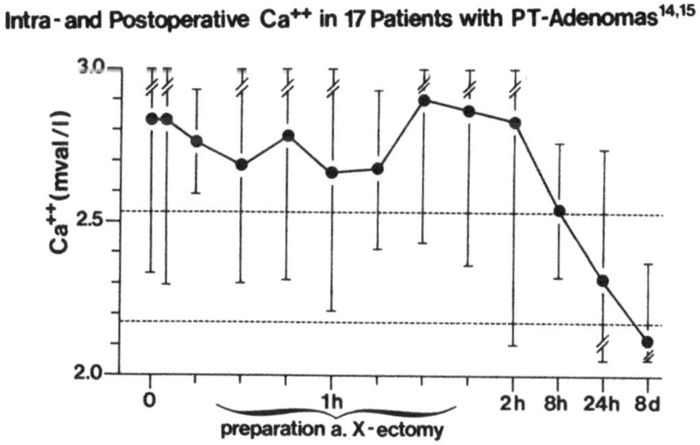

Figure 10.

REFERENCES

1. F. C. McLean and A. B. Hastings, Am. J. Med. Sci. 189:601 (1935).
2. E. R. Yendt, T. B. Connor, and J. E. Howard, Bull. Johns Hopkins Hosp. 96:1 (1955).
3. W. G. Robertson, Clin. Chim. Acta. 20:315 (1968).
4. J. Raaflaub, Z. Physiol. Chem. 288:228 (1951).
5. G. A. Rose, Clin. Chim. Acta. 2:227 (1957).
6. J. W. Ross, Science 156:1378 (1967).
7. Instruction Manual Space-Stat 20 Ionized Calcium Analyzer. Orion Biomedical, Division of Orion Research Inc., Cambridge, Massachusetts (1976).
8. H. Husdan, M. Lenug, D. Oreopoulos, A. Rappaport, Clin. Chem. 23:1775 (1977).
9. K. Paschen, in:"Die Bestimmung des Calciums und Seiner Fraktionen im Serum," Thieme-Verlag, Stuttgart, West Germany (1975).
10. C. Fuchs, D. Dorn, C. McIntosh, and F. Scheler, Clin. Chim. Acta. 67:99 (1976).
11. J. C. Low, M. Schaaf, J. M. Earll, J. T. Plechoki, and T. K. Li, JAMA 152:223 (1973).
12. F. P. Muldowney, R. Freaney, E. A. Spillane, and P. O'Donohoe, Irish J. Med. Sci.142:223 (1973).
13. B. Ulshofer and G. Rodeck, Akt. Urol. 9:43 (1978).
14. B. Ulshofer, K. Joseph and G. Rodeck, Helv. Chir. Acta. 46:399 (1979).
15. E. W. Moore, in:"National Bureau of Standards," R. Durst, ed., Gaithersburg, Maryland (1969).

NEW GLASS CAPILLARY GAS-CHROMATOGRAPHIC METHODS FOR METABOLITES IN URINE AND SERUM

Werner Dosch

Institut für Geowissenschaften, University of Mainz

Mainz, Germany

The analytical system suggested in this paper is a further development of pre-chromatographic methods and of column switching techniques described in previous papers[1,2,3]. In order to use modern gas-chromatographic techniques for the determination of metabolites in urine and serum quick and reliable pre-chromatographic methods for extraction, concentration and derivatization must be developed which give final (dosage) volumes of 5 to 10 µl with starting sample volumes of 0.1 ml of urine or 5 ml of serum as described by Dünges[4].

Complex mixtures of organic compounds in biological samples lead to time consuming gas-chromatographic procedures. Time of analysis can be drastically reduced by column switching techniques according to Deans[5] which additionally improve sensitivity and protect glass capillary columns against damage. The simplest of these methods, which is nevertheless very effective, is backflushing: compounds with retention times greater than those of analytical interest are backflushed while the separation is done. It is also possible to exclude from detection that sample part which appears in front of the compounds to be analyzed, especially the solvent ("heart cutting"). The most sophisticated system allows arbitrary and repeated cuts of the sample stream.

Although its principles are known for some time, column switching is not yet in common laboratory use. The paper shows that simple and low-cost column switching devices can be easily constructed. They can be attached to most commercial gas-chromatographs and are still extremely reliable as the author was able to show.

Pre-chromatographic and column switching methods must be coordinated in such a way that a simple and reliable procedure of

Table 1. Working Instructions for the Determination of Oxalic Acid in Urine

A) Pre-chromatographic method

Series of 12 samples: working time 50 minutes,

total time 12 hours.

1. Adjust 5 ml samples of fresh urine with 5NHCl to a pH of 1-1.5 and add 50 μl of an internal standard*.

2. Pipet 100 μl into 1 ml vessels, shown in Figure 1a, bring to dryness in 12 h in a vacuum desiccator over P_2O_5. If single samples are used, evaporation with a rotary evaporator (30°C) is also possible.

3. Add 100 μl BF_3-methanol (20% in methanol), stir with a vibromix, transfer to 1 ml reacti-vial[6], using a syringe with filter insert, see Figure 1c, rewash residues twice with 50 μl of BF_3-methanol each. Keep the sealed reacti-vials 20 minutes at 80°C, cool in an ice bath.

4. Add 200 μl of water and 200 μl of CH_2Cl_2, agitate with the aid of the vibromix. After the phases have settled, transfer the CH_2Cl_2-phases to the 100 μl micro-flask, Figure 1b.

5. Concentrate to 7 μl under partial reflux. Here part of the solvent evaporates while another part is refluxing. With this method[4], volatile solutes are enriched without losses. Cool in an ice bath.

B) Glass-capillary gc-analyses with packed pre-column (backflush)

Time of analyses for a series of 12 samples: 72 minutes
working time: 11 minutes

1. Inject 1 μl of concentrate

2. Start timer

Gas-chromatographic conditions: see Figure 3.

* 300 mg malonic acid in 100 ml of water, freshly prepared.

analysis is achieved which can be performed even by untrained personnel.

These procedures were optimized for the analysis of oxalic acid and other acidic metabolites after derivatization as methylesters. The methods are not limited however to these compounds.

Advantages of glass-capillary gas-chromatography within this method are: only small amounts of urine or serum are needed; different components are quantitated in one run; large series of analyses can conveniently be carried out in a short time; and high precision, reproducibility and selectivity are achieved.

PRE-CHROMATOGRAPHIC METHOD

Work and time needed for the recommended pre-chromatographic and gas-chromatographic methods are given in the working instruction, Table 1. Special pre-chromatographic devices are shown in Figure 1. The concentration of the solute (dimethyl ester derivatives of oxalic acid and of the internal standard malonic acid) is performed under partial reflux. This concentration step in the microliter range can be done free of loss[4].

BACKFLUSHING IN GAS-CHROMATOGRAPHY

With conventional gas-chromatography, the whole sample is carried through the capillary column. With backflushing the solutes which are to be determined are separated on a main column while unwanted compounds with greater retention times are backflushed from a pre-column. In this way the pre-column is cleaned and prepared for the next analysis while the actual analysis is carried out. The timer required for switching the magnetic valve[7] as well as the necessary fittings to the gas-chromatograph, can be constructed quite easily and inexpensively. For sources of supply and details of the construction please ask the author. A typical gas-chromatogram according to Table 1 is shown in Figure 3. In operating the simple backflush device, as shown in Figure 2, one of five sections of the printed circuit of the multitimer, described in [7], is sufficient for optimal operation. By optimizing the backflush cycle, compounds with retention times greater than that for malonic acid (standard) are suppressed as much as possible without suppressing the standard itself.

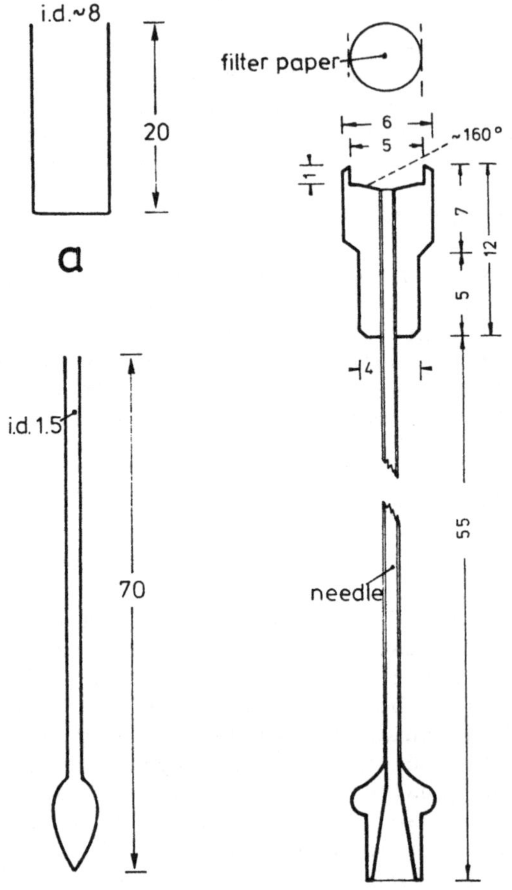

Figure 1. Pre-chromatographic devices: (a) glass evaporation vessel for urine with flat bottom; (b) concentration vessel according to [4]; (c) syringe-needle with filter insert.

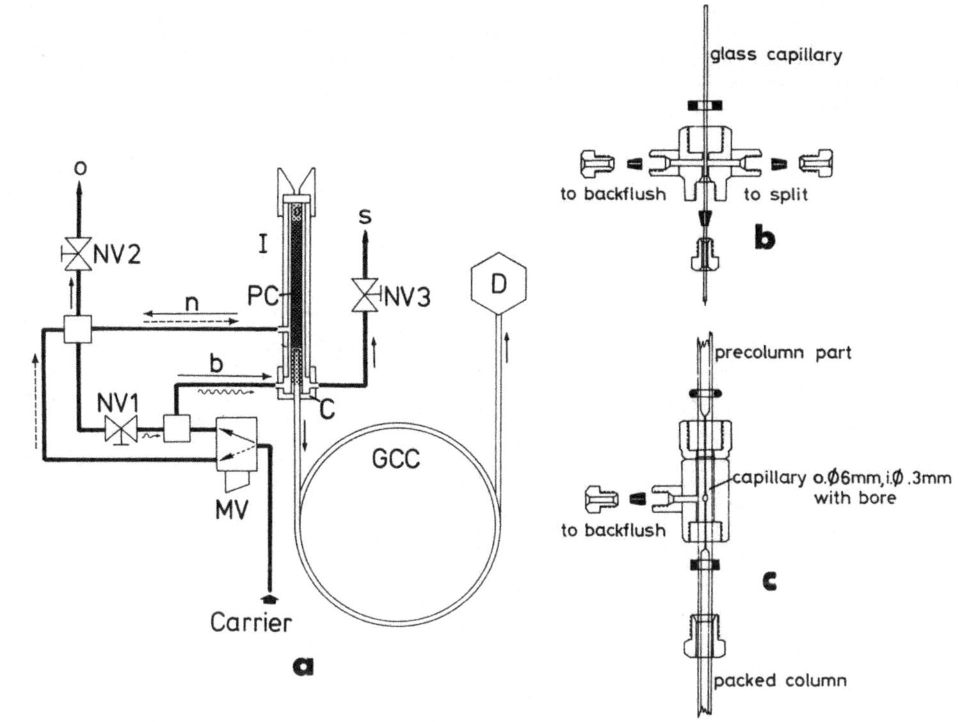

Figure 2. Backflush equipment: (a) Pneumatic system: I = injector, PC = glass precolumn with 25% OV-101 on volasphere 80/100 mesh, GCC = glass capillary column, D = FID-detector, C = adapter (see also figure 2b, c), MV = magnetic valve, operated by the timer[7], NV1, 2, 3 = needle valves, s = split, o = outlet, n = normal entrance of carrier gas to the injector, b = inlet for the backflush stream. Full arrows indicate gas flow if MV is not operated (backflush-phase). Dotted arrows indicate the conventional gas flow for gas-chromatography which works only if MV is switched on.

(b) Construction detail of adapter C, assembled with commercial parts.

(c) With this adapter packed columns can also be used. In this case the pre-column-part is directly connected with the separation column by means of a connecting piece, from a thick-walled capillary, i.d. 0.3 mm, with a 1 mm borehole for the backflush entrance.

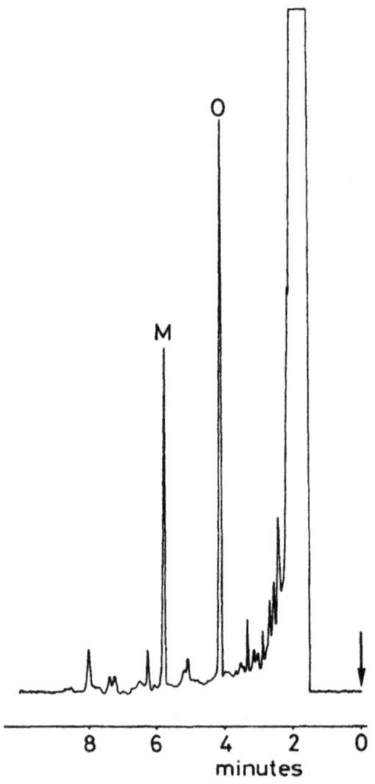

Figure 3. Gas-chromatogram of a urine-extract according to Table 1. Backflushing 8 seconds after injection. Without backflushing two hours are needed for each sample as late peaks are eluted. Here the column is ready for the following analysis after 6 minutes. Glass capillary-column: 20 m FFAP. Oven: 80°C, isotherm. Injector: 250°C, detector: 300°C. FID. Carrier gas: N_2.Gas-chromatograph: Carlo Erba Fractovap 4100.

REFERENCES

1. W. Dosch, Fortschr. Urol. u. Nephrol. 11:199 (1978).
2. W. Dosch, Fortschr. Urol. u. Nephrol. 14:266 (1979).
3. W. Dosch, Urol. Res. 7:227 (1979).
4. W. Dünges, in:"Prä-Chromatographische Mikromethoden," A. Hüthig-Verlag, Heldelberg (1979).
5. D. R. Deans, Chromatographia 1:18 (1968).
6. Pierce Chemical Company, P. O. Box 117, Rockford, IL 61105, USA.
7. W. Dosch, J. High Resolution Chromatography 4:223 (1978).

ACKNOWLEDGMENT

This work was supported by a grant of the Deutsch Forschungsgemeinschaft.

COMPARISON OF X-RAY DIFFRACTION, IR-SPECTROSCOPIC, AND POLARIZING MICROSCOPIC CORE-SHELL ANALYSIS OF URINARY STONES

W. Hicking, A. Hesse, and W. Vahlensieck

Harnsteinforschungsstelle der Urologischen
Universitats-Klinik
Bonn, Venusberg

OBJECTS

Qualitative and quantitative stone analysis is used today to determine specific treatment to prevent stone recurrence. Two-thirds of all urinary stones are mixed stones, so crystal nidi may differ from the remainder of the stone. Stone composition may change in a patient with time. The core and shell of a calculus can be composed of different crystal types. This study compares several methods of stone analysis.

METHODS

Comparison of three analytical methods for the specific stone analysis of core and shell.

1. X-ray diffraction
2. IR-Spectroscopy
3. Polarizing microscopy on thin sections

Twenty-two urinary calculi (diameter 1-2 cm) were selected at random for the investigation.

The whole stone was imbedded into self-hardening plastic (ARALDIT, Fa. Ciba-Geigy). The imbedded stone was sawed into two equal pieces. From one half a sample was taken from core and shell respectively for x-ray diffraction and IR-spectroscopy. The other half was taken for the preparation of thin sections.

Principles of the applied analytical methods:

1. X-ray diffraction

   Identification of crystal phases based on the diffraction of x-rays at a crystal grid

2. IR-spectroscopy

   Identification of the absorption in the infrared spectral color range based on the stimulation of oscillation in molecules and crystals

3. Polarizing microscopy in thin sections

   Identification of the morphology and distribution of crystallites in the cross-section of a calculus based on different properties of double refraction of the crystals.

RESULTS

Table 1 shows the results of x-ray diffraction, IR-spectroscopy, and polarizing microscopy analysis of 22 urinary stones (including one gall-stone).

Figure 1 and Figure 2 show examples of x-ray diagrams.

Figures 3, 4 and 5 show examples of IR-spectra.

CONCLUSIONS

For a core-shell analysis with IR-spectroscopic and x-ray diffractometric methods the stone under investigation must have a diameter of at least 1 cm to ensure that a representative sample can be taken. With polarizing microscopy the zones of growth on even small stones can be evaluated. The main components of core and shell of the stones could be identified with x-ray diffraction and IR-spectroscopy as well as with polarizing microscopy. Only by the identification of minor components were differences seen (stone no. 9 or 18). In 8 stones a different composition of the core and shell was found. E.g. is weddellite mainly in the shell (7 stones). In stone no. 11 besides whewellite and weddellite, brushite was found in the shell; while in the core besides whewellite and weddellite, apatite was found.

The investigation of thin sections in polarized light cannot be regarded as a routine method. In investigations concerning stone growth, thin sections give some further information. Determinable are:

Sample No.	X-ray diffraction	IR-spectroscopy	Polarized light microscopy
1 i	Cystine	Cystine 100%	Cystine
1 o	Cystine	Cys 80% Apa 20%	Cystine Apatite
2 i	-	Cystine 100%	Cystine
2 o	Cys Uadh	Cys 95% Uadh 5%	Cystine
3 i	Uric acid	Uric acid 100%	Uric acid
3 o	Uric acid	U a 90% Uadh 10%	Ua Uadh
4 i	Whe Apa We	Whe 50% Apa 40% We 10%	Whe We (pseudomorphism) Apa
4 o	Whe Apa We	Whe 50% We 35% Apa 15%	Whe We (pseudomorphism) Apa
5 i	Whe We Apa	Whe 50% We 40% Apa 10%	Whe We Apa (pseudomorphism)
5 o	Whe Apa We	Whe 50% Apa 40% We 10%	Whe We Apa (pseudomorphism)
6 i	We Apa	We 60% Apa 40%	We Apa few Whe (=pseudomorphism)
6 o	We Whe	We 80% Apa 20%	We Apa
7 i	Whe We	Whe 80% We 10% Apa 10%	Whe We Apa
7 o	Whe Apa	Apa 40% We 40% Whe 20%	Whe (pseudomorhism) We Apa
8 i	Whe Apa We	Whe 70% Apa 20% We 10%	Whe Apa We
8 o	Whe Apa	Whe 70% Apa 20% We 10%	We Whe Apa
9 i	Whewellite	Whe 80% Apa 20%	Whe Apa
9 o	Whewellite	Whe 80% Apa 20%	Whe (pseudomorphism) Apa We
10 i	Whe Apa	Whe 50% Apa 40% We 10%	Whe Apa
10 o	-	-	Whe Apa
11 i	Whe Apa We	Apa 40% Whe 30% We 30%	We Whe Apa
11 o	Bru Whe We	Bru 80% Whe 20%	We Bru Whe Apa
12 i	Whe Apa	Whe 60% Apa 40%	Whe Apa
12 o	Stru Apa	Struvite 100%	Apa Stru
13 i	Apatite	Apatite 100%	Apatite
13 o	Whe Apa	Whe 50% Apa 50%	Apa Whe (pseudomorphism)
14 i	Str Apa	Struvite 100%	Stru Apa
14 o	Stru Apa	Struvite 100%	Stru Apa
15 i	Apatite	Apatite 100%	Apatite
15 i. o.	Apatite	Apatite 100%	Apatite
15 o	Apatite	Apatite 100%	Apatite
16 i	Stru Apa	Stru 90% Apa 10%	Apatite
16 o	Stru Apa	Stru 90% Apa 10%	Apa Stru
17 i	Stru Apa	Stru 50% Apa 50%	Apatite
17 o	Apatite	Apatite 100%	Apa Stru
18 i	Struvite	Stru 95% Apa 5%	Apa Stru
18 o	Struvite	Stru 90% Apa 10%	Stru Apa
19 i	Whitlockit	Apa (Whi ?)90% Protein 10%	amorph (few Brushite ?)
19 o	Whitlockit	Apa (Whi ?)80% Prot. 10% We 10%	amorph (few Brushite ?)
20 i	We Apa NH_4Urate	Apa 50% NH_4Urate 40% We 10%	Apa We
20 o	Apa NH_4Urate We	NH_4Urate 50% Apa 40% We 10%	Apa We
21 i	Stru Apa	Struvite 100%	Stru Apa
21 o	Apa NH_4Urate	Stru 80% Apa 20%	Stru Apa
22 i	-	Protein 100%	Erythrocytes
22 i. o.	-	Cholesterine	Cholesterine
22 o	-	Cholesterine	Cholesterine

Abbreviations:
Apa = Apatite
Cys = Cystine
Stru = Struvite
We = Weddellite
Whe = Whewellite
Whi = Whitlockit
Ua = Uric acid
Uadh = Uric acid dihydrate

i = inner part, core
o = outer part, shell

Data from x-ray diffraction and polarized light microscopy in succession to percentage.

Table 1. Results of x-ray diffraction, IR-spectroscopy, and polarizing microscopy of 22 urinary stones (including one gall-stone).

Comparison of x-ray diffraction, IR-spectroscopic and polarized microscopy. Core-shell analysis of urinary stones.

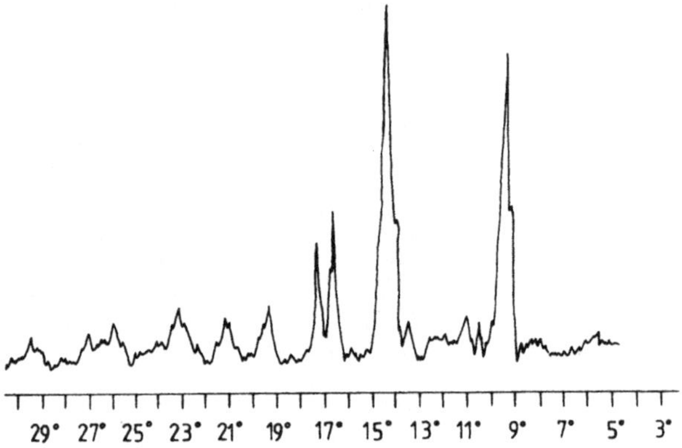

Figure 1. X-ray diffraction diagram from sample no. 1: Cystine. Comparison of x-ray diffraction, IR-spectroscopy, and polarizing microscopy. Core-shell analysis of urinary stone.

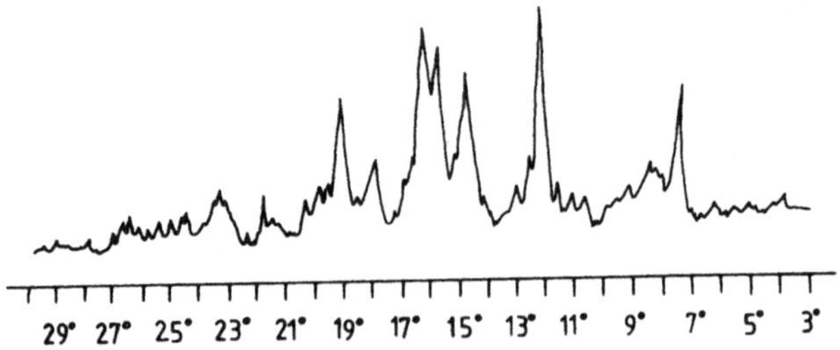

Figure 2. Example of an x-ray diffraction diagram. Whewellite-apatite (Whitlockit) urinary mixed stone. Distribution 1:1. Comparison of x-ray diffraction, IR-spectroscopy, and polarizing microscopy. Core-shell analysis of urinary stones.

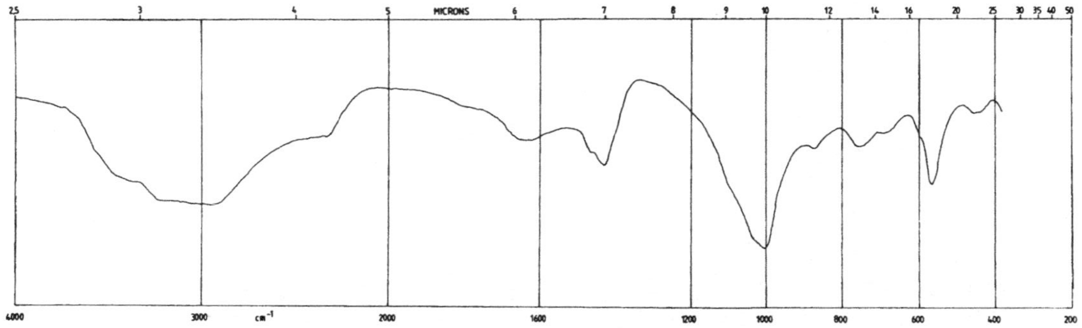

Figure 3. IR-spectroscopic diagram of sample no. 120: Struvite 100%. Comparison of x-ray diffraction, IR-spectroscopy, and polarizing microscopy. Core-shell analysis of urinary stones.

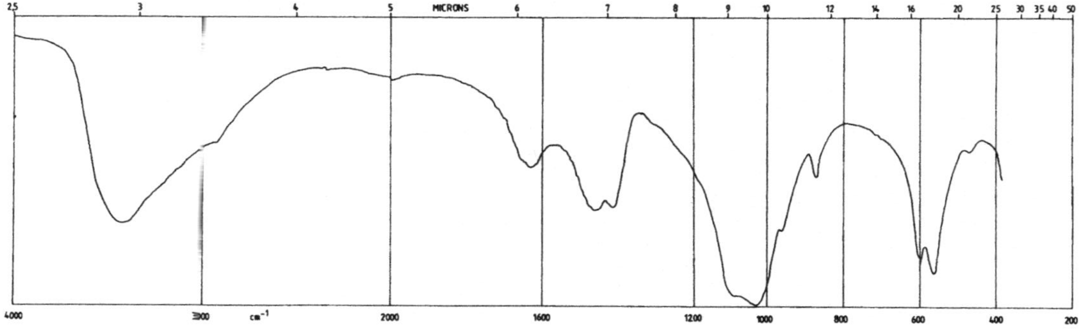

Figure 4. IR-spectroscopic diagram of sample. Carbonate-apatite 100%. Comparison of x-ray diffraction, IR-spectroscopy and polarizing microscopy. Core-shell analysis of urinary stones.

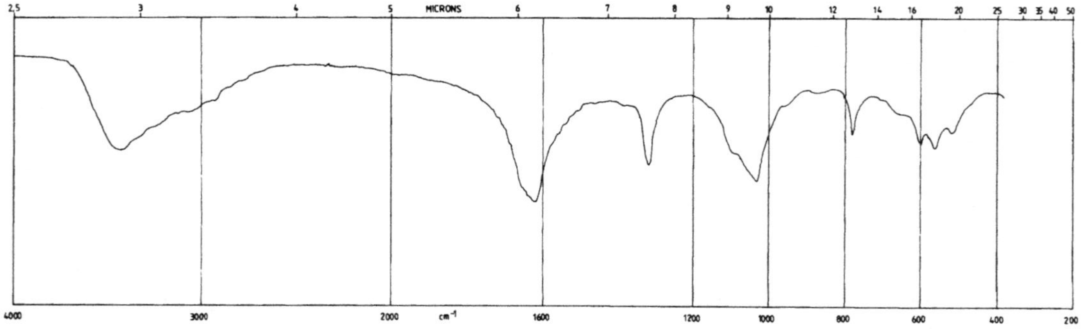

Figure 5. IR-spectroscopic diagram of sample no 51: Whewellite 50%, apatite 40%, weddellite 10%. Comparison of x-ray diffraction, IR-spectroscopy and polarizing microscopy. Core-shell analysis of urinary stones.

1. Centers of crystallization
2. Processes of dissolution and shifting (pseudomorphism)
3. Enclosure of foreign bodies
4. Small portions of different crystal phases
5. Distribution in crystal sizes

For a good qualitative and quantitative routine analysis of urinary stones, x-ray diffractometric and IR-spectroscopic methods are well suited.

EXPERIENCE WITH INFRARED ANALYSIS OF URINARY TRACT CALCULI IN A CLINICAL LABORATORY

M. H. Gault, M. Ahmed, J. Kalra, I. Senciall,
J. Morgan, W. Cohen, and D. Churchill
Memorial University and the General Hospital

St. John's, Newfoundland, A1B 3V6, Canada

Infrared analysis (IR) using the "decision tree" system of interpretation of spectra of Oliver and Sweet[1] was compared with the wet chemical analysis (WC)[2] of calculi from 450 patients. Senior laboratory technicians could be rapidly taught to interpret accurately IR spectra.

Minimum detectable amounts of reference standards measured by IR analysis varied approximately within one order of magnitude, compared with a range of 10^5 for WC. About 6 μg calculus was required for detection of oxalate by IR compared with about 1 mg for WC analysis. Failure to detect oxalate was the most important deficiency of WC procedures.

The reproducibility of IR analysis was superior to that of WC methods. For 720 paired decisions related to IR analysis of 85 calculi, there were <1% disagreements, compared with 8% disagreements for 312 paired decisions related to WC analysis of 42 calculi. Only 1 mg of calculus is required for IR analysis, permitting analysis of many calculi not possible by standard WC methods which require at least 5-10 mg. Twelve percent of calculi were found to weigh between 1 and 5 mg.

The limitations or disadvantages of IR analysis using this system of interpretation[1] include the somewhat greater time and cost compared with WC analysis, difficulty in separating the phosphates of different salts when they occur together (e.g. struvite and carbonate apatite), difficulty in determining carbonate in the presence of the ammonium ion in struvite and the lower sensitivity for struvite than with WC methods. We have found it necessary to use a wet chemical test to detect small amounts of struvite and to distinguish carbonate from ammonium.

The results of IR analysis of 450 calculi from Newfoundland, where there is a very high prevalence of urolithiasis, showed 73% to be entirely or predominantly calcium oxalate (with calcium phosphate as the only other component observed), 9% calcium phosphate alone or exceeding the amount of calcium oxalate, 12% predominantly struvite and/or carbonate apatite, 5% urate or uric acid (frequently with oxalate as a minor component), and 1% cystine, calcium carbonate, artifacts, etc.

Although IR analysis is primarily a qualitative procedure, quantitative or semiquantitative analysis of IR spectra has been proposed as being of value in stone analysis[3,4]. The relatively uniform sensitivity for the detection of phosphate and oxalate with IR, where the lower limit of sensitivity was 4 and 6 μg respectively, permits a semiquantitative approach. We found a linear relationship between the amount of calcium oxalate and calcium phosphate added to potassium bromide, and the log of the ratio of percent transmission at the base of the peak and the lowest point of the peak (Figure 1). Use of these standard curves permits calculation of a ratio of these two compounds, which were the sole constituents observed in 82% of the calculi studied by IR.

To assess the possibility that the stone composition might have value in predicting urine constituents, the calcium oxalate:calcium phosphate (O:P) ratio was calculated in 30 male stone formers seen consecutively and correlated with values for the mean of two 24-h urine collections for calcium, phosphate, and oxalate. Patients were studied on a random diet at home. They were not receiving diuretics. The O:P ratio ranged from 0.05 to 50. Significant correlations were found for calcium ($r = 0.41$, $p < 0.05$) and phosphate ($r = -0.43$, $p < 0.05$), but not for oxalate. When expressed as mg/l, only the significance of the correlation with phosphate changed ($r = -0.43$, $p < 0.02$). Stepwise multiple regression with O:P as the dependent variable and 24-h urinary excretion of oxalate, phosphate, and calcium as independent variables showed that 24-h urine calcium accounted for 15.9% of the variance while phosphate accounted for 12.3%.

Of 10 patients with carbonate-apatite calculi whose records were available for analysis, 8 had significant bacteriuria (10^5 bacteria/ml) and increased leukocyte excretion. Analysis of records from 30 consecutive patients with calculi containing calcium oxalate as the major constituent and calcium phosphate as the only other component showed no patient with significant bacteriuria or increased leukocyte excretion.

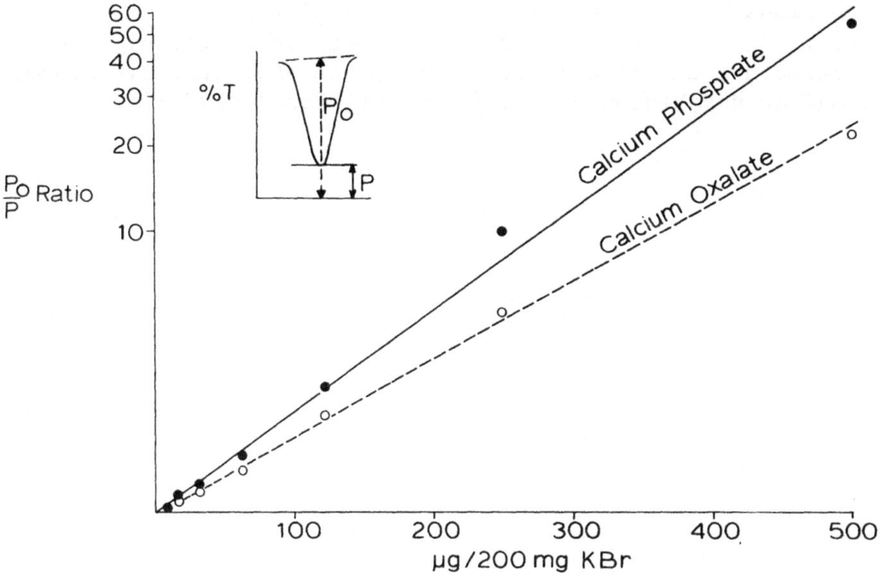

Figure 1. The linear relationship between the concentrations of calcium oxalate and of calcium phosphate and the log of the ratio of the percent transmission at the base of the peak (P_O) and at the lowest point on the peak (P). Calcium oxalate monohydrate and calcium phosphate (as hydroxyapatite) were added in increasing amounts to 200 mg potassium bromide in combination.

In spite of some limitations, IR analysis using the system of interpretation of Oliver and Sweet[1] combined with limited wet chemical analysis, is considered to be a major advance in methodology for analysis of urinary tract calculi in the clinical laboratory compared with WC alone. The reproducibility was greater, the sensitivity more uniform and the requirement for sample size smaller. The potential for semiquantitation of the relative amounts of calcium oxalate and phosphate with IR analysis may prove to be important.

REFERENCES

1. L. K. Oliver and R. V. Sweet, Clin. Chim. Acta. 72:17 (1976).
2. M. H. Gault, M. Ahmed, J. Kalra, I. Senciall, W. Cohen, and D. Churchill, Clin. Chim. Acta. (in press).
3. E. Takasaki, Calc. Tiss. Res. 7:232 (1971).

4. J. Bellanato, L. Cifuentes-Delatte, A. Hidalgo, and M. Santos, in:"Urinary Calculi: Recent Advances in Aetiology, Stone Structure and Treatment," L. Cifuentes-Delatte, A. Rapado, and A. Hodgkinson, eds., S. Karger, Basel (1973).

HIGH VOLTAGE ELECTRON MICROSCOPY OF URINARY CALCULI

M. Spector and J. C. Lilga

Medical University of South Carolina

Charleston, South Carolina

INTRODUCTION

Over the years many different physical and chemical techniques have been employed in investigations of the composition and structure of renal stones. Scanning and transmission electron microscopy (SEM and TEM) have been implemented in studies of the ultrastructure of urinary calculi[1-4]. TEM and associated selected area electron diffraction techniques have the unique potential of providing direct evidence of mechanisms, such as epitaxy, which have been proposed as being the key to stone formation. However, the considerable difficulties associated with ultramicrotomy and TEM of urinary stones have hindered progress in this area. In recent years, high voltage transmission electron microscopy[5] (HVEM; 800-1000kV) has been employed for the study of materials which do not lend themselves to investigation with conventional TEM (e.g. 100kV). The objective of the present study was to implement HVEM in the study of the ultrastructure of urinary calculi.

HVEM has several advantages over conventional TEM that facilitate study of urinary stones. These advantages include: 1) increased electron beam penetration power, 2) decreased electron beam-induced specimen damage, and 3) decreased size of areas selected for electron diffraction. One of the major problems encountered in conventional TEM of hard tissues or concretions is ultramicrotomy (i.e., preparation of thin sections about 100nm in thickness). Since the electron beam penetration power and hence the thickness of specimen which can be examined increase with increasing voltage, thicker sections of urinary stones (>1μm) can be examined by HVEM. In addition to facilitating microtomy of stone specimens, the capability to examine thick sections affords a second benefit of performing stereomicroscopy. Three-dimensional visualization of urinary stone components can provide a better description of their interrelationship in the stone. A second advantage of HVEM over conventional TEM is the reduction of the electron beam-induced specimen damage that results from the decrease in the inelastic scattering at higher voltages. A third advantage of HVEM which facilitates study of urinary stone structure is that electron diffraction analyses can be performed on much smaller selected areas than possible with conventional electron beam voltages. There is only one report in the literature of the use of HVEM to study urinary stone ultrastructure[6].

MATERIALS AND METHODS

Human urinary stones obtained from surgery were either air dried or immediately placed into cacodylate-buffered glutaraldehyde. Individual stones were dissected to provide samples for x-ray diffraction study, SEM, TEM, and HVEM. Stone fragments allocated for TEM and HVEM were embedded in a low viscosity plastic embedding medium in preparation for ultramicrotomy. Thin sections (~100nm) were prepared for conventional TEM, while thicker sections (>1μm) were prepared for HVEM. A variety of trough solutions was utilized during ultramicrotomy to inhibit demineralization of the sections as they floated on the knife trough. Unstained sections and sections stained with uranyl acetate and lead citrate were examined at conventional TEM voltages (80-125kV) and by HVEM (800-1000kV). Electron microscopy specimens were also prepared by depositing powdered samples of selected areas of stone onto carbon coated TEM grids. Selected area electron diffraction was routinely performed on all electron microscopy specimens.

RESULTS

HVEM of calcium oxalate renal stones revealed characteristic morphologies of the whewellite, weddelite, and hydroxyapatite components. Each accounted for discrete areas of the stone structure but some admixture of phases was observed. Whewellite appeared as arrays of thin lath-like crystallites radiating from a central focus. Weddellite crystals were larger than the individual whewellite crystallites and appeared as fragmented plates. Both the monohydrate and dihydrate forms of calcium oxalate were found to undergo changes in the electron beam. Foam-like features appeared within the crystals as exposure to the electron beam increased. A loss of crystalline structure as evidenced by a disappearance of the electron diffraction pattern accompanied the formation of the bubble- and foam-like features. These changes were similar to those observed with conventional TEM but appeared only after prolonged exposure in HVEM (Figure 1).

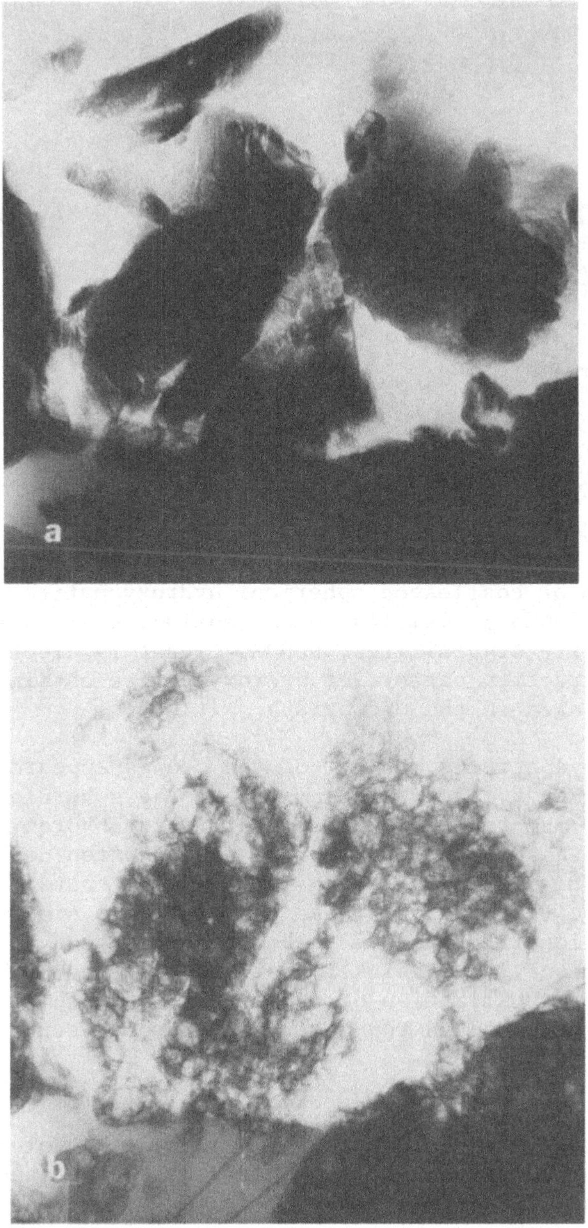

Figure 1. a) HVEM of calcium oxalate crystals in a urinary stone; b) electron beam induced changes in the same crystals after prolonged exposure to the beam. 1600X.

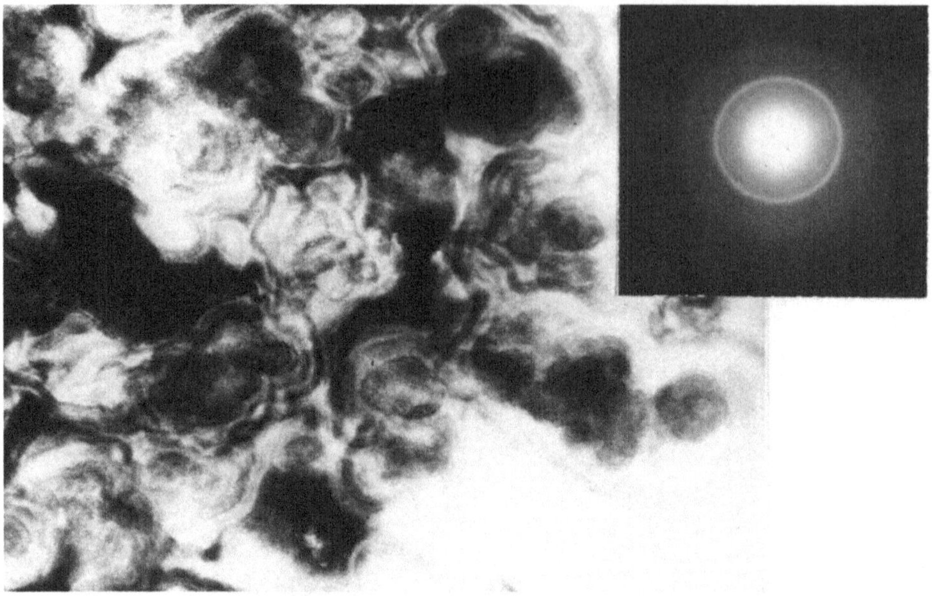

Figure 2. HVEM of coallesced spherical hydroxyapatite aggregates enveloped in lamellae also consisting of hydroxyapatite crystallites, 9000X. Inset is electron diffraction pattern of hydroxyapatite obtained from the area in the micrograph.

The hydroxyapatite component of the stones appeared as spherical bodies consisting of concentric lamellae. The spherules which measured from 0.5μm to 10μm consisted of minute hydroxyapatite crystallites. These smaller spherical bodies often coalesced to form larger lobulated masses which in turn were coated with distinct apatite lamellae (Figure 2). These deposits were similar to those seen in conventional TEM and SEM and often accounted for entire layers of the stone. The thicker sections examined by HVEM provided a more dramatic visualization of the extent to which hydroxyapatite crystallites aggregated in the spherical microstructures.

DISCUSSION

The results of the present study evidence the value of HVEM for the study of urinary stones. The several advantages of HVEM over conventional TEM afford the opportunity to obtain ultrastructural information that complements results yielded by TEM and SEM investigation.

The present study confirms the nature of the electron beam-induced damage that is produced in calcium oxalate crystals as they are exposed to an electron beam[1,7]. The identification of the concentric lamellar morphology of the apatite component of urinary stones by HVEM confirms earlier SEM and conventional TEM studies[3,4].

REFERENCES

1. A. S. Meyer, B. Finlayson, and L. DuBois, Br. J. Urol. 43:154 (1971).
2. R. S. Malek and W. H. Boyce, J. Urol. 117:336 (1977).
3. M. Spector and L. H. Jameson, in:"Scanning Electron Microscopy," O. Johari, ed., IIT Res. Inst. Press, Chicago (1976).
4. M. Spector, N. M. Garden, and S. N. Rous, Br. J. Urol. 50:12 (1978).
5. G. Dupouy, in:"Optical and Electron Microscopy," R. Barer and V. E. Cosslett, ed., Academic Press, New York (1978).
6. K. El-Sayed and V. E. Cosslett, Experimentia 33:919 (1977).
7. L. de Meis, W. Hasselbach, and R. D. Machado, J. Cell Biol. 62:505 (1974).

ACKNOWLEDGMENTS

This research was supported in part by NIH Contract 70-4136 from the Division of Research Resources. Dr. Spector was supported by NIH-NIDR Research Career Development Award DE00067.

PHYSICAL INVESTIGATIONS OF URINARY CALCULI

Bridget E. McConville

Department of Physics, University of Birmingham,

Birmingham B15 2TT, England

INTRODUCTION

Urinary calculi have been analyzed at Birmingham University by three separate techniques: autoradiographic analysis using charged particle activation[1], electron microscopy[2] and a technique hitherto unknown in the field of stone investigations - proton induced characteristic x-ray emission spectroscopy (PIXE). This latter technique has been developed as a method for quantitative analysis of biological material for trace and minor elements[3].

MATERIALS AND METHODS

Birmingham Radiation Centre's Dynamitron, which is a 3 MV High Current Cockroft-Walton Accelerator, Figure 1, was used to produce a beam of protons incident upon calculi sections for the PIXE analyses. The characteristic x-ray yield is proportional to the elemental concentration seen by the proton beam in that region through which it has passed. The yield varies linearly with trace concentrations (< 500 ppm). The x-rays produced were determined using a Si(Li) detector on line to computer and peak recognition was obtained directly.

Charged particle activation analysis was achieved by irradiating cross-sections of stones in the cyclotron. This technique was made quantitative by using standards. The standards contained known amounts of the elements of interest (i.e. carbon, oxygen, sodium, phosphorus and calcium), and were irradiated at the same time as the stone sections. Autoradiographs of standards and stone sections were obtained under identical conditions (on the same film) and percentage elemental compositions obtained from microdensitometer scans taken across the autoradiograph. Elemental identification was made by half-life determination and γ-spectroscopy.

Electron microscopy was undertaken on calculi sections evaporated with gold or carbon using a scanning electron microscopy (S.E.M.) equipped with an energy dispersive x-ray analysis system for routine simultaneous elemental analysis of each specimen.

RESULTS

An interesting illustration of the PIXE technique is shown here, where a so-called "pure" uric acid calculus supplied by University College, London, was shown to contain trace amounts of sulphur, chlorine, potassium, calcium, and iron, Figure 2. This stone was examined autoradiographically using charged particle activation and also on the S.E.M. with accompanying x-ray microanalysis. In both cases no trace elements were determined.

The effectiveness of the activation analysis technique was illustrated by examining a "staghorn" calculus. Carbon, sodium, oxygen and calcium were determined autoradiographically. The geographic distribution intensity of carbon radioactivity, Figure 3, is clearly defined and shows a concentration range of approximately

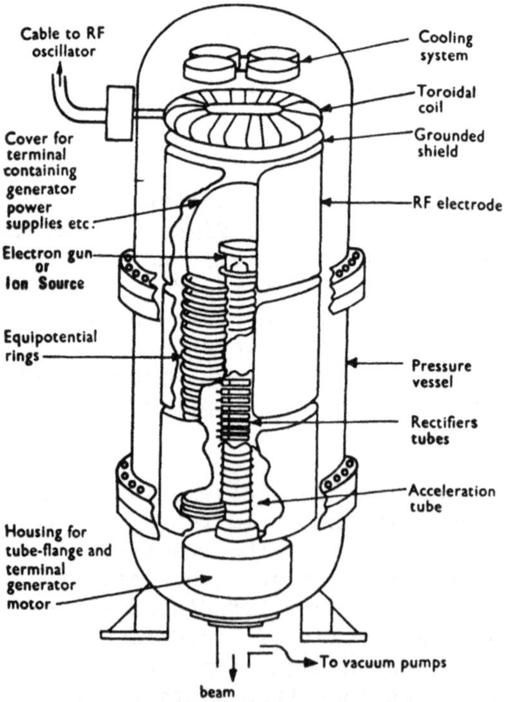

Figure 1. Dynamitron accelerator: 3MV

eleven percent carbon in the lighter area in the autoradiograph to 2% carbon in the other regions. The oxygen autoradiograph was exactly parallel to that of carbon, varying between 55 ± 1% oxygen in the less dense regions. The calcium distribution, Figure 4, was the direct reciprocal to those of carbon and oxygen, showing variations of 21 to 26% calcium in the denser regions.

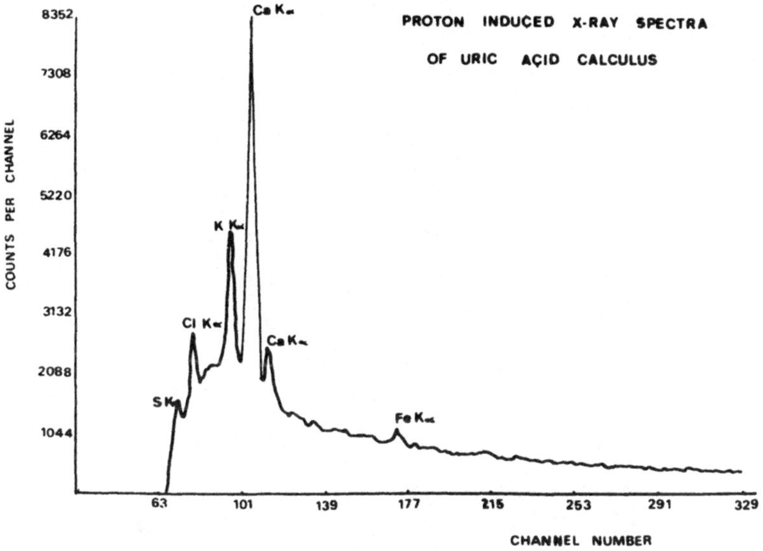

Figure 2. Proton induced x-ray spectra of uric acid calculus.

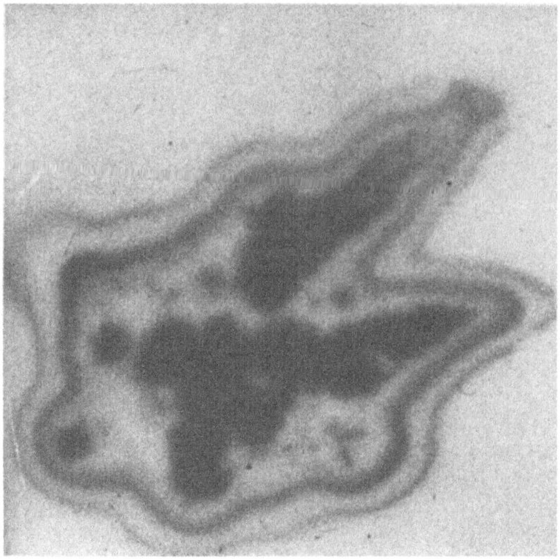

Figure 3. Carbon autoradiograph

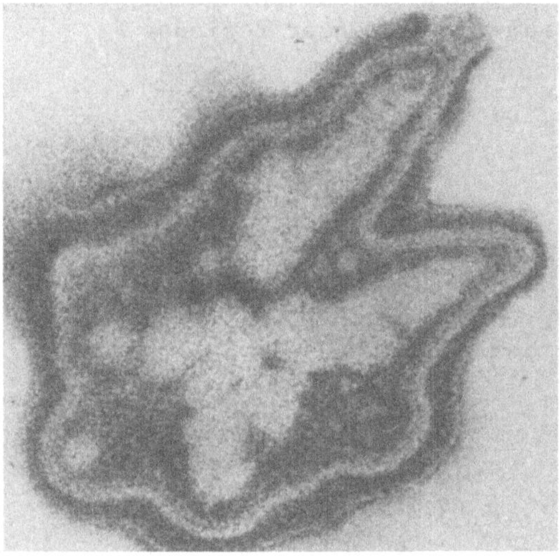

Figure 4. Calcium autoradiograph

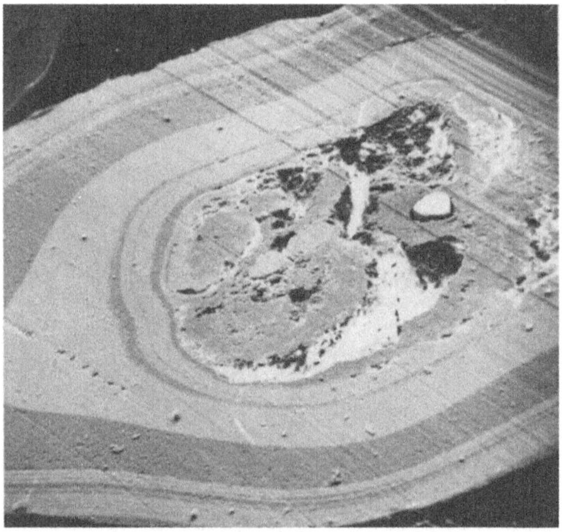

Figure 5. Electron micrograph of uric acid calculus (x35).

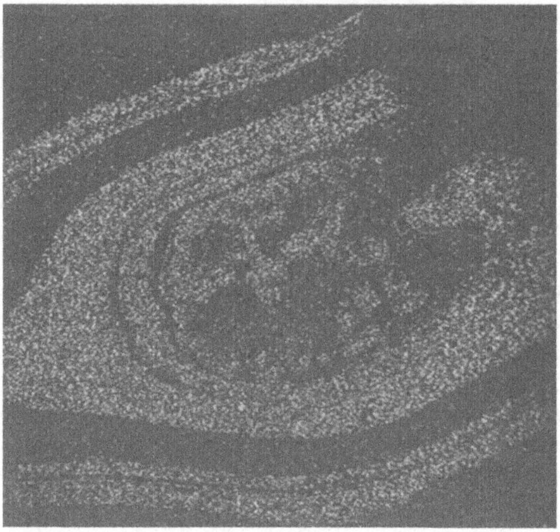

Figure 6. Ca K_α distribution of uric acid calculus (x35).

A chemical analysis was undertaken using a ground-up portion of material taken across the stone and 10.25% calcium and 27.29% oxalate were found.

A staghorn calculus was examined with S.E.M. at very low magnification, the different layers or growth rings of a section of this stone were clearly seen, Figure 5. The complimentary x-ray map, Figure 6, of the Ca K_α distribution across this region identifies the discrete bands of calcium - as demonstrated above by auto-radiographic analysis.

DISCUSSION

Since trace elements are obviously excluded from "ordinary" chemical analysis, the PIXE technique is particularly useful in their determination especially in the region of the nucleus.

The sensitivity of the autoradiographic and the x-ray micro-analysis techniques is of the order of 0.5%, whereas the limits of determination of PIXE are in parts per million. Those low levels of trace elements have been undetectable by previous methods of stone analysis.

The autoradiographic analysis provides visual interpretation of results since areas of intense elemental concentrations are clearly seen. In the results presented, calcium was shown to be present in the staghorn calculus in approximately 50% of the area across the stone and was seen to be present in discrete bands. Since these bands were found to contain between 21 to 26% calcium, the results correlate well with those obtained by the "averaged-out" percentage contribution obtained by chemical analysis.

Ordinary chemical analysis uses ground-up portions taken from specific regions across or within the stone, thus because of sampling errors, it is possible that chemical analysis of stones of mixed composition can give erroneous results. In this respect these techniques of PIXE, autoradiographic analysis and S.E.M. augment existing methods and provide a more reliable representation of the distribution of atomic elements in a stone.

REFERENCES

1. B. E. McConville, Br. J. Urol. (1980) (in press).
2. B. E. McConville, in:"Microbeam Analysis," D. E. Newbury, ed., San Francisco Press, San Francisco (1979).
3. N. A. Dyson and A. E. Simpson, Proc. Analyt. Div. Chem. Soc. 13:198 (1976).

INVESTIGATIONS FOR CHARACTERIZING SINGLE CRYSTAL PHASES IN URINARY STONES BY MEANS OF AN ARRANGEMENT OF LIGHT MICROSCOPY IN COMBINATION WITH SCANNING MICROSCOPY

A. Hesse, W. Hicking, and W. Vahlensieck

Urinary Stone Research Department
Urological University Clinic
Bonn, West Germany

Modern analysis of urinary calculi enables us to determine different structures in a stone, which by chemical analysis could not be identified. The efforts formerly made to discover the genesis of different kinds of stones were based mainly on the classification of stones by their major constituents such as uric acid, calcium oxalate, phosphate, or cystine. Nowadays, stone genesis is investigated in terms of how uric acid, uric acid dihydrate, calcium oxalate monohydrate, as well as dihydrate and the different phosphates such as struvite, carbonate apatite, brushite, and newberyite, develop. But in addition, more attention should be paid to the more difficult problem of the identification of the minor or rare components of urinary calculi. In crystalluria, unusual crystals sometimes appear that are difficult to identify. With sufficient material available, identification by means of x-ray diffraction analysis or IR spectroscopy is no problem. However, with a urinary sediment, crystalline material usually is scarce, although this is not the case when examining urinary calculi. Taking samples from different layers of a stone always represents only an integration over a larger area. Without good spatial resolution, initial nucleation centers of yet unknown components could remain undiscovered. The detection of possible nucleation centers can be carried out on thin sections of urinary calculi. Examination with ordinary light and polarized light microscopy permits localization of the initial phases of stone formation. Based on their double refraction, single crystals in thin sections and urinary sediments can be characterized. But with this method, whenever rare and unknown types of crystals appear, the identification is rendered difficult

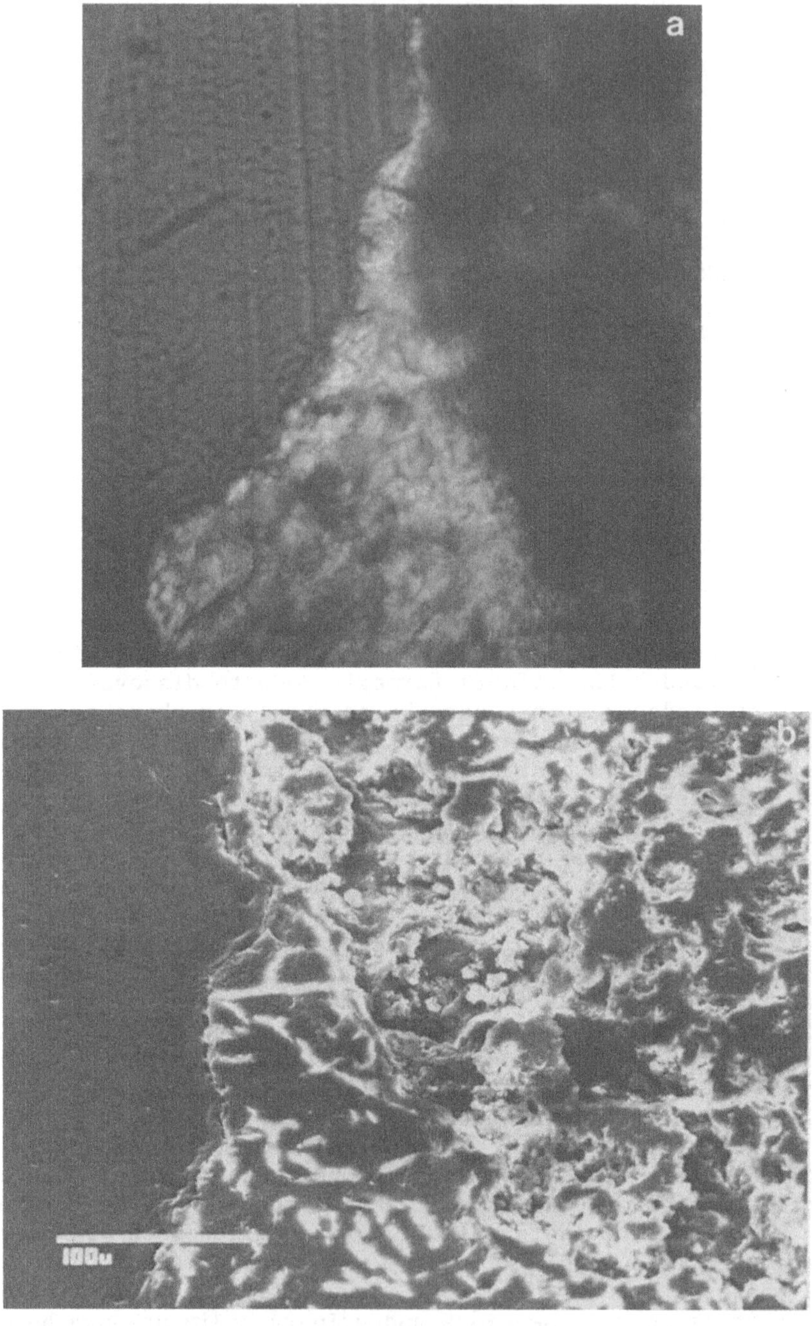

Figure 1. Investigations of thin sections with the arrangement of a light microscope in combinations with scanning electron microscope. a) Light microscopic picture of a whewellite struvite thin section. b) Corresponding SEM picture.

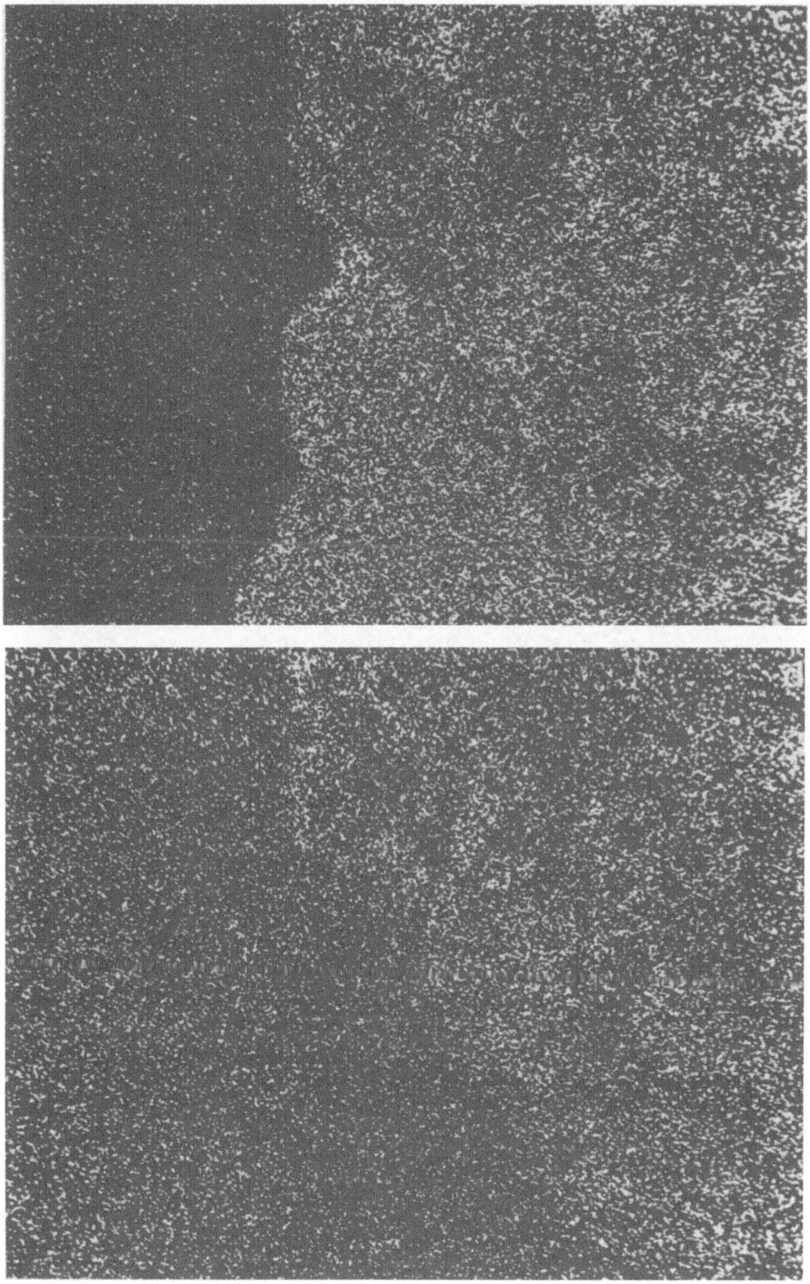

Figure 1. (Continued) c) Elemental analysis of Ca. d) Elemental analysis of P.

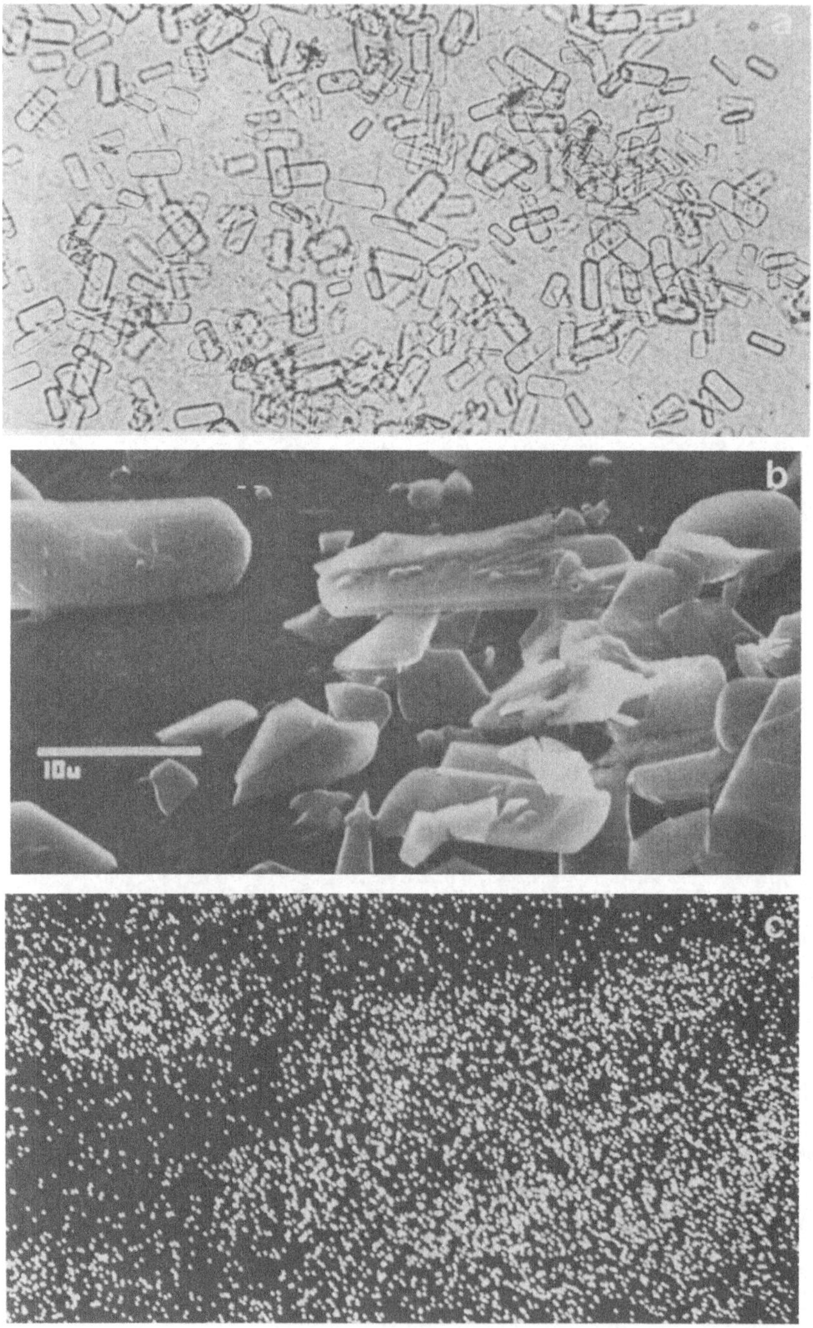

Figure 2 a, b, c.

because it cannot be done repetitively on the same specimens. By using an arrangement of light microscopy combined with scanning electron microscopy (SEM) and an elemental analysis system (EDAX), investigations on the same preparation with different methods can be carried out more easily. For SEM/EDAX analyses, the thin section is dusted with carbon which causes only unimportant changes in the microscopic picture. Granular preparations of urinary stones can be treated in the same way. However, when preparing a urinary sediment for this examination, liquid has to be carefully removed using filter paper and the sediment has to be exposed to air drying before it is dusted with carbon. We examined thin sections of different kinds of stones, mainly mixed stones. In Figure 1a-d, the different techniques of the investigation are demonstrated with a whewellite/ struvite calculi.

The examination of urinary sediments occasionally reveals atypical crystal shapes. Following an oral oxalate load, we found oval-shaped structures (Figure 2a) and the subsequent SEM study (Figure 2b) with elemental analysis showed Ca in the crystals (Figure 2c).

Evidence for the presence of other elements could not be obtained. Thus, the presence of calcium oxalate can be confirmed. Definitive distinction between the two calcium oxalate hydrates is not possible with SEM. Based on their double refraction in the polarized light, we identify these crystals as whewellite.

The significance of the above technique is that it enables the characterization of single structures, as to both their shape and chemical composition. The technique of combining a light microscope with a scanning electron microscope and energy dispersive x-ray analysis will enhance further investigations about the causal chain of events in stone formation, supersaturation of the urine, nucleation, aggregation, fixation, and stone growth.

SYMPOSIUM PARTICIPANTS

Ahmad, Dr. R., Renal Unit, Sefton General Hospital, Liverpool, Merseyside, United Kingdom

Alken, Dr. P., Department of Urology, University Clinic, 6500 Mainz, West Germany

Austin, Mr. Bill, L. C. Herring Co., P. O. Box 2191, Orlando, Florida, 32802, U.S.A.

Bach, Dr. D., Urologische University Klinik Bonn, 53 Bonn-Venusberg, West Germany

Backman, Dr. L., Department of Surgery, Danderyd Hospital, Karolinska Institute, S-18203 Danderyd, Sweden

Backman, Dr. U., Department of Internal Medicine, University Hospital, Uppsala, Sweden

Bellantone, Dr. Nancy, University of Connecticut, School of Pharmacy, U-92, Storrs, Connecticut, 06268, U.S.A.

Bergert, Mr. Jan, Mayo Clinic, Rochester, Minnesota, 55901, U.S.A.

Berlin, Dr. Thomas, Department of Urology, Huddinge Hospital, S-141 86 Huddinge, Sweden

Bichler, Dr. K.-H., University of Tubingen, Calwerstr. 7, 74 Tubingen, West Germany

Blaine, Mr. M. N., Blaine Pharmaceuticals Company, Inc., 2700 Dixie Highway, Ft. Mitchell, Kentucky, 41017, U.S.A.

Blomen, Dr. Leo J. M. J., Clinical Investigation Unit, Department of Endocrinology, Building 19, University Hospital, Leiden, The Netherlands 2333 AA

Brandes, Dr. Lida, The Toronto Western Hospital, Department of Medicine, Toronto, Ontario, Canada

Broadus, Dr. Arthur, Yale University, 333 Cedar Street, New Haven, Connecticut, 06510, U.S.A.

Brockis, Dr. J. G., Department of Urology, University of Western Australia, Perth, Western Australia 6009

Bruce, Dr. Robert, 5923 Bankside, Houston, Texas, 77096, U.S.A.

Burns, Dr. John, Department of Surgery, Division of Urology, University of Florida, Gainesville, Florida, 32610, U.S.A.

Butz, Dr. M., Free Universitat Berlin, D-1000 Berlin 45, West Germany

Carter, Dr. William C., III, Chief Resident in Urology, Medical University of South Carolina, 171 Ashley Avenue, Charleston, South Carolina, 29403, U.S.A.

Churchill, Dr. D. N., Memorial University, The General Hospital, St. John's, Newfoundland A1B 3V6, Canada
Cifuentes Delatte, Dr. Luis, Monte Esquinza, 20, Madrid-4, Spain
Coe, Dr. Fredric L., Michael Reese Medical Center, 29th Street and Ellis Avenue, Chicago, Illinois, 60616, U.S.A.
Cohanim, Dr. M., Etherington Hall, Queen's University, Kingston, Ontario, Canada K7L 3N6
Cole, Dr. Francis E., Alton Ochsner Medical Foundation, 1520 Jefferson Highway, New Orleans, Louisiana, 70121, U.S.A.
Connor, Dr. T. P., University of Maryland Hospital, Baltimore, Maryland, 21201, U.S.A.
Costello, Dr. J., The Irish Stone Foundation, Department of Clinical Medicine, Meath Hospital, Dublin 8, Ireland
Covaliu, Dr. Tina, Clinica a II-a Medicala, Str. Mandinesti nr. 2, Bucuresti, Romania
Cowgill, Dr. U. M., Department of Biologic Sciences, University of Pittsburgh, Pittsburgh, Pennsylvania, 15260, U.S.A.
Cummings, Dr. Nancy B., National Institute of Arthritis, Metabolism, and Digestive Diseases, National Institutes of Health, Room 9A-17, Building 31, Bethesda, Maryland, 20014, U.S.A.
Curreri, Dr. Peter A., 809 Northwest 19 Avenue, Gainesville, Florida, 32601, U.S.A.
Danielson, Dr. B. G., Department of Internal Medicine, University Hospital, Uppsala, Sweden
de Vries, Dr. A., Teva, P. O. Box 1423, Tel-Aviv, Israel
Diaz Gonzalez, Dr. R., c/Brescia n 1-3-B, Madrid-28, Spain
Dirks, Dr. John H., Head, Department of Medicine, 700 West 10 Avenue, Vancouver, British Columbia, Canada V5Z 1M9
Dobbins, Dr. J. W., Yale University, 333 Cedar Street, New Haven, Connecticut, 06510, U.S.A.
Dosch, Dr. W., Institut f. Mineralogie, Universitat Mainz, Saarstr. 21, D-6500 Mainz, West Germany
Dousa, Dr. Thomas P., Mayo Clinic, Rochester, Minnesota, 55901, U.S.A.
Dulce, Dr. H. J., Institute for Clinical Chemistry, Universitat Berlin, Hinderburgdamm 30, D-1000 Berlin, 45 West Germany
Dunham, Dr. Richard, P. O. Box 2091, Rockville, Maryland, 20852, U.S.A.
Eisenberg, Mr. Harry, Willen Drug Company, 18 North High Street, Baltimore, Maryland, 21202, U.S.A.
Eisenberg, Mr. Louis, Willen Drug Company, 18 North High Street, Baltimore, Maryland, 21202, U.S.A.
Erickson, Dr. Stephen, Mayo Clinic, Rochester, Minnesota, 55901, U.S.A.
Ettinger, Dr. B., 2200 O'Farrell Street, San Francisco, California, 94115, U.S.A.
Favus, Dr. Murray, Michael Reese Hospital, Division of Renal Medicine, 29 and Ellis Avenue, Chicago, Illinois, 60616, U.S.A.
Fellstrom, Dr. Bengt, University of Uppsala, Department of Internal Medicine, University Hospital, Uppsala, Sweden S-75014

Finlayson, Dr. Birdwell, Professor, Division of Urology, Department of Surgery, College of Medicine, University of Florida, Gainesville, Florida, 32610, U.S.A.
Fishbein, Dr. William N., Walter Reed Army Medical Center, 14th and Alaska, Building 54, Room 3001, Washington, D.C. 20306, U.S.A.
Fleisch, Dr. Herbert, Universitat Bern, Pathophysiologisches Institut, 3008 Bern, Murtenstr. 35, Switzerland
Furedi-Milhofer, Dr. Helga, Department of Physical Chemistry, Rudjer Boskovic Institute, POB 1016, 41001 Zagreb, Croatia, Yugoslavia
Gaca, Dr. A., Stiftung Deutsche Klinik, Fur Diagnostik GmbH, 62 Wiesbaden, West Germany 6200
Gault, Dr. M. H., Memorial University, The General Hospital, St. John's, Newfoundland A1B 3V6, Canada
Gebhardt, Dr. Manfred, Mineralogisch-Petrologisches Institut, Poppelsdorfer Schloss, D-5300 Bonn, West Germany
Gill, Dr. W. B., The University of Chicago, 950 East 59 Street, Chicago, Illinois, 60637, U.S.A.
Gillenwater, Dr. J. Y., Professor and Chairman, Department of Urology, University of Virginia Hospital, Charlottesville, Virginia, 22901, U.S.A.
Goldberg, Dr. E. P., Department of Materials Science and Engineering, Room MAE 217, University of Florida, Gainesville, Florida, 32611, U.S.A.
Gregory, Dr. J. G., Department of Surgery, Section of Urology, St. Louis University, 1325 South Grand Boulevard, St. Louis, Missouri, 63104, U.S.A.
Griffith, Dr. Donald P., 1200 Moursund, Houston, Texas, 77025, U.S.A.
Haas, Mr. John, Mayo Clinic, Rochester, Minnesota, 55901, U.S.A.
Hackett, Dr. R. L., J. H. Miller Health Center, Department of Pathology, Box J275, Gainesville, Florida, 32610, U.S.A.
Hagmaier, Dr. V., Universitatsklinik Basel, Division of Urology, Basel, Switzerland
Hailey, Dr. Francis J., Norwich-Eaton Laboratories, P. O. Box 191, Norwich, New York, 13815, U.S.A.
Hallwachs, Dr. O., Grafenstr. 9, 61 Darmstadt, West Germany
Halstead, Dr. S. B., Department of Tropical Medicine, University of Hawaii, School of Medicine, Honolulu, Hawaii, U.S.A.
Hautmann, Dr. R., Department of Urology, RWTH Aachen, Goethestr. 27-29, 51 Aachen, West Germany
Hering, Dr. Franz, Department of Urology Medical Faculty, RWTH Aachen, Goethestr. 27-29, D-5100 Aachen, West Germany
Hesse, Dr. A., Urologische Universitatsklinik, 5300 Bonn-Venusberg, West Germany
Hiatt, Dr. Robert, Medical Methods Research Department, The Permanente Medical Group, 3700 Broadway, Oakland, California, 94611, U.S.A.
Hicking, Dr. Wilhelm, Urologische Universitatsklinik Bonn, Sigmund-Freud-Str., 5300 Bonn 1, West Germany

Howard, Dr. John Eager, Professor Emeritus of Medicine, The Union Memorial Hospital, 201 East University Parkway, Baltimore, Maryland, 21205, U.S.A.

Jenkins, Dr. Alan D., University of Virginia School of Medicine, Department of Urology, Charlottesville, Virginia, 22901, U.S.A.

Johansson, Dr. Gunnar, Department of Medicine, University Hospital, S-750 14 Uppsala, Sweden

Johnson, Dr. Paul F., New York State College of Ceramics, Alfred University, Alfred, New York, 14802, U.S.A.

Joost, Dr. J., Department of Urology, University Clinic, Innsbruck, Austria

Khan, Dr. Saeed R., Department of Pathology, Box J-275, University of Florida, Gainesville, Florida, 32610, U.S.A.

Klein, Dr. A. Scott, 8901 South Braeswood Drive, No. 108, Houston, Texas, 77074, U.S.A.

Knox, Dr. Franklyn G., Mayo Clinic, Rochester, Minnesota, 55901, U.S.A.

Kolb, Dr. Felix O., 3580 California Street, San Francisco, California, 94118, U.S.A.

Kraljevich, Zlatica, The University of Arizona, Health Sciences Center, College of Medicine, Section of Urology, Tucson, Arizona, 85724, U.S.A.

Kumar, Dr. S., University of Massachusetts, Medical Center, 55 Lake Avenue North, Worcester, Massachusetts, 01605, U.S.A.

Larsson, Dr. Lasse, Department of Surgery, University of Linkoping, Linkoping, Sweden

Lemann, Dr. Jacob, Jr., Renal Section, The Medical College of Wisconsin, Milwaukee County General Hospital, 8700 West Wisconsin Avenue, Milwaukee, Wisconsin, 53226, U.S.A.

Leskovar, Dr. Peter, Dipl. Ing. Chem., D-8000 Munchen 7, Appenrellerstr 77/2, 8000 Munchen, West Germany

Leusmann, Dr. D. B., Institut fur Medizinische Physik, 44 Munster/Westf, Hufferstrabe 68, West Germany

Levinson, Dr. A. A., Department of Geology, University of Calgary, Calgary, Alberta T2N 1N4, Canada

Linari, Dr. Franco, C.so Q. Sella n 20, 10100 - Torino, Italy

Ljunghall, Dr. Sverker, Department of Internal Medicine, University Hospital, Uppsala, Sweden S-750-14

Lovatt, Dr. G. E., The Wellcome Research Laboratories, Langley Court, Beckenham, Kent BR3 3BS, United Kingdom

Lycklama, Dr. A. A., Afd. Urologie, Academisch Ziekenhuis, Leiden, The Netherlands

McConville, Dr. B. E., Physics Department, University of Birmingham, Birmingham, England

McGeown, Dr. M. G., Department of Nephrology, Belfast City Hospital, Belfast BT9 7AB, Northern Ireland

McSherry, Dr. Elizabeth, University of California, San Francisco, California, 94143, U.S.A.

Maass, Dr. Al, Smith Kline and French Laboratories, P. O. Box 7929, Philadelphia, Pennsylvania, 19101, U.S.A.

Magura, Dr. Christian E., 1429 Downwood Place, Charleston, South Carolina, 29412, U.S.A.

Malluche, Dr. Hartmut, P. O. Box 478, University of Southern California, 1200 North State Street, Los Angeles, California, 90033, U.S.A.

Mandel, Dr. G., Veterans Administration Center, 5000 West National Avenue, Milwaukee, Wisconsin, 53193, U.S.A.

Mandel, Dr. N., Veterans Administration Center, 5000 West National Avenue, Milwaukee, Wisconsin, 53193, U.S.A.

Marangella, Dr. Martino, C.so F. Turati n 41, 10100 Torino, Italy

Marshall, Dr. Villis R., Urology Unit, Department of Surgery, Flinders Medical Center, Bedford Park, South Australia 5042

Mautalin, Dr. Carlos, Centro De Osteopatias Medicas, Saavedra 189, 1083 Buenos Aires, Argentina

Melick, Dr. Roger, Department of Medicine, University of Melbourne, Melbourne, Australia

Menon, Dr. Mani, 3313 Claran Road, Baltimore, Maryland, 21215, U.S.A.

Meyer, Dr. John L., National Institute of Dental Research, Building 30, Room 211, National Institutes of Health, Bethesda, Maryland, 20014, U.S.A.

Modlin, Dr. Monte, 25 Avenue Alexandra, Fresnaye, 8001, Cape Town, South Africa

Monreal, Dr. A., Gottfried Clarenstr. 32, 53 Bonn 3, Germany

Muldowney, Dr. F. P., Department of Metabolism and Renal Disease, St. Vincent's Hospital, Dublin, Ireland

Nancollas, Dr. George H., Professor of Chemistry, State University of New York at Buffalo, Buffalo, New York, 14214, U.S.A.

Nel, Dr. Fred, P. O. Box/Posbus 37287, Overport, Durban 4067, South Africa

Nordenvall, Dr. Bjorn, Department of Surgery, Danderyd Hospital at Karolinska Institute, S-18288 Danderyd, Sweden

Oldroyd, Mr. Norman, L. C. Herring Company, P. O. Box 2191, Orlando, Florida, 32802, U.S.A.

Oreopoulos, Dr. D. G., The Toronto Western Hospital, Department of Medicine, Toronto, Ontario, Canada

Pak, Dr. Charles Y. C., Professor of Internal Medicine, 5323 Harry Hines Boulevard, Southwestern Medical School, Dallas, Texas, 75235, U.S.A.

Pawelchak, Dr. John, ConvaTec Research and Development Laboratories, 25 Cotters Lane, East Brunswick, New Jersey, 08816, U.S.A.

Peacock, Dr. M., MRC Mineral Metabolism Unit, The General Infirmary, Great George Street, Leeds LS1 3EX, England

Pinto, Dr. B., Laboratorio de Exploraciones Metabolicas, Aragon, 420, 1.0, 1.a, Barcelona-13, Spain

Prien, Dr. E. L., Jr., 81 Wyman Street, Newton, Massachusetts, 02168, U.S.A.

Purnell, Dr. Don, Mayo Clinic, Rochester, Minnesota, 55901, U.S.A.

Randolph, Dr. A. D., The University of Arizona, Section of Urology, Tucson, Arizona, 85724, U.S.A.

Rapado, Dr. A., Laboratorio de Urolithiasis, Enfermedades Metabolicas, Fudacion Jimenez Diaz, Madrid, Spain

Rasmussen, Dr. Howard, Yale University, 333 Cedar Street, New Haven, Connecticut, 06510, U.S.A.

Resnick, Dr. M., Department of Surgery, Bowman Gray School of Medicine, Wake Forest University, 300 South Hawthorne Road, Winston-Salem, North Carolina, 27103, U.S.A.

Richardson, Dr. K. E., Department of Physical Chemistry, The Ohio State University College of Medicine, Columbus, Ohio, 43210, U.S.A.

Robertson, Dr. W. G., MRC Mineral Metabolism Unit, The General Infirmary, Great George Street, Leeds LS1 3EX, England

Rodgers, Dr. Allen, Department of Medical Biochemistry, University of Cape Town, Cape Town, Republic of South Africa

Rose, Dr. G. A., St. Peters Hospital, Institute of Urology, Endell Street, London WC2, England

Rugendorff, Dr. E. W., Ludwissplatz 11, D-6300 Giessen, West Germany

Rundquist, Mr. Robert, Mayo Clinic, Rochester, Minnesota, 55901, U.S.A.

Rushton, Dr. H. Gil, 1286 Old Colony Road, Mt. Pleasant, South Carolina, 29464, U.S.A.

Rutishauser, Dr. G., Kantonsspital Basel, Urologische Klinik, Spitalstrabe 21, CH - 4031 Basel, Switzerland

Ryall, Dr. Rosemary L., Department of Surgery, Flinders Medical Centre, Bedford Park, South Australia 5042

Sallis, Dr. John D., Department of Biochemistry, University of Tasmania, HOBART Box 252C G.P.O., Tasmania, Australia

Sarig, Dr. Sara, The Hebrew University of Jerusalem, Casali Institute of Applied Chemistry, Jerusalem, Israel

Scherbenske, Dr. M. J., Director, Extramural Programs, National Institute of Arthritis, Metabolism and Digestive Diseases, National Institutes of Health, Bethesda, Maryland, 20014, U.S.A.

Schmidt, Dr. K., Department of Surgery, University of Tubingen, Calwerstrasse 7, D-7400 Tubingen, West Germany

Schneeberger, Dr. Winfried, Rehabilitationskrankenhaus, Klosterstr. 2, 5303 Bornheim - Merten, West Germany

Schneider, Dr. H.-J., Urologische Klinik und Poliklinik, Schiller-Universitat Jena, DDR - 69 Jena, Lessingstr. 1, Germany, GDR

Scholz, Dr. Donald A., Mayo Clinic, Rochester, Minnesota, 55901, U.S.A.

Scholz, Dr. Dieter, University Hospital, Department of Surgery, Maximiliansplatz, D-8520 Erlangen, West Germany

Schrier, Dr. Eugene E., Professor of Chemistry, State University of New York at Binghamton, Binghamton, New York, 13901, U.S.A.

Schwam, Dr. Harvey, Merck Sharp and Dohme Research Laboratories, West Point, Pennsylvania, 19486, U.S.A.

Schwille, Dr. Paul O., Department of Surgery and Urology, University of Erlangen, 852 Erlangen, West Germany

Scott, Dr. Roy, Consultant Surgeon, Urological Department, Royal Infirmary, Glasgow, G4 OSF, Scotland

Segura, Dr. Joseph W., Mayo Clinic, Rochester, Minnesota, 55901, U.S.A.

Selby, Dr. Theodore, Smith Kline and French Laboratories, P. O. Box 7929, Philadelphia, Pennsylvania, 19101, U.S.A.

Shah, Dr. Julian, Norfolk and Norwich Hospital, St. Stephen's Road, Norwich, Norfolk, England
Shahin, Dr. Salem, 1710 Winnetka Avenue North, Golden Valley, Minnesota, 55427, U.S.A.
Sheehan, Dr. Mary, 62 Fisher Street, Buffalo, New York, 14215, U.S.A.
Simmonds, Dr. H. A., Department of Medicine, Guy's Hospital Medical School, London SE1 9RT, England
Simonelli, Dr. Anthony P., Professor and Chairman, School of Pharmacy, University of Connecticut, Storrs, Connecticut, 06268, U.S.A.
Smith, Dr. Lynwood H., Mayo Clinic, Rochester, Minnesota, 55901, U.S.A.
Smith, Dr. M. J. V., Medical College of Virginia, Virginia Commonwealth University, MCV Station, Richmond, Virginia, 23298, U.S.A.
Spector, Dr. M., Medical University of South Carolina, Charleston, South Carolina, 29401, U.S.A.
Sperling, Dr. O., Metabolic Unit, Tel-Aviv University, Beilinson Medical Center, Petah Tikva, Israel
Starkman, Dr. Martin, Box 160 MCV Station, Medical College of Virginia, Richmond, Virginia, 23298, U.S.A.
Stote, Dr. Robert, University of Pennsylvania Medical Center, 51 North 39 Street, Philadelphia, Pennsylvania, 19104, U.S.A.
Strenge, Dr. Anke, Urologische Universitatsklinik Bonn, Sigmund-Freud-Str., 5300 Bonn 1, West Germany
Sur, Dr. B. K., Professor and Head, Department of Biochemistry, G.S.V.M. Medical College, Kanpur - 208002, India
Sutton, Dr. R. A. L., University of British Columbia, Vancouver General Hospital, Vancouver, British Columbia, Canada V5Z 1M9
Tew, Dr. William, The Johns Hopkins Hospital, 600 North Wolfe Street, Baltimore, Maryland, 21205, U.S.A.
Thind, Dr. S. K., Department of Biochemistry, PGIMER, Chandigarh, U.T., India 160012
Thomas, Dr. William C., Jr., Veterans Administration Hospital, Gainesville, Florida, 32601, U.S.A.
Tiselius, Dr. H. G., University of Linkoping, S-581 85 Linkoping, Sweden
Tomazic, Dr. Branko, State University of New York at Buffalo, Acheson Hall, Buffalo, New York, 14214, U.S.A.
Tschope, Dr. W., Med. Universitatsklinik, Bergheimerstr. 58, D-69 Heidelberg, West Germany
Ulshofer, Dr. B. M., Urologische Universitatsklinik und Poliklinik, 3550 Marburg/Lahn, Germany, FRG
Vahlensieck, Dr. W., Urologische Universitatsklinik, 5300 Bonn-1, West Germany
Valyasevi, Dr. A., Department of Pediatrics, Ramathibodi Hospital, Mahidol University, Bangkok, Thailand
Van Acker, Dr. K. J., Groeningelei 120, 2550 Kontich, Belgium
Van Den Berg, Dr. Christian J., Mayo Clinic, Rochester, Minnesota, 55901, U.S.A.

Van Der Linden, Dr. M., Clinical Investigation Unit, Building 19, University Hospital, Leiden, The Netherlands 2333 AA
van't Reit, Dr. B., Medical College of Virginia, Virginia Commonwealth University, Richmond, Virginia, 23298, U.S.A.
Walker, Dr. Valerie R., Clinical Investigation Unit, Shaughnessy Hospital, 4500 Oak Street, Vancouver, British Columbia, Canada V6H 3N1
Wasserstein, Dr. Alan, Renal Electrolyte Section, 860 States Building, Hospital of the University of Pennsylvania, 34th and Spruce, Philadelphia, Pennsylvania, 19130, U.S.A.
Watson, Dr. L., University College Hospital, Rayne Institute, London WC11 6JJ, England
Weinerth, Dr. John, Duke University, Box 3343, Durham, North Carolina, 27710, U.S.A.
Werness, Dr. Peter G., Mayo Clinic, Rochester, Minnesota, 55901, U.S.A.
White, Mr. Donald, State University of New York at Buffalo, Acheson Hall, Buffalo, New York, 14214, U.S.A.
Wikstrom, Dr. Bjorn, Department of Internal Medicine, University Hospital, S-75014 Uppsala, Sweden
Will, Dr. E. J., Renal Unit, Nottingham City Hospital, Hucknall Road, Nottingham, NG5 1PB, England
Williams, Dr. H. E., Dean, School of Medicine, University of California at Davis, Davis, California, 95616, U.S.A.
Williams, Dr. John, 525 East 68 Street, New York City, New York, 10021, U.S.A.
Wilson, Dr. Mary H., Department of Urology, Baylor College of Medicine, 1200 Moursund, Houston, Texas, 77025, U.S.A.
Wochos, Dr. Daniel, Mayo Clinic, Rochester, Minnesota, 55901, U.S.A.
Yendt, Dr. E. R., Department of Medicine, Queen's University, Kingston, Ontario, Canada
Zackson, Dr. David, 110 East 59 Street, New York, New York, 10023, U.S.A.
Zarembo, Dr. John, Smith Kline and French Laboratories, P. O. Box 7929, Philadelphia, Pennsylvania, 19101, U.S.A.
Zechner, Dr. O., Urologische Universitats-Klinik, 1090 Wien 9, Alserstrasse 4, Austria
Zerwekh, Dr. Joseph, Southwestern Medical School, 5323 Harry Hines Boulevard, Dallas, Texas, 75235, U.S.A.

INDEX

GPSR Compliance

The European Union's (EU) General Product Safety Regulation (GPSR) is a set of rules that requires consumer products to be safe and our obligations to ensure this.

If you have any concerns about our products, you can contact us on ProductSafety@springernature.com

In case Publisher is established outside the EU, the EU authorized representative is:

Springer Nature Customer Service Center GmbH
Europaplatz 3
69115 Heidelberg, Germany

Batch number: 10632798

Printed by Printforce, the Netherlands